# Bipolar Disorder: From Neuroscience to Treatment

# Bipolar Disorder: From Neuroscience to Treatment

Editor: Francisco Watkins

AMERICAN
MEDICAL PUBLISHERS
www.americanmedicalpublishers.com

AMERICAN
MEDICAL PUBLISHERS
www.americanmedicalpublishers.com

**Cataloging-in-Publication Data**

Bipolar disorder : from neuroscience to treatment / edited by Francisco Watkins.
p. cm.
Includes bibliographical references and index.
ISBN 978-1-63927-934-0
1. Manic-depressive illness. 2. Manic-depressive illness--Treatment.
3. Cognitive neuroscience. 4. Depression, Mental. 5. Mania. I. Watkins, Francisco.
RC516 .B57 2023
616.895--dc23



American Medical Publishers,
41 Flatbush Avenue,
1st Floor, New York,
NY 11217, USA

ISBN 978-1-63927-934-0 (Hardback)

# Contents

# Preface

This book aims to highlight the current researches and provides a platform to further the scope of innovations in this area. This book is a product of the combined efforts of many researchers and scientists, after going through thorough studies and analysis from different parts of the world. The objective of this book is to provide the readers with the latest information of the field.

Bipolar disorder refers to a type of mood disorder characterized by cycles of abnormally heightened happiness followed by episodes of depression that can continue from days to weeks. It can be classified into several types including cyclothymic disorder, bipolar I disorder, bipolar II disorder, etc. Mania is an elevated mood that is severe and is linked to psychosis, while hypomania is milder. Manic episodes that last at least a week are the defining symptom of bipolar I disorder, whereas hypomanic episodes characterize cyclothymic and bipolar II disorder. The diagnosis of bipolar disorder can be done using a variety of tools including blood tests, physical examination, a mental health assessment and examination of medical history. Bipolar disorder is treatable with a combination of factors such as adopting a healthy lifestyle, medication, appropriate medical care and talk therapy. This book is a valuable compilation of topics, ranging from the basic to the most complex advancements in the study of bipolar disorder. It strives to provide a fair idea about this medical condition and to help develop a better understanding of the latest advances in its clinical management. Those in search of information to further their knowledge will be greatly assisted by this book.

I would like to express my sincere thanks to the authors for their dedicated efforts in the completion of this book. I acknowledge the efforts of the publisher for providing constant support. Lastly, I would like to thank my family for their support in all academic endeavors.

**Editor**

# 1

# Bipolar depression: a major unsolved challenge

Ross J. Baldessarini[1,2*], Gustavo H. Vázquez[2,3] and Leonardo Tondo[1,2,4]

**Abstract**

Depression in bipolar disorder (BD) patients presents major clinical challenges. As the predominant psychopathology even in treated BD, depression is associated not only with excess morbidity, but also mortality from co-occurring general-medical disorders and high suicide risk. In BD, risks for medical disorders including diabetes or metabolic syndrome, and cardiovascular disorders, and associated mortality rates are several-times above those for the general population or with other psychiatric disorders. The SMR for suicide with BD reaches 20-times above general-population rates, and exceeds rates with other major psychiatric disorders. In BD, suicide is strongly associated with mixed (agitated-dysphoric) and depressive phases, time depressed, and hospitalization. Lithium may reduce suicide risk in BD; clozapine and ketamine require further testing. Treatment of bipolar depression is far less well investigated than unipolar depression, particularly for long-term prophylaxis. Short-term efficacy of antidepressants for bipolar depression remains controversial and they risk clinical worsening, especially in mixed states and with rapid-cycling. Evidence of efficacy of lithium and anticonvulsants for bipolar depression is very limited; lamotrigine has long-term benefit, but valproate and carbamazepine are inadequately tested and carry high teratogenic risks. Evidence is emerging of short-term efficacy of several modern antipsychotics (including cariprazine, lurasidone, olanzapine-fluoxetine, and quetiapine) for bipolar depression, including with mixed features, though they risk adverse metabolic and neurological effects.

**Keywords:** Bipolar disorder, Depression, Disability, Morbidity, Mortality, Suicide, Treatment

## Background: depression in bipolar disorder

### Nosological uncertainties

Debate concerning Kraepelin's broadly inclusive concept of manic-depressive illness (MDI) continued to 1980 with a first formal separation of a distinct *bipolar disorder* (BD) with mania from nonbipolar major depressive disorder (MDD) in DSM-III (Trede et al. 2005; Baldessarini et al. 2015). Tension continues between lumping mood syndromes and separating various depressive and bipolar subtypes, and considering a "spectrum" of disorders ranging from more or less pure depression to archetypical BD, leading to profound therapeutic ambiguities (Cuellar et al. 2005; Goodwin and Jamison 2007; Baldessarini 2013; Yildiz et al. 2015; Tondo et al. 2018).

*Correspondence: rbaldessarini@mclean.harvard.edu
[1] Department of Psychiatry, Harvard Medical School, Boston, MA, USA
Full list of author information is available at the end of the article

### Current status of bipolar depression

Adequate understanding, timely diagnosis, and effective short- and long-term treatment of depressive episodes in BD patients are critically important but remarkably insufficiently resolved (Baldessarini et al. 2010c). Clinical significance of bipolar depression is underscored by strong association with overall morbidity, other co-occurring psychiatric conditions (notably anxiety and substance-abuse disorders), disability, and excess mortality owing largely to suicide in young patients and intercurrent medical illness in older patients (Ösby et al. 2001, 2018; Tondo et al. 2014, 2016; Baldessarini et al. 2020).

### Diagnosis

Clinical challenges include difficult and often long-delayed diagnostic differentiation of depression as an initial presentation of BD vs. a manifestation of nonbipolar MDD. Accurate diagnosis and appropriate treatment typically are delayed by 6–8 years, and even longer following juvenile onset (Post et al. 2010; Bschor et al. 2012; Drancourt et al. 2013; Tondo et al. 2014). Depression is initially considered as unipolar MDD in as many as 40% of patients later diagnosed with BD (Stensland et al. 2008; Shen et al. 2018). Such uncertainty is heightened as depression is the most prevalent presenting polarity in BD, (Goodwin and Jamison 2007; Baldessarini et al. 2014; Yildiz et al. 2015). Moreover, excess future depression in BD can be anticipated by initial episodes of anxiety or mixed-states as well as of depression (Baldessarini et al. 2012, 2014, 2020).

BD patients commonly fear, seek to avoid, to report, and to seek clinical help for depression. Contrarily, they may not recognize moderate increases of mood, energy, activity, or libido as hypomanic symptoms as clinically relevant, and may even prefer such states. Diagnostic uncertainty is especially likely early in the illness-course and without corroborating information from a family member or close friend (Vöhringer and Perlis 2016).

In perhaps 12–17% of cases, BD is not recognized until there is a mood "switch" into hypomania or mania ("[hypo]mania"), either spontaneously or with exposure to a mood-elevating substance (Tondo et al. 2010; Baldessarini et al. 2013; Barbuti et al. 2017). Other indirect factors suggesting a diagnosis of BD include: (a) familial mania, psychosis, "nervous breakdown," or psychiatric hospitalization; (b) early illness-onset, commonly with depression; (c) cyclothymic temperament; (d) multiple recurrences (e.g., ≥4 depressive episodes within 10 years); (e) depression with prominent agitation, anger, insomnia, irritability, talkativeness, other "mixed" or hypomanic features, or psychotic symptoms; (f) clinical "worsening," especially with mixed features during an antidepressant treatment; (g) suicidal ideation and acts; and (h) substance abuse (Tondo et al. 2014; Vöhringer and Perlis 2016).

### Depression in overall morbidity

Of note, overall time in depressive phases of BD, and duration of depressive episodes are much greater than in mania or hypomania ("[hypo]mania") (Kupka et al. 2007; De Dios et al. 2010). Moreover, morbidity has been surprisingly high in BD despite supposedly effective treatment. Indeed, BD patients averaged 45% of time ill during long-term follow-up, and depression accounted for 72% of time-ill, and somewhat more with BD-II (81%) than BD-I (70%) (Forte et al. 2015) (Table 1).

## Morbidity and disability

### Disability

Given the high proportion of time in depression among BD patients, depression is likely to be associated with

**Table 1 Depressive morbidity in clinically treated bipolar disorder subjects. Data adapted from Forte et al. (2015), based on systematic review of studies involving adult patients treated by community standards**

| Measure | Bipolar I | Bipolar II | All bipolar |
|---|---|---|---|
| Studies | 12 | 8 | 15 |
| Subjects | 2760 | 822 | 3582 |
| Exposure (years) | 7.78 [3.53–12.0] | 8.28 [2.18–14.4] | 7.89 [5.47–12.6] |
| %-Time depressed | 30.6 [23.9–37.3] | 35.9 [23.1–48.7] | 31.8 [23.7–39.9] |
| Total %-time ill | 43.7 [37.5–49.4] | 43.2 [35.2–51.1] | 43.6 [37.0–49.8] |
| %-of illness depressed | 69.6 [60.4–78.9] | 81.2 [71.3–91.0] | 72.3 [62.9–81.7] |

Data are means with 95% confidence intervals [CI]. Depression includes major episodes plus dysthymia

dysfunction and disability, including limited academic achievement and decreased employment success. Perhaps 80% of BD patients experience some work-loss, and 30–40% experience prolonged unemployment during adult working years—much of that disability associated with depression (Zimmerman et al. 2010; Arvilommi et al. 2015).

### Co-occurring psychiatric disorders

Psychiatric conditions commonly encountered in BD patients include substance-abuse and anxiety disorders, as well as various personality disorders and temperament types (Goodwin and Jamison 2007; Pavlova et al. 2015; Preti et al. 2016; Messer et al. 2017; Stokes et al. 2017; Vázquez et al. 2017b; Post et al. 2018). Such concomitant conditions may meet standard diagnostic criteria, but whether they should be considered separate, "comorbid" disorders vs. expressions of the range of psychopathology of BD remains unresolved (Yildiz et al. 2015; Vázquez et al. 2017b). Multiple diagnoses risk contributing to complexity and potential incoherence of treatment choices to compromise clinical care.

### General-medical morbidity and mortality

BD patients have increased risk of many general-medical disorders, including vascular conditions, with increased morbidity, disability and diminished longevity (McIntyre et al. 2007; Correll et al. 2017; Fornaro et al. 2017). In addition, obesity, diabetes, migraine, and some infectious diseases are more prevalent among BD patients (McIntyre et al. 2007; Almeida et al. 2018). With BD, risk of myocardial infarction was 37% greater (88% among women), stroke 60%, and congestive heart failure nearly 230% greater than in age-matched general populations (Wu et al. 2015; Fornaro et al. 2017; Tsai et al. 2017). Cardiovascular diseases are particularly frequent in association with BD disorder (Table 2) (Correll et al. 2017). Mediating

**Table 2 Risk of cardiovascular diseases in bipolar disorder patients vs. general population. Data adapted from Correll et al. (2017)**

| Outcome | Studies | Subjects | HR [95% CI] | *p*-value |
|---|---|---|---|---|
| Congestive heart failure | 1 | 1397 | 2.27 [1.49–3.45] | < 0.0001 |
| Cardiovascular mortality | 3 | 179,651 | 1.65 [1.10–2.47] | 0.02 |
| Cerebrovascular disease | 4 | 6,673,266 | 1.60 [0.99–2.57] | 0.05 |
| Any cardiovascular disease | 10 | 7,058,912 | 1.57 [1.28–1.93] | < 0.0001 |
| Coronary artery disease | 4 | 6,808,812 | 1.16 [0.76–1.78] | 0.49 |

Based on longitudinal studies with 8.4 [range: 1.8–30) years of follow-up. Hazard ratio (HR) is adjusted for six potential confounders; ranked by HR

factors include obesity, inactivity, diabetes or metabolic syndrome, and increased inflammatory factors—all with increased prevalence among BD patients (Vancampfort et al. 2013; Halaris 2017; Tsai et al. 2017), and at least in part attributable to treatments which may contribute to these risks (Baldessarini 2013; Correll et al. 2015).

With many general-medical disorders, BD patients have more adverse clinical outcomes and diminished life-expectancy, with all-cause mortality up to 15-times above general population rates, and rising (McIntyre et al. 2007; Ösby et al. 2018; Hällgren et al. 2018; Staudt-Hansen et al. 2019). Life-expectancy with BD is reduced by 12–15 years (Chesney et al. 2014). Factors associated with this decreased longevity include co-occurring substance abuse, smoking, and being overweight, unmarried, and having limited access to adequate medical care (Hjorthøj et al. 2015; Brietzke et al. 2017; Dickerson et al. 2018). The decreased longevity may be particularly associated with depression (Dickerson et al. 2018).

## Bipolar depression and suicide

### Suicidal risks

The reported international annual suicide rate averages 15.4/100,000 (0.015%/year), with wide regional variation (WHO 2018). The standardized mortality ratio (SMR) for suicide in BD is about 20 (Baldessarini et al. 2019a). By diagnosis, suicide risk ranks: bipolar disorders (BD-I = BD-II; especially with mixed or psychotic features) ≥ severe major depressive disorder with hospitalization > moderate depression among outpatients (Bachmann 2018; Hällgren et al. 2018; Baldessarini et al. 2019a). Risk for suicide and attempts is especially high in days following discharge from psychiatric hospitalization, in association with delay or lack of appropriate aftercare (Olfson et al. 2016; Large and Swaraj 2018; Forte et al. 2019).

In mood-disorder patients depressive-dysphoric phases are more associated with suicide than other illness states, especially if accompanied by mixed (hypomanic) features, co-occurring substance abuse, and following previous suicidal acts (Tondo et al. 1999, 2018; Baldessarini et al. 2019b). General population rates of suicide *attempts* average 0.2–0.6% per year, or approximately 36-times the suicide rate, and over 1%/year in BD (Kessler et al. 2005; Nock et al. 2008; Tondo et al. 2016; Baldessarini et al. 2019b). The ratio of suicide attempts/suicides (A/S), an *index of lethality* lower with more lethal intent or method, is only 5–10 in BD and MDD, or about five-times above lower than that for the general population (Tondo and Baldessarini 2015; Baldessarini et al. 2019b).

Among both BD-I and BD-II patients, especially with mixed or psychotic features, risk of suicidal behavior is among the highest of all psychiatric disorders despite supposedly effective treatments (Baldessarini et al. 2019b). This disparity almost certainly reflects great difficulty of treating depressive and mixed states in BD (Baldessarini et al. 2010c; Saunders and Hawton 2013; Forte et al. 2015). The remarkably prolonged delay of recognition and intervention in BD, sometimes for more than a decade, contrasts strikingly with observations that half of long-term risk of suicidal acts among BD patients occurred within the first 2–3 years of illness (Tondo and Baldessarini 2014, 2015).

### Suicide and treatment with antidepressants

Suicide cannot be "treated" but only prevented (Table 3). Research on treatments aimed at suicide prevention, not surprisingly, is very limited because of clinical and ethical problems arising if an inactive or ineffective treatment, such as placebo, were compared to an experimental intervention, with death as a potential outcome. In addition, it is virtually impossible to know when a suicide has been prevented, whereas suicidal acts or surrogate measures can be counted. Rarity of suicide, even among psychiatric patients, encourages research reliance on more prevalent measures related to suicide, including suicidal ideation, threats, self-injurious acts, or emergency interventions. However, the typically distant relationship of such measures to suicide limits their value in testing for therapeutic effects on suicide itself. Relating treatments to suicidal risks is further complicated by uncertain long-term adherence to recommended treatments (Isometsä 2005; Simon and Hales 2012; Baldessarini 2013; Ahmedani et al. 2014). Treatments for BD considered for possible suicide-prevention include antidepressants, anticonvulsants and lithium, antipsychotics, ECT, and psychosocial interventions (Table 3).

**Table 3 Treatments aimed at reducing suicidal risk in bipolar disorder patients**

| Intervention | Timing | Findings | Comments |
|---|---|---|---|
| Antidepressants | Short-term benefits are not clear; long-term effects are virtually untested | Research findings are inconclusive. Suicidal risk may increase with agitation, and in youth but may be lower in older adults | Studies lack long-term randomization with suicidal acts as an explicit outcome measure |
| Antipsychotics | Short-term benefits are not adequately tested. Clozapine is probably beneficial long-term in schizophrenia (with FDA approval) but untested in BD | Except for clozapine, testing remains inadequate and inconclusive | Effects of clozapine rely mainly on a single randomized trial vs. olanzapine, without reduction of mortality |
| Anticonvulsants | Short-term effects are not established; long-term benefits have been proposed | Valproate most studied; anticonvulsants may be less effective than lithium | Studies lack suicidal acts as an explicit outcome |
| Lithium | Very likely effective long-term | Consistent decrease of risk of suicide and attempts in controlled and uncontrolled studies; not clear if effect is via reducing risk of depression, impulsivity, or specific anti-suicidal action | Even randomized trials lack suicidal behavior as explicit outcome measure. Long-term acceptance and tolerance suggests some self-selection; potentially toxic on overdose |
| Other pharmacological treatments | Only short-term effects have been tested | Ketamine can reduce suicidal ideation; effects on suicidal behavior are untested; newer NMDA agents untested | Ketamine has a short-term antidepresant effect in BD |
| Other somatic treatments | If there are benefits, they are probably short-term | ECT, magnetic, vagal nerve, or deep-brain stimulations can benefit depression | Inadequate testing vs. suicidal behavior specifically |
| Psychotherapies | Effects not established, but widely assumed to be helpful clinically | Cognitive-behavioral, dialectic and interpersonal methods best studied, but research results for suicide are inconclusive | Psychotherapy involves self-selection |

References to relevant studies are provided in the text

Strong association of suicidal behavior or acts with depression suggests that treatment with antidepressants might reduce suicidal risk, though most studies have yielded inconsistent evidence. Most were not designed to test for suicidal behavior as an explicit outcome measure rather than as an incidental and passively reported "adverse event" (Möller 2006; Tondo and Baldessarini 2015; Baldessarini et al. 2020). Too, some patients can *worsen* clinically when given an antidepressant, and the treated depressive episode can be accompanied by agitation, dysphoria, restlessness, irritability, anger, insomnia, behavioral disinhibition, or other mixed features, with increased risk of suicidal behavior (Tondo et al. 1999, 2018; Maj et al. 2006; Simon and Hales 2012; Pacchiarotti et al. 2013). In addition, abrupt or rapid discontinuation of antidepressant treatment markedly increases early risk of new depression, and might increase suicidal risk (Baldessarini et al. 2010b).

Several studies have found only minor associations of antidepressant treatment and suicidal behaviors, mainly with MDD (Beasley et al. 1991; Acharya et al. 2006; Möller 2006; Tondo et al. 2008; Khan et al. 2011; Tondo and Baldessarini 2015; Braun et al. 2016). Other findings noted increased risk of suicidal acts in juveniles and young adults but decreased risk in older adults (Hammad et al. 2006; Laughren et al. 2006; Bridge et al. 2007; Barbui et al. 2009; Saunders and Hawton 2013; Braun et al. 2016). However, most such studies lacked explicit, validated, predefined outcome measures pertinent to suicide.

In our experience, emergence of new suicidal behaviors among mood-disordered adults treated with sustained antidepressant treatment in clinical settings was infrequent, involving perhaps 5/1000 patients/year (Tondo et al. 2008). Nevertheless, risks of clinical worsening with antidepressants, as well as the possibility that acute depression may be the initial episode of BD, should be considered and monitored at any age, especially early in antidepressant treatment.

#### Lithium treatment and suicide

An association of reduced risk of suicides and attempts during long-term treatment with lithium in BD is supported consistently by most (Müller-Oerlinghausen et al. 2006; Baldessarini and Tondo 2008; Tondo and Baldessarini 2014, 2015, 2018; Roberts et al. 2017; Smith and Cipriani 2017; Felber et al. 2018), but not all studies (Marangell et al. 2008; Oquendo et al. 2011). At least 10 placebo-controlled, randomized trials not specifically designed with suicide risk as the primary outcome measure, but involving more than 110,000 person-years of risk, found five- to sixfold reductions in suicidal acts (Tondo et al. 1998, 2001; Angst et al. 2005; Cipriani et al. 2005; Baldessarini et al. 2006; Lauterbach et al. 2008; Khan et al. 2011). Based on such studies, several expert reports recommend long-term lithium treatment to limit risk of suicidal behavior in BD patients (Wasserman et al. 2012; Lewitzka et al. 2013; Yatham et al. 2018).

#### Anticonvulsants and suicide

Few studies directly compare suicidal risks during treatment with alternatives to lithium, including anticonvulsants, and findings are largely inconsistent and inconclusive (Thies-Flechtner et al. 1996; Goodwin et al. 2003; Yerevanian et al. 2007; Baldessarini and Tondo 2009; Chen et al. 2019). The FDA (2008) proposed that some anticonvulsants may even be associated with increased risk of suicidal behavior, at least in epilepsy patients, though probably not in psychiatric applications (Yerevanian et al. 2007; Gibbons et al. 2009). Meta-analysis of suicidal behavior with lithium vs. several anticonvulsants (mainly valproate) in six direct comparisons involving over 30,000 patients found nearly three-fold greater reductions with lithium (Baldessarini and Tondo 2009).

#### Antipsychotics and suicide

Antipsychotic drugs remain little-evaluated for effects on suicidal behavior (Simon and Hales 2012). However, one study found no difference in relatively short-term risk of suicides or attempts during treatment of > 10,000 psychotic patients with either first- or second-generation antipsychotics (FGAs or SGAs) vs. placebo (Khan et al. 2001). In addition, mortality risk was not increased in nearly 109,000 schizophrenia subjects given antipsychotic drugs (Schneider-Thoma et al. 2018), but was greater without antipsychotic treatment in another study of over 2200 such patients (Tiihonen et al. 2006). The InterSePT study comparing suicide-related behavior in schizophrenia patients at high risk for suicide provided strong support for an antisuicidal effect of clozapine compared to olanzapine (Meltzer et al. 2003). Clozapine has not been evaluated adequately in the treatment of BD patients, although it may have antimanic or mood-stabilizing effects (Li et al. 2015). Studies of SGAs with antidepressant effects in BD patients, in particular, require assessment for effects on suicide.

#### Other treatments and suicide

Evidence is growing that the glutamate NMDA-receptor antagonist ketamine and its active *S*-enantiomer (esketamine) can exert rapid, short-term reduction of suicidal ideation along with rapid reduction of symptoms of depression, including in BD patients, although effects on suicidal behavior are uncertain (Parsaik et al. 2015; Grunebaum et al. 2017; Wilkinson et al. 2018).

There is considerable uncertainty about how to continue use of racemic or *S*-ketamine following initial benefits, and some concern that its discontinuation may provoke adverse clinical responses (Schatzberg 2019). ECT often appears to be lifesaving in suicidal emergencies but lacks evidence of sustained antisuicidal efficacy (Fink et al. 2014). Other methods of external electrical or magnetic stimulation of brain, vagal nerve stimulation, and deep brain stimulation are being investigated or introduced for the treatment of otherwise treatment-resistant depression but remain to be tested adequately for specific effects on suicidal behavior, particularly in BD.

Additional interventions of potential value include emergency hospitalization (Zalsman et al. 2016) as well as psychotherapies, in particular cognitive-behavioral, dialectic, and interpersonal methods, which can improve depressive symptoms and may reduce suicidal risk (Brown et al. 2005; Zalsman et al. 2016; McCauley et al. 2018; Baldessarini et al. 2020). However, results from studies of psychosocial interventions may be limited by the self-selection of patients who adhere to such prolonged treatments.

## Treatment of bipolar depression

As noted, depressive, dysthymic, and mixed states account for the majority of illness-burden in BD, and are strongly predicted by initial depressive, mixed, or anxious episodes (Goodwin and Jamison 2007; Yildiz et al. 2015; Forte et al. 2015; Baldessarini et al. 2014, 2019a). Remarkably few treatments are proved to be highly and consistently effective in acute episodes of bipolar depression, and there is even less evidence supporting substantial long-term protection from recurrences (Table 4). In particular, there is continued controversy about the value and risks of antidepressant drugs in bipolar depression (Pacchiarotti et al. 2013; McGirr et al. 2016). Lack of highly effective treatments encourages widespread drug-combinations and other off-label treatments largely untested for effectiveness and safety.

Relative paucity of experimental treatment studies for bipolar depression may reflect a broadly accepted view that "major depression" is similar in its clinical characteristics as well as treatment responses in BD and MDD (Baldessarini 2013). Instead, their characteristics differ, e.g., in family history, sex-distribution, onset-age, long-term diagnostic stability, episode duration, recurrence rates, and treatment-responses (Baldessarini et al. 2010a, c). The assumption of similarity probably contributes to the rarity of direct comparisons of treatment responses with depression in BD vs. MDD, and leaves bipolar depression as a leading challenge for psychiatric therapeutics (Goodwin et al. 2016; Baldessarini et al. 2019b, 2020).

**Table 4 Placebo-controlled trials for acute depression in bipolar disorder**

| Treatments | Subjects (n) | Responders/subjects (%) | | RR [95%CI] |
|---|---|---|---|---|
| | | Drug | Placebo | |
| Anticonvulsants [10 trials, 3 agents] | 1281 | 313/657 [47.6%] | 181/624 [29.0%] | 1.61 [1.39–1.87] |
| Antidepressants [12 trials, 11 agents] | 1895 | 383/803 [48.9%] | 419/1092 [38.4%] | 1.32 [1.07–1.62] |
| Antipsychotics [13 trials, 6 agents] | 6044 | 2135/3859 [55.3%] | 904/2185 [41.4%] | 1.28 [1.09–1.51] |
| Lithium [1 trial, 1 agent] | 265 | 85/136 [62.5%] | 72/129 [55.8%] | 1.12 [0.92–1.37] |
| Pooled/totals [36 trials, 21 agents] | 9485 | 2926/5455 [54.4%] | 1576/4030 [39.4%] | 1.37 [1.30–1.44] |

Dropout rates (average: 32.9% [28.0–37.8]) were similar across treatments and with drug or placebo. Response typically involved ≥ 50% improvement in depression symptom ratings. By separate random-effects meta-analysis, antidepressants were statistically more effective than placebo (RR = 1.32 [1.07–1.87]; $z = 2.65$, $p = 0.008$), as were the other agents (RR = 1.34 [1.17–1.53]; $z = 431$, $p < 0.0001$). The overall weighted average drug vs. placebo difference (RR = 1.37) was highly significant ($\chi^2 = 196$, $p < 0.0001$). Antidepressant dose averaged 172 [146–198] mg/day imipramine-equivalent (Baldessarini 2013). Antidepressant monotherapy trials yielded greater drug/placebo differences than with addition to a mood-stabilizer (RR = 1.64 [1.05–2.56] vs. 1.18 [0.96–1.46]). Of note, in 23/36 trials (63.9%) drug was *not* statistically superior to placebo. Results are ranked by drug/placebo Risk Ratios (RR). [References: Nemeroff et al. (2001); Tohen et al. (2003); Shelton and Stahl (2004); Agosti and Stewart (2008); McElroy et al. (2010); McGirr et al. (2016); Yatham et al. (2018); Vázquez et al. (2017a); Baldessarini et al. (2019b)]

### Antidepressants for bipolar depression

Ease and relative safety of treating depressive episodes with modern antidepressants, and strenuous efforts to minimize or avoid depression by BD patients and clinicians, have made antidepressants the leading treatment provided to BD patients (Baldessarini et al. 2008, 2019b). Nevertheless, there is a striking paucity of therapeutic experimentation and inconsistent findings, despite more than a half-century of use of antidepressant drugs to treat "depression," with particularly serious gaps regarding dysthymia and dysphoria, mixed features, and long-term prophylaxis for bipolar depression (Ghaemi et al. 2008, 2010; Sidor and MacQueen 2012; Baldessarini 2013; Pacchiarotti et al. 2013; Fountoulakis et al. 2017; Liu et al. 2017a; Gitlin 2018). Many experts advise caution in using antidepressants, particularly for BD-I patients to avoid potentially dangerous mood-switches, and encourage their use, if necessary, only with mood-stabilizing agents or SGAs, and without current mixed features or agitation (Pacchiarotti et al. 2013; Tondo et al. 2013; Goodwin et al. 2016; Yatham et al. 2018).

Well-designed, controlled, monotherapy trials of antidepressants for acute bipolar depression are surprisingly few, vary in size and quality, and yield inconsistent findings (Table 4) (Vázquez et al. 2011; Tondo et al. 2013; Gitlin 2018; Yatham et al. 2018). Two large trials found no additional improvement in bipolar depression by adding paroxetine or bupropion to mood-stabilizing or antipsychotic drugs (Sachs et al. 2007; McElroy et al. 2010). Two meta-analyses including these and the few other relevant trials supported possible efficacy of various antidepressants in bipolar depression (Gijsman et al. 2004; Vázquez et al. 2013); another did not (Sidor and MacQueen 2012). Several direct comparisons found similar antidepressant responses in depressed BD and MDD patients (Vázquez et al. 2011). Another comparison of clinical responses in large samples of depressed BD-I, BD-II, or MDD patients also found only minor differences in response or remission and low risk of mood-switching in these disorders, provided that subjects with agitation or even minor mixed features were excluded (Tondo et al. 2013).

Impressions that antidepressants may be less effective in acute bipolar depression than in MDD may, to some extent, reflect adverse effects of treatment, including worsening of agitation, anger, or dysphoria, interpreted as failure of depression to respond (Tondo et al. 2013). Our findings from available randomized, controlled trials support the impression that antidepressant treatment has yielded a significant, 32% superiority over placebo for acute bipolar depression, with moderately high heterogeneity of outcomes (Table 4). Despite this limited and inconsistent body of research, it is evidently widely assumed clinically that antidepressants may be appropriate for some BD patients, and especially safe for BD-II depression (Baldessarini et al. 2008; Amsterdam and Shults 2010; Undurraga et al. 2012; Altshuler et al. 2017; Gitlin 2018). Selection of BD candidates for clinical antidepressant treatment may usefully be guided by previous beneficial and tolerated responses, relatively less severe or nonrapidly cycling illness, relatively few previous depressions, lack of switching from depression to mania, or of current agitation or even minor mixed features (Pacchiarotti et al. 2013; Tondo et al. 2013; Baldessarini et al. 2019b). Research on biomarkers associated with response to antidepressants is ongoing and may help in identifying more effective treatments for various types of depression (Gadad et al. 2018).

### Antidepressants and mood switching

There is widespread concern that antidepressant treatment for bipolar depression risks switching into potentially dangerous agitation or mania, especially in BD-I (Bond et al. 2008; Undurraga et al. 2012). Such risk is more associated with the long-term BD course-pattern of depression followed by mania before a stable interval ("DMI") than the opposite ("MDI") (Koukopoulos et al. 2013). However, it is difficult to distinguish spontaneous from antidepressant-associated switching in BD, mean rates of which are similar (13.8% [12.2–15.3] vs. 15.3% [14.5–16.1]) (Tondo et al. 2010). Though it is plausible to expect mood-stabilizing and antipsychotic drugs to prevent mood-switching with antidepressants, required randomized comparisons are lacking (Tondo et al. 2010; Baldessarini et al. 2019b). Trials of antidepressants have found little difference in risk of new mania between antidepressants and placebo, with or without a mood-stabilizer included, although exposure times were short (Liu et al. 2017a). However, one study found that switching in BD was 2.8-times greater within 9 months after adding an antidepressant, but not if a mood-stabilizer also was used (Viktorin et al. 2014), and switching risk was increased in the rare long-term trials with an antidepressant included in treatment (Ghaemi et al. 2008).

An evident clinical consensus is that antidepressants be used for BD only cautiously, with short-acting agents given in moderate, slowly increased doses, briefly, and with effective mood-stabilizing co-treatment, while monitoring for emerging hypomania. It seems prudent that antidepressants, especially tricyclics and some SNRIs, be used very cautiously for bipolar depression, especially in BD-I patients, and perhaps avoided altogether with a history of mood-switching during antidepressant treatment, rapid-cycling without antidepressant treatment, or if mixed symptoms are present (Tondo et al. 2010; Pacchiarotti et al. 2013).

### Mood-stabilizers

Several anticonvulsants have been used widely for BD, based on secure evidence of short-term antimanic effects (carbamazepine and valproate) or long-term reduction of risk of depressive recurrences (lamotrigine) (Baldessarini 2013; Geddes and Miklowitz 2013; Reinares et al. 2013). Such treatment choices are encouraged by seeming simpler than treatment with lithium (Baldessarini 2013; Vázquez et al. 2014). For divalproex monotherapy, 4 small trials suggest possible value in acute bipolar depression (Table 4), but it remains FDA-unapproved for depression or long-term treatment in BD. Evidence that lamotrigine is effective in acute bipolar depression rests on pooling inconsistent data, including from individually failed trials vs. placebo (Table 4) (Solmi et al. 2016). Lamotrigine is FDA-approved only for long-term prophylaxis in BD, with partial effectiveness against recurrences of depression but little efficacy against acute or recurrent mania (Frye et al. 2011; Baldessarini 2013). Moreover, slow dose-increases to avoid potentially serious dermatological reactions limit practicality of off-label use of lamotrigine in acute bipolar depression. Evidence concerning carbamazepine for short- or long-term use for bipolar depression is very limited (Table 4), and controlled trials for other anticonvulsants in BD are lacking (Reinares et al. 2013; Selle et al. 2014).

Despite use of lithium as a fundamental treatment for BD for more than six decades, and its position as a first-line treatment in some expert guidelines (Goodwin et al. 2016; Yatham et al. 2018), it remains virtually untested for acute bipolar depression. Lithium was included as a third-arm of a trial in acute bipolar depression designed primarily to test quetiapine, with little benefit (Table 4) (Young et al. 2010). Nevertheless, lithium has some long-term effectiveness against recurrences of bipolar depression as well as greater prophylactic effects against [hypo] mania (Baldessarini 2013; Bschor 2014; Yatham et al. 2018), and benefits in mixed episodes in BD (Sani and Fiorillo 2019). Moreover, as noted, lithium may reduce risk of suicide substantially in BD patients (Tondo et al. 2001; Baldessarini et al. 2006; Cipriani et al. 2013; Tondo and Baldessarini 2014, 2018; Song et al. 2017).

### Second-generation antipsychotics

SGAs, including cariprazine, lurasidone, olanzapine-fluoxetine, and quetiapine are currently the only FDA-approved medicines for short-term treatment of acute depressive episodes in BD (Baldessarini 2013; Selle et al. 2014; Earley et al. 2019; Ragguett and McIntyre 2019). Of these, only quetiapine has outperformed placebo consistently in several trials, with similar results for doses of 300 vs. 600 mg/day, and only the lower dose is FDA-approved (McElroy et al. 2010). Olanzapine-fluoxetine was superior to placebo, whereas olanzapine alone was less effective (Tohen et al. 2003). Unsurprisingly, as both olanzapine and quetiapine are antimanic, they have yielded somewhat *lower* risks of mood-switching than placebo (Selle et al. 2014). Most of these responses in acute bipolar depression have been modest (Table 4), and possible long-term protective effects require further study. Of note, beneficial effects in bipolar depression are not a class-effect of all SGAs (Taylor et al. 2014). In effective doses, antipsychotics risk adverse effects that include excessive sedation as well as distressing restlessness (akathisia) (Brown et al. 2006; Tamayo et al. 2010). Although risks of tardive dyskinesia with most SGAs are far lower than with FGAs (Tarsy et al. 2010; Carbon et al. 2017), their greatly increasing use and broadening indications may risk increased numbers of cases of even this uncommon adverse outcome (Pompili et al. 2016). Moreover, risks of weight-gain, type-2 diabetes, and other features of metabolic syndrome (hyperlipidemia, hypertension) are encountered with some SGAs (particularly olanzapine and quetiapine), sometimes rapidly (Centorrino et al. 2012; Baldessarini 2013; Vázquez et al. 2015). These medically important adverse effects tend to limit the potential value of SGAs for prophylactic treatment against recurrences of bipolar depression (Vázquez et al. 2014, 2015; Fountoulakis et al. 2017). In summary, cariprazine, lurasidone, and quetiapine, as well as olanzapine-fluoxetine are effective in acute bipolar depression, though with some risks, and they need further testing for long-term, prophylactic effects against bipolar depression.

### Other treatments

Growing numbers of novel pharmacological treatments for depression are under investigation; some may be of value in BD, including drugs that act at synaptic transmission systems mediated by amino acid neurotransmitters glutamate and GABA. They include the NMDA-glutamate receptor antagonist ketamine and newer pharmacologically similar agents (e.g., apimostinel, rapastinel) (Dhir 2017; Garay et al. 2017; Grady et al. 2017; Grunebaum et al. 2017; Ragguett et al. 2019; Wilkinson and Sanacora 2019). Given apparent association of postpartum mood disorders and BD (Liu et al. 2017b), neurosteroids that interact with $GABA_A$ receptors and found effective for postpartum depression (e.g., brexanolone) may be of interest for bipolar depression (Martinez-Botella et al. 2017; Scott 2019). Agents of less certain value include polyunsaturated fatty acids, anti-inflammatory agents, and probiotics (Vázquez et al. 2017a).

Among nonpharmacological treatments, acute bipolar depression is responsive to ECT (Itagaki et al. 2017; Perugi et al. 2017; Bahji et al. 2019), although optimal treatment to follow successful ECT remains uncertain. Other biomedical treatments may be of value in bipolar depression. Intense light therapy and sleep deprivation are plausible candidates that require adequate testing in BD (Tseng et al. 2016; Suzuki et al. 2018). Vagal nerve stimulation (VNS) is FDA-approved for treatment-resistant depression, with evidence of efficacy in depression of BD and MDD (Cimpianu et al. 2017; Conway et al. 2018), though with some risk of inducing mania (Salloum et al. 2017). Repeated transcranial magnetic stimulation (rTMS) and various forms of electrical stimulation of brain from the surface or through stereotaxically placed deep-brain electrodes remain experimental for bipolar depression (Nierenberg et al. 2008; Vázquez et al. 2017a; Widge et al. 2018; Filkowski and Sheth 2019).

Finally, several manual-based, replicable forms of psychotherapy, alone or added to antidepressants, have shown promise for treating BD patients (Bouwkamp et al. 2013; McMahon et al. 2016; Salcedo et al. 2016; Lovas and Schuman-Olivier 2018; Yatham et al. 2018).

**Table 5 Current status of depression in bipolar disorder**

| |
|---|
| Depression in bipolar disorder (BD) is the major residual psychiatric morbidity with available treatments, accounting for three-quarters of the 40–50% long-term time-ill |
| Unresolved morbidity, and especially depression, is associated with excess medical morbidity, including metabolic syndrome and cardiovascular disease, with increased mortality |
| Suicide risk in BD is similar in types I and II BD, greater than in most other psychiatric disorders, ca. 20-times above general population rates, and strongly associated with depression, especially with agitation (mixed-dysphoric states), and in the days–weeks following hospital discharge |
| Predicting suicide in BD clinically is limited regarding individuals and timing |
| Treatments proposed to prevent suicidal behavior in BD include lithium, clozapine, and possibly ketamine and psychotherapies, which all require further study |
| Therapeutics of bipolar depression is far less well developed than for nonbipolar major depression, probably reflecting lack of recognition of differences between bipolar and unipolar depression |
| The short-term value and safety of antidepressant treatment for bipolar depression remains controversial, and long-term value remains virtually untested; it is best avoided with ongoing dysphoric agitation or mixed features |
| Some modern antipsychotics are effective in bipolar depression short-term; lithium and lamotrigine have modest prophylactic value long-term but are not adequately tested short-term; other anticonvulsant mood-stabilizers have very limited evidence of short- or long-term efficacy in bipolar depression |
| All available treatments for bipolar depression have risks of adverse metabolic or neurological effects; valproate and carbamazepine are also highly teratogenic |

## Conclusions

Depression, dysthymia, and dysphoria in BD represent major, only partially solved, clinical challenges (Table 5). As the main unresolved illness in treated BD, bipolar depression is associated with excess morbidity as well as mortality from co-occurring general-medical disorders and very high suicide risk. Suicide risk in BD exceeds general-population rates by 20-fold and is strongly associated with depressive phases, especially with mixed or psychotic features. Treatments proposed to reduce suicide risk notably include lithium. Treatment of bipolar depression is far less well investigated than MDD, and the value and tolerability of standard antidepressants for bipolar depression remain controversial. Evidence of efficacy in bipolar depression of mood-stabilizing agents, including lithium and several anticonvulsants (except lamotrigine, long-term) remains far less substantial than for several SGAs. All available pharmacological treatments used for bipolar depression have limited efficacy and risk adverse metabolic or neurological effects. Overall, we strongly encourage renewed efforts to consider bipolar depression as distinct from depression in MDD and to seek more effective treatments especially for long-term prophylaxis aimed at reducing morbidity and mortality.

**Acknowledgements**

Ms. Rita Burke provided valuable assistance in gathering bibliographic material on which this report is based.

**Authors' contributions**

All authors contributed substantively to the collection and critical assessment of information, writing, and final preparation of this report. All authors read and approved the final manuscript.

**Author details**

[1] Department of Psychiatry, Harvard Medical School, Boston, MA, USA. [2] International Consortium for Bipolar & Psychotic Disorders Research, McLean Hospital, Belmont, MA, USA. [3] Department of Psychiatry, Queen's University School of Medicine, Kingston, ON, Canada. [4] Lucio Bini Mood Disorder Center, Cagliari, Sardinia, Italy.

**References**

Acharya N, Rosen AS, Polzer JP, et al. Duloxetine: meta-analyses of suicidal behaviors and ideation in clinical trials for major depressive disorder. J Clin Psychopharmacol. 2006;26(6):587–94.

Agosti V, Stewart JW. Hypomania with and without dysphoria: comparison of comorbidity and clinical characteristics of respondents from a national community sample. J Affect Disord. 2008;108(1–2):177–82.

Ahmedani BK, Simon GE, Stewart C, et al. Healthcare contacts in the year before suicide death. J Gen Int Med. 2014;29(6):870–7.

Almeida OP, Hankey GJ, Yeap BB, Golledge J, Flicker L. Older men with bipolar disorder: clinical associations with early and late illness. Int J Geriatr Psychiatry. 2018;33(12):1613–9.

Altshuler LL, Sugar CA, McElroy SL, et al. Switch rates during acute treatment for bipolar II depression with lithium, sertraline, or the two combined: randomized, double-blind comparison. Am J Psychiatry. 2017;174(3):266–76.

Amsterdam JD, Shults J. Efficacy and safety of long-term fluoxetine vs. lithium monotherapy of bipolar II disorder: randomized, double-blind, placebo-substitution study. Am J Psychiatry. 2010;167(7):792–800.

Angst J, Angst F, Gerber-Werder R, Gamma A. Suicide in 406 mood-disorder patients with and without long-term medication: a 40 to 44 years' follow-up. Arch Suicide Res. 2005;9(3):279–300.

Arvilommi P, Suominen K, Mantere O, Valtonen H, Leppamaki S, Isometsa E. Predictors of long-term work disability among patients with type I and II bipolar disorder: prospective 18-month follow-up study. Bipolar Disord. 2015;17(8):821–35.

Bachmann S. Epidemiology of suicide and the psychiatric perspective. Int J Environ Res Public Health. 2018;15(7):E1425–47.

Bahji A, Hawken ER, Sepehry AA, Cabrera CA, Vázquez GH. ECT beyond unipolar major depression: systematic review and meta-analysis of electroconvulsive therapy in bipolar depression. Acta Psychiatr Scand. 2019;139(3):214–26.

Baldessarini RJ. Chemotherapy in psychiatry. 3rd ed. New York: Springer Press; 2013.

Baldessarini RJ, Tondo L. Lithium and suicidal risk. Bipolar Disord. 2008;10(1):114–5.

Baldessarini RJ, Tondo L. Suicidal risks during treatment of bipolar disorder patients with lithium versus anticonvulsants. Pharmacopsychiatry. 2009;42(2):72–5.

Baldessarini RJ, Tondo L, Davis P, et al. Decreased risk of suicides and attempts during long-term lithium treatment: meta-analytic review. Bipolar Disord. 2006;8(5):625–39.

Baldessarini RJ, Henk H, Sklar A, Chang J, Leahy L. Psychotropic medications for patients with bipolar disorder in the United States: polytherapy and adherence. Psychiatr Serv. 2008;59(10):1175–83.

Baldessarini RJ, Salvatore P, Khalsa HM, et al. Morbidity in 303 first-episode bipolar I disorder patients. Bipolar Disord. 2010a;12(3):264–70.

Baldessarini RJ, Tondo L, Ghiani C, Lepri B. Illness risk following rapid vs. gradual discontinuation of antidepressants. Am J Psychiatry. 2010b;167(8):934–41.

Baldessarini RJ, Vieta E, Calabrese JR, Tohen M, Bowden C. Bipolar depression: overview and commentary. Harv Rev Psychiatry. 2010c;18(3):143–57.

Baldessarini RJ, Undurraga J, Vázquez GH, et al. Predominant recurrence polarity among 928 adult international bipolar I disorder patients. Acta Psychiatr Scand. 2012;125(4):293–302.

Baldessarini RJ, Faedda GL, Offidani E, et al. Antidepressant-associated mood-switching and transition from unipolar major depression to bipolar disorder. J Affect Disord. 2013;148(1):129–35.

Baldessarini RJ, Tondo L, Visioli C. First-episode types in bipolar disorder: predictive associations with later illness. Acta Psychiatr Scand. 2014;129(5):383–92.

Baldessarini RJ, Pérez J, Salvatore P, Trede K, Maggini C. Chapt 1: History of bipolar manic-depressive disorder. In: Yildiz A, Nemeroff C, Ruiz P, editors. The bipolar book: history, neurobiology, and treatment. New York: Oxford University Press; 2015. p. 3–20.

Baldessarini RJ, Tondo L, Pinna N, Nuñez GH, Vázquez GH. Suicidal risk factors in major affective disorders. Br J Psychiatry. 2019a;215(4):621–6.

Baldessarini RJ, Tondo L, Vázquez GH. Pharmacological treatment of adult bipolar disorder. Mol Psychiatry. 2019b;24(2):198–217.

Baldessarini RJ, Tondo L, Vázquez GH. Chapt 4: Unmet needs in psychiatry: bipolar depression. In: Pompili M, McIntyre RS, Fiorillo A, Sartorius N, editors. New directions in psychiatry. New York: Springer Press; 2020.

Barbui C, Esposito E, Cipriani A. Selective serotonin reuptake inhibitors and risk of suicide: systematic review of observational studies. CMAJ. 2009;180(3):291–7.

Barbuti M, Pacchiarotti I, Vieta E, et al. Antidepressant-induced hypomania/mania in patients with major depression: evidence from the BRIDGE-II-MIX study. J Affect Disord. 2017;219(9):187–92.

Beasley CM Jr, Dornseif BE, Bosomworth JC, et al. Fluoxetine and suicide: meta-analysis of controlled trials of treatment for depression. BMJ. 1991;303(3804):685–92.

Bond DJ, Noronha M, Kauer-Sant'Anna M, Lam RW, Yatham LN. Antidepressant-associated mood elevations in bipolar II disorder compared with bipolar I disorder and major depressive disorder: systematic review and meta-analysis. J Clin Psychiatry. 2008;69(10):1589–601.

Bouwkamp CG, de Kruiff ME, van Troost TM, et al. Interpersonal and social rhythm group therapy for patients with bipolar disorder. Int J Group Psychother. 2013;63:97–115.

Braun C, Bschor T, Franklin J, Baethge C. Suicides and suicide attempts during long-term treatment with antidepressants: meta-analysis of 29 placebo-controlled studies including 6934 patients with major depressive disorder. Psychother Psychosom. 2016;85(3):171–9.

Bridge JA, Iyengar S, Salary CB, et al. Clinical response and risk for reported suicidal ideation and suicide attempts in pediatric antidepressant treatment: meta-analysis of randomized controlled trials. JAMA. 2007;297(15):1683–96.

Brietzke E, Mansur RB, McIntyre RS. Impact of inequalities in healthcare on the mortality risk of individuals with severe mental illnesses. Braz J Psychiatry. 2017;39(3):193–4.

Brown GK, Ten Have T, Henriques GR, Xie SX, Hollander JE, Beck AT. Cognitive therapy for the prevention of suicide attempts: randomized controlled trial. JAMA. 2005;294(5):563–70.

Brown EB, McElroy SL, Keck PE Jr, et al. Seven-week, randomized, double-blind trial of olanzapine/fluoxetine combination versus lamotrigine in the treatment of bipolar I depression. J Clin Psychiatry. 2006;67(7):1025–33.

Bschor T. Lithium in the treatment of major depressive disorder. Drugs. 2014;74(8):855–62.

Bschor T, Angst J, Azorin JM, et al. Are bipolar disorders underdiagnosed in patients with depressive episodes? Results of the multicenter BRIDGE screening study in Germany. J Affect Disord. 2012;142(1–3):45–52.

Carbon M, Hsieh C-H, Kane JM, Correll CU. Tardive dyskinesia prevalence in the period of second-generation antipsychotic use, meta-analysis. J Clin Psychiatry. 2017;78(3):e264–78.

Centorrino F, Masters GA, Talamo A, Baldessarini RJ, Öngür D. Metabolic syndrome in psychiatrically hospitalized patients treated with antipsychotics and other psychotropics. Hum Psychopharmacol. 2012;27(5):521–6.

Chen TY, Kamali M, Chu CS, Yeh CB, Huang M, Mao WC, Lin Y, Chen YW, Tseng PT, Hsu CY. Divalproex and its effect on suicide risk in bipolar disorder: systematic review and meta-analysis of multinational observational studies. J Affect Disord. 2019;245(2):812–8.

Chesney E, Goodwin GM, Fazel S. Risks of all-cause and suicide mortality in mental disorders: meta-review. World Psychiatry. 2014;13(2):153–60.

Cimpianu CL, Strube W, Falkai P, Palm U, Hasan A. Vagus nerve stimulation in psychiatry: systematic review of the available evidence. J Neural Transm. 2017;124(1):145–58.

Cipriani A, Pretty H, Hawton K, Geddes JR. Lithium in the prevention of suicidal behavior and all-cause mortality in patients with mood disorders: systematic review of randomized trials. Am J Psychiatry. 2005;162(10):1805–19.

Cipriani A, Hawton K, Stockton S, Geddes JR. Lithium in the prevention of suicide in mood disorders: updated systematic review and meta-analysis. BMJ Clin Res. 2013;346(6):f3646–59.

Conway CR, Kumar A, Xiong W, Bunker M, Aaronson ST, Rush AJ. Chronic vagus nerve stimulation significantly improves quality of life in treatment-resistant major depression. J Clin Psychiatry. 2018;79(5):52–9.

Correll CU, Detraux J, De Lepeleire J, De Hert M. Effects of antipsychotics, antidepressants and mood stabilizers on risk for physical diseases in people with schizophrenia, depression, or bipolar disorder. World Psychiatry. 2015;14(20):119–36.

Correll CU, Solmi M, Veronese N, et al. Prevalence, incidence and mortality from cardiovascular disease in patients with pooled and specific severe mental illness: a large-scale, meta-analysis of 3,211,768 patients and 113,383,368 controls. World Psychiatry. 2017;16(2):163–80.

Cuellar AK, Johnson SL, Winters R. Distinctions between bipolar and unipolar depression. Clin Psychol Rev. 2005;25(3):307–39.

De Dios C, Ezquiaga E, Garcia A, Soler B, Vieta E. Time spent with symptoms in a cohort of bipolar disorder outpatients in Spain: prospective, 18-month follow-up study. J Affect Disord. 2010;125(1–3):74–81.

Dhir A. Investigational drugs for treating major depressive disorder. Expert Opin Investig Drugs. 2017;26(1):9–24.

Dickerson F, Origoni A, Schroeder J, et al. Natural cause mortality in persons with serious mental illness. Acta Psychiatr Scand. 2018;137(5):371–9.

Drancourt N, Etain B, Lajnef M, Henry C, Raust A, Cochet B, Mathieu F, Gard S, Mbailara K, Zanouy L, Kahn JP, Cohen RF, Wajsbrot-Elgrabli O, Leboyer M, Scott J, Bellivier F. Duration of untreated bipolar disorder: missed opportunities on the long road to optimal treatment. Acta Psychiatr Scand. 2013;127(2):136–44.

Earley W, Burgess MV, Rekeda L, et al. Cariprazine treatment of bipolar depression: randomized double-blind placebo-controlled, phase-3 study. Am J Psychiatry. 2019;176(6):439–48.

FDA (US Food and Drug Administration). Antiepileptic drugs and suicidality 2008. Anticon, https://www.fda.gov/downloads/drugs/drugsafety/postmarketdrugsafetyinformationforpatientsandproviders/ucm192556.pdf. Accessed 22 Dec 2018.

Felber W, Bauer M, Lewitzka U, Müller-Oerlinghausen B. Lithium clinics in Berlin and Dresden: 50-year experience. Pharmacopsychiatry. 2018;51(5):166–71.

Filkowski MM, Sheth SA. Deep brain stimulation for depression: emerging indication. Neurosurg Clin N Am. 2019;30(2):243–56.

Fink M, Kellner CH, McCall WV. Role of ECT in suicide prevention. J ECT. 2014;30(1):5–9.

Fornaro M, Solmi M, Veronese N, et al. Burden of mood-disorder/cerebrovascular disease comorbidity: essential neurobiology, psychopharmacology, and physical activity interventions. Int Rev Psychiatry. 2017;29(5):425–35.

Forte A, Baldessarini RJ, Tondo L, Vázquez G, Pompili M, Girardi P. Long-term morbidity in bipolar-I, bipolar-II, and major depressive disorders. J Affect Disord. 2015;178(6):71–8.

Forte A, Buscaioni A, Fiorillo A, Pompili M, Baldessarini RJ. Suicidal risk following hospital discharge: review. Harv Rev Psychiatry. 2019;27(4):209–16.

Fountoulakis KN, Vieta E, Young A, et al. Unmet needs in the treatment of bipolar disorder and recommendations for future research. Int J Neuropsychopharmacol. 2017;20(2):196–205.

Frye MA, Ha K, Kanba S, et al. International consensus group on depression prevention in bipolar disorder. J Clin Psychiatry. 2011;72(10):1295–310.

Gadad BS, Jha MK, Czysz A, et al. Peripheral biomarkers of major depression and antidepressant treatment response: current knowledge and future outlooks. J Affect Disord. 2018;233(6):3–14.

Garay RP, Zarate CA Jr, Charpeaud T, et al. Investigational drugs in recent clinical trials for treatment-resistant depression. Expert Rev Neurother. 2017;17(6):593–609.

Geddes JR, Miklowitz DJ. Treatment of bipolar disorder. Lancet. 2013;381(9878):1672–82.

Ghaemi SN, Wingo AF, Filkowski MA, Baldessarini RJ. Long-term antidepressant treatment in bipolar disorder: meta-analyses of benefits and risks. Acta Psychiatr Scand. 2008;118(5):347–56.

Ghaemi SN, Ostacher MM, El-Mallakh RS, et al. Antidepressant discontinuation in bipolar depression: randomized clinical trial of long-term effectiveness and safety. J Clin Psychiatry. 2010;71(4):372–80.

Gibbons RD, Hur K, Brown CH, Mann JJ. Relationship between antiepileptic drugs and suicide attempts in patients with bipolar disorder. Arch Gen Psychiatry. 2009;66(12):1354–60.

Gijsman HJ, Geddes JR, Rendell JM, Nolen WA, Goodwin GM. Antidepressants for bipolar depression: systematic review of randomized, controlled trials. Am J Psychiatry. 2004;161(9):1537–47.

Gitlin MJ. Antidepressants in bipolar depression: an enduring controversy. Int J Bipolar Disord. 2018;6(1):25–31.

Goodwin FK, Jamison KR. Manic-depressive illness. 2nd ed. New York: Oxford University Press; 2007.

Goodwin FK, Fireman B, Simon GE, Hunkeler EM, Lee J, Revicki D. Suicide risk in bipolar disorder during treatment with lithium and divalproex. JAMA. 2003;290(11):1467–73.

Goodwin GM, Haddad PM, Ferrier IN, et al. Evidence-based guidelines for treating bipolar disorder: revised third edition recommendations from the British Association for Psychopharmacology. J Psychopharmacol. 2016;30(6):495–553.

Grady SE, Marsh TA, Tenhouse A, Klein K. Ketamine for the treatment of major depressive disorder and bipolar depression: review of the literature. Ment Health Clin. 2017;7(1):16–23.

Grunebaum MF, Ellis SP, Keip JG, et al. Ketamine vs. midazolam in bipolar depression with suicidal thoughts. Bipolar Disord. 2017;19(3):176–83.

Halaris A. Inflammation-associated co-morbidity between depression and cardiovascular disease. Curr Top Behav Neurosci. 2017;31(11):45–70.

Hällgren J, Ösby U, Westman J, Gissler M. Mortality trends in external causes of death in people with mental health disorders in Sweden, 1987-2010. Scand J Public Health. 2018;47(2):121–6.

Hammad TA, Laughren TP, Racoosin JA. Suicide rates in short-term randomized controlled trials of newer antidepressants. J Clin Psychopharmacol. 2006;26(2):203–7.

Hjorthøj C, Drivsholm-Østergaard ML, Eriksen-Benros M, et al. Association between alcohol and substance use disorders and all-cause and cause-specific mortality in schizophrenia, bipolar disorder, and unipolar depression: nationwide, prospective, register-based study. Lancet Psychiatry. 2015;2(9):801–8.

Isometsä ET. Suicide in bipolar I disorder in Finland: psychological autopsy findings from the National Suicide Prevention Project in Finland. Arch Suicide Res. 2005;9(3):251–60.

Itagaki K, Takebayashi M, Shibasaki C, et al. Factors associated with relapse after a response to electroconvulsive therapy in unipolar versus bipolar depression. J Affect Disord. 2017;208(1):113–9.

Kessler RC, Berglund P, Borges G, Nock M, Wang PS. Trends in suicide ideation, plans, gestures, and attempts in the US, 1990–1992 to 2001–2003. JAMA. 2005;293(20):2487–95.

Khan A, Khan SR, Leventhal RM, Brown WA. Symptom reduction and suicide risk among patients treated with placebo in antipsychotic clinical trials: analysis of the FDA database. Am J Psychiatry. 2001;158(9):1449–54.

Khan A, Khan SR, Hobus J, et al. Differential pattern of response in mood symptoms and suicide risk measures in severely ill depressed patients assigned to citalopram with placebo or citalopram combined with lithium: role of lithium levels. J Psychiatr Res. 2011;45(11):1489–96.

Koukopoulos A, Reginaldi D, Tondo L, Visioli C, Baldessarini RJ. Course sequences in bipolar disorder: depressions preceding or following manias or hypomanias. J Affect Disord. 2013;151(1):105–10.

Kupka RW, Altshuler LL, Nolen WA, et al. Three times more days depressed than manic or hypomanic in both bipolar I and bipolar II disorder. Bipolar Disord. 2007;9(5):531–5.

Large M, Swaraj S. Suicide, substance use and natural causes are respectively the most important causes of mortality in the first year post discharge from psychiatric hospitals. Evid Based Ment Health. 2018;21(2):e8–9.

Laughren TP. Proceedings of a meeting of the Psychopharmacology Drug Advisory Committee (PDAC) concerning suicidal risk in trials of antidepressant drugs in juvenile and adult patients, 2006. http://www.fda.gov/ohrms/dockets/ac/06/briefing//2006-4272b1-01-fda.pdf. Accessed 22 Dec 2018.

Lauterbach E, Felber W, Müller-Oerlinghausen B, et al. Adjunctive lithium treatment in the prevention of suicidal behavior in depressive disorders: randomized, placebo-controlled, one-year trial. Acta Psychiatr Scand. 2008;118(6):469–79.

Lewitzka U, Bauer M, Felber W, Müller-Oerlinghausen B. Antisuicidal effect of lithium: current state of research and its clinical implications for the long-term treatment of affective disorders. Nervenärzt. 2013;84(3):294–306.

Li XB, Tang YL, Wang CY, de Leon J. Clozapine for treatment-resistant bipolar disorder: systematic review. Bipolar Disord. 2015;17(3):235–47.

Liu B, Zhang Y, Fang H, et al. Efficacy and safety of long-term antidepressant treatment for bipolar disorders: meta-analysis of randomized controlled trials. J Affect Disord. 2017a;223(12):41–8.

Liu X, Agerbo E, Li J, Meltzer-Brody S, Bergink V, Munk-Olsen T. Depression and anxiety in the postpartum period and risk of bipolar disorder: Danish nationwide register-based cohort study. J Clin Psychiatry. 2017b;78(5):e469–76.

Lovas DA, Schuman-Olivier Z. Mindfulness-based cognitive therapy for bipolar disorder: systematic review. J Affect Disord. 2018;240:247–61.

Maj M, Pirozzi R, Magliano L, Fiorillo A, Bartoli L. Agitated, "unipolar" major depression: prevalence, phenomenology and outcome. J Clin Psychiatry. 2006;67(5):712–9.

Marangell LB, Dennehy EB, Wisniewski SR, et al. Case-control analyses of the impact of pharmacotherapy on prospectively observed suicide attempts and completed suicides in bipolar disorder. J Clin Psychiatry. 2008;69(6):916–22.

Martinez-Botella G, Salituro FG, Harrison BL, et al. Neuroactive steroids: SAGE-217, a clinical next-generation neuroactive steroid positive allosteric modulator of the $GABA_A$ receptor. J Med Chem. 2017;60(18):7810–9.

McCauley E, Berk MS, Asarnow JR, et al. Efficacy of dialectical behavioral therapy for adolescents at high risk for suicide: randomized clinical trial. JAMA Psychiatry. 2018;75(8):777–85.

McElroy SL, Weisler RH, Chan W, et al. Double-blind, placebo-controlled study of quetiapine and paroxetine as monotherapy in adults with bipolar depression (EMBOLDEN II). J Clin Psychiatry. 2010;71(2):163–74.

McGirr A, Vöhringer PA, Ghaemi SN, Lam RW, Yatham LN. Safety and efficacy of adjunctive second generation antidepressant therapy with a mood-stabilizer or an atypical antipsychotic in acute bipolar depression: systematic review and meta-analysis of randomized placebo-controlled trials. Lancet Psychiatry. 2016;3(12):1138–46. https://doi.org/10.1016/s2215-0366(16)30264-4).

McIntyre RS, Soczynska JK, Beyer JL, et al. Medical comorbidity in bipolar disorder: reprioritizing unmet needs. Curr Opin Psychiatry. 2007;20(4):406–16.

McMahon K, Herr NR, Zerubavel N, Hoertel N, Neacsiu AD. Psychotherapeutic treatment of bipolar depression. Psychiatr Clin N Am. 2016;39(1):35–56.

Meltzer HY, Alphs L, Green AI, et al. Clozapine treatment for suicidality in schizophrenia: international suicide prevention trial (InterSePT). Arch Gen Psychiatry. 2003;60(1):82–91.

Messer T, Lammers G, Müller-Siecheneder F, Schmidt RF, Latifi S. Substance abuse in patients with bipolar disorder: systematic review and meta-analysis. Psychiatry Res. 2017;253(7):338–50.

Möller HJ. Is there evidence for negative effects of antidepressants on suicidality in depressive patients? Systematic review. Eur Arch Psychiatry Clin Neurosci. 2006;256(8):476–96.

Müller-Oerlinghausen B, Ahrens B, Felber W. Suicide-preventive and mortality-reducing effect of lithium. In: Bauer M, Grof P, Müller-Oerlinghausen B, editors. Lithium in neuropsychiatry. London: Informa Healthcare; 2006. p. 79–192.

Nemeroff CB, Evans DL, Gyulai L, et al. Double-blind, placebo-controlled comparison of imipramine and paroxetine in the treatment of bipolar depression. Am J Psychiatry. 2001;158:906–12.

Nierenberg AA, Alpert JE, Gardner-Schuster EE, Seay S, Mischoulon D. Vagus nerve stimulation: 2-year outcomes for bipolar versus unipolar treatment-resistant depression. Biol Psychiatry. 2008;64(6):455–60.

Nock MK, Borges G, Bromet EJ, et al. Cross-national prevalence and risk factors for suicidal ideation, plans and attempts. Br J Psychiatry. 2008;192(2):98–105.

Olfson M, Wall M, Wang S, Crystal S, Liu SM, Gerhard T, Blanco C. Short-term suicide risk after psychiatric hospital discharge. JAMA Psychiatry. 2016;73(11):1119–26.

Oquendo MA, Galfalvy HC, Currier D, et al. Treatment of suicide attempters with bipolar disorder: randomized clinical trial comparing lithium and valproate in the prevention of suicidal behavior. Am J Psychiatry. 2011;168(10):1050–6.

Ösby U, Brandt L, Correia N, Ekbom A, Sparén P. Excess mortality in bipolar and unipolar disorder in Sweden. Arch Gen Psychiatry. 2001;58(9):844–50.

Ösby U, Westman J, Hällgren J, Gissler M. Mortality trends in cardiovascular causes in schizophrenia, bipolar and unipolar mood disorder in Sweden 1987–2010. Eur J Pub Health. 2018;26(5):867–71.

Pacchiarotti I, Bond DJ, Baldessarini RJ, et al. International Society for Bipolar Disorders (ISBD) Task-Force report on antidepressant use in bipolar disorders. Am J Psychiatry. 2013;170(11):1249–62.

Parsaik AK, Singh B, Khosh-Chashm D, Mascarenhas SS. Efficacy of ketamine in bipolar depression: systematic review and meta-analysis. J Psychiatr Pract. 2015;21(6):427–35.

Pavlova B, Perlis RH, Uher R. Lifetime prevalence er of anxiety disorders in people with bipolar disorder: systematic review and meta-analysis. Lancet Psychiatry. 2015;2(8):710–7.

Perugi G, Medda P, Toni C, et al. Role of electroconvulsive therapy (ECT) in bipolar disorder: effectiveness in 522 patients with bipolar depression, mixed-state, mania and catatonic features. Curr Neuropharmacol. 2017;15(3):359–71.

Pompili M, Baldessarini RJ, Forte A, et al. Do atypical antipsychotics have antisuicidal effects? A hypothesis-generating overview. Int J Mol Sci. 2016;17(10):E1700–13.

Post RM, Leverich GS, Kupka RW, et al. Early-onset bipolar disorder and treatment delay are risk factors for poor outcome in adulthood. J Clin Psychiatry. 2010;71(7):864–72.

Post RM, Leverich GS, McElroy S, et al. Prevalence of Axis-II comorbidities in bipolar disorder: relationship to mood-state. Bipolar Disord. 2018;20(4):303–12.

Preti A, Vrublevska J, Veroniki AA, Huedo-Medina TB, Fountoulakis KN. Prevalence, impact and treatment of generalized anxiety disorder in bipolar disorder: systematic review and meta-analysis. Evid Based Ment Health. 2016;19(3):73–81.

Ragguett RM, McIntyre RS. Cariprazine for the treatment of bipolar depression: a review. Expert Rev Neurother. 2019;19(4):317–23.

Ragguett RM, Rong C, Kratiuk K, McIntyre RS. Rapastinel: investigational NMDA-R modulator for major depressive disorder: evidence to date. Expert Opin Investig Drugs. 2019;28(2):113–9.

Reinares M, Rosa AR, Franco C, et al. Systematic review on the role of anticonvulsants in the treatment of acute bipolar depression. Int J Neuropsychopharmacol. 2013;16(2):485–96.

Roberts E, Cipriani A, Geddes JR, Nierenberg AA, Young AH. Evidence for lithium in suicide prevention. Br J Psychiatry. 2017;211(6):396–7.

Sachs GS, Nierenberg AA, Calabrese JR, et al. Effectiveness of adjunctive antidepressant treatment for bipolar depression. New Engl J Med. 2007;356(17):1711–22.

Salcedo S, Gold AK, Sheikh S, et al. Empirically supported psychosocial interventions for bipolar disorder: current state of the research. J Affect Disord. 2016;201(9):203–14.

Salloum NC, Walker MC, Gangwani S, Conway CR. Emergence of mania in two middle-aged patients with a history of unipolar, treatment-refractory depression receiving vagus nerve stimulation. Bipolar Disord. 2017;19(1):60–4.

Sani G, Fiorillo A. Use of lithium in mixed states. CNS Spectr. 2019. https://doi.org/10.1017/S1092852919001184. **(in press)**.

Saunders KE, Hawton K. Clinical assessment and crisis intervention for the suicidal bipolar disorder patient. Bipolar Disord. 2013;15(5):575–83.

Schatzberg AF. A word to the wise about intranasal esketamine. Am J Psychiatry. 2019;176(6):422–4.

Schneider-Thoma J, Efthimiou O, Huhn M, et al. Second-generation antipsychotic drugs and short-term mortality: systematic review and meta-analysis of randomized placebo-controlled trials. Lancet Psychiatry. 2018;5(8):653–63.

Scott LJ. Brexanolone: first global approval. Drugs. 2019;79(7):779–83.

Selle V, Schalkwijk S, Vázquez GH, Baldessarini RJ. Treatments for acute bipolar depression: meta-analyses of placebo-controlled, monotherapy trials of anticonvulsants, lithium, and second-generation antipsychotics. Pharmacopsychiatry. 2014;47(2):43–52.

Shelton RC, Stahl SM. Risperidone and paroxetine given singly and in combination for bipolar depression. J Clin Psychiatry. 2004;65:1715–9.

Shen H, Zhang L, Xu C, Zhu J, Chen M, Fang Y. Analysis of misdiagnosis of bipolar disorder in an outpatient setting. Shanghai Arch Psychiatry. 2018;30(2):93–101.

Sidor MM, MacQueen GM. Update on antidepressant use in bipolar depression. Curr Psychiatry Rep. 2012;14(6):696–704.

Simon RI, Hales RE, editors. Textbook of suicide assessment and management. 2nd ed. Washington, DC: American Psychiatric Press; 2012.

Smith KA, Cipriani A. Lithium and suicide in mood disorders: updated meta-review on the scientific literature. Bipolar Disord. 2017;19(7):575–86.

Solmi M, Veronese N, Zaninoto L, et al. Lamotrigine compared to placebo and other agents with antidepressant activity in patients with unipolar and bipolar depression: comprehensive meta-analysis of efficacy and safety outcomes in short-term trials. CNS Spectr. 2016;21(5):403–18.

Song J, Sjolander A, Joas E, et al. Suicidal behavior during lithium and valproate treatment: a within-individual 8-year prospective study of 50,000 patients with bipolar disorder. Am J Psychiatry. 2017;174(8):795–802.

Staudt-Hansen P, Frahm-Laursen M, Grøntved S, Puggard-Vogt-Straszek S, Licht RW, Nielsen RE. Increasing mortality gap for patients diagnosed with bipolar disorder: nationwide study with 20 years of follow-up. Bipolar Disord. 2019;21(3):270–5.

Stensland MD, Schultz JF, Frytak JR. Diagnosis of unipolar depression following initial identification of bipolar disorder: common and costly misdiagnosis. J Clin Psychiatry. 2008;69(5):749–58.

Stokes PRA, Kalk NJ, Young AH. Bipolar disorder and addictions: the elephant in the room. Br J Psychiatry. 2017;211(3):132–4.

Suzuki M, Dallaspezia S, Locatelli C, Uchiyama M, Colombo C, Benedetti F. Does early response predict subsequent remission in bipolar depression treated with repeated sleep deprivation combined with light therapy and lithium? J Affect Disord. 2018;229(3):371–6.

Tamayo JM, Zarate CA Jr, Vieta E, Vázquez GH, Tohen M. Level of response and safety of pharmacological monotherapy in the treatment of acute bipolar I disorder phases: systematic review and meta-analysis. Int J Neuropsychopharmacol. 2010;13(6):813–32.

Tarsy D, Lungu C, Baldessarini RJ. Epidemiology of tardive dyskinesia before and during the era of modern antipsychotic drugs. In: Weiner WJ, Tolosa E, editors. Hyperkinetic movement disorders. In Aminoff MJ, Boller F, Swaab DF, editors. Handbook of clinical neurology. Edinburgh: Elsevier Press; 2010. p. 601–16.

Taylor DM, Cornelius V, Smith L, Young AH. Comparative efficacy and acceptability of drug treatments for bipolar depression: a multiple-treatments meta-analysis. Acta Psychiatr Scand. 2014;130(6):452–68.

Thies-Flechtner K, Müller-Oerlinghausen B, Seibert W, Walther A, Greil W. Effect of prophylactic treatment on suicide risk in patients with major affective disorders: data from a randomized prospective trial. Pharmacopsychiatry. 1996;29(3):103–7.

Tiihonen J, Wahlbeck K, Lönnqvist J, et al. Effectiveness of antipsychotic treatments in a nationwide cohort of patients in community care after first hospitalization due to schizophrenia and schizoaffective disorder: observational follow-up study. BMJ. 2006;333(7561):224–9.

Tohen M, Vieta E, Calabrese J, et al. Efficacy of olanzapine and olanzapine-fluoxetine combination in the treatment of bipolar I depression. Arch Gen Psychiatry. 2003;60(11):1079–88.

Tondo L, Baldessarini RJ. Reduction of suicidal behavior in bipolar disorder patients during long-term treatment with lithium. In: Koslow SH, Ruiz P, Nemeroff CB, editors. Concise guide to understanding suicide: epidemiology pathophysiology and prevention. Cambridge: Cambridge University Press; 2014. p. 217–28.

Tondo L, Baldessarini RJ. Chapt 37: Suicide in bipolar disorder. In: Yildiz A, Nemeroff C, Ruiz P, editors. The bipolar book: history, neurobiology, and treatment. New York: Oxford University Press; 2015. p. 509–28.

Tondo L, Baldessarini RJ. Antisuicidal effects in mood disorders: are they unique to lithium? Pharmacopsychiatry. 2018;51(5):177–88.

Tondo L, Baldessarini RJ, Hennen J, Floris G, Silvetti F, Tohen M. Lithium treatment and risk of suicidal behavior in bipolar disorder patients. J Clin Psychiatry. 1998;59(8):405–14.

Tondo L, Baldessarini RJ, Hennen J, et al. Suicide attempts in major affective disorder patients with comorbid substance use disorders. J Clin Psychiatry. 1999;60(2):63–9.

Tondo L, Hennen J, Baldessarini RJ. Reduced suicide risk with long-term lithium treatment in major affective illness: meta-analysis. Acta Psychiatr Scand. 2001;104(3):163–72.

Tondo L, Lepri B, Baldessarini RJ. Suicidal status during antidepressant treatment in 789 Sardinian patients with major affective disorder. Acta Psychiatr Scand. 2008;118(2):106–15.

Tondo L, Vázquez GH, Baldessarini RJ. Mania associated with antidepressant-treatment: comprehensive meta-analytic review. Acta Psychiatr Scand. 2010;121(6):404–14.

Tondo L, Baldessarini RJ, Vázquez GH, Lepri B, Visioli C. Clinical responses to antidepressants among 1036 acutely depressed patients with bipolar or unipolar major affective disorders. Acta Psychiatr Scand. 2013;127(5):355–64.

Tondo L, Visioli C, Preti A, Baldessarini RJ. Bipolar disorders following initial depression: modeling predictive clinical factors. J Affect Disord. 2014;167(10):44–9.

Tondo L, Pompili M, Forte A, Baldessarini RJ. Suicide attempts in bipolar disorders: comprehensive review of 101 reports. Acta Psychiatr Scand. 2016;133(3):174–86.

Tondo L, Vázquez GH, Pinna M, Vaccotto PA, Baldessarini RJ. Characteristics of depressive and bipolar patients with mixed features. Acta Psychiatr Scand. 2018;138(3):243–52.

Trede K, Salvatore P, Baethge C, Gerhard A, Maggini C, Baldessarini RJ. Manic-depressive illness: evolution in Kraepelin's textbook, 1883–1926. Harv Rev Psychiatry. 2005;13(3):155–78.

Tsai SY, Lee CH, Chen PH, et al. Risk factors for early cardiovascular mortality in patients with bipolar disorder. Psychiatry Clin Neurosci. 2017;71(10):716–24.

Tseng PT, Chen YW, Tu KY, et al. Light therapy in the treatment of patients with bipolar depression: meta-analytic study. Eur Neuropsychopharmacol. 2016;26(6):1037–47.

Undurraga J, Baldessarini RJ, Valenti M, et al. Bipolar depression: clinical correlates of receiving antidepressants. J Affect Disord. 2012;139(1):89–93.

Vancampfort D, Vansteelandt K, Correll CU, et al. Metabolic syndrome and metabolic abnormalities in bipolar disorder: meta-analysis of prevalence rates and moderators. Am J Psychiatry. 2013;170(3):265–74.

Vázquez GH, Tondo L, Baldessarini RJ. Comparison of antidepressant responses in patients with bipolar vs. unipolar depression: meta-analytic review. Pharmacopsychiatry. 2011;44(1):21–6.

Vázquez GH, Tondo L, Undurraga J, Baldessarini RJ. Overview of antidepressant treatment of bipolar depression. Int J Neuropsychopharmacol. 2013;16(7):1673–85.

Vázquez GH, Tondo L, Undurraga J, Zaratiegui R, Selle V, Baldessarini RJ. Pharmacological treatment of bipolar depression. Adv Psychiatr Treatment. 2014;20(1):193–201.

Vázquez GH, Holtzman J, Tondo L, Baldessarini RJ. Efficacy and tolerability of treatments for bipolar depression. J Affect Disord. 2015;183(9):258–62.

Vázquez GH, Camino S, Tondo L, Baldessarini RJ. Potential novel treatments for bipolar depression: ketamine, fatty acids, anti-inflammatory agents, and probiotics. CNS Neurol Disord Drug Targets. 2017a;16(8):858–69.

Vázquez GH, Forte A, Camino S, Tondo L, Baldessarini RJ. Chapt 17: Psychiatric comorbidity in bipolar disorder: treatment implications: anxiety syndromes and substance abuse. In: Carvalho E, Vieta E, editors. The treatment of bipolar disorder: integrative treatment strategies and future directions. New York: Oxford University Press; 2017b. p. 225–54.

Viktorin A, Lichtenstein P, Thase ME, et al. Risk of switch to mania in patients with bipolar disorder during treatment with an antidepressant alone and in combination with a mood stabilizer. Am J Psychiatry. 2014;171(10):1067–673.

Vöhringer PA, Perlis RH. Discriminating between bipolar disorder and major depressive disorder. Psychiatr Clin N Am. 2016;39(1):1–10.

Wasserman D, Rihmer Z, Rujescu D, et al. European Psychiatric Association (EPA) guidance on suicide treatment and prevention. Eur Psychiatry. 2012;27(2):129–41.

WHO (World Health Organization). International suicide rates, 2018. http://www.who.int/gho/mental_health/suicide_rates_crude/en/. Accessed 3 Dec 2018.

Widge AS, Malone DA Jr, Dougherty DD. Closing the loop on deep brain stimulation for treatment-resistant depression. Front Neurosci. 2018;12(3):1–9.

Wilkinson ST, Sanacora G. A new generation of antidepressants: update on the pharmaceutical pipeline for novel and rapid-acting therapeutics in mood disorders based on glutamate/GABA neurotransmitter systems. Drug Discov Today. 2019;24(2):606–15.

Wilkinson ST, Ballard ED, Bloch MH, et al. Effect of a single dose of intravenous ketamine on suicidal ideation: systematic review and individual participant data meta-analysis. Am J Psychiatry. 2018;175(2):150–8.

Wu SI, Chen SC, Liu SI, et al. Relative risk of acute myocardial infarction in people with schizophrenia and bipolar disorder: population-based cohort study. PLoS ONE. 2015;10(8):e013463.

Yatham LN, Kennedy SH, Parikh SV, et al. Canadian Network for Mood and Anxiety Treatments (CANMAT) and International Society for Bipolar Disorders (ISBD) 2018 guidelines for the management of patients with bipolar disorder. Bipolar Disord. 2018;20(2):97–170.

Yerevanian BI, Koek RJ, Mintz J. Bipolar pharmacotherapy and suicidal behavior: lithium, divalproex and carbamazepine. J Affect Disord. 2007;103(1–3):23–8.

Yildiz A, Nemeroff C, Ruiz P, editors. The bipolar book: history, neurobiology, and treatment. New York: Oxford University Press; 2015.

Young AH, McElroy SL, Bauer M, et al. Double-blind, placebo-controlled study (EMBOLDEN I) of quietapine and lithium monotherapy in adults in the acute phase of bipolar depression. J Clin Psychiatry. 2010;71(2):150–62.

Zalsman G, Hawton K, Wasserman D, et al. Suicide prevention strategies revisited: 10-year systematic review. Lancet Psychiatry. 2016;3(7):646–59.

Zimmerman M, Galione JN, Chelminski I, Young D, Dalrymple K, Ruggero CJ. Sustained unemployment in psychiatric outpatients with bipolar disorder: frequency and association with demographic variables and comorbid disorders. Bipolar Disord. 2010;12(7):720–6.

# 2

# Predictors of psychosocial outcome of bipolar disorder: data from the Stanley Foundation Bipolar Network

Francis Bennett[1], Sophie Hodgetts[2], Andrew Close[1], Mark Frye[3], Heinz Grunze[4], Paul Keck[5,6], Ralph Kupka[7], Susan McElroy[7], Willem Nolen[8], Robert Post[9], Lars Schärer[10], Trisha Suppes[11] and Aditya N. Sharma[1,12,13*]

**Abstract**

**Background:** Impairments in psychosocial functioning have been demonstrated in 30–60% of adults with bipolar disorder (BD). However, the majority of studies investigating the effect of comorbid mental health disorders and age at onset outcomes in BD have focused on traditional outcome measures such as mood symptoms, mortality and treatment response. Therefore, this project aimed to investigate the impact of comorbid mental health disorders and age at onset on longitudinal psychosocial outcome in participants with BD.

**Method:** Mixed effects modelling was conducted using data from the Stanley Foundation Bipolar Network. Baseline factors were entered into a model, with Global Assessment of Functioning (GAF) score as the longitudinal outcome measure. Relative model fits were calculated using Akaike's Information Criterion.

**Results:** No individual comorbidities predicted lower GAF scores, however an interaction effect was demonstrated between attention deficit hyperactivity disorder (ADHD) and any anxiety disorder ($t = 2.180$, $p = 0.030$). Participants with BD I vs BD II ($t = 2.023$, $p = 0.044$) and those in the lowest vs. highest income class ($t = 2.266$, $p = 0.024$) predicted lower GAF scores. Age at onset ($t = 1.672$, $p = 0.095$) did not significantly predict GAF scores.

**Conclusions:** This is the first study to demonstrate the negative psychosocial effects of comorbid anxiety disorders and ADHD in BD. This study adds to the growing database suggesting that comorbid mental health disorders are a significant factor hindering psychosocial recovery.

**Keywords:** Bipolar disorder, Social functioning, Comorbidity

## Background

Bipolar disorder (BD) is a mood disorder characterised by recurrent episodes of mania, hypomania, and depression, separated by periods of euthymia. Although not characterised by mood symptoms, psychosocial functioning appears to remain impaired during euthymia (Marangell et al. 2009). Psychosocial functioning is an essential component of a person's quality of life (QoL), and includes social, psychological and occupational domains. In 2001, a landmark review found that between 30 and 60% of adults with BD had significant impairments in occupational and social functioning during periods of euthymia (MacQueen et al. 2001). A possible explanation for pervasive psychosocial dysfunction may be the illness itself or the high prevalence of comorbid mental disorders in BD (Post et al. 2015). However, research into BD has often overlooked the role of psychosocial functioning.

High rates of anxiety disorders (AnxD) comorbid with BD have been found consistently in both epidemiological (Merikangas et al. 2011) and clinical (Otto et al. 2006) samples. A recent review of 25 studies concluded that the lifetime risk of developing a comorbid AnxD was 46.8%, although epidemiological samples put this figure closer to 70% (Vazquez et al. 2014). Comorbid AnxD in subjects with BD are associated with a more severe illness

*Correspondence: aditya.sharma@ncl.ac.uk
[13] Academic Psychiatry, Wolfson Research Centre, Campus for Ageing and Vitality, Newcastle University, Newcastle upon Tyne NE4 5PL, UK
Full list of author information is available at the end of the article

course, including increased number of mood episodes, suicide attempts and hospitalizations, compared to BD alone (Merikangas et al. 2007). Despite this considerable evidence base, a recent review highlighted the current stagnation in AnxD comorbidity research, epitomised by the poor understanding of psychosocial factors, scarcity of treatment studies, and the lack of evidence base on antidepressants treating bipolar depression (Provencher et al. 2012). Although studies have shown associations between comorbid AnxD and poor psychosocial functioning (Scott et al. 2014), the picture is still far from clear.

Comorbid substance use disorders (SUD) are also prevalent the BD population, with epidemiological surveys putting lifetime prevalence of comorbid SUD at as high as 42.3% (Merikangas et al. 2007). However, with the exception of alcohol (Hobbs et al. 2011), the functional impacts and treatment options for individual SUD in BD have yet to be rigorously investigated.

Attention deficit hyperactivity disorder (ADHD) is a neurodevelopmental disorder, and its prevalence in BD varies widely with the age at which it is estimated. Approximately 20% of adult patients with ADHD also have bipolar disorder, while 10–20% of patients with bipolar disorder have adult ADHD (Brus et al. 2014). As with SUD and AnxD, ADHD comorbidity has been associated with increased number of mood episodes, higher rates of suicide attempts (McIntyre et al. 2010) and psychosocial dysfunction (Sentissi et al. 2008).

Mental health comorbidities in BD are more likely to be multiple than singular, with the World Mental Health Survey reporting a 62% lifetime prevalence of 3 or more comorbidities when strict Diagnostic and Statistical Manual of Mental Disorders-IV (DSM-IV) criteria were applied (Merikangas et al. 2011). However, research into the psychosocial effects of multiple comorbidities in BD is limited, often due to lack of power in subgroup analyses (Sentissi et al. 2008). Although there is clear evidence of increased rates of both individual and multiple comorbidities in BD, their impacts on day-to-day functioning of people with BD have yet to be established.

Earlier age at onset (AAO) of BD is consistently linked with poorer clinical outcomes, including rapid cycling, greater number of mood episodes and increased risk of suicide (Leverich et al. 2007). Some studies have linked psychosocial dysfunction with younger (< 18 years) AAO (Perlis et al. 2009), although this finding is not consistent (Martinez-Aran et al. 2007). The studies that have focused on younger AAO suggest that psychosocial impairment is due to earlier disruption in the development of interpersonal skills needed to build and maintain healthy relationships as patients grow older (Levy and Manove 2012). However, while younger AAO is associated with an adverse course of illness in adulthood (Leverich et al. 2007), how these may be related to psychosocial functioning has received little attention (Perlis et al. 2009).

In this post hoc analysis we used data from an established database (Stanley Foundation Bipolar Network) (Post et al. 2001) to estimate the effects of comorbid mental health disorders and AAO on psychosocial outcomes in participants with BD. A novel aspect to this study is the use of statistical modelling techniques, specifically mixed effects modelling (MEM). Modelling has been used extensively in the behavioural sciences (Gerhard et al. 1995), while recognition of its utility in medical fields is growing. The STEP-BD group used MEM in two papers assessing psychosocial outcome measures (Otto et al. 2006; Perlis et al. 2009). Complex data sets, such as the SFBN, often violate the assumptions of general linear modelling; in particular, statistical assumptions relating to independence between observations are violated. In contrast, mixed effects modelling is particularly suited to data sets involving measurements obtained from individual patients that share socioeconomic, demographic or biomedical characteristics. Therefore, a key advantage of MEM is that it calculates how much of the variance in the sample is explained by each factor and, crucially, what residual variance is left. Most clinical studies lack sufficient numbers to run the more complex models, but the longitudinal nature and size of the SFBN cohort makes this a unique opportunity in psychiatric research.

### Aims of the study

Psychosocial functioning is key to understanding the overall impact mental health disorders can have on an individual. In BD research, comorbid mental health disorders and age at onset have both been extensively investigated with traditional outcome measures such as mood symptoms, mortality and treatment response. In this study, we used Mixed-Effects Modelling on data collected by the Stanley Foundation Bipolar Network. The study aimed to demonstrate the effect of comorbid mental health disorders and age of onset on psychosocial functioning in participants with BD.

## Methods

### Baseline assessments

Information on comorbid mental health disorders and AAO was collected utilizing items from Structured Clinical Interview for DSM-IV-Patient (SCID-P) and Patient Questionnaire (PQ). AAO was defined as age at first hypomanic, manic, or depressive symptoms that were associated with functional impairment. AAO for BD was collected from the SCID-P, which a previous SFBN paper showed to be highly correlated with self-report from PQ ($r = 0.80$) (Leverich et al. 2007).

### Longitudinal outcome

The Global Assessment of Functioning (GAF) is a well-validated instrument, which constitutes Axis V of DSM-IV. It has been used extensively in BD research and has good inter-rater reliability (Jones et al. 1995). A criticism of the GAF is that it confounds mood and functioning by including mood symptoms in the scale descriptions. In the SFBN this was addressed by ensuring clinicians only used the GAF to rate functioning. Following an interview, clinicians rated the participant's global functioning on a scale of 0–100. Three scores were recorded: best, worst (since last visit) and current. This study only included current score in order not to introduce a selection bias.

### Data selection

The total sample study size in the original data was n = 648, with 21,993 GAF records. Only participants with complete data were included (see Fig. 1) which left a final sample size of n = 469, with 12,556 GAF records.

### Data analysis

Mixed-effects models (MEMs) were developed using the strategy described by Pinheiro et al. (2017) to examine variation in psychosocial dysfunction among participants at follow-up. A GAF score for each participant was obtained at baseline and at follow-up. We implemented the methodology proposed by Vickers and Altman (2001) and used GAF at baseline in order to control for differences in the mean psychosocial function between sites in Europe (Netherlands and Germany) and USA. The impact of BD subtype of each participant, AAO and the mental health comorbidities on psychosocial outcome were also determined. The influences of demographic characteristics of participants were assessed by including sex and income as independent explanatory variables. Independent explanatory variables were assessed within models additively. The potential impact of multiple interactions between AnxD, SUD and ADHD on psychosocial outcome was also explored. Individuals were grouped according to their respective locations (Europe or USA). Study location was then specified as a random-effect within the model in order to capture potential sources of unmeasured variation in psychosocial outcome. In addition, GAF at baseline within the random-effects structure was incorporated to generate a random intercept and random slope model that controlled for variation in overall mean and gradient between locations. Multi-model inference (Burnham and Anderson 2002) was used to compare models with additive terms to those models that incorporated both additive and interaction actions terms.

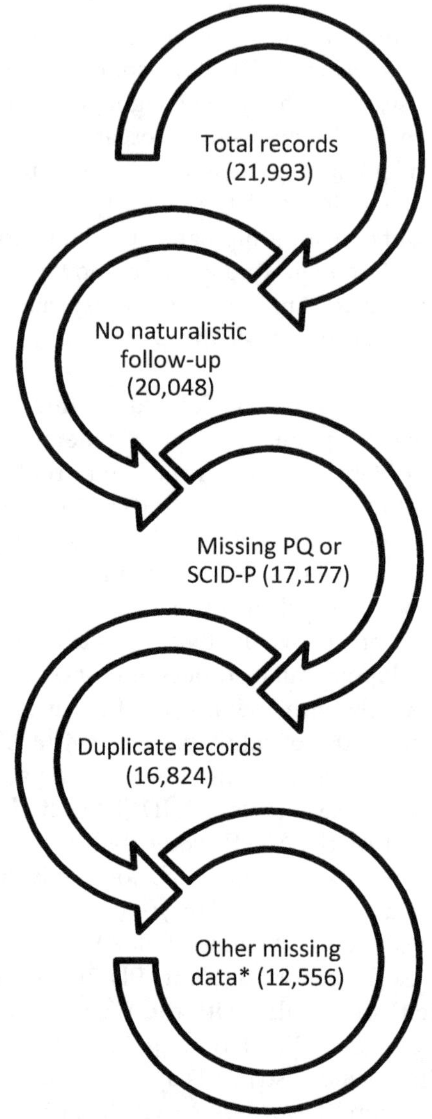


**Fig. 1** Flow-chart of exclusion criteria (GAF record number) *No GAF score/inadequate information, no gender, no income, no education, no age at first treatment for mania, no BD type, no AAO, negative duration of untreated bipolar

A model with the lowest Akaike's Information Criterion (AIC) (Akaike 1973) was considered to be the model that best described variation within data.

## Results

### Preliminary analysis

There were greater numbers of participants included in the final analysis from USA (n = 332) than from Europe (n = 137). However, a Chi-squared test of independence did not find differences in the distribution of genders between USA (female:male, 189:124) and Europe (female:male, 70:63) ($X_2 = 2.17$, $p = 0.141$). In contrast, the distribution of mental health comorbidities, namely

AnxD ($X_2=22.98$, $p=<0.001$), ADHD ($X_2=8.23$, $p=0.004$) and SUD ($X_2=20.29$, $p<0.001$) all differed significantly between locations, and were higher in the US than in Europe. No significant differences in the distribution of BD subtypes ($X_2=0.44$, $p=0.081$), or income classes ($X_2=0.58$, $p=0.748$) was observed between USA and Europe. Demographic information for the whole sample is given in Table 1, while clinical and GAF summaries are given in Table 2.

**Table 1 Demographic characteristics and comorbidity in USA vs Europe**

| | USA (n=332, 70.8%) | Europe (n=137, 29.2%) | Total (n=469, 100%) | $\chi^2$ | *p*-value |
|---|---|---|---|---|---|
| Gender | | | | | |
| Female | 59.9 | 52.6 | 57.8 | | |
| Male | 40.1 | 47.4 | 42.2 | 2.17 | 0.141 |
| Income ($) | | | | | |
| <20,000 | 38.9 | 36.5 | 38.2 | | |
| 20,000–59,999 | 38.6 | 42.3 | 39.7 | | |
| >60,000 | 22.6 | 21.2 | 22.2 | 0.58 | 0.748 |
| BD type | | | | | |
| BD I | 84.3 | 83.2 | 84.0 | | |
| BD II | 13.6 | 15.3 | 14.1 | | |
| BD cyclo-thymic | 2.1 | 1.5 | 1.9 | 0.44 | 0.081 |
| Comorbidity | | | | | |
| AnxD | 52.7 | 28.5 | 45.6 | 22.98 | <0.001 |
| *Panic disorder* | 35.8 | 19.7 | 31.1 | | |
| *Chronic AnxD* | 33.4 | 16.8 | 28.6 | | |
| *OCD* | 22.9 | 4.4 | 17.5 | | |
| ADHD | 16.6 | 6.6 | 13.6 | 8.23 | 0.004 |
| SUD | 47.3 | 24.8 | 40.5 | 20.29 | <0.001 |
| AnxD+SUD | 26.2 | 9.5 | 19.2 | | |
| ADHD+SUD | 9.9 | 2.9 | 7.9 | | |
| ADHD+AnxD | 13.3 | 5.8 | 11.1 | | |

Preliminary analysis undertaken using a Wilcoxon Signed-Rank Test indicated that the location of mean of GAF measured at baseline was significantly different between locations (W=23,472, $p=0.0325$), and higher in Europe. The location of the mean GAF derived at follow-up was also found to be significantly different between locations (W=24,844, $p=0.0012$). It was not possible to explore the impact of educational attainment in the assessment of variation in GAF due to imbalance in sample size between the lower and higher levels of attainment. Similarly, participants with BD NOS were removed from further analyses due to insufficient sample size (n=9). Subsequently, variation in psychosocial function among 446 participants was analysed.

### Statistical analysis of global assessment of functioning (GAF)

The relative fits of MEMs were compared using multi-model inference. A model was considered a plausible fit to data if the difference in AIC between models did not exceed $\Delta_I<2$ (Table 3). The model incorporating an interaction between AnxD and ADHD was considered to be the best candidate model from the specific set of models compared (AIC=3582.256, $\Delta_I=0.000$) (Table 3). The model incorporating comorbidities additively was ranked second within the model set (AIC=3588.113, $\Delta_I=5.361$) and models that examined interactions between ADHD and SUD (AIC=3593.008, $\Delta_I=10.256$) and Anxiety Disorders and SUD (AIC=3594.422, $\Delta_I=11.670$) were ranked third and fourth, respectively.

Results generated by MEMs examining variation in GAF scores at follow-up, and incorporating an interaction between AnxD and ADHD are presented in Table 4.

**Table 2 Sample demographics, mean GAF at baseline, and follow-up by location, sex and BD subtype**

| Location | Sex | DSM-IV bipolar disorder subtype | Mean follow-up attendance (%) | Mean GAF baseline | Mean GAF follow-up | Sample size (%) |
|---|---|---|---|---|---|---|
| Europe | Female | BD I | 30.53 | 63.75 | 66.68 | 57 (12.5) |
| Europe | Female | BD II | 40.85 | 73.08 | 71.62 | 13 (2.9) |
| Europe | Female | BD NOS | 41.00 | 70.00 | 32.50 | 2 (0.40) |
| Europe | Male | BD I | 31.04 | 64.16 | 71.02 | 56 (12.3) |
| Europe | Male | BD II | 38.86 | 67.57 | 80 | 7 (1.5) |
| Europe | Male | BD NOS | NA | NA | NA | NA |
| USA | Female | BD I | 24.22 | 62.84 | 65.25 | 165 (36.3) |
| USA | Female | BD II | 24.08 | 64.33 | 68.46 | 24 (5.3) |
| USA | Female | BD NOS | 11.75 | 54.00 | 62.75 | 4 (0.9) |
| USA | Male | BD I | 28.47 | 61.02 | 65.03 | 104 (22.9) |
| USA | Male | BD II | 26.50 | 63.20 | 67.70 | 20 (4.4) |
| USA | Male | BD NOS | 42.33 | 71.00 | 61.00 | 3 (0.7) |

**Table 3 Multi-model inference indicating that the model incorporating two interactions terms best describes the data**

| Fixed effects structure (comorbidities) | *df* | Log likelihood | AIC | $\Delta_i$ | wt |
|---|---|---|---|---|---|
| Anxiety disorders and ADHD | 24 | − 1762.376 | 3582.752 | 0.000 | 0.928 |
| Additive terms | 25 | − 1769.056 | 3588.113 | 5.361 | 0.064 |
| ADHD and substance use disorder | 23 | − 1773.504 | 3593.008 | 10.256 | 0.006 |
| Anxiety disorder and substance use disorder | 27 | − 1770.211 | 3594.422 | 11.670 | 0.003 |

**Table 4 Mean GAF score at follow-up (intercept) and change with respect to explanatory variables**

| Parameter | Estimate | 95% CI | *se* | *df* | *t*-value | *p*-value |
|---|---|---|---|---|---|---|
| Intercept | 67.757 | 62.225, 73.518 | 2.662 | 431 | 25.456 | ≤0.000 |
| BD: subtype-2 | 3.191 | 0.146, 0.645 | 1.578 | 431 | 2.023 | 0.044 |
| Clinical follow-up attendance | −0.008 | 0.407, 6.908 | 0.029 | 431 | −0.287 | 0.774 |
| GAF baseline | 0.410 | 0.019, 0.308 | 0.114 | 431 | 3.586 | ≤0.000 |
| Age of onset | 0.120 | −4.657, 2.122 | 0.072 | 431 | 1.672 | 0.095 |
| Anxiety disorder | −2.162 | −4.823, 0.498 | 1.354 | 431 | −1.597 | 0.111 |
| ADHD | 1.279 | −2.979, 5.537 | 2.166 | 431 | 0.591 | 0.555 |
| Substance use disorder | 1.552 | −0.869, 3.973 | 1.232 | 431 | 1.260 | 0.208 |
| Sex: male | 0.771 | −1.650, 3.192 | 1.232 | 431 | 0.626 | 0.532 |
| Income-2[a] | −0.551 | −3.261, 2.160 | 1.379 | 431 | −0.399 | 0.690 |
| Income-3[a] | 3.572 | 0.474, 6.670 | 1.576 | 431 | 2.266 | 0.024 |
| BD subtype-2: GAF baseline | −0.265 | −0.518, −0.012 | 0.129 | 431 | −2.059 | 0.040 |
| BD subtype-2: age of onset | −0.244 | −0.518, −0.029 | 0.139 | 431 | −1.758 | 0.080 |
| Anxiety disorder: ADHD | −6.953 | −13.222,−0.683 | 3.190 | 431 | −2.180 | 0.030 |

[a] Income-2: 20,000–59,999 (USD), income-3: >60,000 (USD)

The global mean (Intercept) GAF at follow-up for participants with BDI (reference level) was 67.757 and was significantly different from zero ($t=25.456$, $p\leq 0.000$). Participants with BDII were found to have significantly higher GAF scores at follow-up in comparison to participants with BDI ($t=2.023$, $p=0.044$). Baseline GAF for participants was found to be significantly and positively associated with GAF at follow-up ($t=3.586, =p\leq 0.000$). In addition, a significant negative association was found for participants with BDII and psychosocial function at baseline ($t=-2.059180$, $p=0.017$), suggesting lower psychosocial functioning in BDII patients at baseline. In contrast, there was no significant relationship between BD subtype and AAO and psychosocial function at follow-up. Individuals grouped within the highest income class were significantly associated with higher GAF at follow-up in comparison to participants in the lowest class ($t=2.266$, $p=0.024$). In contrast, there was no significant difference at follow-up between participants within income class-1 and income class-2. Comorbidities included as additive terms within the model, AnxD, SUD and ADHD, did not significantly affect psychosocial function at follow-up. However, when AnxD and ADHD were incorporated as an interaction term, a significant negative effect on GAF at follow-up was observed ($t=2.180$, $p=0.030$). The mean GAF at follow-up was not significantly affected by variation in duration of follow-up, and no significant differences were observed in GAF score at follow-up between females and males.

## Discussion

The aim of this study was to investigate the impact of comorbid mental disorders and AAO on psychosocial functioning in an international sample of participants with BD. These factors were entered into MEM with GAF score as the longitudinal psychosocial outcome measure. The principle finding is that BD comorbid with ADHD and AnxD predicted lower GAF scores, particularly in BDI. Due to the influence of confounding collinearity between explanatory variables, it was not possible to construct a single model that examined the multiplicative effects between all comorbidities simultaneously. Nevertheless, a set of MEMs were developed that first examined the effects of comorbidities additively, in addition to models that examined the multiplicative effects between comorbidities independently. Individual comorbidities were explored independently within the final model, with no single comorbidity reaching statistical significance in predicting psychosocial outcome.

The high rate of comorbid AnxD in BD (45.6%) demonstrated in this study is a well-replicated finding (Simon et al. 2004). BD and comorbid AnxD alone did not predict poorer psychosocial function in the present study. This adds to a limited evidence base, and warrants further investigation. One explanation for this finding could be that the diagnostic criteria used did not capture the full spectrum of anxiety states and their effects.

As discussed earlier, rates of comorbid ADHD and BD vary widely according to age group. In the current study comorbid ADHD (13.6%) was less prevalent than both AnxD (45.6%) and SUD (40.5%). Currently, only two previous papers have looked at psychosocial outcome in comorbid ADHD and BD (Sentissi et al. 2008; Wilens et al. 2003). A study using more specific social functioning measures (SF-36 Health Survey and Social Adjustment Scale) found that poorer scores were predicted by ADHD comorbidity (Sentissi et al. 2008). Another smaller study found only a trend towards poorer global psychosocial functioning (GAF) in the ADHD group (Wilens et al. 2003). Alongside the current results, this may suggest a specific social dysfunction related to ADHD comorbidity, since both studies also found that attention domains were significantly more impaired than hyperactivity domains in the comorbid ADHD group (Sentissi et al. 2008; Wilens et al. 2003). The evidence regarding specific attention deficits and social dysfunction needs further replication, however, it may be that the relationship between ADHD and BD depends upon to specific aspects of attention that are affected.

The current study did not find a predictive effect of comorbid SUD on psychosocial dysfunction in BD. It may have been an over-simplification to analyse all types of SUD together in this study. Alcohol and cannabis were the most widely abused substances in the SFBN sample, but a recent review highlighted the differential impacts of these two SUDs in BD (Cerullo and Strakowski 2007). The current results are especially interesting when looking at the new DSM-5 (American Psychiatric Association 2013) criteria for SUD, which no longer differentiate between substance abuse and dependence. Instead, SUD severity is classified by the number of criteria met. Of the 11 criteria listed three relate to social impairment, making it possible to have a SUD diagnosis without exhibiting any social dysfunction.

To the authors' knowledge, this is the first paper that examines the effect of comorbid ADHD and AnxD on psychosocial outcome in BD. A key similarity between comorbid ADHD and AnxD individually with BD is the persistence of their symptoms during periods of euthymia (Bernardi et al. 2010). This is likely to hinder psychosocial recovery between mood episodes, leading to reduced quality of life. The chronic nature of comorbid ADHD can lead to underreporting the functional impact of symptoms, (Sandra Kooij et al. 2008) although this has yet to be demonstrated in comorbid AnxD. We found that participants within the SFBN cohort with AnxD were significantly more likely to also have ADHD (OR = 5.821, 95% CI 3.00–12.233). This suggests a heavy burden of ADHD in those participants with comorbid AnxD and BD. While the detrimental influence of such a potent combination of mental health disorders is perhaps not surprising, the underlying pathophysiological mechanisms merit further investigation.

The implications for treatment also merit discussion. There is very sparse guidance on treatment of comorbid mental health disorders in BD. The UK National Institute for Health and Care Excellence (NICE) guidelines merely state that clinicians should be "alert to the potential for drug interactions and use clinical judgement" (National Collaborating Centre for Mental Health 2014). American Psychiatric Association guidelines state treatment for comorbid AnxD and BD should "proceed concurrently" (American Psychiatric Association 2002). Canadian/ISBD guidelines state that when ADHD is comorbid with mood disorders then the condition causing most impairment should be treated first (Bond et al. 2012). This scenario can pose challenges for clinicians, as all three conditions are likely to be interacting to worsen the course of the other. In comorbid BD and ADHD, there is evidence in both children and adults to suggest a mood stabiliser and stimulant are effective in treating their respective symptoms (Findling et al. 2007). However, in adults there is also evidence of stimulant associated (hypo)mania (Wingo and Ghaemi 2008). On the other hand, one could also consider psychological treatment for the comorbid ADHD such as CBT or skills' training, which is not likely to harm treatment of BD. The presence of an additional AnxD with ADHD and BD further complicates matters, as dual-action monoamine reuptake inhibitors also risk precipitating a (hypo)manic episode, although again this would not be the case for psychological treatments such as CBT (Goodwin et al. 2016).

Participants with BDII were significantly more likely on average to exhibit higher GAF scores at follow-up than participants with BDI. This is in line with previous findings showing higher GAF scores in BDII patients compared to BDI patients, despite similar illness duration, family history, previous suicide attempts, and overall psychiatric comorbidity (Dell'Osso et al. 2017b). This also indirectly supports the notion that psychotic symptoms that are particularly prevalent in BDI patients, may contribute to the lower GAF scores seen in this group (Dell'Osso et al. 2017a). This finding is also in line with the core criteria for mania as set out in DSM 5, that the mood episode impairs social or occupational functioning. AAO did not significantly influence the mean GAF at follow-up. As discussed previously, there is still sparse literature on the effects of earlier AAO on psychosocial functioning and their conclusions are varied (Martinez-Aran et al. 2007; Perlis et al. 2009). It is important to note that this study used age at first (hypo)manic symptoms or depressive symptoms with dysfunction to define AAO.

Participants in the highest income class were significantly more likely to yield better outcomes than those in the lowest income class. Numerous studies have shown that low socioeconomic status (SES) has significant detrimental impacts on mental health at a population level (Lorant et al. 2003). However, there is little evidence regarding the effects of SES on psychosocial functioning in BD. One study found no association between education levels and functional outcome (Schoeyen et al. 2011), although the outcome was 'disability pension'; a fairly crude measure of psychosocial functioning.

The confounding effect observed between explanatory variables may be an important reason as to why individual assessment of the effects of comorbidities appeared to be spurious. Nevertheless, when we assess the individual effects in conjunction with the interaction term we are able to ascertain the overall effect of mental health comorbidities on psychosocial outcomes. As our results indicate, those with multiple comorbidities (AnxD and ADHD) experience significantly reduced psychosocial function at follow-up.

The present study is not without limitation. First, while it is important that researchers use standardised scoring instruments in order to reduce bias and increase the replicability of their findings, the GAF has several limitations. Indeed, it has been suggested that it lacks the sensitivity to assess longitudinal change in an individual patient (Soderberg et al. 2005). Moreover, the GAF is global measure, and as such fails to capture the contributions of each specific dimension of psychosocial functioning to overall dysfunction. The GAF also specifically excludes functional impairment due to "physical or environmental limitations", yet it is difficult to see how raters can distinguish aetiologically between physical or environmental and psychosocial factors.

A second critical limitation to this study is that it did not control for mood state. The possible impact of mood state on the present findings is two-fold. Firstly, depressive symptoms, even more than manic, are strong predictors of poor psychosocial functioning (Morriss et al. 2013). However, in the present study, it is not possible to replicate this relationship. Secondly, it has been shown that the incidence rates of comorbidities are sensitive to mood state, when assessed cross-sectionally (Post et al. 2018) as in the present study. It is also important to note that this study did not include medical comorbidities. These certainly play a significant role in psychosocial dysfunction but were beyond the scope of the current paper.

A third critical limitation is that the comorbid conditions were characterised by the presence of a lifetime diagnosis, and whether patients continued to manifest these difficulties consistently over their lifetime is not known. This limitation would be of particular importance for ADHD, as a substantial group of patients may have the comorbidity in childhood and/or adolescence, but no longer in adulthood. Similarly, severity of each of the comorbid problems was not assessed. Any anxiety-specific disorder was considered for inclusion in the category, and how individual anxiety disorders or their combination may have affected the relationship to function cannot be determined in this study. In addition, while the incidence of comorbidities in this study population where similar to those reported in the literature, the fact that the population was drawn largely from academic tertiary care facilities may limit the generalizability of the results and conclusions to other populations.

It is also important to challenge some of the assumptions that may be drawn from this paper, including the idea of a unidirectional relationship between the significant predictors and psychosocial dysfunction. As this study was conducted in adults, with data on predictors collected retrospectively, the relationships inferred are not conclusive. Future work should aim to clarify these findings using prospective studies starting in childhood to determine differences between those who do and do not go on to develop BD. This will help to inform the development of interventions aimed specifically at psychosocial dysfunction.

## Conclusion

In summary, this project has demonstrated the negative impact of comorbid AnxD and ADHD on psychosocial functioning in BD. Both inpatient and population studies have demonstrated the alarmingly high prevalence of comorbid disorders in BD, however current guidelines offer little help to clinicians when managing these disorders. Our findings suggest a unique interaction between AnxD and ADHD in BD, which will need further research to both replicate and explore this relationship and ascertain optimal therapeutic interventions. Resolution of clinical symptoms in BD is rarely followed by recovery of psychosocial functioning, and this study has added insights into the role of AnxD and ADHD comorbid disorders in impairing global psychosocial functioning.

**Acknowledgements**
This study was supported by the Stanley Medical Research Institute. We also acknowledge the very substantial contributions of both Gabriele S. Leverich, MSW and the late Lori Altshuler, MD.

**Authors' contributions**
FB, SH and AS developed the study hypothesis and concept of the paper, AC conducted the primary data analysis. Raw data were collected by HG, LS, PK, SME, RP, MF, RK, WN and TS. FB and SH equally contributed to drafting the article which has been edited by AS, AC, HG and RP. All authors read and approved the final manuscript.

**Competing interests**
Mark A. Frye has received grant support from AssureRx, Mayo Foundation, Myriad, National Institute of Alcohol Abuse and Alcoholism (NIAAA), National Institute of Mental Health (NIMH), Pfizer. He has served as a consultant (Mayo) to Janssen, Mitsubishi Tanabe Pharma Corporation, Myriad, Neuralstem Inc., Otsuka American Pharmaceutical, Sunovion, Teva Pharmaceuticals. His employer Mayo Clinic has a financial interest in AssureRX and the technology referenced in this publication/presentation.Heinz Grunze received grants/research support, consulting fees and honoraria within the last 3 years from Gedeon Richter, Janssen-Cilag, Lundbeck, Otsuka, Pfizer and Servier.Dr. Keck has been reimbursed for consulting to Otsuka and Lyndra. He is a co- inventor on United States Patent No. 6387956: Shapira NA, Goldsmith TD, Keck, PE Jr. (University of Cincinnati) Methods of treating obsessive–compulsive spectrum disorder comprises the step of administering an effective amount of tramadol to an individual. Filed March 25, 1999; approved May 14, 2002. Dr. Keck has received no financial gain from this patent.Ralph Kupka has received speakers honoraria over the past 3 years from Lundbeck, Janssen, and Sanofi.W.A. Nolen has received grants from the Netherlands Organisation for Health Research and Development, the European Union; has received honoraria/speaker's fees from Lundbeck and Aristo Pharma, and has served as consultant for Daleco Pharma.Susan McElroy is a consultant to or member of the scientific advisory boards of Bracket, F. Hoffmann-La Roche Ltd., MedAvante, Mitsubishi Tanabe Pharma America, Myriad, Novo Nordisk, Shire, and Sunovion. She is a principal or co-investigator on studies sponsored by the Allergan, Brainsway, Marriott Foundation, Myriad, National Institute of Mental Health, Novo Nordisk, Shire, and Sunovion. She is also an inventor on United States Patent No. 6,323,236 B2, Use of Sulfamate Derivatives for Treating Impulse Control Disorders, and along with the patent's assignee, University of Cincinnati, Cincinnati, Ohio, has received payments from Johnson & Johnson, which has exclusive rights under the patent.Robert Post has received speaker's honoraria over the past 3 years from AstraZeneca, Validus, Sunovion, Takeda, Pamlabs.Lars Schärer received grants/research support from WHO, BMZ, OCHA, WFP, UNICEF, European Commission, IBM, TigerLogic, Omnis.Trisha Suppes in the past 36 months has reported grants from National Institute of Mental Health, Sunovion Pharamaceuticals, Elan Pharma International Limited, VA Cooperative Studies Program, Pathway Genomics, Stanley Medical Research Institute, National Institute of Health, Palo Alto Health Sciences, and National Institute on Drug Abuse; consulting fees from A/S H. Lundbeck, Sunovion, and Merck & Co; honoraria from Medscape Education, Global Medical Education, and CMEology; royalties from Jones and Bartlett and UpToDate; and travel reimbursement from A/S H. Lundbeck, Sunovion Pharmaceuticals, Inc., Global Medication Education, CMEology, and Merck & Co.Aditya Sharma has received research grants from the National Institute for Health Research (UK) and speaker honoraria from the British Association for Psychopharmacology.Sophie Hodgetts, Francis Bennett and Andrew Close declares no competing interests.

**Author details**
[1] Institute of Neuroscience, Newcastle University, Newcastle upon Tyne, UK. [2] School of Psychology, University of Sunderland, Sunderland, UK. [3] Department of Psychiatry & Psychology, Mayo Clinic, Rochester, MN, USA. [4] PMU Nuremberg & Psychiatrie Schwäbisch Hall, Schwäbisch Hall, Germany. [5] Linder Center of Hope, Mason, OH, USA. [6] Biological Psychiatry Program, University of Cincinnati Medical College, Cincinnati, OH, USA. [7] Department of Psychiatry, VU University Medical Center, Amsterdam, The Netherlands. [8] University of Groningen, University Medical Center Groningen, Groningen, The Netherlands. [9] Bipolar Collaborative Network, Bethesda, MD, USA. [10] Department of Psychiatry, and Psychotherapy Medical Center, University of Freiburg, Faculty of Medicine, Freiburg im Breisgau, Germany. [11] School of Medicine and V.A. Palo Alto Health Care System Palo Alto, Stanford University, Palo Alto, CA, USA. [12] Northumberland Tyne and Wear NHS Foundation Trust, Newcastle upon Tyne, UK. [13] Academic Psychiatry, Wolfson Research Centre, Campus for Ageing and Vitality, Newcastle University, Newcastle upon Tyne NE4 5PL, UK.

**References**
Akaike H. Information theory and an extension of the maximum likelihood principle. In: Paper presented at the 2nd international symposium on information theory, Budapest, Akademiai Kiado; 1973.
American Psychiatric Association. Practice guideline for the treatment of patients with bipolar disorder (revision). Am J Psychiatry. 2002;159:1–50.
American Psychiatric Association. Diagnostic and statistical manual of mental disorders. 5th ed. Washington, DC: APA Press; 2013.
Bernardi S, Cortese S, Solanto M, Hollander E, Pallanti S. Bipolar disorder and comorbid attention deficit hyperactivity disorder. A distinct clinical phenotype? Clinical characteristics and temperamental traits. World J Biol Psychiatry. 2010;11:656–66.
Bond DJ, Hadjipavlou G, Lam RW, McIntyre RS, Beaulieu S, Schaffer A, et al. The Canadian network for mood and anxiety treatments (CANMAT) task force recommendations for the management of patients with mood disorders and comorbid attention-deficit/hyperactivity disorder. Ann Clin Psychiatry. 2012;24:23–37.
Brus MJ, Solanto MV, Goldberg JF. ADHD vs. bipolar disorder in the DSM-5 era: a challenging differentiation for clinicians. J Psychiatr Pract. 2014;20:428–37.
Burnham KP, Anderson DR. Model selection and multimodel inference: a practical information-theoretic approach. New York: Springer Sci Bus Media; 2002.
Cerullo MA, Strakowski SM. The prevalence and significance of substance use disorders in bipolar type I and II disorder. Subst Abuse Treat Prev Policy. 2007;2:29.
Dell'Osso B, Camuri G, Cremaschi L, Dobrea C, Buoli M, Ketter TA, et al. Lifetime presence of psychotic symptoms in bipolar disorder is associated with less favorable socio-demographic and certain clinical features. Compr Psychiatry. 2017a;76:169–76.
Dell'Osso B, Dobrea C, Cremaschi L, Buoli M, Miller S, Ketter TA, et al. Italian bipolar II vs I patients have better individual functioning, in spite of overall similar illness severity. CNS Spectr. 2017b;22:325–32.
Findling RL, Short EJ, McNamara NK, Demeter CA, Stansbrey RJ, Gracious BL, et al. Methylphenidate in the treatment of children and adolescents with bipolar disorder and attention-deficit/hyperactivity disorder. J Am Acad Child Adolesc Psychiatry. 2007;46:1445–53.
Gerhard A, Clogg C, Sobel M. Handbook of statistical modeling for the social and behavioral sciences. New York: Springer; 1995.
Goodwin GM, Haddad PM, Ferrier IN, Aronson JK, Barnes T, Cipriani A, et al. Evidence-based guidelines for treating bipolar disorder: revised third edition recommendations from the British Association for Psychopharmacology. J Psychopharmacol. 2016;30:495–553.
Hobbs JDJ, Kushner MG, Lee SS, Reardon SM, Maurer EW. Meta-analysis of supplemental treatment for depressive and anxiety disorders in patients being treated for alcohol dependence. Am J Addict. 2011;20:319–29.
Jones SH, Thornicroft G, Coffey M, Dunn G. A brief mental health outcome scale-reliability and validity of the global assessment of functioning (GAF). Br J Psychiatry. 1995;166:654–9.
Leverich GS, Post RM, Keck PE Jr, Altshuler LL, Frye MA, Kupka RW, et al. The poor prognosis of childhood-onset bipolar disorder. J Pediatr. 2007;150:485–90.
Levy B, Manove E. Functional outcome in bipolar disorder: the big picture. Depress Res Treat. 2012;2012:12.
Lorant V, Deliege D, Eaton W, Robert A, Philippot P, Ansseau M. Socioeconomic inequalities in depression: a meta-analysis. Am J Epidemiol. 2003;157:98–112.
MacQueen GM, Young LT, Joffe RT. A review of psychosocial outcome in patients with bipolar disorder. Acta Psychiatr Scand. 2001;103:163–70.

Marangell LB, Dennehy EB, Miyahara S, Wisniewski SR, Bauer MS, Rapaport MH, et al. The functional impact of subsyndromal depressive symptoms in bipolar disorder: data from STEP-BD. J Affect Disord. 2009;114:58–67.

Martinez-Aran A, Vieta E, Torrent C, Sanchez-Moreno J, Goikolea JM, Salamero M, et al. Functional outcome in bipolar disorder: the role of clinical and cognitive factors. Bipolar Disord. 2007;9:103–13.

McIntyre RS, Kennedy SH, Soczynska JK, Nguyen HT, Bilkey TS, Woldeyohannes HO, et al. Attention-deficit/hyperactivity disorder in adults with bipolar disorder or major depressive disorder: results from the international mood disorders collaborative project. Prim Care Companion J Clin Psychiatry. 2010. https://doi.org/10.4088/PCC.09m00861gry.

Merikangas KR, Akiskal HS, Angst J, Greenberg PE, Hirschfeld RM, Petukhova M, et al. Lifetime and 12-month prevalence of bipolar spectrum disorder in the National Comorbidity Survey replication. Arch Gen Psychiatry. 2007;64:543–52.

Merikangas KR, Jin R, He J, et al. Prevalence and correlates of bipolar spectrum disorder in the world mental health survey initiative. Arch Gen Psychiatry. 2011;68:241–51.

Morriss R, Yang M, Chopra A, Bentall R, Paykel E, Scott J. Differential effects of depression and mania symptoms on social adjustment: prospective study in bipolar disorder. Bipolar Disord. 2013;15:80–91.

National Collaborating Centre for Mental Health. Bipolar disorder: the management of bipolar disorder in adults, children and adolescents, in primary and secondary care. CG185: NICE Guideline. National Institute for Health and Clinical Excellence. 2014.

Otto MW, Simon NM, Wisniewski SR, Miklowitz DJ, Kogan JN, Reilly-Harrington NA, et al. Prospective 12-month course of bipolar disorder in outpatients with and without comorbid anxiety disorders. Br J Psychiatry. 2006;189:20–5.

Perlis RH, Dennehy EB, Miklowitz DJ, DelBello MP, Ostacher M, Calabrese JR, et al. Retrospective age at onset of bipolar disorder and outcome during two-year follow-up: results from the STEP-BD study. Bipolar Disord. 2009;11:391–400.

Pinheiro J, Bates D, DebRoy S, Sarkar D, R Core Team. nlme: linear and nonlinear mixed effects models. R package version 3.1-130. https://CRAN.R-project.org/package=nlme. 2017.

Post RM, Nolen WA, Kupka RW, Denicoff KD, Leverich GS, Keck PE Jr, et al. The Stanley Foundation Bipolar Network. I. Rationale and methods. Br J Psychiatry. 2001;178(S41):s169–76.

Post RM, Altshuler L, Leverich GS, Frye MA, Suppes T, McElroy SL, et al. Relationship of clinical course of illness variables to medical comorbidities in 900 adult outpatients with bipolar disorder. Compr Psychiatry. 2015;56:21–8.

Post RM, Leverich G, McElroy S, Kupka R, Suppes T, Altshuler L, et al. Prevalence of axis II comorbidities in bipolar disorder: relationship to mood state. Bipolar Disorder. 2018;20:303–12.

Provencher MD, Guimond AJ, Hawke LD. Comorbid anxiety in bipolar spectrum disorders: a neglected research and treatment issue? J Affect Disord. 2012;137:161–4.

Sandra Kooij JJ, Marije Boonstra A, Swinkels SH, Bekker EM, de Noord I, Buitelaar JK. Reliability, validity, and utility of instruments for self-report and informant report concerning symptoms of ADHD in adult patients. J Atten Disord. 2008;11:445–58.

Schoeyen HK, Birkenaes AB, Vaaler AE, Auestad BH, Malt UF, Andreassen OA, et al. Bipolar disorder patients have similar levels of education but lower socio-economic status than the general population. J Affect Disord. 2011;129:68–74.

Scott J, Scott EM, Hermens DF, Naismith SL, Guastella AJ, White D, et al. Functional impairment in adolescents and young adults with emerging mood disorders. Br J Psychiatry. 2014;205:362–8.

Sentissi O, Navarro JC, De Oliveira H, Gourion D, Bourdel MC, Bayle FJ, et al. Bipolar disorders and quality of life: the impact of attention deficit/hyperactivity disorder and substance abuse in euthymic patients. Psychiatry Res. 2008;161:36–42.

Simon NM, Otto MW, Wisniewski SR, Fossey M, Sagduyu K, Frank E, et al. Anxiety disorder comorbidity in bipolar disorder patients: data from the first 500 participants in the systematic treatment enhancement program for bipolar disorder (STEP-BD). Am J Psychiatry. 2004;161:2222–9.

Soderberg P, Tungstrom S, Armelius BA. Reliability of global assessment of functioning ratings made by clinical psychiatric staff. Psychiatr Serv. 2005;56:434–8.

Vazquez GH, Baldessarini RJ, Tondo L. Co-occurrence of anxiety and bipolar disorders: clinical and therapeutic overview. Depress Anxiety. 2014;31:196–206.

Vickers AJ, Altman DG. Analysing controlled trials with baseline and follow up measurements. BMJ. 2001;323:1123–4.

Wilens TE, Biederman J, Wozniak J, Gunawardene S, Wong J, Monuteaux M. Can adults with attention-deficit/hyperactivity disorder be distinguished from those with comorbid bipolar disorder? Findings from a sample of clinically referred adults. Biol Psychiatry. 2003;54:1–8.

Wingo AP, Ghaemi SN. Frequency of stimulant treatment and of stimulant-associated mania/hypomania in bipolar disorder patients. Psychopharmacol Bull. 2008;41:37–47.

# 3

# The role of environmental stress and DNA methylation in the longitudinal course of bipolar disorder

Ashley L. Comes[1,2*], Darina Czamara[3], Kristina Adorjan[1,4], Heike Anderson-Schmidt[1,5], Till F. M. Andlauer[3,6], Monika Budde[1], Katrin Gade[5], Maria Hake[1], Janos L. Kalman[1,2,4], Sergi Papiol[1,4], Daniela Reich-Erkelenz[1], Farah Klöhn-Saghatolislam[1,4], Sabrina K. Schaupp[1], Eva C. Schulte[1,4], Fanny Senner[1,4], Georg Juckel[7], Max Schmauß[8], Jörg Zimmermann[9], Jens Reimer[10], Eva Reininghaus[11], Ion-George Anghelescu[12], Carsten Konrad[13], Andreas Thiel[13], Christian Figge[14], Martin von Hagen[15], Manfred Koller[16], Detlef E. Dietrich[17,18,19], Sebastian Stierl[20], Harald Scherk[21], Stephanie H. Witt[22], Sugirthan Sivalingam[23], Franziska Degenhardt[23], Andreas J. Forstner[23,24,25,26], Marcella Rietschel[22], Markus M. Nöthen[23], Jens Wiltfang[5,27,28], Peter Falkai[4], Thomas G. Schulze[1,4†] and Urs Heilbronner[1†]

**Abstract**

**Background:** Stressful life events influence the course of affective disorders, however, the mechanisms by which they bring about phenotypic change are not entirely known.

**Methods:** We explored the role of DNA methylation in response to recent stressful life events in a cohort of bipolar patients from the longitudinal PsyCourse study ($n = 96$). Peripheral blood DNA methylomes were profiled at two time points for over 850,000 methylation sites. The association between impact ratings of stressful life events and DNA methylation was assessed, first by interrogating methylation sites in the vicinity of candidate genes previously implicated in the stress response and, second, by conducting an exploratory epigenome-wide association analysis. Third, the association between epigenetic aging and change in stress and symptom measures over time was investigated.

**Results:** Investigation of methylation signatures over time revealed just over half of the CpG sites tested had an absolute difference in methylation of at least 1% over a 1-year period. Although not a single CpG site withstood correction for multiple testing, methylation at one site (cg15212455) was suggestively associated with stressful life events ($p < 1.0 \times 10^{-5}$). Epigenetic aging over a 1-year period was not associated with changes in stress or symptom measures.

**Conclusions:** To the best of our knowledge, our study is the first to investigate epigenome-wide methylation across time in bipolar patients and in relation to recent, non-traumatic stressful life events. Limited and inconclusive evidence warrants future longitudinal investigations in larger samples of well-characterized bipolar patients to give a complete picture regarding the role of DNA methylation in the course of bipolar disorder.

**Keywords:** DNA methylation, Bipolar disorder, Stressful life events, Longitudinal, Epigenomics, Epigenetic aging

*Correspondence: Ashley.Comes@med.uni-muenchen.de
†Thomas G. Schulze and Urs Heilbronner contributed equally to this work
[1] Institute of Psychiatric Phenomics and Genomics, University Hospital, LMU Munich, Nussbaumstrasse 7, 80336 Munich, Germany
Full list of author information is available at the end of the article

## Background

Bipolar disorder (BD) remains an interesting candidate for neurobiological analyses owing to its heterogenous presentation and both genetic and environmental risk factors (Ludwig and Dwivedi 2016). While genome-wide association studies (GWAS) in BD have identified dozens of associated variants, they have explained only a small fraction of overall disease liability (Stahl et al. 2019). Therefore, the last decade has seen a shift towards investigating the complex interplay between genetic and environmental risk factors (Sharma et al. 2016). Advances in technologies have supported high-throughput investigations of biological markers representative of environmental modulation of the genome. These biomarkers hold promise for stratifying symptom-based phenotypes and assessing the prognosis of individual patients (Kobeissy et al. 2012). Moreover, these biomarkers could contribute to a more accurate multi-level diagnostic framework which relies on biological measures to supplement clinical ratings of symptoms (Meana and Mollinedo-Gajate 2017).

BD is a chronic, disabling, and severe mental illness characterized by recurrent depressive and manic episodes, somatic and psychiatric comorbidities, and functional impairments (Goodwin and Jamison 2007). Considering the high global burden and lifetime prevalence of bipolar spectrum disorders, estimated at approximately 2.4% (Rowland and Marwaha 2018), there is a need to better understand the factors affecting its onset and course. The significance of environment, especially childhood trauma and stressful life events on the trajectories of affective disorders, including vulnerability, onset, relapse and occurrence, has been well established (Aldinger and Schulze 2017; Lex et al. 2017; Johnson 2005; Alloy et al. 2005; Paykel 2003). However, little is known about the mechanisms involved in the consequences of such life events.

Recently, emphasis has been placed on the potential role of epigenetic variation in the etiopathogenesis of BD (Li et al. 2015). Epigenetics is an adaptive mechanism which can modulate the stress response through subtle gene expression modifications (Aas et al. 2016). In particular, DNA methylation (DNAm), the addition of a methyl group to DNA, primarily at cytosine-guanine dinucleotides (CpG), may pose a "mechanism by which life-experiences become 'embedded' in the genome" (Marzi et al. 2018).

Increasing evidence from both animal and human data supports the epigenetic programming of genes in response to trauma and chronic stress. Consistent findings have linked prenatal (Monk et al. 2012; Weaver et al. 2004) and early-life adversities to epigenetic modifications of genes, especially those involved in the hypothalamic–pituitary–adrenal (HPA) axis (Kular and Kular 2018; McGowan et al. 2009; Vinkers et al. 2015; Jaworska-Andryszewska and Rybakowski 2019). While several studies have shown methylation changes associated with trauma during the adult period, few studies have investigated non-traumatic chronic stress (Matosin et al. 2017) or acute stressful life events. Candidate gene approaches in the general population have reported differential methylation of CpGs in the vicinity of *SLC6A4* (Alasaari et al. 2012), *TH* (Myaki et al. 2015), and *BDNF* (Song et al. 2014) in association with sustained work-related stress. One study, which examined *LINE-1* as a proxy for global methylation, found no signification associations with chronic lifestyle stress (Duman and Canli 2015). To the best of our knowledge, not a single study has explored epigenome-wide signatures of DNAm in relation to acute, non-traumatic stress in humans. With regards to BD, studies have investigated methylation differences as both trait and state markers of the disorder in several promoter regions including *SLC6A4, PPIEL31, BDNF, HCG9, KCNQ3, 5HTR1A* and *GPR24* (Ludwig and Dwivedi 2016; Fries et al. 2016; Pishva et al. 2014). Interestingly, evidence supports altered DNAm profiles for high-risk affected and even unaffected offspring of individuals with BD in comparison to low risk controls. Moreover, there seems to be a unique rate of change in DNAm over time for high risk individuals (Duffy et al. 2019). However, despite findings of differential epigenetic profiles, results have been inconsistent and there remains a need for genome-wide methylation studies, especially ones longitudinal in design.

This study aims to gain a better understanding of the role of epigenetic modifications, specifically DNAm, in relation to stress during the course of BD. Using repeated measures over a 1-year period, we explored the relationship between DNAm and stressful life events in chronic BD patients. We took a two-pronged approach, first by interrogating CpGs in the vicinity of candidate genes previously implicated in the stress response and, second, by conducting an exploratory epigenome-wide analysis. Furthermore, we determined whether changes in symptom and stress measures over time were associated with a DNAm-based age estimate and epigenetic aging.

## Methods

### Study sample

The study was conducted using data from the longitudinal PsyCourse cohort. PsyCourse has been described in detail (Budde et al. 2019). Briefly, PsyCourse is a multi-site, naturalistic study, based in the German and Austrian population. Psychopathology, pharmacological treatment, childhood trauma and current stressful life events were among other variables assessed at each of four visits (6-month intervals). Likewise, peripheral blood samples were collected at each visit, paving the way for a detailed analysis of the longitudinal correlation between disease status and peripheral biomarkers. For the purpose of this study, a subset of PsyCourse participants ($n = 96$) was selected according to a DSM-IV diagnosis (American Psychiatric Association 2002) of type I or II BD, availability of genotype data and biomaterial, and completed childhood trauma and stressful life events questionnaires. Demographic and clinical characteristics of these patients are reported in Table 1. The study was approved by the local ethics committee for each study center and was carried out following the rules of the Declaration of Helsinki. All individuals provided written informed consent.

## Measures

### *Stressful life events*

Current stressful life events were assessed with the Life Events Questionnaire (LEQ), a 79-item self-report instrument that has been described in detail (Norbeck 1984; Sarason et al. 1978). The LEQ covers a wide range of stressor exposure related to health, work, school, residence, love and marriage, family and friends, parenting, the personal sphere or social environment, finances, crime and legal matters. At each visit, participants reported whether they experienced any of the listed events in the last 6 months. When the patient experienced a specific event, they rated: (1) the nature of the event (good/bad) and (2) the impact of the event on his/her life (0–3). At each time point, adverse life events were summed to yield a stress score that reflects the impact ratings of all "bad" events. The same was done for the impact ratings of "good" events. A total score was also summed including impact ratings of both "bad" and "good" events. These three LEQ scores were used as outcome measures in our association analyses.

**Table 1 Sample demographic and clinical characteristics**

| | Baseline ($n=96$) | 1-year follow-up ($n=95$) | *p*-value |
|---|---|---|---|
| Sex | | | |
| Female | 50 | 50 | |
| Age, mean ± SD | 45.2 ± 12.4 | 46.17 ± 12.4 | |
| Duration of illness, mean ± SD | 13.52 ± 11.8 | 14.66 ± 11.8 | |
| DSM-IV diagnosis | | | |
| BD-I | 79 | 78 | |
| BD-II | 17 | 17 | |
| Medication | | | |
| Combo therapy | 81 | 75 | |
| Monotherapy | 14 | 16 | |
| No meds | 1 | 4 | |
| Childhood trauma (yes) | 48 | 48 | |
| LEQ scores, mean ± SD | | | |
| Bad events | 10.2 ± 13.8 | 6.3 ± 6.6 | 0.004[b] |
| Good events | 9.7 ± 10.2 | 8.4 ± 7.6 | 0.191[b] |
| Total events | 19.9 ± 18.4 | 14.1 ± 10.7 | 0.001[b] |
| Symptom ratings | | | |
| GAF, mean ± SD | 61.5 ± 12.6 | 65.8 ± 12.4 | 0.032[a] |
| YMRS sum, mean ± SD | 3.9 ± 5.8 | 2.4 ± 3.7 | 0.216[b] |
| IDS-$C_{30}$, mean ± SD | 13.7 ± 11.0 | 10.6 ± 9.7 | 0.124[b] |
| PANSS sum, mean ± SD | 42.8 ± 11.8 | 39.2 ± 9.6 | 0.063[b] |

[a] Paired sample t-test

[b] Wilcoxon signed rank test

### *Childhood trauma*

The Childhood Trauma Screener (CTS) is a German, short version of the Childhood Trauma Questionnaire (Bernstein et al. 1997, 2003; Grabe et al. 2012). The screener includes five questions to assess sexual, physical and emotional abuse, as well as emotional and physical neglect. Validated threshold values (Glaesmer et al. 2013) were used to transform ratings for each item into a dichotomous scale in order to identify individuals with reported childhood trauma (yes/no). Details on reported childhood trauma and thresholds used can be found in Additional file 1: Table S1.

### *Symptom ratings*

The Positive and Negative Syndrome Scale (PANSS) was used as a measure of psychopathology at the time of testing (Kay et al. 1987). A continuous total score of the three subscales, i.e. positive, negative, and general symptoms was used. The Global Assessment of Functioning (GAF) score was used as a measure of psychosocial functioning (Luborsky 1962; Endicott et al. 1976). The Young Mania Rating Scale (YMRS) was used as a measure of manic symptoms in the last 48 h (Young et al. 1978). Lastly, the Inventory of Depressive Symptomatology (IDS-$C_{30}$), a 30-item rating scale, was used to assess the severity of depressive symptoms (Trivedi et al. 2004).

## Analysis of DNA methylation

### *DNA samples*

Genomic DNA was extracted from whole blood using the PerkinElmer Chemagen Kit (chemagic DNA Blood10k prefilling VD120419.che) and all samples were subsequently stored in a Hamilton Bios M system at − 80 °C. DNA quality was assessed using the QIAxcel® system. DNA samples from baseline and 1-year follow-up visits were used to obtain methylation data. Prior to downstream analyses, potential population stratification was evaluated, and an initial step to remove European population outliers was taken (Budde et al. 2019). Thus, our sample consists of an ethnically homogenous population of Caucasians of European descent.

#### *Illumina EPIC chip processing*

Bisulfide conversion of DNA and processing of methylation arrays was accomplished in collaboration with the Institute of Human Genetics, University of Bonn, Germany. Whole-blood genomic DNA diluted with water (50 ng/μl) was treated with sodium bisulfite using the EpiTect® Bisulfite Kit from QIAGEN® following the manufacturer's protocol. DNAm was assessed using the Illumina Infinium Human MethylationEPIC BeadChip array (Illumina Inc., San Diego, CA, USA) according to the manufacturer's instructions. To minimize batch effects during DNAm measurement, an algorithm for sample randomization was used for positioning samples onto 96-well plates according to exposures of interest and confounding variables (see Additional file 1).

### Quality control and normalization

#### *Quality control*

The Bioconductor R package *minfi* was used to read raw intensity data files (.idat files) into R and for the subsequent quality control and normalization of methylation data (Aryee et al. 2014). Concordance between methylation-predicted and reported sex was confirmed. Filtering of poor-performing samples and probes was performed (see Additional file 1: Table S2). Probes with low detection *p*-values ($>0.05$ in $>10\%$ of samples) were excluded. Using the function dropLociWithSnps(), SNPs inside the probe body and at the nucleotide extension were removed according to a minor allele frequency $\geq 5\%$ based on dbSNP. To prevent a possible gender effect, X and Y chromosomes were removed. According to a list previously published (Chen et al. 2013), non-specific probes i.e. probes on the EPIC array that co-hybridize to alternate genomic sequences, were removed. Lastly, probes with a bead count $< 3$ were removed.

#### *Normalization*

Data were normalized using functional normalization (FunNorm), an extension of quantile normalization. FunNorm uses internal control probes present on the array to infer between-array technical variation, by default using the first two principal components of the control probes (Fortin et al. 2014). Density plots were used to evaluate the distribution of *M*-values before and after functional normalization (see Additional file 1: Fig. S1).

Technical batch effects were then identified using linear regressions to inspect the association of principal components of the methylation values with possible technical batches. Additionally, the R package *shinyMethyl* was used for visual inspection of principle component analysis (PCA) plots. Identified batch effects (i.e., array and slide) were removed using the Empirical Bayes' method *ComBat* (Johnson et al. 2007). Batch corrected *M*-values after *ComBat* were used for downstream analyses (see Additional file 1: Fig. S2). According to inspection of PCA plots, a single sample remained an outlier after batch correction and was excluded.

#### *Confounders*

Considering cell-type composition is a confounding factor in epigenome-wide association studies (EWAS), the *minfi* function estimateCellcounts() was used to estimate the cell type composition for our samples. This function uses a modified version of the Houseman algorithm to obtain a cell counts vector for the six cell-types (i.e., CD4T, CD8T, NK, B cells, monocytes, and granulocytes) for each sample (Houseman et al. 2012).

Active smoking is another established modifier of DNA methylation (Lee and Pausova 2013). Methylation-based smoking scores were calculated based on the methylation profile of the 187 CpG sites identified in Zeilinger et al. (2013). First, raw beta values were normalized using the Teschendorff et al. beta-mixture quantile dilation (BMIQ) strategy (Teschendorff et al. 2013). Adjusted beta-values were then used for calculation of methylation-based smoking scores using methods previously described (Elliott et al. 2014). The correlation between self-reported number of cigarettes smoked yearly and methylation-based smoking scores was assessed (Spearman's $\rho = 0.64$; $p < 0.001$).

To rule out possible confounding effects of medication, 5 samples were excluded in sensitivity analyses. These samples were participants who were not taking psychotropic drugs at the time of testing. All other participants were taking at least one (monotherapy) or a combination (combo therapy) of the following (1) antidepressants, (2) antipsychotics, (3) mood stabilizers, (4) tranquilizers, or (5) other psychiatric medications.

### Statistical analyses

All statistical analyses were performed in R version 3.4.4 (http://www.r-project.org/) (R Core Team 2014).

#### *Change in methylation over time*

The general "stability" of methylation over time was investigated. First, the absolute change in methylation $\beta$-values between baseline and 1-year follow-up visits were calculated across all CpG sites. To determine whether differential methylation between visits remained significant after adjusting for known confounders, the package *lme4* (Bates et al. 2015) was used to fit a linear mixed-effects model (LMM) with the dependent variable "*M*-value" and the independent variable "time", adjusting for age, sex, DNAm smoking scores, and cell composition estimates. Patient ID was included as the random effect term.

***Candidate gene analysis***

The association between LEQ scores and the interaction between CT and total LEQ scores with DNAm was assessed via LMMs, adjusting for covariates as described above. We interrogated DNAm in the vicinity of genes previously implicated in the HPA-axis (i.e. *BDNF, FKBP5, IL6, SLC6A4*, and *OXTR*). All probes on the EPIC array annotated to each of these five genes were identified. The number of probes per gene ranged from 22 to 124. We corrected for multiple testing on a gene-level by applying the false discovery (FDR) correction (Benjamini and Hochberg 1995) per gene, with FDR-corrected $p$-values $\leq 0.05$ deemed significant. Afterwards, Bonferroni-correction was used to correct overall for the number of candidate-genes tested.

***Exploratory EWAS***

An exploratory EWAS was conducted. As a means of noise reduction, the top 10% of the most variable CpGs of the normalized, batch corrected $M$-values were extracted according to median absolute deviation (MAD) scores i.e. the median of the absolute deviations from the data's median. Associations between the most variable sites and LEQ scores and the interaction between childhood trauma and total LEQ scores were then tested using LMMs, adjusting for covariates as described above.

***Epigenetic aging***

DNAm-based age prediction was performed using the Horvath age estimation algorithm (Horvath 2013) with a freely available online tool (https://dnamage.genetics.ucla.edu/home) which predicts DNAm-age based on the methylation of 353 CpGs using an elastic net penalized regression model. The difference between the estimated epigenetic age and chronological age (Δage) and a measure of epigenetic age acceleration (AA), i.e., the residual from regressing DNAm age on chronological age, were calculated. LMMs were used to determine the effect of LEQ scores on Δage, adjusting for chronological age, sex, DNAm smoking scores, cell composition estimates, and technical batch effects (sample slide and array). Additionally, the difference in symptom ratings and stress scores between visits were calculated. The association between the change in symptoms and LEQ scores between baseline and 1-year follow-up with AA at 1-year follow-up was determined via linear regression models, again controlling for chronological age, sex, DNAm smoking scores, cell composition estimates and technical batch effects.

***Additional analyses***

Nominally significant CpGs (unadjusted $p < 0.05$) associated with total LEQ scores were used for gene-based enrichment analysis using the *GOmeth* function from the Bioconductor package *missMethyl*. *GOmeth* maps a vector of CpG sites to Entrez Gene IDs, and tests for gene ontology (GO) term pathway enrichment using a hypergeometric test (Geeleher et al. 2013). Additionally, the correlation between DNAm in blood and four brain regions was explored for the most suggestive CpGs associated with total LEQ scores (see Additional file 1).

## Results

### Change in methylation over time

The mean absolute difference in methylation (β) between visits 1 and 3 ($|\Delta\beta|$) was calculated across all samples for all CpG sites (Fig. 1). Over the 1-year period, $|\Delta\beta|$ ranged from $< 0.001$ to 0.299 with an average change of 0.014. Of 753,251 CpG sites, only 68 had an $|\Delta\beta|$ of 0.10 or more, while 8454 sites differed by at least 0.05 between visits. Just over half of the sites (428,610) showed an absolute difference in methylation of at least 1%. Investigation of the functional genomic distribution of the least stable CpGs over time ($|\Delta\beta| \geq 0.10$) revealed the majority of CpGs fell within Open Seas, while 12 fell within CpG Islands, and the remaining in CpG Shores and Shelves (Fig. 2). In summary, 34,776 CpG sites showed a nominally significant difference over time (unadjusted $p$-value $< 0.05$), after correcting for age, sex, smoking and cell composition estimates. However, not a single locus withstood correction for multiple testing (FDR-corrected $p$-value $< 0.05$).

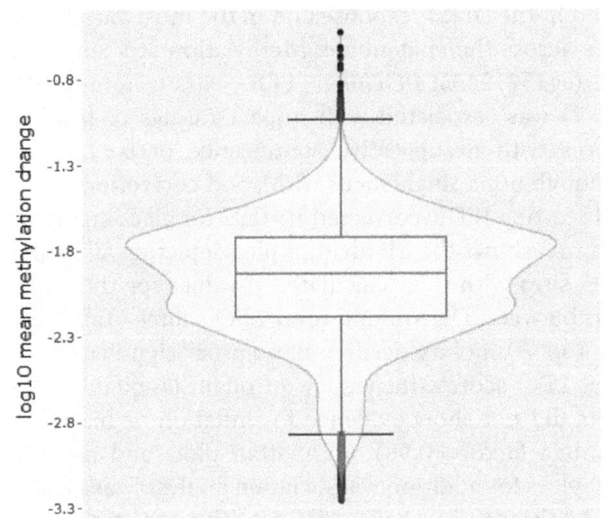


**Fig. 1** Boxplot depicting the log10 mean change in methylation (β) between baseline and 1-year follow-up visit

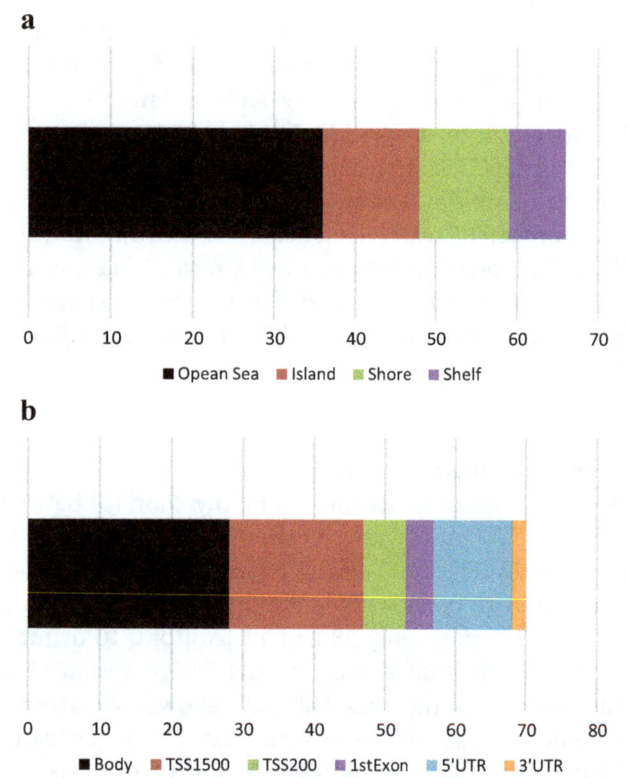


**Fig. 2** Functional genomic distribution for the least stable CpG sites over 1-year period ($|\Delta\beta| \geq 0.10$). **a** Depicts the distribution of probes that fell within CpG Islands (12/66), Shelves (7/66), Shores (11/66) and the Open Sea (36/66). **b** Depicts the distribution of probes that fell within the gene body (28), 5′ UTR (11), 3′ UTR (2), 1st Exon (4), TSS 1500 (19) and TSS 200 (6)

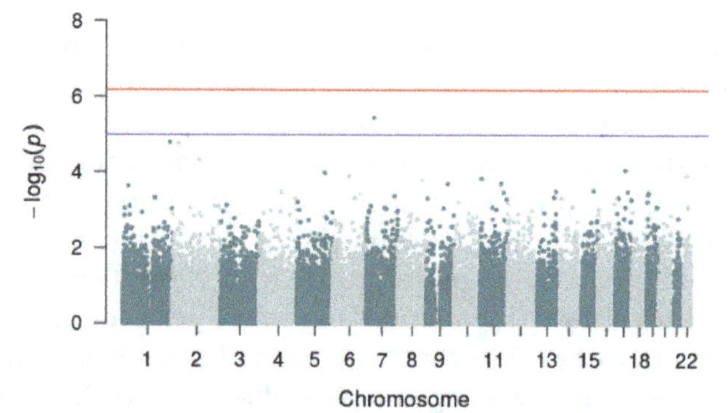


**Fig. 3** Manhattan plot for association between DNA methylation and total LEQ scores. The horizontal red line represents the epigenome-wide significant threshold for this study ($p < 6.6 \times 10^{-7}$) and the blue line represents a suggestive significance threshold ($p < 1.0 \times 10^{-5}$)

#### Methylation association analysis

We performed an exploratory analysis looking for associations between LEQ scores and DNAm in individual CpG probes in the vicinity of candidate genes previously implicated in the stress response and in the most variable CpG sites across the epigenome. Methylation at a single CpG site (cg15212455; *POU6F2*; "POU class 6 homeobox 2"; chr 7) was associated with impact ratings of total LEQ scores with a suggestive significance of $p < 1.0 \times 10^{-5}$, although not a single locus withstood correction for multiple testing (FDR-corrected $p > 0.05$ for all comparisons). Figure 3 shows the Manhattan plot depicting all analyzed CpG sites with their calculated $p$-values for the association between DNAm and total LEQ scores. Table 2 lists the top 20 loci associated at nominal significance with total LEQ scores. Inspection of quantile–quantile (QQ) plots did not show evidence for inflation or bias (Fig. 4; Lambda factor = 0.98). Manhattan plots and associated QQ plots for additional association analyses can be found in Additional file 1: Fig. S3–S8. The sensitivity analysis, excluding subjects who did not take psychotropic drugs at the time of testing, did not yield signification associations. These results, specific to modeling the association between DNAm and total LEQ scores, are presented in Additional file 1: Figs. S9 and S10.

#### Epigenetic aging

As expected, there was a strong positive correlation between individuals' DNAm age and chronological age ($r = 0.941$, $p < 0.001$; see Additional file 1: Fig. S11). According to Horvath's estimate, the mean (SD, range) AA was − 0.23 years (3.71, range − 9.94 to 9.86 years) at baseline and 0.25 years (3.95, range − 8.12 to 9.43 years) at the 1-year follow-up. Between visits, the mean (SD, range) change in AA was 0.50 years (4.97, range − 10.72 to 13.85 years). Overall, no statistically significant associations between epigenetic aging and symptom or stress measures were detected.

#### Additional analyses

We included genes mapped by the top CpG sites (unadjusted $p < 0.05$) associated with total LEQ scores in an enrichment analysis. No biological processes survived FDR correction (see Additional file 1: Table S3). Blood brain correlation coefficients for methylation of the top 20 loci associated with total LEQ scores (overlapping with the 450 K Beadchip array) are presented in Table 3. Eight of the top 20 most differentially methylated loci associated with total LEQ scores showed a significant correlation between methylation in the blood and methylation in at least one brain region. Methylation of the CpG site that was most strongly associated with total LEQ scores was significantly correlated with methylation in all four brain regions ($p < 0.001$; see Additional file 1: Fig. S12).

**Table 2 Top 20 CpG sites associated with total LEQ scores**

| Probe | t value | *p*-value | FDR-corrected *p*-value | Chr | Relation to island | Annotated gene |
|---|---|---|---|---|---|---|
| cg15212455 | − 4.87 | 3.56E−06 | 0.263 | chr7 | Open Sea | *POU6F2* |
| cg05335886 | − 4.55 | 1.02E−05 | 0.263 | chr16 | Island | *TMC5* |
| cg09725915 | 4.54 | 1.05E−05 | 0.263 | chr2 | Island | |
| cg24511004 | 4.43 | 1.62E−05 | 0.263 | chr1 | Open Sea | |
| cg18110277 | − 4.50 | 1.74E−05 | 0.263 | chr2 | Open Sea | |
| cg21516302 | − 4.24 | 4.58E−05 | 0.575 | chr2 | Open Sea | |
| cg05180443 | − 4.04 | 8.61E−05 | 0.927 | chr17 | Island | *CHAD;ACSF2* |
| cg01440452 | − 3.97 | 1.03E−04 | 0.946 | chr5 | N Shore | *PURA* |
| cg26730347 | − 4.00 | 1.20E−04 | 0.946 | chr22 | N Shore | *SLC5A1* |
| cg15869582 | 3.94 | 1.26E−04 | 0.946 | chr6 | S Shore | *IBTK* |
| cg05919744 | 3.95 | 1.44E−04 | 0.977 | chr11 | S Shore | *SLC22A18AS;SLC22A18* |
| cg26822318 | 3.86 | 1.61E−04 | 0.977 | chr8 | Open Sea | *FER1L6* |
| cg27296293 | − 3.80 | 1.98E−04 | 0.977 | chr11 | Island | *RP11-748H22.1;TRPC6* |
| cg06334363 | 3.82 | 2.01E−04 | 0.977 | chr9 | S Shore | *RP11-235C23.5;FKTN* |
| cg00356897 | − 3.79 | 2.30E−04 | 0.977 | chr1 | Open Sea | *RP4-594I10.2* |
| cg24795825 | 3.72 | 2.98E−04 | 0.977 | chr15 | N Shore | *MORF4L1* |
| cg17984201 | 3.69 | 3.17E−04 | 0.977 | chr13 | Open Sea | |
| cg18002447 | − 3.67 | 3.20E−04 | 0.977 | chr17 | Island | |
| cg07349208 | − 3.66 | 3.36E−04 | 0.977 | chr4 | Island | *RP11-380D23.2* |
| cg05705044 | 3.65 | 3.38E−04 | 0.977 | chr11 | S Shore | *RBM7* |

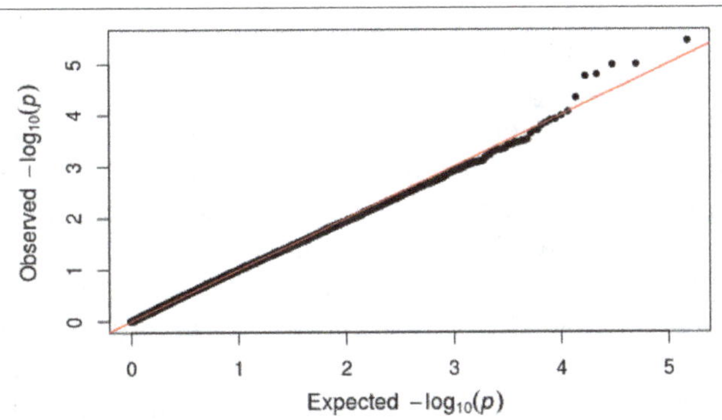


**Fig. 4** QQ plot. The plot shows no evidence for inflation or bias in the association analysis of DNA methylation with total LEQ scores (Lambda = 1.04)

## Discussion

To the best of our knowledge, our study is the first to investigate epigenome-wide methylation changes over time in BD patients. Moreover, it is the first to explore methylation changes related to non-traumatic stressful life events on an epigenome-wide scale. Although no locus withstood correction for multiple testing, our suggestive findings and secondary analyses provide limited evidence supporting a role of DNAm in association with non-traumatic life events in chronic BD patients.

We identified a single, suggestively significant, CpG site associated with total LEQ scores, mapping to *POU6F2*, which has been associated with several psychiatric traits as well as intelligence and educational attainment. More specifically, genome-wide association studies have identified *POU6F2* risk variants associated with psychological distress (Koshimizu et al. 2019), feeling emotionally hurt (Nagel et al. 2018), schizophrenia (Goes et al. 2015), autism (Anney et al. 2010), educational attainment (Lee et al. 2018; Okbay et al. 2016) and intelligence (Hill et al. 2018; Davies et al. 2018). Additionally, in a longitudinal investigation of DNAm changes preceding adolescent psychotic experiences, DNAm of the CpG site cg11604728 (*POU6F2*) measured at age 15–17 was among the top 20 CpG sites indicative of psychotic experiences at age 18 (Roberts et al. 2019). Furthermore, *POU6F2* is highly expressed in the brain with the highest expression found in the frontal cortex (Additional file 1: Fig. S13) and methylation of our suggestive CpG site in blood is correlated with methylation in brain tissue across multiple brain regions. Interestingly, another of our top 20 CpG sites (cg26822318) falls in proximity to the *FER1L6* gene, of which a variant (rs4870888) has been associated with suicide attempts in a meta-analysis of major depressive disorder, schizophrenia and BD (Mullins et al. 2019). Furthermore, another GWAS reported a *FER1L6*

**Table 3 Blood-brain methylation correlation for top differentially methylated CpGs associated with total LEQ scores**

| Probe | Blood-PFC | *p*-value | Blood-EC | *p*-value | Blood-STG | *p*-value | Blood-CER | *p*-value |
|---|---|---|---|---|---|---|---|---|
| cg15212455 | *0.721* | *4.16E−13* | *0.731* | *4.64E−13* | *0.747* | *1.48E−14* | *0.631* | *3.71E−09* |
| cg05335886 | − 0.086 | 0.467 | − 0.101 | 0.404 | − 0.145 | 0.213 | − 0.155 | 0.196 |
| cg09725915 | *0.576* | *7.86E−08* | *0.532* | *1.76E−06* | *0.626* | *1.96E−09* | *0.489* | *1.49E−05* |
| cg21516302 | *0.373* | *0.001* | *0.522* | *3.01E−06* | *0.507* | *3.46E−06* | *0.307* | *0.009* |
| cg05180443 | 0.204 | 0.081 | *0.336* | *0.004* | *0.298* | *0.009* | 0.175 | 0.144 |
| cg01440452 | − 0.097 | 0.413 | 0.062 | 0.606 | − 0.119 | 0.309 | 0.020 | 0.870 |
| cg26730347 | *0.499* | *6.05E−06* | *0.568* | *2.33E−07* | *0.562* | *1.51E−07* | *0.493* | *1.27E−05* |
| cg27296293 | 0.131 | 0.265 | − 0.214 | 0.073 | 0.037 | 0.755 | *0.236* | *0.048* |
| cg24795825 | 0.016 | 0.894 | *0.299* | *0.011* | *0.247* | *0.033* | 0.121 | 0.317 |
| cg18002447 | 0.038 | 0.749 | 0.034 | 0.776 | 0.042 | 0.720 | *− 0.262* | *0.028* |
| cg07349208 | 0.167 | 0.156 | 0.095 | 0.431 | − 0.112 | 0.338 | 0.068 | 0.571 |

*PFC* prefrontal cortex, *EC* entorhinal cortex, *STG* superior temporal gyrus, *CER* cerebellum

Significant correlations in italics

variant (rs10481151) suggestively associated with cognitive performance (Need et al. 2009).

At the current sample size, our study provides only minimal evidence supporting an association between methylation of individual CpGs and non-traumatic, recent stressful life events in BD. These findings, however, corroborate other reports of a limited role of DNAm with non-traumatic stress (Marzi et al. 2018). Noteworthy, a recent study reported hypermethylation of *KITLG* associated with childhood trauma in healthy controls ($n=91$) but not in bipolar patients ($n=50$) (He et al. 2018). Although the mechanistic role of DNAm in the phenotypic expression of early life adversities is well established in the literature, other mechanisms may be responsible in adulthood and in association with subsequent events. This notion aligns with theories such as Post's kindling hypothesis and the decay model which suggest a higher impact of life events on first episode than on subsequent episodes in BD (Aldinger and Schulze 2017; Kemner et al. 2015; Hillegers et al. 2004). Furthermore, it must be considered whether positive epigenetic associations with life events could be disorder-specific, genotype-dependent, associated with specific trauma exposure, age groups, sex and/or tissues measured (Marzi et al. 2018; Vinkers et al. 2015; Uddin et al. 2010; Boks et al. 2015; Smith et al. 2011; Mehta et al. 2017). While there is no gold standard for life stress measurements, differences in how to quantify stress may also have a major effect on findings (Johnson 2005; Bender and Alloy 2011; Monroe 2008; Dohrenwend 2010; Brown and Harris 2012).

The main strength of our study is its longitudinal design, allowing for repeated measures within individuals and to investigate methylation changes over time and in relation to symptomatology and stressful life events. To the best of our knowledge, this is the first study to collect repeated epigenome-wide methylation measures in bipolar patients. Furthermore, our study paid attention to critical confounding factors which often lead to spurious findings. For example, the use of methylation-based smoking scores better controls for the extent of smoking throughout the lifetime than the use of self-reported smoking measures (Elliott et al. 2014; Shenker et al. 2013). Finally, in contrast to most other studies, we have included an exploratory epigenome-wide approach.

Despite the strengths of our study, several limitations need to be addressed. First, our study was limited by our small sample size which makes identifying subtle differences in methylation difficult. Taking power into consideration, and as an attempt to address the inherent multiple testing problem associated with EWAS, we limited our EWAS to only the most variable CpG sites according to MAD scores. While the fact that not a single site-specific association in DNAm survived correction for multiple testing could reflect the limited statistical power of our small sample, it may also be related to an overly conservative multiple testing correction considering the lack of variability in methylation at many CpGs and spatial correlation of methylation with nearby sites (Walker et al. 2016; Lunnon et al. 2015). A recent study estimated there are approximately 530,000 independent tests in a whole blood EPIC array DNAm study. Accordingly, they proposed a corrected significance threshold of $9.42 \times 10^{-8}$ to be used as a standard threshold for future EWAS based on the EPIC array (Mansell et al. 2019). Furthermore, the study introduced a freely available online tool which allows users to perform power calculations to guide sample sizes, accounting for the individual properties of each DNAm site and using their empirically derived significance threshold. According to their tool, an effect size of just

1% difference between cases and controls would require a sample of 1000 participants, for only a third of methylation sites to have > 80% power. We observed an effect size below 5% in our study (based on median split) for our most significantly associated site, indicating that our study is nevertheless underpowered. Future studies should take advantage of this tool to assess, a priori, required sample sizes according to their expected effect sizes. Furthermore, complementary systems biology approaches such as weighted gene co-methylation network analysis (WGCNA) could be beneficial for studies with limited sample sizes, providing more insight into the functional role of altered DNAm (Langfelder and Horvath 2008).

Another limitation is in relation to the fact that our sample represents a cohort of chronic BD patients which likely influenced our investigation of epigenetic aging related to symptom ratings over time. The chronicity of patients may also confound our findings with regards to the heterogenous treatments patients have received over the years. To acknowledge this critical factor, we conducted a sensitivity analysis excluding those subjects not taking psychotropic drugs at the time of testing, however, this also did not lead to significant results. One must also consider the possible recall and desirability biases associated with self-rating questionnaires like the LEQ and CTS. Lastly, little is known about the temporal stability of epigenetic markers (Byun et al. 2012; Talens et al. 2010). We cannot be sure whether the time interval of 1 year was too long or short to observe dramatic methylation changes or at what time window following exposure to stressful life events one might observe changed methylation profiles.

## Conclusions

BD is a multifactorial psychiatric illness, and for many patients full interepisodic remission never occurs (Sam et al. 2019). Stressful life events have been associated with a worse course of BD (Aldinger and Schulze 2017) and there remains a need to better understand the mechanisms which allow these stressors to bring about phenotypic change. Our study provides limited evidence supporting an association between DNAm and recent, non-traumatic stressful life events in BD patients. As findings in clinical populations have been inconsistent, there is still much to be understood especially with regards to the temporal nature of environmentally induced DNA modifications. Future larger studies of well-characterized patients, longitudinal in design, are warranted.

## Supplementary information

**Additional file 1.** Supporting methods, Figures S1-S13, and Tables S1-S3.

#### Abbreviations

BD: bipolar disorder; GWAS: genome-wide association studies; DNAm: DNA methylation; CpG: cytosine-guanine dinucleotides; HPA: hypothalamic–pituitary–adrenal; LEQ: Life Events Questionnaire; CTS: Childhood Trauma Screener; PANSS: Positive and Negative Syndrome Scale; GAF: Global Assessment of Functioning; YMRS: Young Mania Rating Scale; IDS-$C_{30}$: Inventory of Depressive Symptomatology; FunNorm: functional normalization; EWAS: epigenome-wide association analysis; BMIQ: beta-mixture quantile dilation; LMM: linear mixed-effects model; FDR: false discovery rate; MAD: median absolute deviation; AA: age acceleration; GO: gene ontology; QQ: quantile-quantile; WGCNA: weighted gene co-methylation network analysis.

#### Acknowledgements

The Genotype-Tissue Expression (GTEx) Project was supported by the Common Fund of the Office of the Director of the National Institutes of Health, and by NCI, NHGRI, NHLBI, NIDA, NIMH, and NINDS. The data used for the gene tissue expression analysis described in the this manuscript and reported in Additional file 1 were obtained from the GTEx portal: GTEx Analysis Release V8 (dbGaP Accession phs000424.v8.p2) on 09/24/19.

#### Authors' contributions

All authors made substantial contributions to the conception or design of the work, or the acquisition, analysis or interpretation of data. Authors ALC and TGS designed the study. Authors TGS and UH provided supervision. Author ALC conducted the analysis in consultation with UH, SS, DC and TA. Author ALC wrote the first draft of the manuscript. All authors contributed to the manuscript. All authors read and approved the final manuscript.

#### Funding

Thomas G. Schulze and Peter Falkai are supported by the German Research Foundation (Deutsche Forschungsgemeinschaft; DFG) within the framework of the projects http://www.kfo241.de and http://www.PsyCourse.de (SCHU 1603/4-1, 5-1, 7-1; FA241/16-1). The genotyping was in part funded by the German Federal Ministry of Education and Research (BMBF) through the Integrated Network IntegraMent (Integrated Understanding of Causes and Mechanisms in Mental Disorders), under the auspices of the e:Med Program with grants awarded to Thomas G. Schulze (01ZX1614K), Marcella Rietschel (01ZX1614G), and Markus M. Nöthen (01ZX1614A). Thomas G. Schulze received additional support from the German Federal Ministry of Education and Research (BMBF) within the framework of the BipoLife network (01EE1404H) and the Dr. Lisa Oehler Foundation (Kassel, Germany). Sergi Papiol was supported by a 2016 NARSAD Young Investigator Grant (25015) from the Brain and Behavior Research Foundation. Marcella Rietschel and Markus M. Nöthen received funding from the German Research Foundation (DFG, grant FOR2107; RI 908/11-2 to Marcella Rietschel, NO 246/10-2 to Markus M. Nöthen). Franziska Degenhardt received support from the BONFOR Programme of the University of Bonn, Germany. Jens Wiltfang is supported by an Ilídio Pinho professorship and iBiMED (UID/BIM/04501/2013), at the University of Aveiro.

#### Author details

[1] Institute of Psychiatric Phenomics and Genomics, University Hospital, LMU Munich, Nussbaumstrasse 7, 80336 Munich, Germany. [2] International Max Planck Research School for Translational Psychiatry (IMPRS-TP), 80804 Munich, Germany. [3] Department of Translational Research in Psychiatry, Max Planck Institute of Psychiatry, 80804 Munich, Germany. [4] Department of Psychiatry and Psychotherapy, University Hospital, LMU Munich, 80336 Munich, Germany. [5] Department of Psychiatry and Psychotherapy, University Medical Center Göttingen, 37075 Göttingen, Germany. [6] Department of Neurology, Klinikum rechts der Isar, School of Medicine, Technical University of Munich,

81675 Munich, Germany. Department of Psychiatry, Ruhr University Bochum, LWL University Hospital, 44791 Bochum, Germany. [8] Department of Psychiatry and Psychotherapy, Bezirkskrankenhaus Augsburg, University of Augsburg, 86156 Augsburg, Germany. [9] Psychiatrieverbund Oldenburger Land gGmbH, Karl-Jaspers-Klinik, 26160 Bad Zwischenahn, Germany. [10] Department of Psychiatry and Psychotherapy, University Medical Center Hamburg-Eppendorf, 20246 Hamburg, Germany. [11] Department of Psychiatry and Psychotherapeutic Medicine, Research Unit for Bipolar Affective Disorder, Medical University of Graz, 8036 Graz, Austria. [12] Department of Psychiatry, Dr. Frontheim-Mental Health, 38704 Liebenburg, Germany. [13] Department of Psychiatry and Psychotherapy, Agaplesion Diakonieklinikum, 27356 Rotenburg, Germany. [14] Karl-Jaspers Clinic, European Medical School Oldenburg-Groningen, 26160 Oldenburg, Germany. [15] Clinic for Psychiatry and Psychotherapy, Clinical Center Werra-Meißner, 37269 Eschwege, Germany. [16] Asklepios Specialized Hospital, 37081 Göttingen, Germany. [17] AMEOS Clinical Center Hildesheim, 31135 Hildesheim, Germany. [18] Center für Systems Neuroscience (ZSN) Hannover, 30559 Hannover, Germany. [19] Department of Psychiatry, Medical School of Hannover, 30625 Hannover, Germany. [20] Psychiatric Hospital Lüneburg, 21339 Lüneburg, Germany. [21] AMEOS Clinical Center Osnabrück, 49088 Osnabrück, Germany. [22] Department of Genetic Epidemiology in Psychiatry, Central Institute of Mental Health, Medical Faculty Mannheim, University of Heidelberg, 68159 Mannheim, Germany. [23] Institute of Human Genetics, University of Bonn, School of Medicine & University Hospital Bonn, 53127 Bonn, Germany. [24] Center for Human Genetics, University of Marburg, 35033 Marburg, Germany. [25] Department of Biomedicine, University of Basel, 4031 Basel, Switzerland. [26] Department of Psychiatry (UPK), University of Basel, 4002 Basel, Switzerland. [27] German Center for Neurodegenerative Diseases (DZNE), 37075 Göttingen, Germany. [28] iBiMED, Medical Sciences Department, University of Aveiro, 3810-193 Aveiro, Portugal.

### References


Aas M, Henry C, Andreassen OA, Bellivier F, Melle I, Etain B. The role of childhood trauma in bipolar disorders. Int J Bipolar Disord. 2016;4:2.

Alasaari JS, Lagus M, Ollila HM, Toivola A, Kivimäki M, Vahtera J, et al. Environmental stress affects DNA methylation of a CpG rich promoter region of serotonin transporter gene in a nurse cohort. PLoS ONE. 2012;7(9):e45813.

Aldinger F, Schulze TG. Environmental factors, life events, and trauma in the course of bipolar disorder. Psychiatry Clin Neurosci. 2017;71(1):6–17.

Alloy LB, Abramson LY, Urosevic S, Walshaw PD, Nusslock R, Neeren AM. The psychosocial context of bipolar disorder: environmental, cognitive, and developmental risk factors. Clin Psychol Rev. 2005;25(8):1043–75.

American Psychiatric Association. Diagnostic and statistical manual of mental disorders. 4th ed. Washington, DC: American Psychiatric Association; 2002.

Anney R, Klei L, Pinto D, Regan R, Conroy J, Magalhaes TR, et al. A genome-wide scan for common alleles affecting risk for autism. Hum Mol Genet. 2010;19(20):4072–82.

Aryee MJ, Jaffe AE, Corrada-Bravo H, Ladd-Acosta C, Feinberg AP, Hansen KD, et al. Minfi: a flexible and comprehensive bioconductor package for the analysis of infinium DNA methylation microarrays. Bioinformatics. 2014;30(10):1363–9.

Bates D, Maechler M, Bolker B, Walker S. Fitting linear mixed-effects models using lme4. J Stat Softw. 2015;67(1):1–48.

Bender RE, Alloy LB. Life stress and kindling in bipolar disorder: review of the evidence and integration with emerging biopsychosocial theories. Clin Psychol Rev. 2011;31(3):383–98.

Benjamini Y, Hochberg Y. Controlling the false discovery rate: a practical and powerful approach to multiple testing. J R Stat Soc B. 1995;57(1):289–300.

Bernstein DP, Ahluvalia T, Pogge D, Handelsman L. Validity of the Childhood Trauma Questionnaire in an adolescent psychiatric population. J Am Acad Child Adolesc Psychiatry. 1997;36(3):340–8.

Bernstein DP, Stein JA, Newcomb MD, Walker E, Pogge D, Ahluvalia T, et al. Development and validation of a brief screening version of the Childhood Trauma Questionnaire. Child Abuse Negl. 2003;27(2):169–90.

Boks MP, van Mierlo HC, Rutten BP, Radstake TR, De Witte L, Geuze E, et al. Longitudinal changes of telomere length and epigenetic age related to traumatic stress and post-traumatic stress disorder. Psychoneuroendocrinology. 2015;51:506–12.

Brown GW, Harris T. Social origins of depression: a study of psychiatric disorder in women. New York: Routledge; 2012.

Budde M, Anderson-Schmidt H, Gade K, Reich-Erkelenz D, Adorjan K, Kalman JL, et al. A longitudinal approach to biological psychiatric research: the PsyCourse study. Am J Med Genet B Neuropsychiatr Genet. 2019;180(2):89–102.

Byun HM, Nordio F, Coull BA, Tarantini L, Hou L, Bonzini M, et al. Temporal stability of epigenetic markers: sequence characteristics and predictors of short-term DNA methylation variations. PLoS ONE. 2012;7(6):e39220.

Chen YA, Lemire M, Choufani S, Butcher DT, Grafodatskaya D, Zanke BW, et al. Discovery of cross-reactive probes and polymorphic CpGs in the Illumina Infinium HumanMethylation450 microarray. Epigenetics. 2013;8(2):203–9.

Davies G, Lam M, Harris SE, Trampush JW, Luciano M, Hill WD, et al. Study of 300,486 individuals identifies 148 independent genetic loci influencing general cognitive function. Nat Commun. 2018;9(1):2098.

Dohrenwend BP. Toward a typology of high-risk major stressful events and situations in posttraumatic stress disorder and related psychopathology. Psychol Inj Law. 2010;3(2):89–99.

Duffy A, Goodday SM, Keown-Stoneman C, Scotti M, Maitra M, Nagy C, et al. Epigenetic markers in inflammation-related genes associated with mood disorder: a cross-sectional and longitudinal study in high-risk offspring of bipolar parents. Int J Bipolar Disord. 2019;7(1):17.

Duman EA, Canli T. Influence of life stress, 5-HTTLPR genotype, and SLC6A4 methylation on gene expression and stress response in healthy Caucasian males. Biol Mood Anxiety Disord. 2015;5:2.

Elliott HR, Tillin T, McArdle WL, Ho K, Duggirala A, Frayling TM, et al. Differences in smoking associated DNA methylation patterns in South Asians and Europeans. Clin Epigenet. 2014;6(1):4.

Endicott J, Spitzer RL, Fleiss JL, Cohen J. The Global Assessment Scale: a procedure for measuring overall severity of psychiatric disturbance. Arch Gen Psychiatry. 1976;33(6):766–71.

Fortin J-P, Labbe A, Lemire M, Zanke BW, Hudson TJ, Fertig EJ, et al. Functional normalization of 450k methylation array data improves replication in large cancer studies. Genome Biol. 2014;15(11):503.

Fries GR, Li Q, McAlpin B, Rein T, Walss-Bass C, Soares JC, et al. The role of DNA methylation in the pathophysiology and treatment of bipolar disorder. Neurosci Biobehav Rev. 2016;68:474–88.

Geeleher P, Hartnett L, Egan LJ, Golden A, Raja Ali RA, Seoighe C. Gene-set analysis is severely biased when applied to genome-wide methylation data. Bioinformatics. 2013;29(15):1851–7.

Glaesmer H, Schulz A, Hauser W, Freyberger HJ, Brahler E, Grabe HJ. The childhood trauma screener (CTS)—development and validation of cut-off-scores for classificatory diagnostics. Psychiatr Prax. 2013;40(4):220–6.

Goes FS, McGrath J, Avramopoulos D, Wolyniec P, Pirooznia M, Ruczinski I, et al. Genome-wide association study of schizophrenia in Ashkenazi Jews. Am J Med Genet Part B Neuropsychiatr Genet. 2015;168(8):649–59.

Goodwin FK, Jamison KR. Manic-depressive illness: bipolar disorders and recurrent depression. 2nd ed. New York: Oxford University Press; 2007.

Grabe HJ, Schulz A, Schmidt CO, Appel K, Driessen M, Wingenfeld K, et al. Ein Screeninginstrument für Missbrauch und Vernachlässigung in der Kindheit: der Childhood Trauma Screener (CTS). Psychiatr Prax. 2012;39(03):109–15.

He Y, Vinkers CH, Houtepen LC, de Witte LD, Boks MP. Childhood adversity is associated with increased KITLG methylation in healthy individuals but not in bipolar disorder patients. Front Psychiatry. 2018;9:743.

Hill WD, Marioni RE, Maghzian O, Ritchie SJ, Hagenaars SP, McIntosh AM, et al. A combined analysis of genetically correlated traits identifies 187 loci and a role for neurogenesis and myelination in intelligence. Mol Psychiatry. 2018;24(2):169–81.

Hillegers MH, Burger H, Wals M, Reichart CG, Verhulst FC, Nolen WA, et al. Impact of stressful life events, familial loading and their interaction on the onset of mood disorders: study in a high-risk cohort of adolescent offspring of parents with bipolar disorder. Br J Psychiatry. 2004;185:97–101.

Horvath S. DNA methylation age of human tissues and cell types. Genome Biol. 2013;14(10):R115.

Houseman EA, Accomando WP, Koestler DC, Christensen BC, Marsit CJ, Nelson HH, et al. DNA methylation arrays as surrogate measures of cell mixture distribution. BMC Bioinform. 2012;13:86.

Jaworska-Andryszewska P, Rybakowski JK. Childhood trauma in mood disorders: neurobiological mechanisms and implications for treatment. Pharmacol Rep. 2019;71(1):112–20.

Johnson SL. Life events in bipolar disorder: towards more specific models. Clin Psychol Rev. 2005;25(8):1008–27.

Johnson WE, Li C, Rabinovic A. Adjusting batch effects in microarray expression data using empirical Bayes methods. Biostatistics. 2007;8(1):118–27.

Kay SR, Fiszbein A, Opler LA. The positive and negative syndrome scale (PANSS) for schizophrenia. Schizophr Bull. 1987;13(2):261–76.

Kemner SM, van Haren NE, Bootsman F, Eijkemans MJ, Vonk R, van der Schot AC, et al. The influence of life events on first and recurrent admissions in bipolar disorder. Int J Bipolar Disord. 2015;3:6.

Kobeissy F, Alawieh A, Mondello S, Boustany RM, Gold MS. Biomarkers in psychiatry: how close are we? Front Psychiatry. 2012;3:114.

Koshimizu H, Nogawa S, Asano S, Ikeda M, Iwata N, Takahashi S, et al. Genome-wide association study identifies a novel locus associated with psychological distress in the Japanese population. Transl Psychiatry. 2019;9(1):52.

Kular L, Kular S. Epigenetics applied to psychiatry: clinical opportunities and future challenges. Psychiatry Clin Neurosci. 2018;72(4):195–211.

Langfelder P, Horvath S. WGCNA: an R package for weighted correlation network analysis. BMC Bioinform. 2008;9(1):559.

Lee KWK, Pausova Z. Cigarette smoking and DNA methylation. Front Genet. 2013;4:132.

Lee JJ, Wedow R, Okbay A, Kong E, Maghzian O, Zacher M, et al. Gene discovery and polygenic prediction from a genome-wide association study of educational attainment in 1.1 million individuals. Nat Genet. 2018;50(8):1112–21.

Lex C, Bazner E, Meyer TD. Does stress play a significant role in bipolar disorder? A meta-analysis. J Affect Disord. 2017;208:298–308.

Li Y, Camarillo C, Xu J, Arana TB, Xiao Y, Zhao Z, et al. Genome-wide methylome analyses reveal novel epigenetic regulation patterns in schizophrenia and bipolar disorder. Biomed Res Int. 2015;2015:201587.

Luborsky L. Clinicians' judgments of mental health: a proposed scale. Arch Gen Psychiatry. 1962;7(6):407–17.

Ludwig B, Dwivedi Y. Dissecting bipolar disorder complexity through epigenomic approach. Mol Psychiatry. 2016;21(11):1490–8.

Lunnon K, Smith RG, Cooper I, Greenbaum L, Mill J, Beeri MS. Blood methylomic signatures of presymptomatic dementia in elderly subjects with type 2 diabetes mellitus. Neurobiol Aging. 2015;36(3):1600.e1–e4.

Mansell G, Gorrie-Stone TJ, Bao Y, Kumari M, Schalkwyk LS, Mill J, et al. Guidance for DNA methylation studies: statistical insights from the Illumina EPIC array. BMC Genomics. 2019;20(1):366.

Marzi SJ, Sugden K, Arseneault L, Belsky DW, Burrage J, Corcoran DL, et al. Analysis of DNA methylation in young people: limited evidence for an association between victimization stress and epigenetic variation in blood. Am J Psychiatry. 2018;175(6):517–29.

Matosin N, Cruceanu C, Binder EB. Preclinical and clinical evidence of DNA methylation changes in response to trauma and chronic stress. Chronic Stress. 2017. https://doi.org/10.1177/2470547017710764.

McGowan PO, Sasaki A, D'Alessio AC, Dymov S, Labonte B, Szyf M, et al. Epigenetic regulation of the glucocorticoid receptor in human brain associates with childhood abuse. Nat Neurosci. 2009;12(3):342–8.

Meana JJ, Mollinedo-Gajate I. Biomarkers in psychiatry: between myth and clinical reality. Revista de Psiquiatría y Salud Mental. 2017;10(4):183–4 **(English Edition)**.

Mehta D, Bruenig D, Carrillo-Roa T, Lawford B, Harvey W, Morris CP, et al. Genomewide DNA methylation analysis in combat veterans reveals a novel locus for PTSD. Acta Psychiatr Scand. 2017;136(5):493–505.

Monk C, Spicer J, Champagne FA. Linking prenatal maternal adversity to developmental outcomes in infants: the role of epigenetic pathways. Dev Psychopathol. 2012;24(4):1361–76.

Monroe SM. Modern approaches to conceptualizing and measuring human life stress. Annu Rev Clin Psychol. 2008;4:33–52.

Mullins N, Bigdeli TB, Borglum AD, Coleman JRI, Demontis D, Mehta D, et al. GWAS of suicide attempt in psychiatric disorders and association with major depression polygenic risk scores. Am J Psychiatry. 2019;176(8):651–60.

Myaki K, Suzuki T, Song Y, Tsutsumi A, Kawakami N, Takahashi M, et al. Epigenetic changes caused by occupational stress in humans revealed through noninvasive assessment of DNA methylation of the tyrosine hydroxylase gene. J Neurol Neurol Disord. 2015;2(2):201.

Nagel M, Watanabe K, Stringer S, Posthuma D, van der Sluis S. Item-level analyses reveal genetic heterogeneity in neuroticism. Nat Commun. 2018;9(1):905.

Need AC, Attix DK, McEvoy JM, Cirulli ET, Linney KL, Hunt P, et al. A genome-wide study of common SNPs and CNVs in cognitive performance in the CANTAB. Hum Mol Genet. 2009;18(23):4650–61.

Norbeck JS. Modification of life event questionnaires for use with female respondents. Res Nurs Health. 1984;7(1):61–71.

Okbay A, Beauchamp JP, Fontana MA, Lee JJ, Pers TH, Rietveld CA, et al. Genome-wide association study identifies 74 loci associated with educational attainment. Nature. 2016;533(7604):539–42.

Paykel ES. Life events and affective disorders. Acta Psychiatr Scand. 2003;108(s418):61–6.

Pishva E, Kenis G, van den Hove D, Lesch KP, Boks MP, van Os J, et al. The epigenome and postnatal environmental influences in psychotic disorders. Soc Psychiatry Psychiatr Epidemiol. 2014;49(3):337–48.

R Core Team. R: a language and environment for statistical computing. Vienna: R Foundation for Statistical Computing; 2014. https://www.R-project.org/.

Roberts S, Suderman M, Zammit S, Watkins SH, Hannon E, Mill J, et al. Longitudinal investigation of DNA methylation changes preceding adolescent psychotic experiences. Transl Psychiatry. 2019;9(1):69.

Rowland TA, Marwaha S. Epidemiology and risk factors for bipolar disorder. Ther Adv Psychopharmacol. 2018;8(9):251–69.

Sam SP, Nisha A, Varghese PJ. Stressful life events and relapse in bipolar affective disorder: a cross-sectional study from a tertiary care center of southern India. Indian J Psychol Med. 2019;41(1):61–7.

Sarason IG, Johnson JH, Siegel JM. Assessing the impact of life changes: development of the Life Experiences Survey. J Consult Clin Psychol. 1978;46(5):932–46.

Sharma S, Powers A, Bradley B, Ressler KJ. Gene × environment determinants of stress- and anxiety-related disorders. Annu Rev Psychol. 2016;67:239–61.

Shenker NS, Polidoro S, van Veldhoven K, Sacerdote C, Ricceri F, Birrell MA, et al. Epigenome-wide association study in the European Prospective Investigation into Cancer and Nutrition (EPIC-Turin) identifies novel genetic loci associated with smoking. Hum Mol Genet. 2013;22(5):843–51.

Smith AK, Conneely KN, Kilaru V, Mercer KB, Weiss TE, Bradley B, et al. Differential immune system DNA methylation and cytokine regulation in post-traumatic stress disorder. Am J Med Genet B Neuropsychiatr Genet. 2011;156b(6):700–8.

Song Y, Miyaki K, Suzuki T, Sasaki Y, Tsutsumi A, Kawakami N, et al. Altered DNA methylation status of human brain derived neurotrophis factor gene could be useful as biomarker of depression. Am J Med Genet B Neuropsychiatr Genet. 2014;165b(4):357–64.

Stahl EA, Breen G, Forstner AJ, McQuillin A, Ripke S, Trubetskoy V, et al. Genome-wide association study identifies 30 loci associated with bipolar disorder. Nat Genet. 2019;51(5):793–803.

Talens RP, Boomsma DI, Tobi EW, Kremer D, Jukema JW, Willemsen G, et al. Variation, patterns, and temporal stability of DNA methylation: considerations for epigenetic epidemiology. FASEB J. 2010;24(9):3135–44.

Teschendorff AE, Marabita F, Lechner M, Bartlett T, Tegner J, Gomez-Cabrero D, et al. A beta-mixture quantile normalization method for correcting probe design bias in Illumina Infinium 450k DNA methylation data. Bioinformatics. 2013;29(2):189–96.

Trivedi MH, Rush AJ, Ibrahim HM, Carmody TJ, Biggs MM, Suppes T, et al. The Inventory of Depressive Symptomatology, Clinician Rating (IDS-C) and Self-Report (IDS-SR), and the Quick Inventory of Depressive Symptomatology, Clinician Rating (QIDS-C) and Self-Report (QIDS-SR) in public sector patients with mood disorders: a psychometric evaluation. Psychol Med. 2004;34(1):73–82.

Uddin M, Aiello AE, Wildman DE, Koenen KC, Pawelec G, de Los Santos R, et al. Epigenetic and immune function profiles associated with posttraumatic stress disorder. Proc Natl Acad Sci USA. 2010;107(20):9470–5.

Vinkers CH, Kalafateli AL, Rutten BP, Kas MJ, Kaminsky Z, Turner JD, et al. Traumatic stress and human DNA methylation: a critical review. Epigenomics. 2015;7(4):593–608.

Walker RM, Sussmann JE, Whalley HC, Ryan NM, Porteous DJ, McIntosh AM, et al. Preliminary assessment of pre-morbid DNA methylation in individuals at high genetic risk of mood disorders. Bipolar Disord. 2016;18(5):410–22.

Weaver IC, Cervoni N, Champagne FA, D'Alessio AC, Sharma S, Seckl JR, et al. Epigenetic programming by maternal behavior. Nat Neurosci. 2004;7(8):847–54.

Young RC, Biggs JT, Ziegler VE, Meyer DA. A rating scale for mania: reliability, validity and sensitivity. Br J Psychiatry. 1978;133:429–35.

Zeilinger S, Kühnel B, Klopp N, Baurecht H, Kleinschmidt A, Gieger C, et al. Tobacco smoking leads to extensive genome-wide changes in DNA methylation. PLoS ONE. 2013;8(5):e63812.

4

# Blood pressure in bipolar disorder: evidence of elevated pulse pressure and associations between mean pressure and mood instability

Niall M. McGowan[1*], Molly Nichols[2], Amy C. Bilderbeck[1], Guy M. Goodwin[1,3] and Kate E. A. Saunders[1,3,4]

**Abstract**

**Background:** Bipolar disorder (BD) is associated with excess and premature cardiovascular mortality. Elevated blood pressure (BP) is a leading contributor to cardiovascular risk. However, few studies have examined BP in BD in comparison to other psychiatric disorders. Furthermore, the association between BP and mood instability is not presently clear despite increasing interest in repurposing existing antihypertensive medications as possible novel BD treatments. Thus we examined BP differences between BD and borderline personality disorder (BPD), a disorder with a similar symptom profile through chronic mood instability.

**Methods:** A total of 106 adults (38 BD, 25 BPD, and 43 healthy controls), evaluated in the Automated Monitoring of Symptom Severity (AMoSS) study, completed a week-long home blood pressure monitoring assessment and ecological momentary assessment of mood. We examined group-wise differences in mean BP and BP variability and their association with mood instability.

**Results:** BD individuals had a significantly wider resting pulse pressure ($40.8 \pm 7.4$, mmHg) compared to BPD ($35.7 \pm 5.3$, mmHg, $P = 0.03$) and control participants ($37.3 \pm 6.3$, mmHg, $P = 0.036$). Systolic BP was negatively associated with sad mood instability, and all measures of mean BP (systolic, diastolic, and mean arterial pressure) were negatively associated with positive mood instability.

**Conclusions:** This study demonstrates BP differences between BD and healthy and clinical controls that are within a normotensive range. Early pulse pressure widening may be a modifiable pathophysiological feature of BD that confers later cardiovascular risk. BP may be an important transdiagnostic predictor of mood instability and a potential explicit treatment target.

**Keywords:** Blood pressure, Mood instability, Bipolar disorder, Borderline personality disorder, Ecological momentary assessment

## Background

Bipolar disorder (BD) is a severe affective disorder associated with substantial physical co-morbidity and excess mortality. Life expectancy for those with BD is reduced by 8–12 years compared to the general population (Laursen 2011; Crump et al. 2013; Kessling et al. 2015a).

*Correspondence: niall.mcgowan@psych.ox.ac.uk
[1] Department of Psychiatry, University of Oxford, Warneford Hospital, Oxford OX3 7JX, UK
Full list of author information is available at the end of the article

Cardiovascular disease (CVD) is the leading cause of premature death in BD, accounting for over one-third of deaths in people with the disorder (Osby et al. 2001; Westman et al. 2013). A striking feature of CVD risk in BD is the early age of incidence; CVD occurs up to 17 years earlier in individuals with BD compared to the general population, and those aged younger than 40 years have an eightfold higher risk of CVD mortality (Goldstein et al. 2015; Westman et al. 2013). Several factors may contribute to this elevated risk. Prevalence rates of conditions that confer greater CVD risk such as diabetes and metabolic syndrome are increased in BD compared to the general population (Coello et al. 2019a; Charles et al. 2016). Lifestyle factors such as smoking, alcohol consumption, and physical inactivity, are also more common in BD (Brown et al. 2013). However, accounting for these risk factors does not fully explain excess CVD risk in BD (Hayes et al. 2017). Antipsychotic and mood stabiliser medications are also associated with cardiovascular risk factors but there is no direct association with excess CVD mortality (Osborn et al. 2015). Moreover, elevated CVD mortality had been documented in BD before such drugs were widely used for its treatment (Weiner et al. 2011).

Hypertension, persistent high resting blood pressure (BP), is the leading single contributor to all-cause mortality and disability worldwide (Forouzanfar et al. 2016). It is normally defined by a clinic systolic blood pressure (SBP) > 140 mmHg or diastolic blood pressure (DBP) > 90 mmHg. Importantly, the association between BP and CVD is continuous so that even increased BP in the normotensive range is associated with greater risk (Oparil et al. 2018; Whelton et al. 2020). Several studies have demonstrated greater prevalence of hypertension in BD (Ayerbe et al. 2018). The UK National Institute for Health and Care Excellence (NICE) guidelines recommend hypertension screening for those with BD at the earliest opportunity (NICE 2014). However, psychiatric inpatient service audit reveals inconsistent and sub-optimal BP screening practices in patients with BD (Kelbrick and Abdaldayim 2014). Prevalence of hypertension is known to increase dramatically from middle-age onwards (Pinto et al. 2007; Wolf-Maier et al. 2003), but as a consequence, excess cardiovascular risk may be underappreciated in younger patients with BD (Osby et al. 2016; Kessling et al. 2015b), so measurement of BP assumes great importance.

Home blood pressure monitoring (HBPM) at regular intervals over several days is recommended to confirm clinic detection of hypertension. As a research tool it provides an ecologically valid measure of BP and is easy to monitor. Importantly, as HBPM assesses BP at several time-points it can also quantify blood pressure variability (BPV) over a mid to long-term assessment period (Chadachan et al. 2018). Although the mechanisms producing BPV are incompletely understood it is assumed to arise from the interaction of environmental and behavioural factors with intrinsic actions of the autonomic nervous system and circadian timing system (Parati et al. 2013; Grassi et al. 2012). Several studies have shown that greater BPV is a risk factor for poor cardiovascular outcomes and mortality independent of the effect of mean BP (Stevens et al. 2016). As far as we are aware BPV has not been examined previously in BD.

Elevated BP has been linked to several other psychiatric disorders (Stein et al. 2014). Thus a clinical comparison group with similar symptoms is desirable to draw conclusions specific to BD. Borderline personality disorder (BPD) has a very similar clinical phenotype to BD, involving overlapping symptoms such as abrupt mood lability and impulsivity (Ghaelmi et al. 2014). Accumulating evidence suggests that BPD has an underappreciated hypertensive and CVD risk similar to BD (Roininen et al. 2019). BPD is therefore an interesting comparator group for BD in addition to healthy control subjects.

Mood episode frequency of mania/hypomania and severity of depression appear to be associated with excess cardiovascular mortality (Fiedorowicz et al. 2009, 2014). Little is known about the association between elevated BP as an isolated cardiovascular risk factor and subsyndromal mood symptoms which are common between episodes in BD. Recent evidence also indicates that antihypertensive medications may confer treatment benefits for people with mood disorders. In particular angiotensin antagonists and calcium channel blockers have been suggested as promising candidates for repurposing for future BD treatment (Shaw et al. 2019; Cipriani et al. 2016). The therapeutic mechanisms of each are incompletely understood but hypothesised to involve abnormalities in renin-angiotensin system and altered L-type calcium channel signalling in BD (Barbosa and Ferreira 2020; Cipriani et al. 2016). However, given their primary indication is for BP management, a basic gap in the knowledge exists regarding the association between BP and mood disorder symptoms. Mood instability is characteristic of both BD and particularly BPD (Tsanas et al. 2016) and is a continuous variable, present to varying degrees in the general population and a transdiagnostic feature of several psychiatric conditions (Harrison et al. 2018). Elucidating the association between BP and a core dimension of the BD phenotype such as mood instability is fundamental to developing further the theoretical basis for emerging repurposed treatments.

Here, we examine differences in BP and BPV between participants with BD, BPD and healthy controls (HC) who took part in the Automated Monitoring of Symptom Severity (AMoSS) study. We assess group-wise differences in resting pulse rate (HR), SBP, DBP, and two BP derived measures with superior predictive strength of CVD risk: pulse pressure (PP) and mean arterial pressure (MAP) (Franklin et al. 2009). Based on previous hypertension studies in BD, we hypothesised that BP and BPV would be greater in BD than BPD and HC. Additionally, we performed exploratory analyses to examine the association of BP/BPV measures with BD symptom measures and mood instability, assessed via parallel digital ecological momentary assessment, as a means to expand on the role for explicit antihypertensive treatment potential for mood disorders.

## Methods

### Participants

Participants consisted of 106 individuals recruited to take part in the Automated Monitoring of Symptom Severity (AMoSS) study at the University of Oxford. In total 141 participants were originally recruited, with 113 participants undergoing a week of 'high-intensity' behavioural digital monitoring during which participants' mood and blood pressure were monitored daily. Five participants were excluded due to non-completion of the monitoring phase and a further two were excluded due to technical error or missing data.

Participants were recruited from the community in the case of HC, or from the community, out-patient services or from study registration lists in the case of BD and BPD participants. Diagnoses were confirmed prior to study admission by psychiatric interview using the Structured Clinical Interview for DSM-IV and the BPD module of the International Personality Disorders Examination. Individuals with comorbid diagnosis of BD and BPD were excluded from participation. Exclusion criteria for HCs were a history of neurological disorder or head injury, psychiatric diagnosis or having a first degree relative with BD or BPD. Ethical approval for this study was granted by the NRES Committee East of England—Norfolk (13/EE/0288) and informed consent was obtained from all participants taking part.

### Blood pressure

Blood pressure recordings were obtained for each participant over a seven-day HBPM period. Participants used an electronic blood pressure monitor (UA787 Digital Blood Pressure Monitor, A&D Medical) to measure their resting BP. Participants were instructed to take measurements seated upright, wearing the correctly adjusted cuff on their upper left arm, supported, and at heart level (mid-sternal). Participants measured their BP three times each day, once in the morning, afternoon, and evening. At each time-point participants' recorded three measurements. SBP, DBP and pulse rate were recorded by the device and transferred via Bluetooth to the study smartphone application.

PP (SBP–DBP) and MAP (DBP + 1/3 · PP) were calculated for each time-point offline. The daily mean of each participant's BP data was used to assess mid-term BPV between days with the grand averages used as inter-individual measures of BP. To overcome the inherent correlation between standard deviation and mean BP values we used the coefficient of variation (CV) expressed as percentage as a measure of day-to-day BPV.

### Questionnaire assessments

The Quick Inventory of Depressive Symptomatology—Self Report (QIDS) is a 16 item scale that reflects 9 constituent components of depression that participants report on over the previous week. Total QIDS scores range from 0 to 27. The suggested clinical ranges are 5 or less denoting normal, 6–10 denoting mild depression, 11–15 denoting moderate depression, 16–20 denoting severe depression, and 21–27 denoting very severe depression (Rush et al. 2003).

Altman Self Rating Mania Scale (ASRM) is a five-item scale examining severity of manic symptoms arranged across domains of elevated mood, self-confidence, sleep disturbance, speech patterns and amount, and activity level over the previous week. Items are scored on a 0 (symptom-free) to 4 (present nearly all the time) scale, with total scores ranging from 0 to 20. A score of 6 or higher is indicative of mania, or hypomania, with symptom severity indicated by increasing scores (Altman et al. 1997).

Participants completed both questionnaires at the end of the HBPM week period using the True Colours remote monitoring mood system (www.truecolours.nhs.uk).

### Mood Zoom

Mood Zoom (MZ) is a 6-item questionnaire that was designed as part of the AMoSS study to enable a compact ecological momentary assessment of mood instability using participants' smartphone devices. MZ consists of six mood items arranged in three factors: negative ('anxious', 'sad'), positive ('elated', 'energetic'), and irritable ('irritable', 'angry'). Previous work has demonstrated strong correlation between MZ components and standardised measures of depression, anxiety and mental health (Tsanas et al. 2016). Parallel to the HBPM period during the 'high intensity' study week, participants were asked to rate 10-times each day to what extent each of the six mood items reflected their current mood on a 7-point Likert scale ranging from 'Not at all' to 'Very much. Digital prompts for participants to provide their mood rating were delivered at equally spaced intervals throughout each day, between 1000 and 2000 h (i.e. approx. every hour).

To quantify mood instability for each of the six MZ items we used the root mean square of successive differences (RMSSD) over the week of mood monitoring. The RMSSD is a measure of variability reflecting both the temporal order and amplitude of the data (Ebner-Priemer et al. 2009) and is a commonly used measure of mood instability in studies using ecological momentary assessment. Mood diary entries with missing data were excluded pair-wise and the next adjacent case was used for the calculation of RMSSD.

### Data analysis

Normal distribution of data was assessed using Shapiro–Wilk tests of normality and visual inspection of Q-Q plots. BP and BPV variables were normally disturbed but questionnaire and MZ RMSSD values were skewed. Sample descriptive data were analysed using chi-square tests of independence for categorical data and one-way ANOVAs (mean ± SD) or Kruskal–Wallis non-parametric tests (median ± IQR) for continuous data that were normally distributed or non-normally distributed, respectively. Group-wise comparisons of BP measures were analysed using ANCOVAs with participant age and BMI inserted as covariates. All post-hoc tests were conducted using Bonferroni correction for multiple comparisons. Exploratory correlations between questionnaire/mood outcomes and BP/BPV variables were performed using Spearman's rank coefficient with the Benjamini–Hochberg false discovery rate applied to P-values. Adjusted P-values less than 0.05 were considered statistically significant. All analyses were conducting using SPSS v25 (IBM) and R v3.6.3 (R core team).

## Results

### Demographic characteristics

Demographic characteristics of participants are shown in Table 1. After exclusion of five participants for incompletion or technical errors, the final sample analysed consisted of 38 participants with BD (63% female), 25 participants with BPD (88% female), and 43 HC (67% female), aged between 18 and 64 years. There was a greater number of female participants among the BPD group compared with BD and HC groups. Groups were well matched for age and ~ 80% of the sample was younger than 50 years. The mean BMI of clinical groups was only slightly higher than controls. The proportion of smokers was greater in both clinical groups compared to HCs. Groups did not differ by the proportion of alcohol drinkers.

Symptom assessments in this sub-sample of participants were congruent with previously reported findings of the full AMoSS study: depressive symptomatology was significantly greater in both clinical groups compared to HC, and in BPD compared to BD. Manic symptoms were greater in clinical groups compared to HC. Mood instability characterised by MZ assessment revealed greater variability for anxious and sad items in both clinical groups compared to HC; greater variability of elated mood in BPD compared to HC, and greater variability of energetic mood in BPD compared with both HC and BD; for anger and irritability, both clinical groups were significantly more variable than HC, and BPD was significantly more variable compared to BD.

Psychotropic medication use differed between BD and BPD with a larger proportion of BD participants taking medication. Lithium use was exclusive to the BD group, anticonvulsant and antipsychotic use was more common in BD compared to BPD. Antidepressant and anxiolytic use was more common in BPD compared to BD. Four of the BPD group had prescriptions for propranolol to take as required for anxiety: since their use was uncertain, patients are included in the analysis.

### Blood pressure

Out of 106 participants monitored, 91 (86%) were normotensive, and 15 (14%) were hypertensive (2 SBP/DBP hypertension, 1 isolated systolic hypertension, 12 isolated diastolic hypertension based on the 2018 ESH/ESC guideline definitions for HBPM hypertension; ≥ 135 mmHg SBP and/or ≥ 85 mmHg DBP) (Williams et al. 2018).

Expectedly, BP measures were significantly positively associated with age and BMI (Additional file 1: Table S1), thus both variables were retained as covariates in ANCOVA analyses. Group-wise comparisons did not show a significant effect of diagnosis on mean HR, SBP or DBP (Table 2, Fig. 1a, b). The effect of diagnosis on PP was significant, $F(1, 100) = 4.71$, $P = 0.011$, $\eta_P^2 = 0.085$. Post-hoc comparisons revealed that BD had significantly higher PP values (40.8 ± 7.4, mmHg) compared to BPD (35.7 ± 5.3, mmHg, P = 0.03) and HC (37.3 ± 6.3, mmHg, P = 0.036) (Table 2, Fig. 1c). There was no significant effect of diagnosis on MAP (Table 2, Fig. 1d) or BPV estimated by the day-to-day coefficient of variation (Table 2, Additional file 1: Figure S1).

Exploratory group-wise assessments and sensitivity analyses were conducted to determine the effects of potential confounding influences on BP. Alcohol use was associated with significantly wider PP (Additional file 1: Table S2) and smoking with significantly higher pulse-rate (Additional file 1: Table S3). However, controlling for each as additional covariates did not explain the effect of diagnosis on PP (Additional file 1: Tables S4 and S5), and when controlling for smoking status significant between group differences in SBP emerged (Additional file 1: Table S5; Bonferroni post-hoc BD > BPD, P = 0.028). Neither lithium nor anticonvulsant use was associated with BP differences among BD participants (Additional file 1: Tables S6 and S7). Among BD and BPD, antipsychotic use was associated with higher SBP (Additional file 1: Table S8) and antidepressant use with lower PP (Additional file 1: Table S9), partly reflecting the differing medication rates between both diagnoses. Hypnotic and anxiolytic users numbered

**Table 1 Demographic and clinical characteristics of sample**

| | BD ($n=38$) | BPD ($n=25$) | HC ($n=43$) | Test statistic | *P* | *Post-hoc* |
|---|---|---|---|---|---|---|
| Gender | | | | | | |
| Female n (%) | 24 (63.2) | 22 (88) | 29 (67.4) | $\chi^2=4.881$ | 0.087 | – |
| Age, year ± SD | 39.0 ± 13.1 | 34.1 ± 11.2 | 39.84 ± 12.9 | $F=1.794$ | 0.171 | – |
| BMI, kg/m$^2$ ± SD | 26.8 ± 4.1 | 27.4 ± 6.3 | 24.5 ± 4.3 | $F=3.657$ | *0.029* | n.s |
| Smoker, n (%) | 7 (21.9) | 7 (30.4)) | 2 (5) | $\chi^2=7.818$ | *0.022* | BD > HC<br>BPD > HC |
| Drinks Alcohol, n (%) | 28 (77.8) | 14 (58.3) | 31 (72) | $\chi^2=2.691$ | 0.260 | – |
| Questionnaire assessment | | | | | | |
| QIDS, mdn ± IQR | 5.5 ± 6.5 | 12 ± 12.5 | 2 ± 1.5 | $\chi^2=50.586$ | *< 0.001* | BD > HC<br>BPD > HC<br>BPD > BD |
| ASRM, mdn ± IQR | 1 ± 2 | 1 ± 3.5 | 0 ± 0 | $\chi^2=11.663$ | *< 0.003* | BD > HC<br>BPD > HC |
| Mood Zoom Items | | | | | | |
| anx RMSSD ± IQR | 0.87 ± 0.54 | 1.39 ± 0.58 | 0.55 ± 0.65 | $\chi^2=42.81$ | *< 0.001* | BD > HC<br>BPD > HC<br>BPD > BD |
| sad RMSSD ± IQR | 0.72 ± 0.71 | 1.40 ± 0.43 | 0.31 ± 0.75 | $\chi^2=41.662$ | *< 0.001* | BD > HC<br>BPD > HC<br>BPD > BD |
| elt RMSSD ± IQR | 0.67 ± 0.73 | 1.14 ± 1.06 | 0.67 ± 0.88 | $\chi^2=10.489$ | *0.005* | BPD > HC |
| enr RMSSD ± IQR | 0.93 ± 0.70 | 1.22 ± 0.90 | 0.79 ± 0.51 | $\chi^2=11.558$ | *0.003* | BPD > HC<br>BPD > BD |
| ang RMSSD ± IQR | 0.71 ± 0.58 | 1.24 ± 0.97 | 0.31 ± 0.49 | $\chi^2=36.695$ | *< 0.001* | BD > HC<br>BPD > HC<br>BPD > BD |
| irr RMSSD ± IQR | 0.91 ± 0.71 | 1.53 ± 1.05 | 0.48 ± 0.78 | $\chi^2=39.167$ | *< 0.001* | BD > HC<br>BPD > HC<br>BPD > BD |
| Medication | | | | | | |
| Using psychotropic medication, n (%) | 36 (94.7) | 19 (87.3) | – | $\chi^2=4.775$ | *0.029* | – |
| Lithium | 16 (42.1) | 0 (0) | – | $\chi^2=14.11$ | *< 0.001* | – |
| Anticonvulsant | 15 (39.5) | 1 (4) | – | $\chi^2=10.015$ | *0.002* | – |
| Antipsychotic | 25 (65.8) | 5 (20) | – | $\chi^2=12.675$ | *< 0.001* | – |
| Antidepressant | 13 (34.2) | 19 (76) | – | $\chi^2=10.536$ | *0.001* | – |
| Hypnotic | 3 (7.9) | 1 (1.5) | – | $\chi^2=0.339$ | 0.561 | – |
| Anxiolytic | 1 (2.6) | 6 (24) | – | $\chi^2=6.971$ | *0.008* | – |

F test statistic denotes univariate ANOVA result; $\chi^2$ test statistic denotes chi-square test of independence (for categorical data) or Kruskal–Wallis non-parametric test (comparing the medians of continuous variable). *IQR* interquartile range, *mdn* median, *SD* standard deviation

too few to compare statistically. Thus, we conducted a sensitivity analysis on the differences detected between BD, BPD and HC, while additionally controlling for any psychotropic medication use and found the effect of diagnosis on PP was preserved ($P=0.043$; Additional file 1: Table S10). There was insufficient representation of males among the BPD group to adequately include gender as a covariate but a sub-group sensitivity analysis between BD and HC that additionally controlled for gender revealed the same pattern of greater PP in BD ($P=0.029$; Additional file 1: Table S11).

**Association with mood instability**

Associations between BP mean values and MZ items (RMSSD) are shown in Fig. 2a. SBP was negatively associated with instability on the sad mood item and the positive mood items, elated and energetic (higher SBP, lower mood instability). Positive mood items were also negatively associated with DBP, and MAP (higher BP metric, lower mood instability). No significant associations were detected between BP values and angry and irritable mood items, and BPV measures (CV of each BP measure) were not correlated with any MZ items (Fig. 2b).

**Table 2 Group-wise comparisons of BP and BPV measures**

| Variable | BD ($n=38$) | BPD ($n=25$) | HC ($n=43$) | ANCOVA | | |
|---|---|---|---|---|---|---|
| | | | | $F_{(2, 100)}$ | $P$ | $\eta_P^2$ |
| *BP metric* | | | | | | |
| HR, BPM ± SD | 69.3 ± 10.8 | 75 ± 8.9 | 67.57 ± 8.8 | 2.576 | 0.081 | 0.049 |
| SBP, mmHg ± SD | 117.7 ± 11 | 112 ± 7.3 | 113.6 ± 9 | 2.671 | 0.074 | 0.050 |
| DBP, mmHg ± SD | 76.9 ± 8.1 | 76.4 ± 6.8 | 76.3 ± 6.6 | 0.126 | 0.881 | 0.002 |
| PP, mmHg ± SD | *40.8 ± 7.4* | *35.7 ± 5.3* | *37.3 ± 6.3* | *4.711* | *0.011* | *0.085* |
| MAP, mmHg ± SD | 90.5 ± 8.5 | 88.3 ± 6.5 | 88.7 ± 6.9 | 0.494 | 0.612 | 0.010 |
| *BPV metric* | | | | | | |
| cvHR, % ± SD | 10.6 ± 3.6 | 10.5 ± 3.5 | 10.5 ± 3.3 | 0.056 | 0.945 | 0.001 |
| cvSBP, % ± SD | 6.2 ± 1.7 | 6.5 ± 2.2 | 6.4 ± 2 | 1.537 | 0.220 | 0.030 |
| cvDBP, % ± SD | 7.2 ± 2.3 | 7.9 ± 2.3 | 7.8 ± 2.2 | 1.427 | 0.245 | 0.028 |
| cvPP, % ± SD | 13.6 ± 3.7 | 14.1 ± 4 | 14.6 ± 5.3 | 0.586 | 0.559 | 0.012 |
| cvMAP, % ± SD | 6.2 ± 1.9 | 6.8 ± 2.2 | 6.6 ± 1.9 | 2.458 | 0.091 | 0.047 |

ANCOVA results are reported with age and BMI inserted as covariates

Higher resting heart rate correlated with greater instability of negative mood items, anxiety and sad. There was no association between mean BP and BPV metrics and QIDS and ASRM scores (Additional file 1: Figure S2a, b). The inverse correlation between mean BP and negative/positive mood instability was similar for all groups in direction and magnitude (Additional file 1: Figure S3).

## Discussion

Participants with BD exhibited significantly wider PP than HCs and participants with BPD but groups did not differ in terms of resting measures of HR, SBP, DBP or MAP. BP measures and mood instability measures were inversely related. Higher resting HR was associated with greater mood instability on negative MZ items.

### Blood pressure

In most adults both SBP and DBP rise continuously from the age of 30 years. This linear trend continues into old-age for SBP whereas DBP typically plateaus during the fifth decade of life (Franklin et al. 1997). Consequently, PP (SBP–DBP) widens markedly during middle-age. Additionally, BP increases with higher BMI (Kang et al. 2017). Our findings, corrected for age and BMI, suggest a premature elevation of PP in BD.

Increased PP denotes an increase in arterial stiffness and is a correlate of several markers of sub-clinical CVD (Winston et al. 2013). It is an important predictor of CVD risk and cardiovascular mortality, with evidence supporting a stronger association with PP in normotensive individuals compared to those with hypertension (Hadaegh et al. 2012; Benetos et al. 1998; Benetos et al. 1997; Blacher et al. 2000). Additionally, PP may have superior predictive ability for certain cardiovascular outcomes. Data from the Framingham Heart Study suggest that PP is a better predictor of coronary heart disease than SBP and DBP (Franklin et al. 1999). Similar findings have been described for congestive heart failure and myocardial infarction in individuals aged > 65 years (Chae et al. 1999; Vaccarino et al. 2000). In a primarily normotensive cohort such as the current sample, elevated PP in BD may indicate greater sub-clinical risk of adverse cardiovascular outcome compared to healthy and clinical controls. The use of dopamine antagonist drugs and lithium was more common in BD than BPD. Elevated risk for hypertension has been described with antipsychotic use in BD but weight gain may be the main mediator (Correll et al. 2015; Vancampfort et al. 2015) and BMI was controlled in the present comparison. Over 40% of BD participants in this study used lithium. Lithium has been described in one small sample-size study to elevate blood pressure when used as monotherapy (Johnstone et al. 1990), but we did not detect differences between lithium users and non-users. Future studies with greater power are necessary to interrogate further the effects of psychotropic medication and polypharmacy on BP risk and how it relates to BD.

Previous work has focused on the association between BD and hypertension (Johannessen et al. 2006; Goldstein et al. 2009; Chien et al. 2013). Our findings highlight the importance of considering BP as a continuous variable and examining sub-clinical BP differences. This is particularly important given that CVD risk is also related to higher BP well within the normotensive range (Whelton et al. 2020) and excess CVD

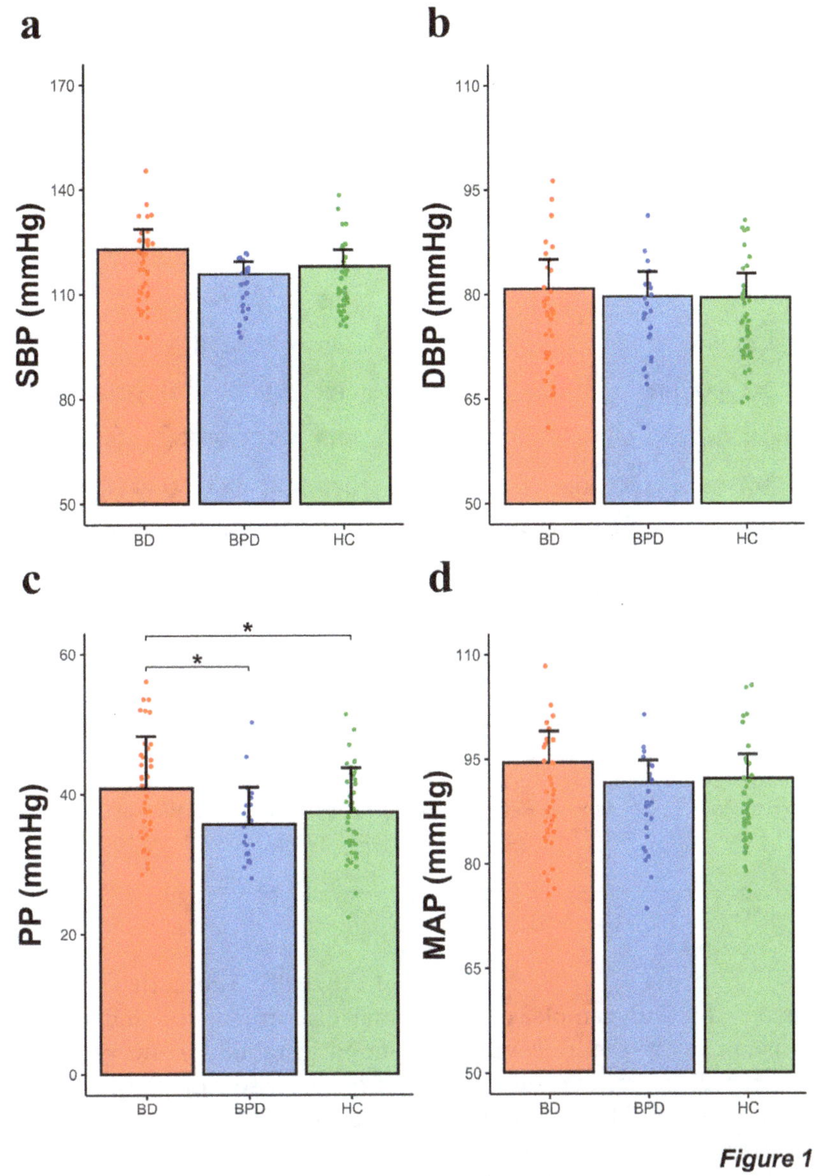


**Fig. 1** Group-wise comparison of mean blood pressure variables. Bars represent group means with error bars indicating standard deviation. Variables plotted are as follows **a** systolic blood pressure (SBP); **b** diastolic blood pressure (DBP); **c** pulse pressure (PP); **d** mean arterial pressure (MAP). All comparisons control for age and BMI as covariates with Bonferroni post-hoc correction applied. *denotes $P < 0.05$

mortality is described in BD before the age where hypertension is normally screened (Osby et al. 2016; Kessling et al. 2015b).

CVD risk is not unique to BD among the psychiatric disorders (Foguet-Boreu et al. 2016). The reasons for this association are multifactorial and include elevated blood pressure, which has been described across several psychiatric disorders (Stein et al. 2014). However, BPD failed to show any differences compared to control participants. Recent evidence suggests a genetic component to CVD in BD, with a higher prevalence of cardiovascular risk factors and increased Framingham risk score present among unaffected siblings/first-degree relatives of individuals with BD (Tsao et al. 2019; Coello et al. 2019b). Furthermore, several overlapping pleiotropic genes have been implicated with both CVD and BD (Amare et al. 2017). The heritability of BPD is probably lower than BD (Skoglund et al. 2019). Dysfunctional behaviour may be more likely to mediate the association of BPD with CVD risk (Grove et al. 2017; Moran et al. 2007). Therefore, treatment effects of recommended psychological therapies that remodel behaviour and improve interpersonal functioning may reduce the risk in BPD.

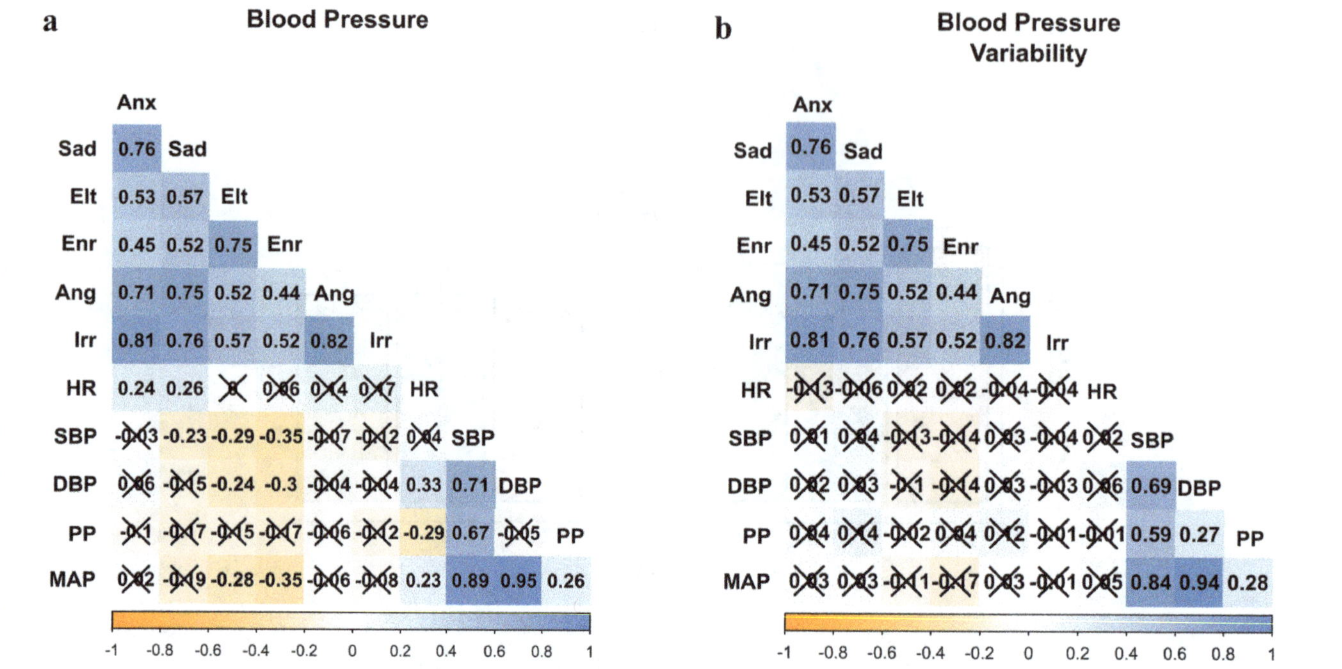


**Fig. 2** Correlations between blood pressure and mood instability. Correlation plot shows Spearman rank-order correlation matrix of mood instability variables from MZ digital questionnaire and **a** mean BP variables and **b** BPV variables measured via the coefficient of variation. Mood instability of each MZ item is estimated by the RMSSD of mood ratings. Strength and direction of correlation is indicated by colour legend. Abbreviations are as follows: Anx = anxious, Elt = elated; Enr = energetic; Ang = angry; Irr = irritable; HR = pulse rate; SBP = systolic blood pressure; DBP = diastolic blood pressure; PP = pulse pressure; MAP = mean arterial pressure. Crossed-out coefficients represent non-significant correlations ($P > 0.05$, FDR correction applied)

### Mood instability

Mood instability findings in this sub-sample of the AMoSS study were consistent with the full sample (Tsanas et al. 2016). Taken transdiagnostically, our findings reveal interesting associations with HBPM variables. Mean SBP was negatively correlated with instability of MZ item sad, and all measures of mean BP (SBP, DBP, and MAP) were negatively associated with instability of positive MZ items elated and energetic. The direction of these associations is unexpected. The hypothesis that emotional distress and elevated BP are positively linked originates from over a century ago (Hildrum et al. 2008). However, few studies have demonstrated prospective evidence to support it; anger shows the strongest association with limited support for depression and anxiety (Rutledge and Hogan 2002). Conversely, several studies report an association between lower BP and depression and anxiety (Hildrum et al. 2008, 2011; Speerforck et al. 2019). That BP was inversely associated with instability of sadness in the current sample is consistent with these trends. However, we did not observe any association with instability among anger or irritability items. An association between emotional reactivity in remitted BD and elevated SBP/DBP has been described previously (Dargel et al. 2018). The authors suggested that BP differences may discriminate BD individuals with high inter-episode mood instability. However, the present findings suggest strongest associations with lower instability among energetic and elated mood components, respectively. Several aspects of our assessment of mood might account for different findings. Our experience sampling methods reflect mood changes in daily life, whereas previous studies have used retrospective self-report instruments often reporting psychological traits rather than current mood per se. Notably, we did not detect any association between BP and manic symptoms. Thus the inverse association between mean BP and mood instability for energetic and elated items may emerge from causes other than subsyndromal mood elevation (e.g. low mean activity and consequently more stable energy ratings for individuals with high BP). Furthermore, only the BPD group showed significant mood instability on these items and thus the generalisability of BP findings and association with more severe mood alterations in remitted BD is unclear. Higher resting HR was associated with greater mood instability of negative MZ items. A higher resting HR (and lower inter-beat-interval heart rate variability) is consistent with lower parasympathetic nervous system activity, which in turn is associated with greater mood instability and difficulties in emotion regulation (Koval et al. 2013; Williams et al. 2015).

The current findings are cross-sectional and thus any potential causal association between BP and mood instability is unclear. However, the associations we describe between BP and mood have implications for future predictive modelling studies and the search for intervention targets. Prospective longitudinal monitoring of BP changes and mood may facilitate the use of this biomarker for identifying individuals at increased risk of residual mood symptoms and episode recurrence. Furthermore, the integration of contemporaneous BP monitoring within antihypertensive experimental medicine studies may clarify their therapeutic role as proposed for BD. Large-scale cohort data suggest that some antihypertensives (e.g. angiotensin antagonists) may be associated with decreased risk of mood disorders, while others (e.g. beta-blockers) are associated with increased risk (Shaw et al. 2019; Boal et al. 2016). Given the associations between BP and mood described here, future healthcare record studies and experimental studies addressing antihypertensive drugs should examine the mediating influence of BP on mood in order to disentangle potential therapeutic mechanism behind their purported effects on mood.

### Blood pressure variability

We did not detect any differences for BPV between groups or any meaningful associations with mood instability. The study demonstrated good tolerability of HBPM monitoring in BD and BPD. Importantly, we assessed mid-term BPV and thus our observations are interpreted within the context of day-to-day changes, limited to waking hours only. Short-term BPV can be measured through ambulatory blood pressure monitoring (ABPM) and better captures BPV over the course of the 24-h day in 15–30 min intervals (Chadachan et al. 2018). Future studies that employ higher frequency BPV sampling methods such as via ABPM are required to thoroughly assess normal circadian fluctuation and finer scale autonomic oscillations of BP in psychiatric groups. This is particularly relevant in the context of previous findings of differential circadian function and autonomic regulation and their influence upon mood instability in BD and BPD (Carr et al. 2018; McGowan et al. 2019, 2020).

### Limitations

There was a preponderance of female participants in the BPD group compared to BD and HC, consistent with its greater prevalence in women (APA 2013). Importantly, age by sex BP differences have been described previously (Reckelhoff 2001); BP is normally higher in men than women until menopause, after which this trend reverses. However, our analyses controlled for age and elevated PP in BD was observed versus a gender equivalent healthy control group and also with gender entered as a covariate. However, future longitudinal studies are required to understand how age and sex interactions may be different among clinical groups (for example post-menopause in women). Although we controlled for psychotropic drug use in our sensitivity analysis, other limitations are differing medication across the clinical samples and their potential interacting influence via polypharmacy. The current sample sizes are too small to fully examine this effect. Future longitudinal studies that harness digital health records will be informative for understanding the long-term effects of medication on BP in mood disorders. However, a clear strength of our approach was monitoring of BP over multiple days to quantify its variability, which was feasible due to our sample size. HBPM was performed at multiple daily time-points in line with ESH/ESC guidelines but its duration/frequency is limited by participant effort. Studies that use ABPM would have the advantage of better capturing BPV and relating this to intra-daily mood changes. Finally, as described above, our data are cross-sectional and thus we cannot determine a cause-effect relation between BP and mood instability or vice versa.

## Conclusions

The results of a week-long HBPM assessment show an elevated resting pulse pressure in BD relative to BPD and HCs while BPV measures did not differ between groups. Mean BP metrics and resting HR correlated with mood instability monitored via ecological momentary assessment. Together, the results demonstrate subtle BP differences in BD subjects within a normotensive range and that mean BP is associated with mood instability in a transdiagnostic group. Despite the high prevalence of cardiovascular mortality in BD, a focus on prevention and risk management in BD is regrettably lacking (Goldstein et al. 2020). Yet, BP is a highly modifiable risk factor. Our findings identify pulse pressure as potential target for risk management and that BP may be associated with mood instability.

## Supplementary Information

**Additional file 1.** Supplementary Tables and Figures.

### Abbreviations

ABPM: Ambulatory Blood Pressure Monitoring; AMoSS: Automated Monitoring of Symptom Severity; APA: American Psychiatric Association; ASRM: Altman Self-Rating Mania Scale; BD: Bipolar Disorder; BP: Blood Pressure; BPD:

Borderline Personality Disorder; BPV: Blood Pressure Variability; CV: Coefficient of Variation; CVD: Cardiovascular Disease; DBP: Diastolic Blood Pressure; ESH/ESC: European Society of Cardiology (ESC) and the European Society of Hypertension (ESH); HBPM: Home Blood Pressure Monitoring; HC: Healthy Controls; MAP: Mean Arterial Pressure; MZ: Mood Zoom; NICE: National Institute for Health and Care Excellence; PP: Pulse Pressure; QIDS: Quick Inventory of Depressive Symptomatology (Self-Report); RMSSD: Root Mean Square of Successive Differences; SBP: Systolic Blood Pressure.

**Acknowledgements**
We thank the participants who took part in this study and members of the AMoSS study team who assisted with data collection.

**Authors' contributions**
GMG, ACB, and KEAS designed and conceived the study. ACB and KEAS recruited the participants and obtained the study data. NMMcG and MN extracted the data, performed statistical analyses and interpreted the data. NMMcG wrote the draft manuscript. All authors had substantial contributions to interpretation of results, and participated in manuscript drafting. All authors read and approved the final manuscript.

**Author details**
[1] Department of Psychiatry, University of Oxford, Warneford Hospital, Oxford OX3 7JX, UK. [2] Academic Centre, John Radcliffe Hospital, Oxford University Clinical School, Oxford OX3 9DU, UK. [3] Oxford Health NHS Foundation Trust, Warneford Hospital, Oxford OX3 7JX, UK. [4] NIHR Oxford Health Biomedical Research Centre, Oxford OX3 7JX, UK.

**References**

Altman EG, Hedeker D, Peterson JL, Davis JM. The Altman self-rating mania scale. Biol Psychiat. 1997;42(10):948–55.

Amare AT, Schubert KO, Klingler-Hoffmann M, Cohen-Woods S, Baune BT. The genetic overlap between mood disorders and cardiometabolic diseases: a systematic review of genome wide and candidate gene studies. Transl Psychiatry. 2017;7(1):1007.

American Psychiatric Publishing. Diagnostic and statistical manual of mental disorders. 5th ed (DSM-5). Arlington: American Psychiatric Publishing; 2013.

Ayerbe L, Forgnone I, Addo J, Siguero A, Gelati S, Ayis S. Hypertension risk and clinical care in patients with bipolar disorder or schizophrenia; a systematic review and meta-analysis. J Affect Disord. 2018;1(225):665–70.

Barbosa IG, Ferreira GC, Ferreira AJD, Januário CR, Belisário AR, Bauer ME, Cristina SEA. The renin angiotensin system and bipolar disorder: a systematic review. Protein Peptide Lett. 2020. https://doi.org/10.2174/0929866527666200127115059.

Benetos A, Safar M, Rudnichi A, Smulyan H, Richard JL, Ducimetieere P, Guize L. Pulse pressure: A predictor of long-term cardiovascular mortality in a French male population. Hypertension. 1997;30:1410–5.

Benetos A, Rudnichi A, Safar M, Guize L. Pulse pressure and cardiovascular mortality in normotensive and hypertensive subjects. Hypertension. 1998;32(3):560–4.

Blacher J, Staessen JA, Girerd X, Gasowski J, Thijs L, Liu L, Wang JG, Fagard RH, Safar ME. Pulse pressure not mean pressure determines cardiovascular risk in older hypertensive patients. Arch Intern Med. 2000;160(8):1085–9.

Boal AH, Smith DJ, McCallum L, Muir S, Touyz RM, Dominiczak AF, Padmanabhan S. Monotherapy with major antihypertensive drug classes and risk of hospital admissions for mood disorders. Hypertension. 2016;68(5):1132–8.

Brown S, Ramesh R, Newson S, Isaacs R. Lifestyle-related cardiovascular risk factors in patients with bipolar disorder. Progress Neurol Psychiatry. 2013;17(4):28–33.

Carr O, de Vos M, Saunders KE. Heart rate variability in bipolar disorder and borderline personality disorder: a clinical review. Evid Based Mental Health. 2018;21(1):23–30.

Chadachan VM, Ye MT, Tay JC, Subramaniam K, Setia S. Understanding short-term blood-pressure-variability phenotypes: from concept to clinical practice. Int J General Med. 2018;11:241.

Chae CU, Pfeffer MA, Glynn RJ, Mitchell GF, Taylor JO, Hennekens CH. Increased pulse pressure and risk of heart failure in the elderly. JAMA. 1999;281(7):634–43.

Charles EF, Lambert CG, Kerner B. Bipolar disorder and diabetes mellitus: evidence for disease-modifying effects and treatment implications. Int J Bipolar Disord. 2016;4(1):13.

Chien IC, Lin CH, Chou YJ, Chou P. Risk of hypertension in patients with bipolar disorder in Taiwan: a population-based study. Compr Psychiatry. 2013;54(6):687–93.

Cipriani A, Saunders K, Attenburrow MJ, et al. A systematic review of calcium channel antagonists in bipolar disorder and some considerations for their future development. Mol Psychiatry. 2016;21(10):1324–32.

Coello K, Vinberg M, Knop FK, Pedersen BK, McIntyre RS, Kessing LV, Munkholm K. Metabolic profile in patients with newly diagnosed bipolar disorder and their unaffected first-degree relatives. Int J Bipolar Disord. 2019;7(1):8.

Coello K, Kjærstad HL, Stanislaus S, Melbye S, Faurholt-Jepsen M, Miskowiak KW, McIntyre RS, Vinberg M, Kessing LV, Munkholm K. Thirty-year cardiovascular risk score in patients with newly diagnosed bipolar disorder and their unaffected first-degree relatives. Aust NZ J Psychiatry. 2019;53(7):651–62.

Correll CU, Detraux J, De Lepeleire J, De Hert M. Effects of antipsychotics, antidepressants and mood stabilizers on risk for physical diseases in people with schizophrenia, depression and bipolar disorder. World Psychiatry. 2015;14(2):119–36.

Crump C, et al. Comorbidities and mortality in bipolar disorder: A Swedish National Cohort Study. JAMA Psychiatry. 2013;70(9):931–9.

Dargél AA, Roussel F, Volant S, Etain B, Grant R, Azorin JM, M'Bailara K, Bellivier F, Bougerol T, Kahn JP, Roux P. Emotional hyper-reactivity and cardiometabolic risk in remitted bipolar patients: a machine learning approach. Acta Psychiatr Scand. 2018;138(4):348–59.

Ebner-Priemer UW, Eid M, Kleindienst N, Stabenow S, Trull TJ. Analytic strategies for understanding affective (in) stability and other dynamic processes in psychopathology. J Abnormal Psychol. 2009;118:195.

Fiedorowicz JG, Solomon DA, Endicott J, Leon AC, Li C, Rice JP, et al. Manic/hypomanic symptom burden and cardiovascular mortality in bipolar disorder. Psychosom Med. 2009;71:598–606.

Fiedorowicz JG, Jancic D, Potash JB, Butcher B, Coryell WH. Vascular mortality in participants of a bipolar genomics study. Psychosomatics. 2014;55:485.

Foguet-Boreu Q, San Martin MI, Mateo GF, del Olmo EZ, Garcia-Morzon LA, López MP, Martin-López LM, Hidalgo JM, Violán C. Cardiovascular risk assessment in patients with a severe mental illness: a systematic review and meta-analysis. BMC Psychiatry. 2016;16(1):141.

Forouzanfar MH, et al. Global, regional, and national comparative risk assessment of 79 behavioural, environmental and occupational, and metabolic risks or clusters of risks, 1990–2015: a systematic analysis for the Global Burden of Disease Study. Lancet. 2016;2015(388):1659–724.

Franklin SS, Gustin W, Wong ND, Larson MG, Weber MA, Kannel WB, Levy D. Hemodynamic patterns of age-related changes in blood pressure: the Framingham Heart Study. Circulation. 1997;96:308–15.

Franklin SS, Khan SA, Wong ND, Larson MG, Levy D. Is pulse pressure useful in predicting risk for coronary heart disease? The Framingham Heart Study. Circulation. 1999;100:354–60.

Franklin SS, Lopez VA, Wong ND, Mitchell GF, Larson MG, Vasan RS, Levy D. Single versus combined blood pressure components and risk for cardiovascular disease: The Framingham Heart Study. Circulation. 2009;119(2):243.

Ghaemi SN, Dalley S, Catania C, Barroilhet S. Bipolar or borderline: a clinical overview. Acta Psychiatr Scand. 2014;130(2):99–108.

Goldstein BI, Fagiolini A, Houck P, Kupfer DJ. Cardiovascular disease and hypertension among adults with bipolar I disorder in the United States. Bipolar Disord. 2009;11(6):657–62.

Goldstein BI, Schaffer A, Wang S, et al. Excessive and premature new-onset cardiovascular disease among adults with bipolar disorder in the US NESARC cohort. J Clin Psychiatry. 2015;76:163–9.

Goldstein BI, Baune BT, Bond DJ, Chen PH, Eyler L, Fagiolini A, Gomes F, Hajek T, Hatch J, McElroy SL, McIntyre RS. Call to action regarding the vascular-bipolar link: a report from the vascular task force of the international society for bipolar disorders. Bipolar Disord. 2020. https://doi.org/10.1111/bdi.12921.

Grassi G, Bombelli M, Brambilla G, Trevano FQ, Dell'oro R, Mancia G. Total cardiovascular risk, blood pressure variability and adrenergic overdrive in hypertension: evidence, mechanisms and clinical implications. Curr Hypertens Rep. 2012;14(4):333–8. https://doi.org/10.1007/s11906-012-0273-8.

Grove JL, Smith TW, Crowell SE, Williams PG, Jordan KD. Borderline personality features, interpersonal correlates, and blood pressure response to social stressors: implications for cardiovascular risk. Personality Individ Differ. 2017;15(113):38–47.

Hadaegh F, Shafiee G, Hatami M, Azizi F. Systolic and diastolic blood pressure, mean arterial pressure and pulse pressure for prediction of cardiovascular events and mortality in a Middle Eastern population. Blood Press. 2012;21(1):12–8.

Harrison PJ, Geddes JR, Tunbridge EM. The emerging neurobiology of bipolar disorder. Trends Neurosci. 2018;41(1):18–30.

Hayes JF, Marston L, Walters K, King MB, Osborn DP. Mortality gap for people with bipolar disorder and schizophrenia: UK-based cohort study 2000–2014. Br J Psychiatry. 2017;211(3):175–81.

Hildrum B, Mykletun A, Holmen J, Dahl AA. Effect of anxiety and depression on blood pressure: 11-year longitudinal population study. Br J Psychiatry. 2008;193(2):108–13.

Hildrum B, Romild U, Holmen J. Anxiety and depression lowers blood pressure: 22-year follow-up of the population based HUNT study, Norway. BMC Public Health. 2011;11(1):601.

Johannessen L, Strudsholm U, Foldager L, Munk-Jørgensen P. Increased risk of hypertension in patients with bipolar disorder and patients with anxiety compared to background population and patients with schizophrenia. J Affect Disord. 2006;95(1–3):13–7.

Johnstone EC, Owens DG, Lambert MT, Crow TJ, Frith CD, Done DJ. Combination tricyclic antidepressant and lithium maintenance medication in unipolar and bipolar depressed patients. J Affect Disord. 1990;20(4):225–33.

Kang MG, Kim KH, Koh JS, Park JR, Hwang SJ, Hwang JY, Ahn JH, Jang JY, Jeong YH, Kwak CH, Park HW. Association between pulse pressure and body mass index in hypertensive and normotensive populations in the Korea National Health and Nutrition Examination Survey V, 2010–2012. J Clin Hypertens. 2017;19(4):395–401.

Kelbrick M, Abdaldayim S. Blood pressure monitoring in psychiatric inpatients with bipolar affective disorder. Prog Neurology Psychiatry. 2014;18(4):11–5.

Kessing LV, Vradi E, Andersen PK. Life expectancy in bipolar disorder. Bipolar Disord. 2015;17(5):543–8.

Kessing LV, Vradi E, McIntyre RS, et al. Causes of decreased life expectancy over the life span in bipolar disorder. J Affect Disord. 2015b;180:142–7.

Koval P, Ogrinz B, Kuppens P, Van den Bergh O, Tuerlinckx F, Sütterlin S. Affective instability in daily life is predicted by resting heart rate variability. PLoS ONE. 2013;8(11):e81536.

Laursen TM. Life expectancy among persons with schizophrenia or bipolar affective disorder. Schizophrenia Res. 2011;131(1–3):101–4.

McGowan NM, Goodwin GM, Bilderbeck AC, Saunders KE. Circadian rest-activity patterns in bipolar disorder and borderline personality disorder. Transl Psychiatry. 2019;9(1):1–1.

McGowan NM, Goodwin GM, Bilderbeck AC, Saunders KE. Actigraphic patterns, impulsivity and mood instability in bipolar disorder, borderline personality disorder, and healthy controls. Acta Psychiatr Scand. 2020. https://doi.org/10.1111/acps.13148.

Moran P, Stewart R, Brugha T, Bebbington P, Bhugra D, Jenkins R, Coid JW. Personality disorder and cardiovascular disease: results from a national household survey. J Clin Psychiatry. 2007;68:69–74.

NICE. Bipolar disorder: Assessment and Management CG185. London: NICE; 2014.

Oparil S, Acelajado M, Bakris G, et al. Hypertension Nat Rev Dis Primers. 2018;4:18014.

Osborn DP, Hardoon S, Omar RZ, Holt RI, King M, Larsen J, Marston L, Morris RW, Nazareth I, Walters K, Petersen I. Cardiovascular risk prediction models for people with severe mental illness: results from the prediction and management of cardiovascular risk in people with severe mental illnesses (PRIMROSE) research program. JAMA Psychiatry. 2015;72(2):143–51.

Osby U, Brandt L, Correia N, Ekbom A, Sparén P. Excess mortality in bipolar and unipolar disorder in Sweden. Arch Gen Psychiatry. 2001;58(9):844-850. https://doi.org/10.1001/archpsyc.58.9.844.

Osby U, Westman J, Hällgren J, Gissler M. Mortality trends in cardiovascular causes in schizophrenia, bipolar and unipolar mood disorder in Sweden 1987–2010. Eur J Public Health. 2016;26(5):867–71.

Parati G, Ochoa JE, Lombardi C, Bilo G. Assessment and management of blood-pressure variability. Nat Rev Cardiol. 2013;10(3):143.

Pinto E. Blood pressure and ageing. Postgrad Med J. 2007;83(976):109–14.

Reckelhoff JF. Gender differences in the regulation of blood pressure. Hypertension. 2001;37(5):1199–208.

Roininen SM, Cheetham M, Mueller BU, Battegay E. Unmet challenges in treating hypertension in patients with borderline personality disorder: a systematic review. Medicine. 2019;98(37):17101.

Rush AJ, Trivedi MH, Ibrahim HM, Carmody TJ, Arnow B, Klein DN, Markowitz JC, Ninan PT, Kornstein S, Manber R, Thase ME. The 16-Item Quick Inventory of Depressive Symptomatology (QIDS), clinician rating (QIDS-C), and self-report (QIDS-SR): a psychometric evaluation in patients with chronic major depression. Biol Psychiat. 2003;54(5):573–83.

Rutledge T, Hogan BE. A quantitative review of prospective evidence linking psychological factors with hypertension development. Psychosom Med. 2002;64(5):758–66.

Shaw RJ, Mackay D, Pell JP, Padmanabhan S, Bailey DS, Smith DJ. The relationship between antihypertensive medications and mood disorders: analysis of linked healthcare data for 1.8 million patients. Psychol Med. 2019. https://doi.org/10.1017/S0033291719004094.

Skoglund C, Tiger A, Rück C, Petrovic P, Asherson P, Hellner C, Mataix-Cols D, Kuja-Halkola R. Familial risk and heritability of diagnosed borderline personality disorder: a register study of the Swedish population. Mol Psychiatry. 2019;3:1.

Speerforck S, Dodoo-Schittko F, Brandstetter S, Apfelbacher C, Hapke U, Jacobi F, Grabe HJ, Baumeister SE, Schomerus G. 12-year changes in cardiovascular risk factors in people with major depressive or bipolar disorder: a prospective cohort analysis in Germany. Eur Arch Psychiatry Clin Neurosci. 2019;269(5):565–76.

Stein DJ, Aguilar-Gaxiola S, Alonso J, Bruffaerts R, De Jonge P, Liu Z, Caldas-de-Almeida JM, O'Neill S, Viana MC, Al-Hamzawi AO, Angermeyer MC. Associations between mental disorders and subsequent onset of hypertension. Gen Hosp Psychiatry. 2014;36(2):142–9.

Stevens SL, Wood S, Koshiaris C, Law K, Glasziou P, Stevens RJ, McManus RJ. Blood pressure variability and cardiovascular disease: systematic review and meta-analysis. BMJ. 2016;9(354):i4098.

Tsanas A, Saunders KE, Bilderbeck AC, Palmius N, Osipov M, Clifford GD, Goodwin GM, De Vos M. Daily longitudinal self-monitoring of mood variability in bipolar disorder and borderline personality disorder. J Affect Disord. 2016;15(205):225–33.

Tsao W-Y, Hsu J-W, Huang K-L, Bai Y-M, Su T-P, Li C-T, et al. Risk of cardiometabolic diseases among siblings of patients with bipolar disorder. J Affect Disord. 2019;253:171–5.

Vaccarino V, Holford TR, Krumholz HM. Pulse pressure and risk for myocardial infarction and heart failure in the elderly. J Am Coll Cardiol. 2000;36(1):130–8. https://doi.org/10.1016/s0735-1097(00)00687-2.

Vancampfort D, Stubbs B, Mitchell AJ, De Hert M, Wampers M, Ward PB, Rosenbaum S, Correll CU. Risk of metabolic syndrome and its components in people with schizophrenia and related psychotic disorders, bipolar disorder and major depressive disorder: a systematic review and meta-analysis. World Psychiatry. 2015;14(3):339–47.

Weiner M, et al. Cardiovascular morbidity and mortality in bipolar disorder. Ann Clin Psychiatry. 2011;23(1):40–7.

Westman J, Hällgren J, Wahlbeck K, et al. Cardiovascular mortality in bipolar disorder: a population-based cohort study in Sweden. BMJ Open. 2013;3(4):e002373.

Whelton SP, McEvoy JW, Shaw L, Psaty BM, Lima JA, Budoff M, Nasir K, Szklo M, Blumenthal RS, Blaha MJ. Association of normal systolic blood pressure level with cardiovascular disease in the absence of risk factors. JAMA Cardiol. 2020. https://doi.org/10.1001/jamacardio.2020.1731.

Williams DP, Cash C, Rankin C, Bernardi A, Koenig J, Thayer JF. Resting heart rate variability predicts self-reported difficulties in emotion regulation: a focus on different facets of emotion regulation. Frontiers in psychology. 2015;10(6):261.

Williams B, Mancia G, Spiering W, Agabiti Rosei E, Azizi M, Burnier M, Clement DL, Coca A, De Simone G, Dominiczak A, Kahan T. 2018 ESC/ESH Guidelines for the management of arterial hypertension: The Task Force for the management of arterial hypertension of the European Society of Cardiology (ESC) and the European Society of Hypertension (ESH). Eur Heart J. 2018;39(33):3021–104.

Winston GJ, Palmas W, Lima J, Polak JF, Bertoni AG, Burke G, Eng J, Gottesman R, Shea S. Pulse pressure and subclinical cardiovascular disease in the multi-ethnic study of atherosclerosis. Am J Hypertens. 2013;26(5):636–42.
Wolf-Maier K, Cooper RS, Banegas JR, Giampaoli S, Hense HW, Joffres M, Kastarinen M, Poulter N, Primatesta P, Rodríguez-Artalejo F, Stegmayr B. Hypertension prevalence and blood pressure levels in 6 European countries, Canada, and the United States. JAMA. 2003;289(18):2363–9.

# 5

# Role of endogenous ouabain in the etiology of bipolar disorder

Rif S. El-Mallakh[1*], Yonglin Gao[1] and Pan You[2]

**Abstract**

**Background:** Bipolar disorder is a severe psychiatric illness with poor prognosis and problematic and suboptimal treatments. Understanding the pathoetiologic mechanisms may improve treatment and outcomes.

**Discussion:** Dysregulation of cationic homeostasis is the most reproducible aspect of bipolar pathophysiology. Correction of ionic balance is the universal mechanism of action of all mood stabilizing medications. Recent discoveries of the role of endogenous sodium pump modulators (which include 'endogenous ouabain') in regulation of sodium and potassium distribution, inflammation, and activation of key cellular second messenger systems that are important in cell survival, and the demonstration that these stress-responsive chemicals may be dysregulated in bipolar patients, suggest that these compounds may be candidates for the coupling of environmental stressors and illness onset. Specifically, individuals with bipolar disorder appear to be unable to upregulate endogenous ouabain under conditions that require it, and therefore may experience a relative deficiency of this important regulatory hormone. In the absence of elevated endogenous ouabain, neurons are unable to maintain their normal resting potential, become relatively depolarized, and are then susceptible to inappropriate activation. Furthermore, sodium pump activity appears to be necessary to prevent inflammatory signals within the central nervous system. Nearly all available data currently support this model, but additional studies are required to solidify the role of this system.

**Conclusion:** Endogenous ouabain dysregulation appears to be a reasonable candidate for understanding the pathophysiology of bipolar disorder.

**Keywords:** Bipolar disorder, Calcium, Endogenous ouabain, Ouabain, Pathophysiology, Sodium, Sodium pump

## Background

Bipolar disorder is a severe psychiatric illness that manifests as extreme variations in mood and energy, usually labelled as mania and depression, interspersed over an euthymic or dysthymic baseline (Ketter and Calabrese 2002). The disorder afflicts approximately 1% of people (Clemente et al. (2015); Grande et al. 2016), with documented suboptimal treatments and a host of undesirable outcomes related to both the disease and its treatment (Cipriani et al. 2017; Dome et al. 2019). Despite over 60 years of directed effort, the pathoetiology of the illness remains unknown (Grande et al. 2016). Nonetheless, multiple clues have emerged that continue to inform ongoing research. The illness is viewed as multifactorial with elements of development and neuroplasticity, inflammation, and aberrant modulation of brain function and circuitry, that are mediated by gene and environment interaction through multiple inherited genes and multiple altered epigenetic changes (Grande et al. 2016; Belvederi Murri et al. 2016; Nestler et al. 2016; Takaesu 2018). Due to the absence of a centralized unifying model, pathophysiologic research continues in a fragmented, siloed fashion. A proposed mechanism of pathophysiology that incorporates much of the translational and clinical data, might help focus and thus accelerate research efforts.

*Correspondence: rselma01@louisville.edu
[1] Mood Disorders Research Program, Depression Center, Department of Psychiatry and Behavioral Sciences, University of Louisville School of Medicine, 401 East Chestnut Street, Suite 610, Louisville, KY 40202, USA
Full list of author information is available at the end of the article

Among the most reproducible findings in bipolar illness has been dysregulation of control of electrically important ions: sodium ($Na^+$), potassium ($K^+$), hydrogen (proton, $H^+$), and calcium ($Ca^{2+}$) (El-Mallakh et al. 1076). Ion regulation spans across all of the proposed mechanisms of pathogenesis of abnormal moods in bipolar illness and across all successful treatment options. For example, in an analysis of susceptibility loci, Askland found that approximately 74% of known loci involve genes related to ion regulation, or what she refers to as neuroelectrical genes (Askland 2006). By comparison, genes involved in any neurotransmitter pathway account for only about 58% of the susceptibility loci, and the monoamines account to only 31% (10). A similar conclusion is reached when genome wide association studies (GWAS) are explored (Judy and Zandi 2013). The only animal models of bipolar illness that meet all validity criteria create ion transport abnormalities (Mack et al. 2019; Valvassori et al. 2019). Additionally, nearly all interventions that are effective in mania or mood stabilization reduce intracellular sodium either directly or indirectly (El-Mallakh and Huff 2001; El-Mallakh and Paskitti 2001; Roberts et al. 2010). A model in which a primary ion abnormality can produce the symptoms of bipolar illness has been proposed (El-Mallakh and Wyatt 1995) but the question remains how are environmental stressors that may lead to mood recurrence translated into pathophysiologic abnormalities that cause mood symptoms?

The authors propose that endogenous cardiac steroids may be the factors that transduce the consequences of stressors to produce syndromes of mania or depression via abnormal neural function (Fig. 1). This paper will review the evidence that endogenous cardiac steroids, such as endogenous ouabain, may be involved in the pathogenesis of bipolar illness, and how these stress-responsive compounds may lead to periods of illness.

## Methods

PubMed and Google Scholar were interrogated with the search words of "digoxin mood," "digoxin bipolar," "ouabain mood," "ouabain bipolar," "cardenolide mood," and "cardenolide bipolar." Only the first 100 titles of each search were reviewed by two authors, because the utility declined quickly after that, and articles that informed the topic were specifically read.

## Results

The possible involvement of ion dysregulation and endogenous cardiac steroids in BD was recently reviewed (El-Mallakh et al. 1076; Mack et al. 2019; Valvassori et al. 2019; Lichtstein et al. 2018). "Digoxin mood" yielded 507 items on Pubmed and 11,000 on Google Scholar. "Digoxin bipolar" yielded 17 items on Pubmed and 9720 on Google Scholar. Similarly, "ouabain mood" yielded 1288 and 580, respectively; and "ouabain bipolar" yielded 108 and 5890. "Cardenolide mood" and "cardenolide bipolar" yielded 1329, 230, 101, and 216 items.

## Discussion

### Endogenous cardiac steroids and the sodium pump

Endogenous cardiac steroids include digoxin-like, ouabain-like, and bufadienolide-like molecules. These molecules were first identified in plants (Foxglove, *Digitalis,* for digoxin (Kaul et al. 2013), twisted flower, *Strophanthus,* for ouabain (Fürstenwerth 2019)) and toads (*Rhinella* and other for bufadienolides (Krenn and Kopp 1998; Abdelfatah et al. 2019)). These agents have been used for centuries for treating congestive heart failure, atrial fibrillation, and appear to have a positive inotropic effect on cardiac muscle (Norn and Kruse 2004).

Cardiac steroids effects are mediated by multiple mechanisms. They are known to bind to specific sites on the α subunit of the sodium and potassium-activated adenosine triphosphatase (Na,K-ATPase) or sodium pump. The discovery of the sodium pump resulted in a 1997 Noble Prize to Jens C. Skou, the Danish scientist who documented its existence in 1957 (Skou (1957)). It is usually composed of two subunits, α and β. The α subunit has the sodium, potassium, adenosine triphosphatase (ATP), magnesium, and cardiac glycoside binding sites, while the β subunit is needed for membrane localization of the catalytic αsubunit and cellular adhesion. There are four different isoforms of the α subunit, and mRNA of all four can be found in nearly all human tissues. Protein expression of α1 isoform is ubiquitous in all human tissues. The α2, α3, and α4 are found in human brain, heart, and to a lesser extent, breast and reproductive tissues (GeneCards Human Gene Database 2020). The pump is additionally regulated by a small peptide that binds to the β subunit that was initially called γ, but is now referred to as FXYD domain containing ion transport regulator (Geering 2005). FXYD1 in muscle and FXYD2 in the kidney generally reduce sodium pump activity, FXYD7 in the brain also does so by reducing the affinity of the potassium binding site to extracellular potassium (Geering 2005; Clausen et al. 2020).

In the last 20 years, acceptance that cardiac glycosides are synthesized in the adrenal and hypothalamus of mammals has increased (El-Masri et al. 2002; Lichtstein et al. 1998; Blaustein 2018), but is still not universal (Baecher et al. 2014). It is known that cholesterol (which may be reduced in the brains of patients with bipolar illness (Beasley et al. 2005)) is needed for endogenous ouabain production (Blaustein 2018); and the pathway may involve pregnenolone and progesterone as intermediate steps, (Baecher et al. 2014). (Interestingly, pregnenolone

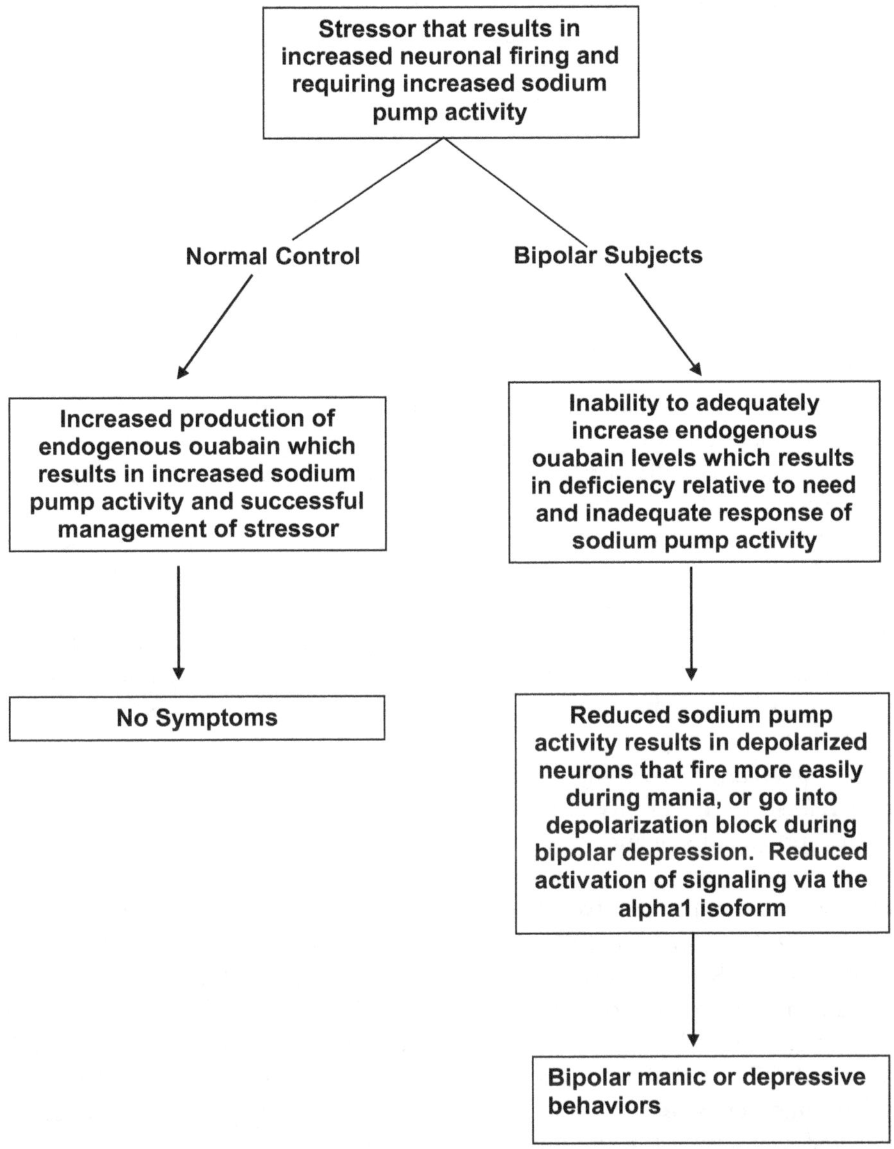


**Fig. 1** Proposed model of role of endogenous ouabain in pathophysiology of bipolar disorder

levels may be reduced in the cerebrospinal fluid of individuals with a diagnosis of mood disorder *and* in relation to the severity of their symptoms (George et al. 1994).) Once synthesized, endogenous bufadienolides in toads (Lichtstein et al. 1993; Butler et al. 1996), and endogenous cardenolides in mammals (Antolovic et al. 1998) may circulate bound to a plasma protein. Rapid elevations in plasma levels of endogenous cardiac glycosides, as occurs with exhaustive exercise (Valdes et al. 1988), may occur due to release of bound glycosides from this carrier protein (Antolovic et al. 2000). The structure of the endogenous glycosides strongly resembles their plant-derived or toad-derived namesakes (Goto et al. 1989; Hamlyn et al. 1991; Komiyama et al. 2000). There is a large and reproducible literature that finds the endogenous glycosides play a significant role in regulation of fluid and electrolytes in animals and humans (Hamlyn and Manunta 2011) and have been associated with a multitude of diseases that involve expanded volume (El-Mallakh et al. 2019).

### Physiological actions of endogenous glycosides

Plants manufacture glycosides for the purpose of protection. The concentrations of glycosides in plant tissues are toxic to animals and reduce herbivory. That means that at the concentrations in plants glycosides are at superphysiologic concentrations. Different glycosides have different actions. For example, marinbufagenin, which has higher affinity with preferential inhibition of the α1 isoform (Feraille and Doucet 2001; Dvela et al. 2007) and greater constriction of vascular smooth muscle (Dvela et al. 2007). Administration of ouabain may increase blood pressure, while digoxin would actually lower it (Huang et al. 1999; Manunta et al. 2000), and endogenous compounds appear to have a similar effect (Balzan et al. 2007). For understanding bipolar disorder, endogenous ouabain appears to be most important (El-Mallakh et al. 2010).

At concentrations found in plants or used experimentally, glycosides inhibit the activity of the Na, K-ATPase and have served as the major experimental purpose of cardenolides, particularly ouabain (Noël et al. 2018). Recently it has been demonstrated that in physiologic mammalian fluids the concentrations of endogenously produced ouabain are quite low (El-Mallakh et al. 2010; Manunta et al. 2006; Dvela et al. 2012). At these physiologic picomolar to nanomolar concentrations glycosides *increase* sodium pump activity in heart, smooth muscle, kidney, and brain (Ghysel-Burton and Godfraind 1979; Gao et al. 2002; Dvela-Levitt et al. 2015; Lichtstein et al. 1985). Even when disease increases the plasma levels of endogenous ouabain, the total levels remain below concentrations that inhibit sodium pump activity (Holthouser et al. 2010). The ouabain-induced increase of sodium pump activity is related to the affinity of the glycoside-binding site to the endogenous ligand, so that α3 appears more susceptible to inhibition with lower concentrations, followed by α2 and α1 at progressively higher concentrations (Balzan et al. 2007; Gao et al. 2002; Holthouser et al. 2010; Saunders and Scheiner-Bobis 2004). This effect may not be a direct effect on the sodium pump but may be secondary to signal transduction on α1, and possibly α 3, and α 4. Specifically, ouabain may increase sodium pump activity through activation of Src kinase-, ERK1/2-, and Akt-mediated pathway or the sodium-proton exchanger 1 (NHE1) (Holthouser et al. 2010; Liang et al. 2006; Khundmiri et al. 2007, 2008).

More recently, it has been discovered that endogenous glycosides can activate second messenger signals through phosphorylation of the Src protein (Thomas and Brugge 1997; Cui and Xie 2017). This discovery has been very exciting because it ties in endogenous glycosides with many cell regulatory processes that occur at physiologic, low nM concentrations of endogenous ouabain (Lichtstein et al. 2018; Touza et al. 2011). The effect on cellular signaling may be of particular importance for the pathophysiology of mood disorders, in general, and bipolar disorder, in particular (Lichtstein et al. 2018). Specifically, activation of extracellular signal-regulated kinase (ERK), protein kinase B (AKT), and nuclear factor kappa-light-chain-enhancer of activated B cells (NFkB) result from the interaction of endogenous ouabain with its receptor on the α 1 isoform which phosphorylate the Src intracellular protein (Lichtstein et al. 2018). These systems are important in calcium signaling and neurotransmitter regulation (Lichtstein et al. 2018). ERK and Raf–mitogen-activated protein kinase (MAPK) are involved in cell survival and proliferation (Kim and Choi 2010), which may be important in cell loss in bipolar patients (Chen and Manji 2006; Yuan et al. 2010; Schroeder et al. 2016).

Activation of the sodium pump appears to be an essential feature to reduce central nervous system inflammation (Kinoshita et al. 2017). Sterile inflammation appears to be a characteristic of bipolar disorder pathophysiology (Rosenblat and McIntyre 2016). If sodium pump activity is blocked in glial cells, inflammatory pathways are activated in the presence of lipopolysaccharides (Kinoshita et al. 2017).

Because the sodium pump activating effect of ouabain occurs at physiologic (low) concentrations (Holthouser et al. 2010), this effect is probably more important to understanding physiologic actions of endogenous ouabain than studies using pharmacologic (high) doses of the plant-derived form of this compound.

The concentrations of endogenous ouabain in the brain may be particularly important in understanding the differential roles of control of ion regulation and control of signal transduction. The α1 isoform is clearly involved in signal transduction (Cui and Xie 2017; Madan et al. 2017), even though all isoforms have highly conserved sequences important in regulating that interaction (Cui and Xie 2017). Alpha2 does not appear to activate ERK, but α3 and α4 appear to do so with at lower doses of ouabain (Pierre et al. 2008). In studies in which cells are designed to express only the α3 isoform, the Src protein does not appear to be phosphorylated, but the ERK system is still activated (Madan et al. 2017), which may occur due to increases of intracellular calcium or other disruption of cellular function (Balasubramaniam et al. 2015; Ghilardi et al. 2020). Similarly, mice without a functional α3 protein show increased calcium signaling in cultured cortical neurons and phospho-activation of ERK and Akt in the hippocampus (Kirshenbaum et al. 2011a), suggesting that increased intracellular calcium may play a role in signal transduction independent of α3. If these differences in isoform involvement in the Src/ERK/MAPK signaling pathway apply in human brains, and given that the affinity of α3 glycoside receptor site greatly exceeds that of α1 (Pierre et al. 2008), activation of ion transport activity will occur via α3 before activation via α1.

### Glycoside induced behavior changes in animal models

Creating an animal model for psychiatric illnesses is always difficult. Bipolar illness may be particularly hard since an adequate animal model would manifest both mania *and* depression *and* response *and* prevention of both with medications like lithium (Fineberg et al. 2011). The only animal models of mania that achieve face validity, construct validity, and predictive validity are ionic models (Mack et al. 2019). One of these models utilizes administration of high doses of ouabain by intracerebroventricular (ICV) injection in rats (El-Mallakh et al. 2003).

Direct ICV ouabain administration will reduce sodium pump activity in the brain (Hamid et al. 2009), induce both depressive and manic symptoms which can be treated and prevented with lithium (Valvassori et al. 2019; El-Mallakh et al. 1995; Li et al. 1997). The model attempts to mimic the reduced sodium pump activity that has been reported in bipolar illness, not changes in endogenous ouabain. The outcome of both a deficiency of endogenous ouabain (which is expected to increase Na, K-ATPase activity), or an excess of exogenous ouabain (which reduces Na, K-ATPase activity), would be expected to be the same—a reduction in sodium pump activity.

However, there are animal models of depression that suggest that reducing sodium pump activity may be antidepressive. Specifically, ICV administration of anti-ouabain antibodies to normal rats has been shown to reduce depressive behaviors (Goldstein et al. 2006). Additionally, in animal models of depression such as Flinders Sensitive Line of genetically sensitized rats to diisopropyl fluorophosphate (DFP, which inhibit organophosphorus cholinesterase (Overstreet 1993)), or lipopolysaccharide-treated rats, treatment with ICV anti-ouabain antibodies also improves depressive symptoms (Goldstein et al. 2006, 2012). Similarly, a three-fold increase of brain endogenous glycoside occurs in the amphetamine model of mania, but the hyperactivity is prevented with ICV administration of anti-ouabain antibodies (Hodes et al. 2016).

It is not clear which brain area and how many degrees of the reduction of sodium pump activity are associated with manic or depressive behaviors.

### Endogenous ouabain aberration in bipolar disorder subjects

Before the discovery of the sodium pump in 1957, John Cade in Australia described the antimanic effect of lithium treatment (Cade 1949). By the mid-1950s the efficacy of lithium treatment had been well-established in Europe (Schou et al. 1954; Rice 1956). This created an initial focus on ion regulation in bipolar illness and led to early studies in this area. Most importantly were a large number of studies that documented a mood-state related reduction in sodium pump activity (Looney and El-Mallakh 1997). These changes were seen in both bipolar depression and mania. Furthermore, whole body intracellular sodium was also increased in both mania and depression and normalizes with treatment or euthymia (Coppen et al. 1966; Shaw 1966; Coppen 1967). Since intracellular sodium concentration is a major determinant of intracellular calcium concentrations (Blaustein 1993), it is not surprising that free intracellular calcium is also elevated in mania and normalizes with treatment or euthymia (Dubovsky et al. 1989, 1992). Postmortem brain studies of the sodium pump in patients with bipolar illness report that the expression of the α2 isoform is reduced in the temporal cortex of patients with bipolar illness compared to non-bipolar controls (Rose et al. 1998), and the expression of the α3 subunit is increased overall but reduced in GABAergic neurons in several brain regions of patients with bipolar illness versus non-psychiatrically ill controls (Hodes et al. 2019). There are specific haplotypes of the α2 subunit that have been associated with bipolar illness in a small sample of unrelated subjects (Goldstein et al. 2009). In the periphery, regulation of the α1 of both red cells (Looney and El-Mallakh 1997; Nurnberger et al. 1982) and immortalized white cells (Huff et al. 2010; Li and El-Mallakh 2004; Cherry and Swann 1994) is impaired in bipolar individuals. These findings served as some of the basis of the Na, K-ATPase hypothesis for bipolar illness, in which it is proposed that increases of these ions depolarized neurons and make them more likely to fire and lead to mania, while more substantial increases of intracellular sodium would lead to depolarization block and depression (El-Mallakh and Wyatt 1995). Genetic associations to both the α1 and α3 subunit genes of the Na, K-ATPase have been reported (Goldstein et al. 2009; Mynett-Johnson et al. 1998), but have not been reliably reported (Philibert et al. 2001). The later study examined a population of Old Order Amish individuals that have been genetically isolated for nearly two centuries (Philibert et al. 2001; Crowley 1978). Animal models, which can be used to test hypotheses, reveal that heterozygote α2 knockout (KO) mice may have a partial manic-like picture [108, but heterozygote α3 KO mice have a more complete bipolar-like picture with both manic (Kirshenbaum et al. 2011a, 2014, 2011b). These data are compatible with the interpretation that the decline of sodium pump activity associated with abnormal moods in bipolar patients is secondary to another process, such as differential elaboration of endogenous ouabain.

A non-specific antibody for endogenous glycosides was used to demonstrate that these agents are present in reduced concentrations in manic individuals versus normal controls (Li and El-Mallakh 2004). Furthermore, subjects with bipolar illness lacked the seasonal variation in circulating glycosides found in controls (low in winter and higher during the rest of the year), with similar levels during winter (the most stable time for bipolar patients) but lower levels for the rest of the year (Li and El-Mallakh 2004). These findings suggested that bipolar illness may be characterized by inability to upregulate endogenous ouabain production in response to environmental needs. Since endogenous glycoside synthesis is known to increase in response to exercise to exhaustion (Valdes et al. 1988), an experiment was performed with bipolar patients and non-athletic controls. Euthymic patients with bipolar illness did not increase endogenous ouabain levels when exercised to exhaustion compared to non-bipolar controls (El-Mallakh et al. 2010). This may have led to a reduced exercise duration of patients with bipolar illness (Cherry and Swann 1994). All of these measures were in peripheral blood; in postmortem brain tissue, endogenous glycoside levels were higher in the parietal cortex of patients who had bipolar illness compared to those with major depressive disorder and non-mentally ill controls, but not compared to those with schizophrenia (Goldstein et al. 2006). However, tissue measurements are limited by the fact that they are expressed per unit amount of protein, and so endogenous glycosides may appear higher in a group of patients whose illness manifests in tissue loss (Mynett-Johnson et al. 1998). Moreover, different brain tissues may have different affinity of endogenous ouabain binding, also it is possible that endogenous ouabain concentration of brain and peripheral blood may not synchronously change.

Release of endogenous ouabain from the adrenals appears to be under the control of adrenocortical trophic hormone (ACTH) (Philibert et al. 2001; Crowley 1978). Hypothalamic-pituitary axis (HPA) disruption is associated with ill phases of bipolar illness (Belvederi Murri et al. 2016) as are stressors that may predispose to affective recurrence, such as sleep deprivation (Gao et al. 2013). Sleep deprivation in mice is associated with increased corticosterone and endogenous ouabain (Gao et al. 2013). Similarly, experimental sleep deprivation increases cortisol levels and manic symptoms in men (Kirshenbaum et al. 2014). Even 24 h of sleep deprivation is enough to increase serum cortisol (Kirshenbaum et al. 2011b; Grider et al. 1999; Shah et al. 2007), though this finding is not universal (Moorhead et al. 2007). Rats that receive anti-ouabain antibodies microinjections into the locus coeruleus have a significant reduction in rapid eye movement (REM) sleep (Goto et al. 1996). Conversely, rats undergoing REM deprivation had a decrease in affinity to ouabain (Hinson et al. 1998). ICV ouabain enhanced wakefulness in rats (Gao et al. 2017) which is consistent with its manic-like effects (El-Mallakh et al. 2003, 1995; Hamid et al. 2009; Li et al. 1997), but did not induce any other lasting changes. No studies measuring endogenous glycosides in humans after sleep deprivation have been performed. However, it is expected that circulating endogenous ouabain would increase parallel to cortisol in humans. If observations that individuals with bipolar illness are unable to upregulate endogenous ouabain in response to need are correct, then one would predict, that sleep deprivation in bipolar subjects would not result in endogenous ouabain secretion.

### Proposed endogenous ouabain model of pathogenesis of bipolar disorder

Endogenous ouabain has the highest affinity of all the endogenous glycosides to the α3 isoform of the sodium pump. The α3 isoform has its greatest distribution in neurons in the central nervous system. At physiologic concentrations, endogenous ouabain increases sodium pump activity, and may or may not activate cellular signaling through the α1 isoform receptor. Under certain circumstances that include season of year and exhaustive exercise (and possibly sleep deprivation), endogenous ouabain levels increase in non-bipolar subjects, but do not appear to respond in people with bipolar illness (Fig. 1). The hypothesis argues that these are stressors in which increased sodium pump activity is needed, and since physiologic concentrations of endogenous ouabain increase pump activity, increased ouabain production is needed to deal with the stress. Patients with bipolar illness are not able to upregulate endogenous ouabain production, and so enter the stress with a relative deficiency of endogenous ouabain, resulting in a relative reduction in sodium pump activity, and excessively depolarized resting potential, and expected abnormalities in neural function that result in both mania and bipolar depression.

## Conclusions

Recent work has highlighted the potential role of endogenous glycosides, particularly endogenous ouabain-like factor, in the pathophysiology and possible pathogenesis of bipolar illness. It is purported that individuals with bipolar disorder appear to be unable to upregulate endogenous ouabain under conditions mandating the action of that hormone. This leaves patients with neural tissues that is unable to maintain adequate depolarization, and leads to symptoms of mania or bipolar depression. Nearly all available data currently support this model, but additional studies are required to solidify the role of this system. Endogenous ouabain dysregulation appears to be a reasonable candidate for understanding the pathophysiology of bipolar disorder.

**Abbreviations**

ACTH: Adrenocortical trophic hormone; AKT: Protein kinase B; ATP: Adenosine triphosphatase; DFP: Diisopropyl fluorophosphate; ERK: Extracellular signal-regulated kinase; GABA: Gamma-Aminobutyric acid,; HPA: Hypothalamic-pituitary axis; ICV: Intracerebroventricular; Na,K-ATPase: Sodium- and potassium-activated adenosine triphosphatase; NFkB: Nuclear factor kappa-light-chain-enhancer of activated B cells; NHE1: Sodium-proton exchanger 1; MAPK: Mitogen-activated protein kinase.

**Acknowledgements**

None.

**Authors' contributions**

RSE-M performed the literature search, and most of the writing and final editing. YG was involved in the synthesis of the findings and providing her expertise on sodium homeostasis and second messenger signaling. PY performed his own literature search and screening of articles for inclusion into the review. He was involved in the writing and editing of the manuscript.

**Author details**

[1] Mood Disorders Research Program, Depression Center, Department of Psychiatry and Behavioral Sciences, University of Louisville School of Medicine, 401 East Chestnut Street, Suite 610, Louisville, KY 40202, USA. [2] Xiamen Xianyue Hospital, 399 Xianyue Road, Xiamen, China.

**References**

Abdelfatah S, Lu X, Schmeda-Hirschmann G, Efferth T. Cytotoxicity and antimitotic activity of *Rhinella schneideri* and *Rhinella marina* venoms. J Ethnopharmacol. 2019;242:112049. https://doi.org/10.1016/j.jep.2019.112049.

Antolovic R, Kost H, Mohadjerani M, Linder D, Linder M, Schoner W. A specific binding protein for cardiac glycosides exists in bovine serum. J Biol Chem. 1998;273(26):16259–64.

Antolovic R, Bauer N, Mohadjerani M, Kost H, Neu H, Kirch U, Grünbaum EG, Schoner W. Endogenous ouabain and its binding globulin: effects of physical exercise and study on the globulin's tissue distribution. Hypertens Res. 2000;23(Suppl):S93–8.

Askland KD. Toward a biaxial model of "bipolar" affective disorders: further exploration of genetic, molecular and cellular substrates. J Affect Disord. 2006;94(1–3):35–66.

Baecher S, Kroiss M, Fassnacht M, Vogeser M. No endogenous ouabain is detectable in human plasma by ultra-sensitive UPLC-MS/MS. Clin Chim Acta. 2014;431:87–92. https://doi.org/10.1016/j.cca.2014.01.038.

Balasubramaniam SL, Gopalakrishnapillai A, Gangadharan V, Duncan RL, Barwe SP. Sodium-calcium exchanger 1 regulates epithelial cell migration via calcium-dependent extracellular signal-regulated kinase signaling. J Biol Chem. 2015;290(20):12463–73. https://doi.org/10.1074/jbc.M114.629519.

Balzan S, D'Urso G, Nicolini G, Forini F, Pellegrino M, Montali U. Erythrocyte sodium pump stimulation by ouabain and an endogenous ouabain-like factor. Cell Biochem Funct. 2007;25(3):297–303. https://doi.org/10.1002/cbf.1387.

Beasley CL, Honer WG, Bergmann K, Falkai P, Lütjohann D, Bayer TA. Reductions in cholesterol and synaptic markers in association cortex in mood disorders. Bipolar Disord. 2005;7(5):449–55. https://doi.org/10.1111/j.1399-5618.2005.00239.x.

Belvederi Murri M, Prestia D, Mondelli V, Pariante C, Patti S, Olivieri B, Arzani C, Masotti M, Respino M, Antonioli M, Vassallo L, Serafini G, Perna G, Pompili M, Amore M. The HPA axis in bipolar disorder: systematic review and meta-analysis. Psychoneuroendocrinology. 2016;63:327–42. https://doi.org/10.1016/j.psyneuen.2015.10.014.

Blaustein MP. Physiological effects of endogenous ouabain: control of intracellular $Ca^{2+}$ stores and cell responsiveness. Am J Physiol. 1993;264(6 Pt 1):C1367–87.

Blaustein MP. The pump, the exchanger, and the holy spirit: Origins and 40-year evolution of ideas about the ouabain-$Na^{+}$ pump endocrine system. Am J Physiol Cell Physiol. 2018;314(1):C3–26. https://doi.org/10.1152/ajpcell.00196.2017

Butler VP Jr, Morris JF, Akizawa T, Matsukawa M, Keating P, Hardart A, Furman I. Heterogeneity and lability of endogenous digitalis-like substances in the plasma of the toad, *Bufo marinus*. Am J Physiol. 1996;271(2 Pt 2):R325–32.

Cade JF. Lithium salts in the treatment of psychotic excitement. Med J Aust. 1949;2(10):349–52.

Chen G, Manji HK. The extracellular signal-regulated kinase pathway: an emerging promising target for mood stabilizers. Curr Opin Psychiatry. 2006;19(3):313–23.

Cherry L, Swann AC. Cation transport mediated by Na+, K(+)-adenosine triphosphatase in lymphoblastoma cells from patients with bipolar I disorder, their relatives, and unrelated control subjects. Psychiatry Res. 1994;53(2):111–8. https://doi.org/10.1016/0165-1781(94)90102-3.

Cipriani G, Danti S, Carlesi C, Cammisuli DM, Di Fiorino M. Bipolar disorder and cognitive dysfunction: a complex link. J Nerv Ment Dis. 2017;205(10):743–56. https://doi.org/10.1097/NMD.0000000000000720.

Clausen MV, Hilbers F, Poulsen H. The structure and function of the Na, K-ATPase isoforms in health and disease. Front Physiol. 2017;8:371. https://doi.org/10.3389/fphys.2017.00371.

Clemente AS, Diniz BS, Nicolato R, Kapczinski FP, Soares JC, Firmo JO, Castro-Costa É. Bipolar disorder prevalence: a systematic review and meta-analysis of the literature. Braz J Psychiatry. 2015;37(2):155–61. https://doi.org/10.1590/1516-4446-2012-1693.

Coppen A. The biochemistry of affective disorders. Br J Psychiatry. 1967;113(504):1237–64.

Coppen A, Shaw DM, Malleson A, Costain R. Mineral metabolism in mania. Br Med J. 1966;1(5479):71–5.

Crowley WK. Old Order Amish settlement: diffusion and growth. Ann Assoc Am Geographers. 1978;68(2):250–1. https://doi.org/10.1111/j.1467-8306.1978.tb01194.x.

Cui X, Xie Z. Protein interaction and Na/K-ATPase-mediated signal transduction. Molecules. 2017;22(6):990. https://doi.org/10.3390/molecules22060990.

Dome P, Rihmer Z, Gonda X. Suicide risk in bipolar disorder: a brief review. Medicina. 2019;55(8):E403. https://doi.org/10.3390/medicina55080403.

Dubovsky SL, Christiano J, Daniell LC, Franks RD, Murphy J, Adler L, Baker N, Harris RA. Increased platelet intracellular calcium concentration in patients with bipolar affective disorders. Arch Gen Psychiatry. 1989;46(7):632–8.

Dubovsky SL, Murphy J, Thomas M, Rademacher J. Abnormal intracellular calcium ion concentration in platelets and lymphocytes of bipolar patients. Am J Psychiatry. 1992;149(1):118–20.

Dvela M, Rosen H, Feldmann T, Nesher M, Lichtstein D. Diverse biological responses to different cardiotonic steroids. Pathophysiology. 2007;14(3–4):159–66. https://doi.org/10.1016/j.pathophys.2007.09.011.

Dvela M, Rosen H, Ben-Ami HC, Lichtstein D. Endogenous ouabain regulates cell viability. Am J Physiol Cell Physiol. 2012;302:C442–52.

Dvela-Levitt M, Ben-Ami HC, Rosen H, Ornoy A, Hochner-Celnikier D, Granat M, Lichtstein D. Reduction in maternal circulating ouabain impairs offspring growth and kidney development. J Am Soc Nephrol. 2015;26(5):1103–14.

El-Mallakh RS, Huff MO. Mood stabilizers and ion regulation. Harv Rev Psychiatry. 2001;9:23–32.

El-Mallakh RS, Paskitti ME. The ketogenic diet may have mood-stabilizing properties. Med Hypoth. 2001;57:724–6.

El-Mallakh RS, Wyatt RJ. The Na, K-ATPase hypothesis for bipolar illness. Biol Psychiatry. 1995;37:235–44.

El-Mallakh RS, Yff T, Gao Y. Ion Dysregulation in the pathogenesis of bipolar illness. Ann Depress Anxiety 2016;3(1):1076. https://austinpublishinggroup.com/depression-anxiety/fulltext/depression-v3-id1076.php.

El-Mallakh RS, Harrison LT, Li R, Changaris DG, Levy RS. An animal model for mania: preliminary results. Prog Neuro-Psychopharmacol Biol Psychiatry. 1995;19:955–62.

El-Mallakh RS, El-Masri MA, Huff MO, Li X-P, Decker S, Levy RS. Intracerebroventricular administration of ouabain to rats models human mania. Bipolar Disord. 2003;5:362–5.

El-Mallakh RS, Stoddard M, Jortani SA, El-Masri MA, Sephton S, Valdes R Jr. Aberrant regulation of endogenous ouabain-like factor in bipolar subjects. Psychiatry Res. 2010;178(1):116–20.

El-Mallakh RS, Brar KS, Yeruva RR. Cardiac glycosides in human physiology and disease: update for entomologists. Insects. 2019;10:102. https://doi.org/10.3390/insects10040102.

El-Masri MA, Clark BJ, Qazzaz HM, Valdes R Jr. Human adrenal cells in culture produce both ouabain-like and dihydroouabain-like factors. Clin Chem. 2002;48(10):1720–30.

Feraille E, Doucet A. Sodium-potassium-adenosine triphosphatase-dependent sodium transport in the kidney: Hormonal control. Physiol Rev. 2001;81:345–418.

Fineberg NA, Chamberlain SR, Hollander E, Boulougouris V, Robbins TW. Translational approaches to obsessive-compulsive disorder: from animal models to clinical treatment. Br J Pharmacol. 2011;164(4):1044–61. https://doi.org/10.1111/j.1476-5381.2011.01422.x.

Fürstenwerth H. Comment on endogenous ouabain and related genes in the translation from hypertension to renal diseases, International Journal of Molecular Science 2018;19:1948. Int J Mol Sci. 2019;20:505. https://doi.org/10.3390/ijms20030505.

Gao J, Wymore RS, Wang Y, Gaudette GR, Krukenkamp IB, Cohen IS, Mathias RT. Isoform-specific stimulation of cardiac Na/K pumps by nanomolar concentrations of glycosides. J Gen Physiol. 2002;119:297–312.

Gao Y, Jhaveri M, Lei Z, Chaneb BL, Lingrel J, El-Mallakh RS. Glial-specific gene alterations associated with manic behaviors. Int J Bipolar Disord. 2013;1(1):33. https://doi.org/10.1186/2194-7511-1-20.

Gao Y, Akers B, Roberts MB, El-Mallakh RS. Corticosterone response in sleep deprivation and sleep fragmentation. J Sleep Disord Manage. 2017;3:018. https://doi.org/10.23937/2572-4053.1510018.

GeneCards Human Gene Database. https://www.genecards.org/Search/Keyword?queryString=atp1a1. Accessed 10 Oct 2020.

Geering K. Function of FXYD proteins, regulators of Na. K-ATPase J Bioenerg Biomembr. 2005;2005(37):387–92. https://doi.org/10.1007/s10863-005-9476-x.

George MS, Guidotti A, Rubinow D, Pan B, Mikalauskas K, Post RM. CSF neuroactive steroids in affective disorders: pregnenolone, progesterone, and DBI. Biol Psychiatry. 1994;35(10):775–80. https://doi.org/10.1016/0006-3223(94)91139-8.

Ghilardi SJ, O'Reilly BM, Sgro AE. Intracellular signaling dynamics and their role in coordinating tissue repair. Wiley Interdiscip Rev Syst Biol Med. 2020;12(3):e1479. https://doi.org/10.1002/wsbm.1479.

Ghysel-Burton J, Godfraind T. Stimulation and inhibition of the sodium pump by cardioactive steroids in relation to their binding sites and their inotropic effects on guinea-pig isolated atria. Br J Pharmacol. 1979;66:175–84.

Goldstein I, Levy T, Galili D, Ovadia H, Yirmiya R, Rosen H, Lichtstein D. Involvement of $Na^+$, $K^+$-ATPase and endogenous digitalis-like compounds in depressive disorders. Biol Psychiatry. 2006;60(5):491–9.

Goldstein I, Lerer E, Laiba E, Mallet J, Mujaheed M, Laurent C, Rosen H, Ebstein RP, Lichtstein D. Association between sodium- and potassium-activated adenosine triphosphatase alpha isoforms and bipolar disorders. Biol Psychiatry. 2009;65(11):985–91.

Goldstein I, Lax E, Gispan-Herman I, Ovadia H, Rosen H, Yadid G, Lichtstein D. Neutralization of endogenous digitalis-like compounds alters catecholamines metabolism in the brain and elicits anti-depressive behavior. Eur Neuropsychopharmacol. 2012;22(1):72–9.

Goto A, Yamada K, Ishii M, Yoshioka M, Ishiguro T, Eguchi C, Sugimoto T. Existence of a polar digitalis-like factor in mammalian hypothalamus. Biochem Biophys Res Commun. 1989;161(3):953–8.

Goto A, Yamada K, Hazama H, Uehara Y, Atarashi K, Hirata Y, Kimura K, Omata M. Ouabain like compound in hypertension associated with ectopic corticotropin syndrome. Hypertension. 1996;28:421–5.

Grande I, Berk M, Birmaher B, Vieta E. Bipolar disorder. Lancet. 2016;387(10027):1561–72. https://doi.org/10.1016/S0140-6736(15)00241-X.

Grider G, El-Mallakh RS, Huff MO, Buss TJR, Miller J, Valdes R Jr. Endogenous digoxin-like immunoreactive factor (DLIF) serum concentrations are decreased in manic bipolar patients compared to normal controls. J Affect Disord. 1999;54:261–7.

Hamid H, Gao Y, Lei Z, Hougland MT, El-Mallakh RS. Effect of ouabain on sodium pump alpha-isoform expression in an animal model of mania. Prog Neuro Psychopharmacol Biol Psychiatry. 2009;33(7):1103–6.

Hamlyn JM, Manunta P. Endogenous ouabain: a link between sodium intake and hypertension. Curr Hyperten Rep. 2011;13(1):14–20. https://doi.org/10.1007/s11906-010-0161-z.

Hamlyn JM, Blaustein MP, Bova S, DuCharme DW, Harris DW, Mandel F, Mathews WR, Ludens JH. Identification and characterization of a ouabain-like compound from human plasma. Proc Natl Acad Sci USA. 1991;88(14):6259–6263. Erratum in: Proc Natl Acad Sci USA 1991;88(21):9907.

Hinson JP, Harwood S, Dawnay AB. Release of ouabain-like compound (OLC) from the intact perfused rat adrenal gland. Endocr Res. 1998;24(3–4):721–4. https://doi.org/10.3109/07435809809032675.

Hodes A, Rosen H, Deutsch J, Lifschytz T, Einat H, Lichtstein D. Endogenous cardiac steroids in animal models of mania. Bipolar Disord. 2016;18:451–9. https://doi.org/10.1111/bdi.12413.

Hodes A, Rosen H, Cohen-Ben Ami H, Lichtstein D. $Na^+$, $^K$+-ATPase a3 isoform in frontal cortex GABAergic neurons in psychiatric diseases. J Psychiatr Res. 2019;115:21–8. https://doi.org/10.1016/j.jpsychires.2019.04.014.

Holthouser KA, Mandal A, Merchant ML, Schelling JR, Delamere NA, Valdes R Jr, Tyagi SC, Lederer ED, Khundmiri SJ. Ouabain stimulates Na-K-ATPase through a sodium/hydrogen exchanger-1 (NHE-1)-dependent mechanism in human kidney proximal tubule cells. Am J Physiol Renal Physiol. 2010;299(1):F77–90. https://doi.org/10.1152/ajprenal.00581.2009.

Huang BS, Kudlac M, Kumarathasan R, Leenen FH. Digoxin prevents ouabain and high salt intake-induced hypertension in rats with sinoaortic denervation. Hypertension. 1999;34:733–8.

Huff MO, Li XP, Ginns E, El-Mallakh RS. Effect of ethacrynic acid on the sodium- and potassium-activated adenosine triphosphatase activity and expression in Old Order Amish bipolar individuals. J Affect Disord. 2010;123(1–3):303–7. https://doi.org/10.1016/j.jad.2009.09.018.

Judy JT, Zandi PP. A review of potassium channels in bipolar disorder. Front Genet. 2013;4:105. https://doi.org/10.3389/fgene.2013.00105.

Kaul S, Ahmed M, Zargar K, Sharma P, Dhar MK. Prospecting endophytic fungal assemblage of *Digitalis lanata* Ehrh. (foxglove) as a novel source of digoxin: a cardiac glycoside. 3 Biotech. 2013;3(4):335–40. https://doi.org/10.1007/s13205-012-0106-0.

Ketter TA, Calabrese JR. Stabilization of mood from below versus above baseline in bipolar disorder: a new nomenclature. J Clin Psychiatry. 2002;63(2):146–51.

Khundmiri SJ, Amin V, Henson J, Lewis J, Ameen M, Rane MJ, Delamere NA. Ouabain stimulates protein kinase B (Akt) phosphorylation in opossum kidney proximal tubule cells through an ERK-dependent pathway. Am J Physiol Cell Physiol. 2007;293(3):C1171–80.

Khundmiri SJ, Ameen M, Delamere NA, Lederer ED. PTH-mediated regulation of $Na^+$-$K^+$-ATPase requires Src kinase-dependent ERK phosphorylation. Am J Physiol Renal Physiol. 2008;295(2):F426–37.

Kim EK, Choi E-J. Pathological roles of MAPK signaling pathways in human diseases. Biochim Biophys Acta. 2010;1802(4):396–405. https://doi.org/10.1016/j.bbadis.2009.12.009.

Kinoshita PF, Yshii LM, Orellana AMM, Paixão AG, Vasconcelos AR, de Sá Lima L, Kawamoto EM, Scavone C. Alpha 2 Na+, K+-ATPase silencing induces loss of inflammatory response and ouabain protection in glial cells. Sci Rep. 2017;7:4894. https://doi.org/10.1038/s41598-017-05075-9.

Kirshenbaum GS, Clapcote SJ, Duffy S, Burgess CR, Petersen J, Jarowek KJ, Yücel YH, Cortez MA, Snead OC 3rd, Vilsen B, Peever JH, Ralph MR, Roder JC. Mania-like behavior induced by genetic dysfunction of the neuron-specific $Na^+$, $^K$+-ATPase a3 sodium pump. Proc Natl Acad Sci USA. 2011a;108(44):18144–9. https://doi.org/10.1073/pnas.1108416108.

Kirshenbaum GS, Saltzman K, Rose B, Petersen J, Vilsen B, Roder JC. Decreased neuronal $Na^+$, $^K$+-ATPase activity in *Atp1a3* heterozygous mice increases susceptibility to depression-like endophenotypes by chronic variable stress. Genes Brain Behav. 2011b;10(5):542–50. https://doi.org/10.1111/j.1601-183X.2011.00691.x.

Kirshenbaum GS, Burgess CR, Déry N, Fahnestock M, Peever JH, Roder JC. Attenuation of mania-like behavior in $Na^+$, $^K$+-ATPase a3 mutant mice by prospective therapies for bipolar disorder: Melatonin and exercise. Neuroscience. 2014;260:195–204. https://doi.org/10.1016/j.neuroscience.2013.12.011.

Komiyama Y, Nishimura N, Dong XH, Hirose S, Kosaka C, Masaki H, Masuda M, Takahashi H. Liquid chromatography mass spectrometric analysis of ouabain like factor in biological fluid. Hypertens Res. 2000;23(Suppl):S21–7.

Krenn L, Kopp B. Bufadienolides from animal and plant sources. Phytochemistry. 1998;48(1):1–29.

Li R, El-Mallakh RS. Differential response of bipolar and normal control lymphoblastoid cell sodium pump to ethacrynic acid. J Affect Disord. 2004;80(1):11–7. https://doi.org/10.1016/S0165-0327(03)00044-2.

Li R, El-Mallakh RS, Harrison L, Changaris DG, Levy RS. Lithium prevents ouabain-induced behavioral changes: Toward an animal model for manic-depression. Mol Chem Neuropathol. 1997;31:65–72.

Liang M, Cai T, Tian J, Qu W, Xie ZJ. Functional characterization of Src-interacting Na/K-ATPase using RNA interference assay. J Biol Chem. 2006;281(28):19709–21919.

Lichtstein D, Samuelov S, Bourrit A. Characterization of the stimulation of neuronal $Na^+$, $K^+$-ATPase activity by low concentrations of ouabain. Neurochem Int. 1985;7(4):709–15. https://doi.org/10.1016/0197-0186(85)90069-5.

Lichtstein D, Gati I, Samuelov S, Berson D, Rozenman Y, Landau L, Deutsch J. Identification of digitalis-like compounds in human cataractous lenses. Eur J Biochem. 1993;216(1):261–8.

Lichtstein D, Steinitz M, Gati I, Samuelov S, Deutsch J, Orly J. Biosynthesis of digitalis-like compounds in rat adrenal cells: hydroxycholesterol as possible precursor. Life Sci. 1998;62(23):2109–26.

Lichtstein D, Ilani A, Rosen H, Horesh N, Singh SV, Buzaglo N, Hodes A. $Na^+$, $^K$+-ATPase signaling and bipolar disorder. Int J Mol Sci. 2018;19(8):2314. https://doi.org/10.3390/ijms19082314.

Looney SW, El-Mallakh RS. Meta-analysis of erythrocyte Na, K-ATPase activity in bipolar illness. Depres Anxiety. 1997;5:53–65.

Mack A, Gao Y, Kakar S, Ratajczak M, El-Mallakh RS. Review of animal models of bipolar disorder that alter ion regulation. Neurosci Biobehav Rev. 2019;107:208–14.

Madan N, Xu Y, Duan Q, Banerjee M, Larre I, Pierre SV, Xie Z. Src-independent ERK signaling through the rat α3 isoform of Na/K-ATPase. Am J Physiol Cell Physiol. 2017;312(3):C222–32.

Manunta P, Hamilton J, Rogowski AC, Hamilton BP, Hamlyn JM. Chronic hypertension induced by ouabain but not digoxin in the rat: antihypertensive effect of digoxin and digitoxin. Hypertens Res. 2000;23(suppl):S77–85.

Manunta P, Hamilton BP, Hamlyn JM. Salt intake and depletion increase circulating levels of endogenous ouabain in normal men. Am J Physiol Regul Integr Comp Physiol. 2006;290(3):R553–9.

Moorhead TWJ, McKirdy J, Sussmann JED, Hall J, Lawrie SM, Johnstone EC, Mcintosh AM. Progressive gray matter loss in patients with bipolar disorder. Biol Psychiatry. 2007;62(8):894–900. https://doi.org/10.1016/j.biopsych.2007.03.005.

Mynett-Johnson L, Murphy V, McCormack J, Shields DC, Claffey E, Manley P, McKeon P. Evidence for an allelic association between bipolar disorder and a $Na^+$, $K^+$ adenosine triphosphatase alpha subunit gene (*ATP1A3*). Biol Psychiatry. 1998;44(1):47–51.

Nestler EJ, Peña CJ, Kundakovic M, Mitchell A, Akbarian S. Epigenetic basis of mental illness. Neuroscientist. 2016;22(5):447–63. https://doi.org/10.1177/1073858415608147.

Noël F, Azalim P, do Monte FM, Quintas LEM, Katz A, Karlish SJD. Revisiting the binding kinetics and inhibitory potency of cardiac glycosides on Na+, K+-ATPase(α1β1): Methodological considerations. J Pharmacol Toxicol Methods. 2018;94(Pt 2):64–72. https://doi.org/10.1016/j.vascn.2018.09.001.

Norn S, Kruse PR. Cardiac glycosides: From ancient history through Withering's foxglove to endogeneous cardiac glycosides [Article in Danish]. Dan Medicinhist Arbog 2004:119–132.

Nurnberger J Jr, Jimerson DC, Allen JR, Simmons S, Gershon E. Red cell ouabain-sensitive Na+-K+-adenosine triphosphatase: a state marker in affective disorder inversely related to plasma cortisol. Biol Psychiatry. 1982;17(9):981–92.

Overstreet DH. The Flinders Sensitive Line Rats: A genetic animal model of depression. Neurosci Biobehav Rev. 1993;17(1):51–68. https://doi.org/10.1016/s0149-7634(05)80230-1.

Philibert RA, Cheung D, Welsh N, Damschroder-Williams P, Thiel B, Ginns EI, Gershenfeld HK. Absence of a significant linkage between $Na^+$, $^K$+-ATPase subunit (*ATP1A3* and *ATP1B3*) genotypes and bipolar affective disorder in the Old-Order Amish. Am J Med Genet. 2001;105(3):291–4.

Pierre SV, Sottejeau Y, Gourbeau JM, Sánchez G, Shidyak A, Blanco G. Isoform specificity of Na-K-ATPase-mediated ouabain signaling. Am J Physiol Renal Physiol. 2008;294(4):F859–66. https://doi.org/10.1152/ajprenal.00089.2007.

Rice D. The use of lithium salts in the treatment of manic states. J Ment Sci. 1956;102(428):604–11.

Roberts RJ, Repass R, El-Mallakh RS. Effect of dopamine on intracellular sodium: a common pathway for pharmacologic mechanism of action in bipolar illness. World J Biol Psychiatry. 2010;11(2 Pt 2):181–167.

Rose AM, Mellett BJ, Valdes R Jr, Kleinman JE, Hermann MM, Li R, El-Mallakh RS. Alpha2 isoform of the Na, K-ATPase is reduced in temporal cortex of bipolar individuals. Biol Psychiatry. 1998;44:892–7.

Rosenblat JD, McIntyre RS. Bipolar disorder and inflammation. Psychiatr Clin North Am. 2016;39(1):125–37. https://doi.org/10.1016/j.psc.2015.09.006.

Saunders R, Scheiner-Bobis G. Ouabain stimulates endothelin release and expression in human endothelial cells without inhibiting the sodium pump. Eur J Biochem. 2004;271(5):1054–62.

Schou M, Juel-Nielsen N, Stromgren E, Voldby H. The treatment of manic psychoses by the administration of lithium salts. J Neurol Neurosurg Psychiatry. 1954;17(4):250–60.

Schroeder E, Gao Y, Lei Z, Roisen F, El-Mallakh RS. The gene *BRAF* is underexpressed in bipolar subject olfactory neuroepithelial progenitor cells undergoing apoptosis. Psychiatry Res. 2016;236:130–5. https://doi.org/10.1016/j.psychres.2015.12.018.

Shah A, Alshaher M, Dawn B, Siddiqui T, Longaker RA, Stoddard MF, El-Mallakh RS. Exercise tolerance is reduced in bipolar illness. J Affect Disord. 2007;104(1–3):190–5.

Shaw DM. Mineral metabolism, mania, and melancholia. Br Med J. 1966;2(5508):262–7.

Skou JC. The influence of some cations on an adenosine triphosphatase from peripheral nerves. Biochim Biophys Acta. 1957;23(2):394–401. https://doi.org/10.1016/0006-3002(57)90343-8.

Takaesu Y. Circadian rhythm in bipolar disorder: A review of the literature. Psychiatry Clin Neurosci. 2018;72(9):673–82. https://doi.org/10.1111/pcn.12688.

Thomas SM, Brugge JS. Cellular functions regulated by Src family kinases. Annu Rev Cell Dev Biol. 1997;13:513–609.

Touza NA, Pôças ES, Quintas LE, Cunha-Filho G, Santos ML, Noël F. Inhibitory effect of combinations of digoxin and endogenous cardiotonic steroids on $Na^+/K^+$-ATPase activity in human kidney membrane preparation. Life Sci. 2011;88(1–2):39–42.

Valdes R Jr, Hagberg JM, Vaughan TE, Lau BWC, Seals DR, Ehsani AA. Endogenous digoxin-like immunoreactivity in blood is increased during prolonged strenuous exercise. Life Sci. 1988;42:103–10.

Valvassori SS, Dal-Pont GC, Resende WR, Varela RB, Lopes-Borges J, Cararo JH, Quevedo J. Validation of the animal model of bipolar disorder induced by Ouabain: face, construct and predictive perspectives. Transl Psychiatry. 2019;9(1):158. https://doi.org/10.1038/s41398-019-0494-6.

Yuan P, Zhou R, Wang Y, Li X, Li J, Chen G, Guitart X, Manji HK. Altered levels of extracellular signal-regulated kinase signaling proteins in post- mortem frontal cortex of individuals with mood disorders and schizophrenia. J Affect Disord. 2010;124(1–2):164–9.

6

# Deficits in explicit emotion regulation in bipolar disorder

Marcel Kurtz[1*], Pia Mohring[1], Katharina Förster[1], Michael Bauer[2] and Philipp Kanske[1,3]

**Abstract**

**Background:** This study aimed to compile and synthesize studies investigating explicit emotion regulation in patients with bipolar disorder and individuals at risk of developing bipolar disorder. The importance of explicit emotion regulation arises from its potential role as a marker for bipolar disorders in individuals at risk and its potent role in therapy for bipolar disorder patients.

**Methods:** To obtain an exhaustive compilation of studies dealing specifically with explicit emotion regulation in bipolar disorder, we conducted a systematic literature search in four databases. In the 15 studies we included in our review, the emotion-regulation strategies *maintenance*, *distraction*, and *reappraisal* (self-focused and situation-focused) were investigated partly on a purely behavioral level and partly in conjunction with neural measures. The samples used in the identified studies included individuals at increased risk of bipolar disorder, patients with current affective episodes, and patients with euthymic mood state.

**Results:** In summary, the reviewed studies' results indicate impairments in explicit emotion regulation in individuals at risk for bipolar disorder, patients with manic and depressive episodes, and euthymic patients. These deficits manifest in subjective behavioral measures as well as in neural aberrations. Further, our review reveals a discrepancy between behavioral and neural findings regarding explicit emotion regulation in individuals at risk for bipolar disorders and euthymic patients. While these groups often do not differ significantly in behavioral measures from healthy and low-risk individuals, neural differences are mainly found in frontostriatal networks.

**Conclusion:** We conclude that these neural aberrations are a potentially sensitive measure of the probability of occurrence and recurrence of symptoms of bipolar disorders and that strengthening this frontostriatal route is a potentially protective measure for individuals at risk and patients who have bipolar disorders.

**Keywords:** Explicit emotion regulation, Bipolar disorder, Systematic review, Frontostriatal network, Reappraisal

## Background

The primary characteristics of bipolar disorders (BD) are aberrations of mood and emotion (American Psychiatric Association 2013; Gruber 2011; Phillips 2003; Townsend and Altshuler 2012). These aberrations manifest in episodes of euphoric and excessively elevated mood (i.e., manic and hypomanic episodes), with manic episodes indicating type 1 bipolar disorder (BD-I) and hypomanic episodes indicating type 2 (BD-II). Typically, episodes of excessive negative affect (i.e., depressive episodes) accompany both types of BD. Further, patients with BD exhibit aberrations in the processing of emotional stimuli (Mercer and Becerra 2013; Rosen and Rich 2010; Townsend and Altshuler 2012; Wessa et al. 2014; Wessa and Linke 2009), which are at least partly due to deficits in the regulation of emotions (Aldao et al. 2010; Dodd et al. 2019; Green et al. 2011; Gruber et al. 2013b; Phillips 2003; Phillips et al. 2008; Townsend and Altshuler, 2012). Deviations in patients with BD occur in everyday, spontaneous, and automatic ER (i.e., implicit

*Correspondence: marcel.kurtz@tu-dresden.de
[1] Clinical Psychology and Behavioral Neuroscience, Faculty of Psychology, Technische Universität Dresden, Chemnitzer Str. 46, 01187 Dresden, Germany
Full list of author information is available at the end of the article

ER) and explicit ER, which describes conscious, planned processes. Explicit ER is trainable and can be volitionally integrated into everyday life and is therefore of particular interest because of its high potential as a treatment target in therapeutic intervention. Because of this potential, our aim in the present article is to review and integrate studies that investigate explicit ER in BD. Furthermore, as recent studies addressed the neural correlates of such explicit ER, we also aim to summarize this literature to conclude implications for the treatment of BD and identify open questions regarding the neural processes underlying different ER strategies.

## Rational

ER denotes processes that enable us to modulate the experience and the expression of our emotions (Gross 1998b). Strategies of ER have been classified, for instance, according to their explicitness (Phillips et al. 2008), motivational aspects (Koole, 2009), or the chronological order of regulation (Gross 1998a, 1998b, 2013, 2015).

### *Antecedent-focused and response-focused emotion regulation*

The influential classification of Gross (1998a) distinguishes two categories, depending on whether the regulation of emotions takes place in anticipation of, or response to, emotions.

Antecedent-focused regulation strategies involve selecting and modifying the situation in which we experience emotions and modify emotions via cognition (Gross 1998a, 2013; Phillips et al. 2008). Cognitive processes can be further differentiated into subprocesses on a continuum between pure attentional processes and processes of cognitive change (Ochsner and Gross, 2005). An example of an attentional strategy is *distraction,* which describes the detachment of attention from a stimulus that evokes emotions to other, non-emotional aspects of the situation, away from the situation entirely, or non-emotional thoughts (Gross, 2013). In contrast to simple attentional processes, cognitive change includes higher cognitive abilities that lead to an alternative evaluation of a situation that evokes emotions. Cognitive change can either be caused by concentrating on one's coping strategies or an alternative interpretation of the situation (i.e., reappraisal). Reappraisal can be further distinguished in self-focused and situation-focused reappraisal (Ochsner et al. 2004). While self-focused reappraisal describes the modification of the degree of personal involvement in an emotionally loaded situation, situation-focused reappraisal describes the reinterpretation of the situation itself.

Response-focused strategies include the suppression or alteration of behavioral, experiential, and physiological responses that accompany emotions. They further include processes that enable us to prolong or maintain the experience of emotions (Gross 1998b; Tugade and Fredrickson 2007). To accomplish emotion maintenance, an individual has to express the behavioral response associated with an emotion (Izard 1990), for example, yelling in case of anger. Further, an individual can maintain an emotion in a working-memory system specialized for emotions (Mikels et al. 2008). Notably, the listed ER strategies are not valence specific; both negative and positive emotions can be regulated.

### *Neural basis of emotion regulation*

Neurally, emotion regulation is accomplished through the interaction of two systems. (Ochsner and Gross 2014). One system is responsible for the experience and the contextual valuation of emotions, consisting of the amygdala, insula, ventral striatum, and medial areas of the prefrontal cortex (PFC). A control system acts on this system, consisting of the dorsal anterior cingulate cortex (dACC), dorsal posterior medial PFC, dorsolateral PFC (DLPFC), inferior parietal cortex, and ventrolateral prefrontal cortex (VLPFC). In part, specific cognitive processes are associated with specific areas within this network. For example, the DLPFC, the dorsal posterior mPFC, and the inferior parietal cortex are associated with the control of attention to relevant stimuli and the maintenance of goals during emotion regulation. The ventrolateral PFC is associated with inhibiting inappropriate behaviors, and the dACC is associated with monitoring conflicts between desirable and actual actions. For the involvement of most of the mentioned areas, meta-analytical evidence has been accumulated (Kohn et al. 2014). While the model of Ochsner and Gross (2014) is characterized by a high level of detail, including the attribution of cognitive processes to specific areas, it does not distinguish between explicit and implicit ER, concepts whose importance to ER more recently has been demonstrated and which are the focus of the next section.

### *Implicit and explicit emotion regulation*

In recent research, ER strategies have been classified according to how voluntarily they occur (Braunstein et al. 2017; Gross, 2013; Gyurak et al. 2011; Phillips et al. 2008). While implicit ER runs spontaneously, automatically, and unconsciously, explicit ER operates planned, consciously, and volitionally. A further distinction can be made between whether the goal of the ER is explicit or implicit and how automatic or controlled the ER process itself is (Braunstein et al. 2017). In the present review, we adhere to a strict definition of explicit ER in which both the goal of ER is explicit (which is ensured in experimental setups by instruction), and the required processes are controlled.

Explicit and implicit ER are further distinguishable by their demands on different neural networks. The neural model by Phillips et al. (2008) postulates a hierarchical organization of implicit and explicit ER (Fig. 1). On the lowest level, areas involved in emotion reactivity (i.e., ventral striatum, thalamus, and amygdala) are embedded in a network, together with areas involved in automatic ER (i.e., rostral anterior cingular cortex (rACC), subgenual anterior cingular cortex, orbitofrontal cortex (OFC), and a hippocampus-parahippocampus region). On the highest level, explicit ER is primarily realized by prefrontal areas (dorsolateral prefrontal cortex (DLPFC) and the ventrolateral prefrontal cortex (VLPFC)) but mediated by areas associated with implicit ER (such as the OFC) that, in turn, have direct connections to subcortical areas associated with emotion reactivity. According to the model, the dorsomedial prefrontal cortex (DMPFC) and dorsal anterior cingulate cortex fulfill functions in explicit and implicit ER.

In addition to the consideration of explicit and implicit ER, the model of Phillips et al. (2008) has the advantage that it includes findings on the ER of patients with bipolar disorders. Based on previous results (Elliott et al. 2004; Wessa et al. 2007), the researchers concluded that inefficient use of the DLPFC and VLPFC results in increased activity in these regions and is, thus, a probable cause for deficit regarding explicit ER in patients with BD. However, due to the model's hierarchical structure, aberrations in areas associated with implicit ER or emotion reactivity could also impair explicit ER. For this reason, an alternative explanation is that hyperactivity in DLPFC and VLPFC may represent a compensatory mechanism for aberrations in areas associated with implicit ER and emotion reactivity.

Taken together, the model of Phillips et al. (2008) provides essential insights into the neural basis of ER deficits in patients with BD. However, the model is based on only a few studies, especially for explicit ER, which leads to limitations since the results are derived from homogeneous samples and low diversity tasks.

Patients who have BD show aberrations not only at the neural level but also in the experience of emotions and associated behavior. Studies sampling experiences in everyday life found an increased frequency of attempts to regulate emotions in BD patients (Gruber et al. 2013b). However, these spontaneous emotion-regulation attempts are less successful compared to healthy subjects (Gruber et al. 2012), which is partly due to the more frequent use of maladaptive strategies (e.g., rumination) by patients with BD (Becerra et al. 2013; Dodd et al. 2019; Green et al. 2011; Gruber et al. 2012; Gruber et al. 2013b). Interestingly, in laboratory settings, differences

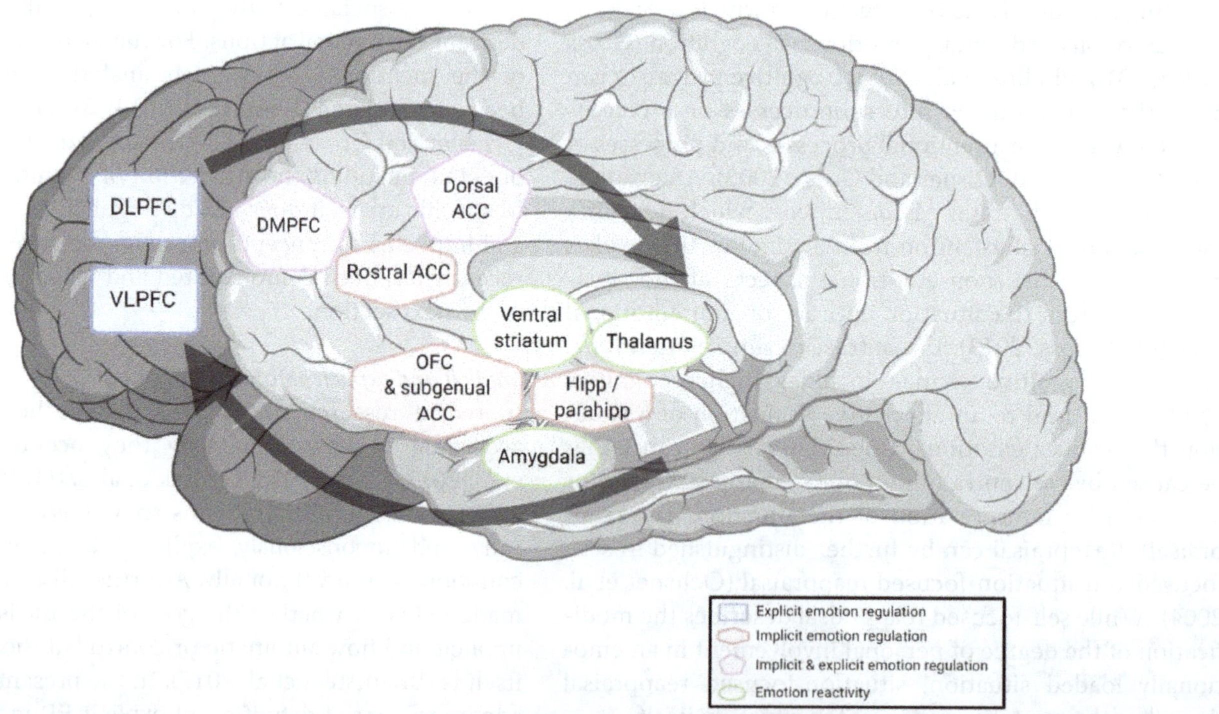


**Fig. 1** Simplified neural model of emotion regulation. Illustration of areas involved in emotion reactivity, implicit emotion regulation, and explicit emotion regulation. Black arrows indicate feedforward and feedback mechanisms of these subsystems. Adapted from "A neural model of voluntary and automatic emotion regulation: implications for understanding the pathophysiology and neurodevelopment of bipolar disorder" by Phillips et al. (2008). Created with BioRender.com

between BD patients and healthy controls (HC) are less pronounced (Dodd et al. 2019). A possible explanation for this phenomenon could be that participants in laboratory settings are often explicitly instructed to use ER; that is, they initiate ER voluntarily, which could positively affect their success. This positive effect makes explicit ER strategies an exciting topic for research as explicit ER strategies might be a resource to build on in psychotherapeutic interventions.

### Objectives

Contrary to implicit processes, which are difficult to influence by an individual, explicit ER strategies allow for the volitional integration into everyday life. Most importantly, it has been pointed out that implicit ER processes can be altered via extensive training of explicit ER (Denny and Ochsner 2014; Gyurak et al. 2011). Due to training, explicit ER may then become habitual, implicit, and automatic. This hypothesis is supported by findings that suggest an overlap of the neural circuits underlying explicit and implicit ER (Phillips et al. 2008). In summary, due to their trainability, explicit ER strategies are of particular interest in the development of therapeutic approaches and interventions related to ER in BD.

Recent studies also stress the importance of early detection of BD risk in individuals for early intervention and prophylactic treatment (Malhi et al. 2017; Almeida and Phillips 2013; Phillips and Kupfer 2013). For this topic, studies investigating explicit ER in risk groups could be particularly revealing since risk groups may have ER aberrations even before the development of BD, making explicit ER a potential marker for early detection of the disorder. In contrast to this trait marker hypothesis (Rohde et al. 1990), the scar hypothesis (Rohde et al. 1990) claims that impairments in ER of BD patients are more likely a consequence of an experienced affective episode. If alterations in explicit ER already appear in risk groups, another interesting question is how specific these aberrations are for BD, given that these aberrations are also characteristic of other mental disorders. For example, aberrations in ER also occur in schizophrenia (Khoury and Lecomte 2012) and patients with depression (Rive et al. 2013). Due to depression and BD's similarity in their characterization by affective episodes, the distinction between these two disorders is particularly challenging. Recently it has been shown that unipolar patients can be distinguished from bipolar patients based on valence-specific aberrations in emotion reactivity (Bürger et al. 2017; Surguladze et al. 2010; Grotegerd et al. 2013; Lawrence et al. 2004). Accordingly, the question arises whether individuals with BD risk also show valence-specific aberrations specific for BD.

In the present review, we aim to provide an overview of what behavioral and neural aberrations are present in individuals at risk for BD, patients with current affective episodes, and euthymic patients during explicit ER. From this, we aim to conclude the suitability of explicit ER as a potential marker for BD or as a marker for relapse into affective episodes. Furthermore, we aim to draw implications for the use of ER in the treatment of BD.

## Methods

To obtain an exhaustive compilation of studies addressing specifically explicit ER in BD, we conducted a systematic literature search. We used a systematic approach to identify relevant papers in the Medline, PsycINFO, PubMed, and Web of Science databases. The search was conducted in December 2018. A criterion regarding the publication date was not included. According to our criteria, all abstracts of the identified papers were read and included or excluded for the further review process. Our search included all studies in which the title or abstract contained the words Bipolar Disorder, Bipolar Affective Disorder, or Bipolar Mood Disorder, together with the words Emotion Regulation, Affect Regulation, Emotion Control, or Affect Control. The search term was ("Bipolar Disorder" OR "Bipolar Affective Disorder" OR "Bipolar Mood Disorder") AND ("Emotion Regulation" OR "Affect Regulation" OR "Emotion Control" OR "Affect Control"). Our search revealed 487 studies. To these studies, we applied further inclusion criteria. First, we exclusively included studies in which explicit ER was instructively induced. This criterion is consistent with the strict definition of explicit ER that we base the review on because instruction ensures that ER goals are deliberate and planned, and the specific processes take place in a controlled manner. The second inclusion criterion was that the studies used subjects with a diagnosed BD and/or a proven propensity and/or genetic vulnerability corresponding to these disorders. Fifteen studies met the inclusion criteria. The full text of all included studies was inspected.

## Results

Studies we identified in our literature search investigated the ER strategies maintenance, distraction, and reappraisal (self-focused as well as situation-focused). Figure 2 shows the selection steps of the literature search. The results of these studies are summarized in the section below. We grouped the studies depending on ER strategies. Within the sections on strategies, we have further subdivided the studies according to which the patient or risk group was investigated. As both terms, *euthymic* and *remitted*, describe patients who have been diagnosed with BD but who did not have a manic, depressive or

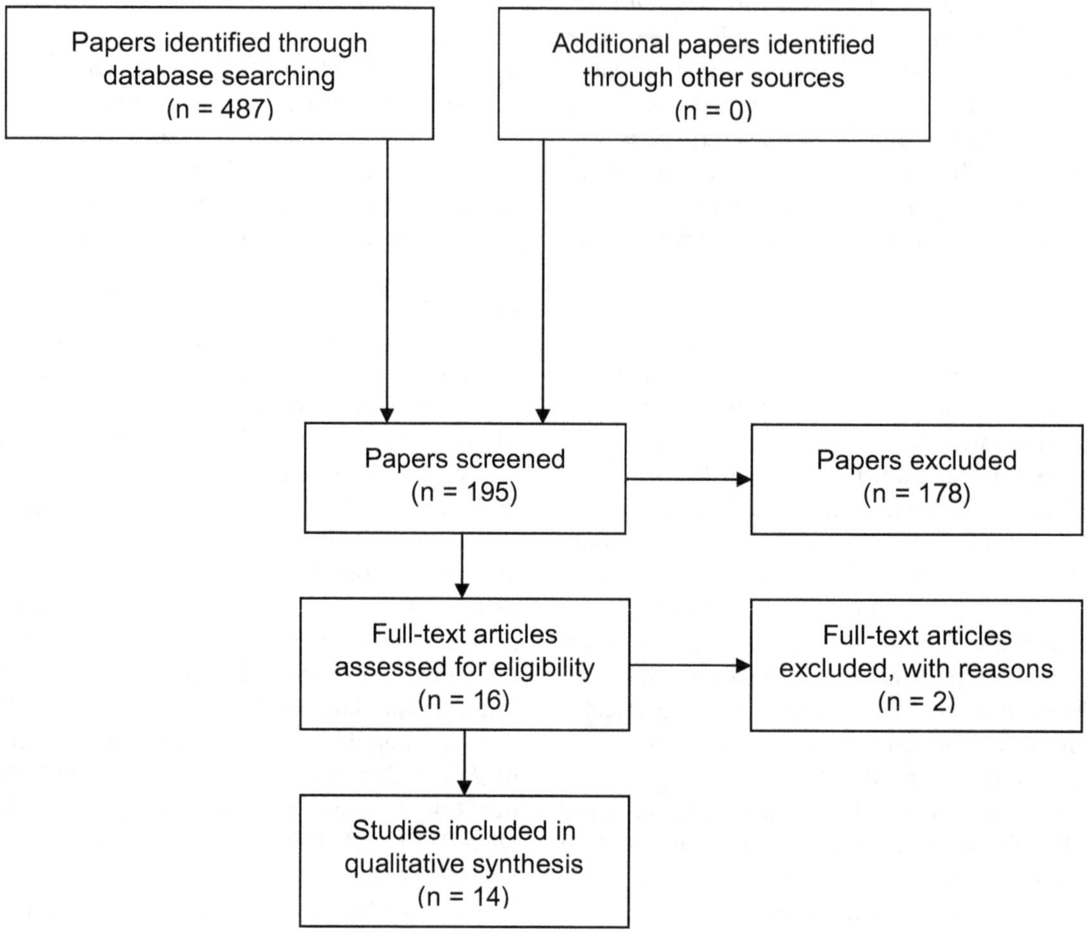


**Fig. 2** Prisma flow diagram of the selection of papers

mixed mood at the time of the study, we will not further differentiate between these states.

### Maintenance of emotions

Only one study investigated processes concerning the maintenance of emotions in BD (Gruber et al. 2013a). The results are shown in Table 1. Maintenance of emotion refers to sustaining an emotion that contributes to goal-oriented behavior beyond the presence of the emotion-triggering stimulus. In this study, the authors tested subjects with BD-I in euthymic mood state and HC in an emotional working memory task (Larkin and Cartensen 2005; Mikels et al. 2008). Participants received the instruction to maintain an emotion evoked by a picture during a delay phase. At the end of the delay phase, participants saw a second picture and compared the two pictures' emotional intensity. Afterward, participants rated each picture regarding emotional intensity. This

**Table 1** Studies that investigated the maintenance of emotions in euthymic BD patients

| Study | Age | Medication | Paradigm | Dependent variables | Results behavioral | Results neural |
|---|---|---|---|---|---|---|
| Gruber et al. (2013a, b) | Adults | Yes | Task:<br>Emotional working memory task<br>Valence:<br>Negative, positive<br>Participants:<br>BD-I, remitted (n = 29)<br>HC (n = 30) | Behavioral:<br>Performance in the emotion working memory task | Maintaining negative emotions:<br>BD-I < HC<br>Maintaining positive emotions:<br>NS | X |

*BD* bipolar disorder, *HC* healthy controls, UD, *NS* not significant study's dependent variable represents the degree of concordance between the comparison task and the subsequent ratings. Euthymic BD-I patients did not differ from HC in the maintenance of positive emotions. However, patients with BD-I were less able to maintain negative emotions than HC. In sum, the study revealed deficits in maintaining negative emotions in euthymic patients with BD-I.

### Regulating emotions via distraction

Six studies that we identified investigated distraction as ER strategy in BD (Caseras et al. 2015; Heissler et al. 2014; Kanske et al. 2013, 2015; Ladouceur et al. 2013; Lois et al. 2017). An overview of the findings on distraction in risk groups can be found in Table 2, Table 3 shows an overview of the findings on distraction in euthymic patients.

Note, Heissler et al. (2014) and Kanske et al. (2015) also investigated reappraisal as an ER strategy in addition to distraction. In this section, we only address their results regarding distraction. Lois et al. (2017) explicitly compared reappraisal and distraction as ER strategies, which we, therefore, review in another corresponding section. Tasks used to measure distraction have in common that they contain a cognitive task and emotional stimuli presentation. Interestingly, the studies investigating distraction in BD can be distinguished by their independent variables: while some studies focus on the self-ratings of emotion and associated neural activity as independent variables (Heissler et al. 2014; Kanske et al. 2015), others focus on the influence of emotion on the performance in cognitive tasks and associated neural activity as independent variables (Kanske et al. 2013; Ladouceur et al. 2013). For the study of attentional ER in BD, both measures are of interest since both cognitive task losses and increased emotional ratings indicate impaired distraction from emotional content. In the following section, we grouped studies according to their task rather than their independent variables.

#### *Distraction in people at risk for BD*

Ladouceur et al. (2013) used an emotional n-back task to investigate alterations of voluntary, attentional ER and its neural correlates. In this task's 0-back condition, the attention demand is low (a simple keystroke is requested for a specific stimulus). In the 2-back condition, the demand is high (a keystroke is required when a stimulus is the same as in the second last trial). In some of the task's trials, task-irrelevant pictures, either emotional or neutral faces, are presented. Participants show the ER by controlling their attention to focus on the n-back task and ignoring the emotional distractors. Therefore, a heightened error rate and an extended response time (RT) in the n-back task during the presence of emotional distractors indicate failures in ER.

Interestingly, the authors chose to investigate healthy offspring of patients with BD compared to healthy low-risk controls (i.e., offspring of parents, neither of whom had been diagnosed with an axis 1 disorder). The n-back task performance in healthy offspring of BD patients and low-risk controls did not differ significantly. However, in the high demanding 2-back condition, both groups differed in neural activity evoked by emotional distractors. BD patients' healthy offspring showed hyperactivity in the VLPFC in the presence of happy but not fearful distractors. In the presence of both types of emotional distractors, the healthy offspring of BD patients showed a reduced modulation of the amygdala by the VLPFC. Additionally, in the presence of happy distractors, healthy offspring of BD patients showed a reduced modulation of the DLPFC by the VLPFC.

Heissler et al. (2014) examined individuals with an increased risk for BD (indicated by high scores in the Hypomanic Personality Scale (HPS; (Eckblad and Chapman 1986) and compared their performance in a picture viewing task (positive, negative, and neutral stimuli) with a low-risk group. In the picture viewing task, participants look at pictures with emotional content (Heissler et al. 2014; Kanske et al. 2013, 2015). They receive either the instruction to simply view the pictures or to regulate their emotions. In this particular version of the task, participants could distract themselves from emotions by solving an arithmetical task presented in addition to the pictures.

During the processing of emotions in the passive viewing condition, the risk group exhibited increased amygdala activity in response to negative stimuli compared to the control group. Behaviorally, the risk group showed no significant impairments in ER. However, participants with increased risk for BD exhibited enhanced amygdala activity in the passive viewing condition and increased activity in the left inferior parietal cortex in the distraction condition.

Kanske et al. (2015) used the same setup. Individuals at risk for BD did not significantly differ from HC concerning behavioral and neural measures during distraction. Kanske et al. (2013) used a similar setup and partly the same sample as Kanske et al. (2015), examining two risk groups. For the first, an increased risk was indicated by high HPS scores. The second risk group consisted of unaffected first-degree relatives of patients with BD. This study investigated the activity of the neural network to emotional stimuli during the arithmetic task. No significant losses or aberrations concerning neural measures were observed in the risk groups.

**Table 2** Studies that investigated distraction in risk groups

| Study | Age | Medication | Paradigm | Dependent variables | Results behavioral | Results neural |
|---|---|---|---|---|---|---|
| Ladouceur et al. (2013) | Adolescents | No | Task:<br>N-back task with emotional distractors<br>Valence:<br>Negative, positive<br>Participants:<br>HBO (n = 15)<br>HC (n = 16) | Behavioral:<br>Performance in n-back task<br>Neural:<br>fMRI, PPI<br>Regions of interest:<br>Amygdala, Ventral Striatum, ventrolateral prefrontal cortex (VLPFC), DLPFC, and anterior cingulate cortex (ACC)<br>PPI seed:<br>VLPFC<br>PPI targets:<br>Amygdala, DLPFC | Distraction from emotional distractors:<br>NS | During distraction from emotional distractors:<br>Right VLPFC: happy: Risk group > HC<br>Right VLPFC: fearful: NS<br>PPI during distraction from emotional distractors:<br>VLPFC – Amygdala (positive connectivity)<br>Fearful: HC > Risk group (right amygdala)<br>Happy: HC > Risk group (left amygdala)<br>Neutral: HC vs. Risk group: NS<br>Right VLPFC – left DLPFC (positive connectivity)<br>Fearful: HC vs. Risk group: NS<br>Happy: HC > Risk group<br>Neutral: HC vs. Risk group: NS |
| Kanske et al. (2013) | Adults | No | Task:<br>Picture viewing task<br>Valence:<br>Negative, positive<br>Participants:<br>High HPS scores (n = 22)<br>FDR (n = 17)<br>HC (n = 22, n = 17) | Behavioral:<br>Performance in the distraction task<br>Neural:<br>fMRI | RT (mental arithmetic task):<br>NS | During distraction:<br>HC vs. Risk groups: NS |
| Heissler et al. (2014) | Young adults | No | Task:<br>Picture viewing task<br>Valence:<br>Negative, positive<br>Participants:<br>High HPS scores (n = 22)<br>HC (n = 24) | Behavioral:<br>Self-report (during and after the task)<br>Neural:<br>fMRI<br>Regions of interest:<br>Emotions reactivity:<br>Amygdala, subgenual ACC, VMPFC, occipital and ventral temporal cortices, thalamus<br>Emotion regulation:<br>OFC, DLPFC, DMPFC, dACC, parietal cortex, precuneus | Rating after the experiment:<br>Risk group > HC<br>Viewing condition:<br>NS<br>Emotion regulation:<br>NS<br>Performance in the mental arithmetic task:<br>NS | Viewing:<br>Negative vs. neutral:<br>Right Amygdala: Risk group > HC<br>Positive vs. neutral: NS<br>Distraction vs. viewing:<br>Negative: NS<br>Positive: left inferior parietal cortex: Risk group > HC |
| Kanske et al. (2015) | Adults | No | Task:<br>Picture viewing task<br>Valence:<br>Negative, positive<br>Participants:<br>FDR (n = 17)<br>HC (n = 17) | Behavioral:<br>Self-report during and after the task<br>Neural:<br>fMRI<br>Regions of interest:<br>Bilateral OFC, dorsolateral (DLPFC, middle frontal) and dorsomedial prefrontal (DMPFC, superior medial), anterior cingulate (ACC), and parietal cortex (inferior, superior) | Rating after the experiment:<br>Risk group > HC (all pictures more positive)<br>Viewing:<br>Positive: Risk group < HC<br>Negative: NS<br>Distraction:<br>NS | Viewing:<br>NS<br>Distraction vs. viewing:<br>NS |

*ACC* anterior cingulate cortex, *dACC* dorsal anterior cingulate cortex, *DLPFC* dorsolateral prefrontal cortex, *DMPFC* dorsomedial prefrontal cortex, *fMRI* functional magnetic resonance imaging, *FDR* first-degree relatives, *HBO* healthy bipolar offspring, *HC* healthy controls, *HPS* hypomanic personality scale, *NS* not significant, *OFC* orbitofrontal cortex, *PFC* prefrontal cortex, *PPI* psychophysiological interaction, *VLPFC* ventrolateral prefrontal cortex, *VMPFC* ventromedial prefrontal cortex

**Table 3** Studies that investigated distraction in euthymic BD patients

| Study | Age | Medication | Paradigm | Dependent variables | Results behavioral | Results neural |
|---|---|---|---|---|---|---|
| Caseras et al. (2015) | Adults | Yes | Task:<br>N-back task with emotional distractors<br>Valence:<br>Negative, positive<br>Participants:<br>BD-I, euthymic (n = 16)<br>BD-II, euthymic (n = 19)<br>HC (n = 20) | Behavioral:<br>Performance in n-back task<br>Neural:<br>fMRI, PPI, DTI<br>Regions of interest:<br>DLPFC, amygdala, and accumbens<br>PPI seed:<br>DLPFC<br>PPI targets:<br>Amygdala, accumbens | RT (2-back vs. 0-back):<br>BD-I > BD-II and HC<br>Slowing due to distractors in 2-back task:<br>BD-I > BD-II and HC<br>RT in 2-back without distractors:<br>BD-I > HC<br>BD-II vs. HC: NS<br>RT in the 2-back task (no distractor vs. emotional distractor):<br>BD-I:<br>Fear > no distractor<br>Happy > no distractor<br>BD-II:<br>NS<br>HC:<br>Fear > no distractor<br>Neutral > no distractor | 2-back (no distractor) vs. 0-back (no distractor):<br>Working memory network: BD-I > BD-II and HC<br>2-back task (distractor vs. no distractor):<br>DLPFC:<br>Fear: BD-II > BD-I > HC<br>Happy: BD-I > BD-II and HC<br>Neutral: HC > BD-I<br>Amygdala:<br>Fear: BD-II > BD-I > HC<br>Happy: BD-I > BD-II > HC<br>Neutral: BD-I > HC<br>Accumbens:<br>Fear: BD-I and BD-II > HC<br>Happy: BD-I > BD-II and HC<br>Neutral: BD-I > HC<br>Functional connectivity:<br>DLPFC-Amygdala<br>Fear: BD-II > BD-I and HC<br>DLPFC-Accumbens<br>NS<br>Structural integrity:<br>Left uncinate fasciculus: NS<br>Right uncinate fasciculus: BD-I < BD-II and HC |
| Kanske et al. (2013) | Adults | Yes | Task:<br>Picture viewing task<br>Valence:<br>Negative, positive<br>Participants:<br>BD-I, euthymic (n = 22)<br>HC (n = 22) | Behavioral:<br>Performance in the distraction task<br>Neural:<br>fMRI | RT in the mental arithmetic task:<br>BD-I > HC | During distraction:<br>Right parietal cortex: BD-I > HC |
| Kanske et al. (2015) | Adults | Yes | Task:<br>Picture viewing task<br>Valence:<br>Negative, positive<br>Participants:<br>BD-I, euthymic (n = 22)<br>HC (n = 22) | Behavioral:<br>Self-report during and after the task<br>Neural:<br>fMRI<br>Regions of interest:<br>Bilateral OFC, dorsolateral (DLPFC, middle frontal) and dorsomedial prefrontal (DMPFC, superior medial), anterior cingulate (ACC), and parietal cortex (inferior, superior) | Self-report:<br>Rating after the experiment:<br>NS<br>Viewing:<br>Positive: NS<br>Negative: NS<br>Distraction:<br>NS | Viewing:<br>NS<br>Distraction vs. viewing:<br>NS |

*ACC* anterior cingulate cortex, *BD* bipolar disorder, *DLPFC* dorsolateral prefrontal cortex, *DMPFC* dorsomedial prefrontal cortex, *DTI* diffusion tensor imaging; fMRI, functional magnetic resonance imaging, *HC* healthy controls, *NS* not significant, *OFC* orbitofrontal cortex, *PFC* prefrontal cortex, *PPI* psychophysiological interaction, *VLPFC* ventrolateral prefrontal cortex, *VMPFC* ventromedial prefrontal cortex

In sum, there was no evidence on the behavioral level that people at risk for BD differ significantly from HC in distracting themselves from negative or positive emotions (Heissler et al. 2014; Kanske et al. 2013, 2015; Ladouceur et al. 2013). Concerning neural measures, patients at risk for BD showed increased neural activity while distracting themselves from positive emotional stimuli in the VLPFC (Ladouceur et al. 2013) and the inferior parietal cortex (Heissler et al. 2014). Despite increased activity in the VLPFC, connectivity analyses revealed a lower modulation of the amygdala (for positive and negative stimuli) and the DLPFC (for positive stimuli) by the VLPFC in the risk group (Ladouceur et al. 2013) during distraction. These findings contrast with studies that found no significant differences regarding neural measures between people at risk for BD and HC (Kanske et al. 2013, 2015).

#### *Distraction in euthymic patients*

Caseras et al. (2015) investigated differences in distraction in euthymic patients with BD-I, euthymic patients with BD-II, and HC assessed in an emotional n-back task. Particularly patients with BD-I exhibited impairments. First, this group showed inferior performance in the 2-back condition. Additionally, in the 2-back condition, BD-I patients showed slower RT due to distractors than the other groups. In contrast to the other groups, especially the distraction from happy distractors was impaired. Regarding the neural correlates of ER, patients with BD-I compared to other groups exhibited increased activity in the DLPFC, amygdala, and accumbens when happy distractors were present. In the presence of fear distractors, activity in these areas was highest in patients with BD-II. BD-II patients also showed a higher (inverse) functional connectivity between DLPFC and amygdala when fearful distractors were present. For patients with BD-I, results indicate lower structural integrity in the uncinate fasciculus, a white matter association tract that connects frontal regions with subcortical regions. In contrast, no significant structural aberrations were found for patients with BD-II.

Euthymic patients with BD-I in Kanske et al. (2015) did not significantly differ from HC regarding self-reports of emotions or neural activity during distraction. However, in Kanske et al. (2013), the same patient group solved the arithmetic task slower than HC when emotional pictures were present. In the presence of emotionally background pictures, patients with BD-I, compared to HC, exhibited increased activity in the right parietal cortex.

Regarding distraction in patients with BD, it is essential to note that all patients examined in the cited studies were in a euthymic state. While the self-report of emotions in euthymic BD patients provides no evidence of significant impairment (Kanske et al. 2015), the cognitive measures show the opposite (Kanske et al. 2013; Caseras et al. 2015). Regarding neural measures, patients with BD-I exhibited hyperactivity in DLPFC, amygdala, and nucleus accumbens during distraction from happy pictures and aberrations in structural integrity between frontal areas and the amygdala (Caseras et al. 2015). In contrast, patients with BD-II exhibited heightened activity in these areas and increased inverse functional connectivity between DLPFC and amygdala during the distraction from fearful stimuli (Caseras et al. 2015). Other results indicate no such aberrations in areas associated with emotion reactivity and regulation, but instead aberrations in areas associated with the cognitive distraction task (Kanske et al. 2013).

### Regulating emotions via reappraisal

Our search identified three studies investigating reappraisal abilities of patients with BD without using imaging methods (Ajaya et al. 2016; Gruber et al. 2014; Kjærstad et al. 2016). Seven studies investigated neural correlates in addition to behavioral measures (Corbalán et al. 2015; Heissler et al. 2014; Kanske et al. 2015; Morris et al. 2012; Rive et al. 2015; Townsend et al. 2013; Zhang et al. 2018). The majority of studies that examined reappraisal used a picture viewing task to evoke emotions. Exceptions are Gruber et al. (2014) and Ajaya et al. (2016). Gruber et al. (2014) presented emotional movie clips to participants and instructed them to carefully view the clips or reappraise to regulate their emotions. In the study of Ajaya et al. (2016), a manipulation of the keyboard with which participants navigated in a video game was supposed to induce anger. Three studies investigated reappraisal in participants at risk for BD [indicated by HPS scores (Ajaya et al. 2016; Heissler et al. 2014) and genetic predisposition (Kanske et al. 2015)]. Table 4 shows the results of these studies. Two studies included samples with a current affective episode (Table 5). Patients in Morris et al. (2012) consisted partly of euthymic individuals and partly of hypomanic individuals. Rive et al. (2015) examined patients with BD in a euthymic and depressive state. In seven studies, patients were in a euthymic state (Corbalán et al. 2015; Gruber et al. 2014; Kanske et al. 2015; Kjærstad et al. 2016; Rive et al. 2015; Townsend et al. 2013; Zhang et al. 2018). An overview of these studies is given in Table 6.

#### *Reappraisal in individuals at risk for BD*

Heissler et al. (2014) did not find significant differences in behavioral measures of reappraisal in HC and participants at risk for BD. However, individuals at risk for BD exhibited hyperactivity in the amygdala during the reappraisal of negative emotions, indicating deficits in reappraisal, which did not manifest in behavioral measures.

Kanske et al. (2015) were able to clarify the role of frontal areas in the reappraisal of participants at risk for BD and euthymic patients with BD-I using the same setup as Heissler et al. (2014). In contrast to Heissler et al. (2014), differences in ER abilities were found for the high-risk group compared to their controls, with the high-risk group showing a decreased downregulation of positive emotions during reappraisal. Regarding neural measures, the high-risk group exhibited increased activity of the amygdala during reappraisal compared to HC. Most importantly, further analyses revealed that this was due

**Table 4** Studies that investigated reappraisal in risk groups

| Study | Age | Medication | Paradigm | Dependent variables | Results behavioral | Results neural |
|---|---|---|---|---|---|---|
| Heissler et al. (2014) | Young adults | No | Task: Picture viewing task Valence: Negative, positive Participants: High HPS scores (n = 22) HC (n = 24) | Behavioral: Self-report during and after the task Neural: fMRI Regions of interest: Emotions reactivity: Amygdala, subgenual ACC, VMPFC, occipital and ventral temporal cortices, thalamus; Emotion regulation: OFC, DLPFC, DMPFC, dACC, parietal cortex, precuneus | Rating after the experiment: Arousal: Risk group > HC Viewing condition: NS Reappraisal: NS | Viewing: Negative vs. neutral: Right Amygdala: Risk group > HC Positive vs. neutral: NS Reappraisal vs. viewing: Negative: Right Amygdala: Risk group > HC Positive: NS |
| Kanske et al. (2015) | Adults | No | Task: Picture viewing task Valence: Negative, positive Participants: FDR (n = 17) HC (n = 17) | Behavioral: Self-report during and after the task Neural: fMRI, PPI Regions of interest: Bilateral OFC, dorsolateral (DLPFC, middle frontal) and dorsomedial prefrontal (DMPFC, superior medial), anterior cingulate (ACC), and parietal cortex (inferior, superior) PPI seed: Amygdala PPI targets: OFC, dorsolateral (DLPFC, middle frontal) and dorsomedial prefrontal (DMPFC, superior medial), anterior cingulate (ACC) and parietal cortex (inferior, superior) | Rating after the experiment: Risk group > HC (all pictures more positive) Viewing: Positive: Risk group < HC Negative: NS Reappraisal: Risk group < HC | Viewing: NS Reappraisal vs. viewing: Amygdala: Risk group > HC PPI: Left amygdala/bilateral OFC: HC, negative connectivity; Risk group, positive connectivity Right amygdala/right OFC: HC, negative connectivity; Risk group, positive connectivity |
| Ajaya et al. (2016) | Young adults | No | Task: Videogame task Valence: Negative Participants: Undergraduates (n = 66) | Behavioral: self-reported affect, facial expressions Psychophysiology: Respiratory sinus arrhythmia (RSA) | Higher HPS scores increased RSA during ER (only in the deliberated reappraisal condition) | X |

*ACC* anterior cingulate cortex, *dACC* dorsal anterior cingulate DLPFC, dorsolateral prefrontal cortex, *DMPFC* dorsomedial prefrontal cortex, *fMRI* functional magnetic resonance imaging, *HC* healthy controls, *HPS* hypomanic personality scale, *OFC* orbitofrontal cortex, *PFC* prefrontal cortex, *PPI* psychophysiological interaction, *VLPFC* ventrolateral prefrontal cortex, *VMPFC* ventromedial prefrontal cortex

to an impaired downregulation of the amygdala by OFC in the reappraisal condition.

Like Heissler et al. (2014), Ajaya et al. (2016) measured the risk for BD with the HPS. The authors were particularly interested in the effect of explicit and implicit instruction on reappraisal in individuals at risk for BD. Subjects in the video game task either received the instruction to concentrate on the game, were implicitly primed with the sentence-unscrambling task (Mauss et al. 2007) to apply reappraisal, or were explicitly instructed to apply reappraisal. Increased expression of anger indicated aberrant emotion reactivity in individuals with higher HPS scores. Interestingly, in Ajaya et al. (2016), HPS scores were correlated with respiratory sinus arrhythmia (RSA) deviations from baseline during ER after explicit instruction. This effect

**Table 5** Studies that investigated reappraisal in patients with a current affective episode

| Study | Age | Medication use | Paradigm | Dependent variables | Results behavioral | Results neural |
|---|---|---|---|---|---|---|
| Rive et al. (2015) | Adults | No | Task:<br>Picture viewing task<br>Valence:<br>Negative, positive<br>Participants:<br>BD-I/BD-II, currently depressed (n = 9)<br>BD-I/BD-II, remitted (n = 26)<br>HC (n = 36) | Behavioral:<br>Self-report<br>Neural:<br>fMRI<br>Regions of interest:<br>Amygdala, thalamus, insula, DLPFC, ACC, medial PFC, and hippocampus | ER success in depressed groups:<br>Happy: UDd < HC<br>BDd vs. HC: n.s. differences<br>Happy vs. sad:<br>BDd: happy > sad<br>HC: happy vs. sad: NS | Depressive state:<br>Reappraisal of happiness vs. reappraisal of sadness:<br>rACC: BDd > UDd |
| Morris et al. (2012) | Adults | Yes | Task:<br>Picture viewing task<br>Valence:<br>Negative<br>Participants:<br>BD-I (n = 13)<br>(six BD patients met criteria for euthymia and five met criteria for hypomania)<br>HC (n = 15) | Behavioral:<br>Self-report<br>Neural:<br>fMRI<br>Regions of interest:<br>Amygdala, cortico-lymbic areas with activity during ER<br>Coupling seed:<br>Amygdala<br>Coupling targets:<br>Whole brain | Self-report of emotions:<br>HC: Increase > Maintain > Decrease<br>BD: Increase > Maintain<br>BD: Maintain v.s. Decrease: NS | Down regulation:<br>Right VLPFC: BD > HC<br>Up regulation:<br>Right VLPFC: BD > HC<br>Rostral ACC: BD > HC<br>Inverse coupling of left PFC (especially left IFG) and amygdala found in HC did not occur in BD |

*ACC* anterior cingulate cortex, *BD* bipolar disorder, *DLPFC* dorsolateral prefrontal cortex, *fMRI* functional magnetic resonance imaging, *HC* healthy controls, *PFC* prefrontal cortex, *PPI* psychophysiological interaction, *rACC* rostral anterior cingulate cortex

was absent when the instruction was implicitly primed or when participants received no instruction. Because RSA is an ER indicator, the authors conclude that these results suggest that explicit instruction enabled participants with higher HPS scores to successfully control their emotions. A characteristic of this analog study that has to bear in mind is the sample whose members were undergraduates and on a wide range of HPS scores. Thus, it differs from the strict definition of risk groups in the other studies reviewed in this section.

Taken together, the results of studies investigating reappraisal in participants at risk for BD revealed aberrations in emotion reactivity as well as in the ability to reappraise emotions. Regarding reappraisal, aberrations were found on behavioral (Kanske et al. 2015), as well as on neural levels (Heissler et al. 2014; Kanske et al. 2015). Neurally, aberrant emotion reactivity of negative emotions is reflected by hyperactivity in the amygdala (Heissler et al. 2014; Kanske et al. 2015). In participants at risk for BD, amygdala hyperactivity was associated with aberrant connectivity between the OFC and the amygdala during reappraisal (Kanske et al. 2015). While in HC, both areas were inversely coupled, they were positively associated with the risk group. The studies provide equivocal findings regarding the extent to which neural aberrations also affect the behavioral level. In two of three studies investigating reappraisal in people at risk for BD, no significant impairments at the behavioral level were found (Ajaya et al. 2016; Heissler et al. 2014).

#### *Reappraisal in patients with current manic and depressive episodes*

Rive et al. (2015) investigated ER in a mixed sample, which included patients who had BD-I, patients who had BD-II, and HC in a picture viewing task with negative and positive stimuli in an fMRI setting. Patient groups were further divided into two subgroups depending on whether they were currently remitted (BDr) or depressed (BDd). In this section, we review the results of BD patients with a depressive episode; the results regarding remitted patients are reviewed in a corresponding section below. A notable characteristic of this study is that exclusively self-focused reappraisal was used. In healthy individuals, self-focused reappraisal has been shown to be less effective than situation-focused reappraisal (Willroth and Hilimire 2016). However, because situation-focused reappraisal is a relatively complex cognitive process, it has been argued that self-focused reappraisal for patients with affective disorders is more comfortable to apply (Rive et al. 2015). For BD-patients in a depressed state, the reappraisal of sad emotions compared to the reappraisal of happy emotions was compromised. Neurally, this patient group showed a decreased activity in rACC during the regulation of happy and hyperactivity during the regulation of sad emotions.

A distinguishing feature of Morris et al. (2012) is the BD-patient sample, which includes euthymic patients and patients who currently suffered from hypomanic episodes. Subjects were instructed to either use situation- or self-focused reappraisal, intensify, or maintain their emotions in a picture viewing task. The subjective affect rating revealed no significant differences between the patients and the group across all conditions. However, while the control group reported lower affect after the decrease condition than the maintain condition, affect ratings of patients who suffered from BD did not differ significantly between these conditions. Regarding the upregulation of emotions, both groups were able to increase their emotions compared to the maintenance of emotions. At the neural level, BD patients, as compared to HC, showed aberrant hyperactivity in the right VLPFC during up- and downregulation. Additionally, hyperactivity in rACC was found in BD patients during upregulation. Patients who suffered from BD differed from HC in the functional connectivity between areas in the frontal cortex and the amygdala. A negative correlation between activity in the left IFG and activity in the amygdala, found in HC during the downregulation of emotions, was absent in BD patients.

The studies investigating reappraisal in patients with current affective episodes show an affect-congruent impairment of reappraisal in the depressed state associated with hypoactivity in the rACC. Further, the opposite pattern was found in patients with a hypomanic episode. Here, affect-incongruent deviations in reappraisal were shown. These were associated with hyperactivity in the rACC and aberrations in fronto-limbic connectivity. A different approach to investigate reappraisal in BD was taken in the following studies. In these studies, reappraisal in patients with euthymic mood state was investigated.

#### *Reappraisal in euthymic patients*

In four studies we identified in our literature search, reappraisal abilities of patients with BD at a euthymic state were investigated (Corbalán et al. 2015; Kanske et al. 2015; Townsend et al. 2013; Zhang et al. 2018). Three further studies described the patient group's mood state as remitted (Gruber et al. 2014; Kjærstad et al. 2016; Rive et al. 2015).

In the study of Gruber et al. (2014), euthymic subjects that suffered from BD-I and HC saw movie clips that induced neutral, positive, or negative emotions. Instructions were to either observe these clips or to use reappraisal to modify emotions. Emotions were assessed by self-report, facial expression, and physiological measures (skin conductivity and respiratory sinus arrhythmia). Both groups were successful in reappraisal, implying intact reappraisal in euthymic patients.

Kjærstad et al. (2016) investigated reappraisal in patients with BD (a mixed group that contained BD-I patients and patients with BD-II) and HC. Patients were in a partly or fully remitted state. Two different ER paradigms were used in this study. First, in a social scenario task, participants read fictional social scenarios and corresponding self-beliefs. The scenarios could either be positive, negative, or neutral. Participants were instructed to either typically react to the scenarios or to dampen their emotions. Second, participants applied reappraisal in a picture viewing task. The authors assumed that the social scenarios task evokes stronger emotions due to patients' higher personal involvement. Indeed, in the social scenarios task, patients with BD were less able to downregulate negative emotions than HC.

In contrast, in the picture viewing task, patients with BD did not significantly differ from HC in reappraising negative emotions. It is difficult to conclude the divergent findings in both tasks since both tasks differ not only in the stimulus material but also in the instruction. The instruction to dampen emotions in the social scenarios task may be more challenging to implement than clearly defined reappraisal. Nevertheless, like Gruber et al. (2014), Kjærstad et al. (2016) did not found indications for significant deficits in reappraisal in euthymic patients with BD. However, it is not clear from either study whether euthymic patients and HC differ in their neural activity regarding reappraisal. Fortunately, the following studies addressed this question.

Euthymic patients in Rive et al. (2015) showed impaired self-focused reappraisal of happy and sad emotions. Neurally, patients with BD in a euthymic state did not significantly differ from HC during self-focused reappraisal.

Regarding neural measures, euthymic patients with BD-I in Kanske et al. (2015) showed amygdala hyperactivity during reappraisal compared to HC. Further analyses revealed aberrations in functional connectivity between the amygdala and the OFC, and the ventral ACC. While in HC, the connection between these areas was reverse, in euthymic patients, the connection was positive.

Corbalán et al. (2015) investigated differences in the reappraisal of euthymic patients with BD-I and HC during a picture viewing task. Self-report of emotions indicated that euthymic BD-I patients and HC were able to regulate their emotions successfully. Regarding self-report measurement, tests between the two groups did not reveal significant differences. However, both groups differed concerning neural activity. BD-I patients showed no reduction in amygdala activity during the reappraisal of negative emotions that healthy control participants exhibited. Further, in contrast to HC, patients with BD-I showed an involvement of the VLPFC in the neutral reappraisal condition and the negative viewing condition.

While Corbalán et al. (2015) give insights into neural activity during reappraisal, Townsend et al. (2013) primarily focused on differences in functional connectivity

**Table 6** Studies that investigated reappraisal in euthymic BD patients

| Study | Age | Medication use | Paradigm | Dependent variables | Results behavioral | Results neural |
|---|---|---|---|---|---|---|
| Kanske et al. (2015) | Adults | Yes | Task:<br>Picture viewing task<br>Valence:<br>Negative, positive<br>Participants:<br>BD-I, euthymic (n = 22)<br>HC (N = 22) | Behavioral:<br>Self-report during and after the task<br>Neural:<br>fMRI, PPI<br>Regions of interest:<br>Bilateral OFC, dorsolateral (DLPFC, middle frontal) and dorsomedial prefrontal (DMPFC, superior medial), anterior cingulate (ACC), and parietal cortex (inferior, superior)<br>PPI seed:<br>Amygdala<br>PPI targets:<br>OFC, dorsolateral (DLPFC, middle frontal) and dorsomedial prefrontal (DMPFC, superior medial), anterior cingulate (ACC) and parietal cortex (inferior, superior) | Rating after the experiment:<br>NS<br>Viewing:<br>NS<br>Reappraisal:<br>NS | Viewing:<br>NS<br>Reappraisal vs. viewing:<br>Amygdala: BD-I > HC<br>Parahippocampal: BD-I > HC<br>PPI during reappraisal:<br>Left amygdala/right OFC<br>HC negative connectivity, BD-I positive connectivity<br>Left amygdala/ventral ACC:<br>HC negative connectivity, BD-I positive connectivity<br>Right amygdala/right OFC<br>HC negative connectivity, BD-I positive connectivity |
| Corbalán et al. (2015) | Adults | Yes | Task:<br>Picture viewing task<br>Valence:<br>Negative<br>Participants:<br>BD-I, euthymic (n = 19)<br>HC (n = 17) | Behavioral:<br>Self-report<br>Behavioral<br>fMRI<br>Regions of interest:<br>Whole brain | NS | Viewing negative:<br>VLPFC: BD-I > HC<br>Reappraisal negative:<br>VLPFC: BD-I > HC<br>Reappraisal negative vs. viewing negative:<br>Amygdala: BD-I > HC |
| Townsend et al. (2013) | Adults | Yes | Task:<br>Picture viewing task<br>Valence:<br>Negative<br>Participants:<br>BD-I, euthymic (n = 30)<br>HC (n = 26) | Neural:<br>fMRI<br>Regions of interest:<br>Bilateral amygdala<br>PPI seed:<br>Bilateral amygdala<br>PPI target:<br>Whole brain (and a priori VLPFC) | No affect related behavioral data was reported | Viewing negative vs. viewing neutral:<br>HC vs. BD-I: NS<br>Reappraisal Negative vs. Viewing Negative:<br>Amygdala: HC vs. BD-I: n.s. differences<br>Bilateral VLPFC: HC > BD-I<br>Insula: HC > BD-I<br>Bilateral MFG: HC > BD-I<br>Bilateral cingulate: HC > BD-I<br>pre-SMA: HC > BD-I<br>PPI Seed: Left amygdala<br>Negative Functional connectivity<br>Left VLPFC: HC > BD-I<br>Left occipital gyrus: HC > BD-I<br>Right posterior cingulate: HC > BD-I<br>PPI Seed: Right amygdala:<br>Negative functional connectivity<br>Right MFG: BD-I > HC |

**Table 6** (continued)

| Study | Age | Medication use | Paradigm | Dependent variables | Results behavioral | Results neural |
|---|---|---|---|---|---|---|
| Zhang et al. (2018) | Adults | Yes | Task:<br>Picture viewing task<br>Valence:<br>Negative<br>Participants:<br>BD patients,euthymic (n = 23), (2 currently depressed)<br>HC (n = 17) | Behavioral:<br>Self-report<br>Neural:<br>fMRI, DCM<br>VOI:<br>DLPFC, left VLPFC, and left amygdala | ER and emotion reactivity:<br>NS | GLM contrasts:<br>NS<br>DCM:<br>DLPFC to Amygdala during reappraisal:<br>BD < HC |
| Gruber et al. (2014) | Adults | Yes | Task:<br>Film clips<br>Valence:<br>Negative, positive<br>Participants:<br>BD-I, remitted (n = 23)<br>HC (n = 23) | Behavioral:<br>Self-report, analysis of facial expression<br>Physiological measures:<br>Skin conductivity and Respiratory sinus arrhythmia | Uninstructed vs. Reappraisal:<br>NS | X |
| Kjærstad et al. (2016) | Adults | Yes | Tasks:<br>Social scenarios task, Picture viewing task<br>Valence:<br>Negative<br>Participants:<br>BD-I, full or partial remitted (n = 9)<br>BD-II, full or partial remitted (n = 11)<br>Depression, full or partial remitted (n = 20)<br>HC (n = 20) | Behavioral:<br>Self-report | Emotion reactivity:<br>NS<br>Social Scenarios/dampen:<br>Negative: BD < HC<br>Positive: NS<br>Picture task/reappraisal:<br>NS | X |
| Rive et al. (2015) | Adults | No | Task:<br>Picture viewing task<br>Valence:<br>Negative, positive<br>Participants:<br>BD-I/BD-II, remitted (n = 26)<br>HC (n = 36) | Behavioral:<br>Self-report<br>Neural:<br>fMRI<br>Regions of interest:<br>Amygdala, thalamus, insula, DLPFC, ACC, medial PFC, and hippocampus | ER success in remitted groups across all emotions:<br>BDr < HC | Regulate vs. viewing across emotions:<br>DLPFC: NS |

*ACC* anterior cingulate cortex, *BD* bipolar disorder, *DCM* dynamic causal modeling, *DLPFC* dorsolateral prefrontal cortex, *DMPFC* dorsomedial prefrontal cortex, *fMRI* functional magnetic resonance imaging, *HC* healthy controls, *HPS* hypomanic personality scale, *OFC* orbitofrontal cortex, *PFC* prefrontal cortex, *PPI* psychophysiological interaction, *VLPFC* ventrolateral prefrontal cortex

between the amygdala and frontal regions in euthymic patients with BD-I. This group showed reduced activity in bilateral VLPFC, insula, bilateral middle frontal gyrus (MFG), cingulate, and pre-supplementary motor area (SMA). Most importantly, reduced negative connectivity between the left amygdala and left VLPFC, left occipital gyrus, and right posterior cingulate was found in the patient group during reappraisal. In contrast, negative connectivity between the right amygdala and the right MFG was enhanced in BD-I patients. The results of Townsend et al. (2013) do not allow any conclusions about the causal direction of aberrant connectivity between the amygdala and other regions in patients with BD. This causal direction was addressed by Zhang et al. (2018).

Zhang et al. (2018) investigated causal connectivity between frontal areas (namely DLPFC and VLPFC) and the amygdala. Participants in this study were euthymic BD-I patients who had experienced past psychotic symptoms and a control group. Regarding the self-report of emotions, no evidence was found that both groups differ in their ability to regulate emotions. However, regarding neural measures, the influence of reappraisal on the connectivity from the left DLPFC to the left amygdala was weaker in patients with BD. No significant differences were found for the connectivity of the VLPFC and the amygdala.

Taken together, most studies that investigated reappraisal in euthymic patients reveal no significant behavioral differences in patients with BD and HC (Corbalán et al. 2015; Gruber et al. 2014; Kanske et al. 2015; Kjærstad et al. 2016; Townsend et al. 2013; Zhang et al. 2018). However, one study contrasts with these findings; Rive et al. (2015) did find deficits in the ability to use self-focused reappraisal in euthymic patients with BD-I. Regarding neural measures, amygdala hyperactivity of euthymic and euthymic patients suggests less effective reappraisal (Corbalán et al. 2015; Kanske et al. 2015). Analyses of functional connectivity revealed aberrations in the connectivity between the amygdala and OFC and ACC (Kanske et al. 2015), VLPFC, occipital gyrus, posterior cingulate, right middle frontal gyrus (Townsend et al. 2013), and DLPFC (Zhang et al. 2018).

#### Comparing distraction and reappraisal

In three of the studies we identified, participants applied both distraction and reappraisal. Therefore, these studies allow us to compare both strategies with each other.

Regarding behavioral measures, Heissler et al. (2014) neither found significant differences between people at risk for BD and HC in the distraction condition nor the reappraisal condition. Regarding neural measures, participants at risk for BD showed a heightened activity of the amygdala during the reappraisal of negative emotions compared to HC. During distraction from positive emotions, participants at risk for BD exhibited increased activity in the left inferior parietal cortex.

Kanske et al. (2015) found distraction and reappraisal for BD-I patients to be an effective strategy to regulate positive and negative emotions at the behavioral level. However, for people at risk for BD compared to HC, they found reappraisal to be more effective than distraction. Regarding neural measures, neither patients with BD-I nor individuals at risk for BD differed significantly from HC.

Lois et al. (2017) investigated neural network connectivity during reappraisal and distraction in euthymic patients with BD-I and HC. The patient groups showed aberrantly increased intra-network and inter-network connectivity in the default mode network during distraction compared to the reappraisal condition, which indicates that distraction and reappraisal in patients with BD can be distinguished by specific activity patterns in large-scale brain networks.

Taken together, the findings of studies investigating reappraisal and distraction show that the two ER strategies can be distinguished based on their use of large scale networks. Impairments can occur for both strategies in BD. A direct comparison suggests that reappraisal has an advantage over distraction.

## Discussion

Aberrant emotion reactivity (Mercer and Becerra 2013; Rosen and Rich 2010; Townsend and Altshuler 2012; Wessa and Linke 2009) and regulation of emotions are predominant features of bipolar disorder (Aldao et al. 2010; Dodd et al. 2019; Green et al. 2011; Gruber et al. 2013a; Phillips 2003; Phillips et al. 2008; Townsend and Altshuler 2012). The present article reviews studies that examined explicit ER in patients with BD and/or individuals at risk for BD. The compilation of the results leads to a threefold conclusion: First, we highlight the potential role of neural activity during explicit ER as a specific marker indicating the risk for the development of BD. Second, we highlight the role of ventral-rostral regions of the ACC in patients with current affective episodes, and third, we describe possible neural mechanisms that prevent euthymic patients from showing behavioral deficits in ER.

We identified 15 studies investigating explicit ER via maintenance, distraction, situation-focused reappraisal, and self-focused reappraisal of emotions. On a subjective level, self-report measures of valence or arousal were used. Objective measures included the analysis of facial expression and physiological parameters (skin conductivity, respiratory sinus arrhythmia, and MRI). Different patient and risk groups were tested; most diversely, reappraisal was investigated in participants at risk for BD, euthymic patients, and patients in a depressed or hypomanic state. Maintenance of emotions was studied in euthymic patients. Studies on distraction examined participants at risk for BD and euthymic patients. A specific characteristic of the distraction studies is that impairments can manifest in either reduced down-regulation of emotional sensitivity through distraction or in hampered performance in the task that is intended to provide a distraction (e.g., a cognitively demanding task) (van Dillen et al. 2009; Wessa et al. 2013). In the following, we discuss and synthesize these studies along the different participant groups to carve out the potential etiological role of ER deficits in BD.

#### The potential role of explicit emotion regulation as a marker for bipolar disorder

Recent research has highlighted the importance of identifying specific markers that indicate the risk of BD for early intervention and prophylactic treatment (Malhi et al. 2017). Risk groups are particularly well suited to identify such markers.

##### *Explicit emotion regulation in risk groups*

In terms of behavioral measures, the reviewed studies suggest a relatively intact ER of risk groups. Regarding distraction, no impairments were found. Regarding reappraisal, two of three studies that investigated reappraisal in individuals at risk for BD revealed no significant impairments at the behavioral level (Ajaya et al. 2016; Heissler et al. 2014).

In contrast, the third study revealed reduced reappraisal effects in the risk group (Kanske et al. 2015). A crucial difference between these studies is the selection of risk groups. The studies that found no behavioral differences in reappraisal selected participants based on personality traits. In contrast, the study that examined first degree relatives of BD patients showed impaired reappraisal. Because the experimental setup of Kanske et al. (2015) and Heissler et al. (2014) was identical, the different selection of risk groups could cause contradictory findings. However, given that the difference between these risk groups was not systematically investigated, a conclusive interpretation of these findings is difficult. Previous studies have shown that both genetic risk and personality traits are highly predictive of the development of BD (Craddock and Sklar, 2013; Johnson et al. 2015; Kwapil et al. 2000; Rasic et al. 2014; Walsh et al. 2015).

***Neural deviations in risk groups during explicit emotion regulation***

Because risk groups showed sustained ER in most studies, the underlying neural activity of explicit ER is particularly interesting. Regarding distraction, this group exhibited aberrations in neural networks associated with emotion reactivity and ER (Heissler et al. 2014; Ladouceur et al. 2013). Individuals at risk exhibited VLPFC hyperactivity and reduced positive functional connectivity between VLPFC and the amygdala and the DLPFC during distraction from positive emotional stimuli (Ladouceur et al. 2013). During the distraction from positive emotional stimuli in an arithmetic task, individuals at risk showed hyperactivity in the left inferior parietal cortex, an area related to arithmetical operations (Heissler et al. 2014). Taken together with the behavioral results, these findings suggest that while individuals at risk can distract themselves from emotional stimuli at a level comparable to HC, this ability may be associated with increased cognitive effort, as indicated by hyperactivity in the corresponding areas. Please note, however, not all studies found significant neural aberrations in risk groups during distraction (Kanske et al. 2013, 2015). Regarding reappraisal, individuals at personality-based risk show hyperactivity in the amygdala (Heissler et al. 2014), which is also present in first-degree relatives, where aberrant positive functional connectivity between the amygdala and parts of the regulation network were demonstrated (Kanske et al. 2015).

***Deviations in risk groups: implications for theories on the etiology of bipolar disorders***

These findings in risk groups provide information on whether aberrations in emotion reactivity and regulation of individuals with affective disorders are vulnerability factors that exist before the development of a disorder as claimed by the trait marker hypothesis (Rohde et al. 1990), or the consequence of affective episodes that occur during an affective disorder as claimed by the scar hypothesis (Rohde et al. 1990). Concerning these opposing hypotheses, the behavioral findings of the reviewed studies do not provide a definite conclusion. While one study revealed behavioral impairments in the explicit ER of individuals at risk for BD (Kanske et al. 2015), the majority of studies found no significant differences between risk groups and HC regarding behavioral measures (Heissler et al. 2014; Kanske et al. 2013; Ladouceur et al. 2013). However, in contrast to behavioral impairments, most studies revealed aberrations in frontostriatal areas (Heissler et al. 2014; Kanske et al. 2015; Ladouceur et al. 2013). Given that the reviewed studies' risk groups did not experience any preceding affective episodes, aberrations in explicit ER provide evidence for the trait marker hypothesis. These aberrations often cannot be detected in behavioral measures of explicit ER but are initially only visible in more sensitive neural measures. Interestingly, however, in a study that examined individuals at genetic risk, impairments in reappraisal were revealed on the behavioral level. In this sample, the additional activity alterations in areas involved in implicit ER (i.e., OFC and ventral ACC) may have led to additional behavioral impairments, which underlines the role of areas associated with implicit ER in explicit ER.

Concerning the use of explicit ER as a marker for the BD risk, neural aberrations during explicit ER seem to be promising due to their high sensitivity relative to behavioral measures. Most importantly, especially the regulation of positive emotions seems to be associated with neural aberrations (Heissler et al. 2014; Ladouceur et al. 2013). This detail is essential because valence-specific aberrations potentially distinguish bipolar disorders from other affective disorders, especially depression. Recently, it has been shown that patients with BD and UD can be distinguished based on structural and (valence-specific) functional neural aberrations associated with altered ER. (Bürger et al. 2017; Redlich et al. 2014; Repple et al. 2017). Concerning prophylactic treatment, in particular, the differentiation during the early course of the disorder could be critical. Although research on explicit ER of positive emotions in patients with major depression disorder and especially in risk groups is relatively rare, there is evidence to suggest that individuals at risk for unipolar depression (UD) differ from individuals at risk for BD regarding neural changes during explicit ER. For example, patients with UD exhibit decreased activity in the VLPFC during explicit ER of positive emotions (Canli et al. 2004; Kanske et al. 2012), which is the opposite of what was found for individuals at risk for BD during distraction from positive emotions (Ladouceur et al. 2013). To our knowledge, only one study investigated neural aberrations in individuals at risk for UD during ER of positive emotions (Simsek et al. 2017). This study revealed no significant aberrations. However, these studies' results cannot be regarded as conclusive, especially as there are, to our knowledge, no studies that have directly compared both risk groups.

Also, longitudinal studies are indispensable to investigate if, in BD risk groups, neural activity in areas associated with implicit and explicit ER is predictive and specific of developing BD later on. Nevertheless, the results in risk groups provide essential information about neural changes underlying BD since the results are not possibly confounded by medication or treatment effects. Studying medicated participants can lead to results that are challenging to interpret because it is difficult to determine whether differences between patients and HC are due to medication, the disorder, or an interaction of both. Additionally, patients—especially euthymic/remitted ones—have mostly undergone some form of psychotherapy that often specifically trains explicit emotion regulation, a factor that should be considered when interpreting the results in patient samples. However, recent tools such as the tracking software chronocord (Bauer et al. 2019; Pilhatsch et al. 2018) can be used to determine mood, sleep, and medication more specifically and can investigate their effects on emotion regulation and neural activity in patient groups.

### The role of the rACC in emotion regulation during affective episodes

The literature search revealed a lack of studies investigating patients with current depressive, manic, and hypomanic episodes.

Only one study investigated reappraisal in BD patients with a depressive episode (Rive et al. 2015). This patient group exhibited valence-specific aberrations during reappraisal. Reappraisal of sad emotions was accompanied by hyperactivity in the rACC, and the reappraisal of happy emotions was associated with decreased activity in this area. In previous studies, the rACC has been associated with resolving emotional conflicts (Etkin et al. 2006). Rive et al. (2015) hypothesize from valence-specific aberrations in the rACC that the reappraisal of mood-congruent emotions for BD patients with a depressive episode represents an emotional conflict. This hypothesis raises whether aberrant activity in the rACC is also evident for patients in a manic or hypomanic episode regulating mood-congruent emotions.

Likewise, only one study that we identified in our literature search investigated hypomanic patients; however, they were part of a mixed sample, including euthymic patients (Morris et al. 2012). Unfortunately, the authors did not investigate positive, that is, mood-congruent emotions for hypomanic patients. However, BD patients exhibited hyperactivity in rACC during the upregulation of negative emotions, but not during downregulation. While these findings do not contrast with the hypothesis of Rive et al. (2015), according to which an emotional conflict arises in the downregulation of emotions corresponding to the current mood, these findings indicate a further emotional conflict in patients with BD, which may contribute to difficulties in the emotional regulation of this patient group.

In sum, the findings of studies that investigated patients with current affective episodes suggest that the downregulation of mood-congruent and the upregulation of mood-incongruent emotions is associated with aberrant activity in the rACC. With reciprocal connections to the DLPFC, VLPFC, other parts of the ACC, and the amygdala, the rACC takes a prominent role within the ER network (Etkin et al. 2006, 2011; Phillips et al. 2008; Tang et al. 2019). The consistent reporting of aberrations in the rACC in BD patients with affective episodes suggests that this area is of particular relevance for the deficit ER of BD patients. Interestingly, aberrant activity in the rACC is also a neural differentiator between individuals at risk for BD and patients with current episodes. While both groups exhibit hyperactivity in the amygdala and the VLPFC and aberrant functional connectivity between these areas (Heissler et al. 2014; Kanske et al. 2015; Ladouceur et al. 2013), hyperactivity in the rACC seems to be exclusive for patients with current affective episodes (Morris et al. 2012; Rive et al. 2015). Revisiting the scar hypothesis, an interesting question is whether this aberrant rACC activity can also be found in remitted/euthymic patients. Since no aberrations were found in the rACC of risk groups, this would indicate that the aberrant rACC activity is more a consequence of the disorder than a risk factor, which would provide evidence for the scar hypothesis.

### Impairments of explicit emotion regulation in euthymic individuals

As outlined above, impairments in distraction can manifest in two ways. First, in impairments in the cognitive distraction task, and second in the experience of emotions as measured via self-report. Therefore, the results for distraction in euthymic BD patients are challenging to interpret. While in euthymic patients, measures concerning the distraction task's performance suggest impaired distraction (Caseras et al. 2015; Kanske et al. 2013), self-report measures of emotions revealed no significant differences between euthymic patients and HC (Kanske et al. 2015). Thus, taken together, the results suggest that euthymic patients may regulate their emotions successfully but at the expense of performance in cognitive tasks. In other words, distraction may require a higher cognitive effort in euthymic patients.

Regarding behavioral measures of reappraisal, the majority of studies did not find evidence for deficits in euthymic patients (Corbalán et al. 2015; Gruber et al. 2014; Kanske et al. 2015; Kjærstad et al. 2016; Townsend et al. 2013; Zhang et al. 2018). The only study that revealed impaired reappraisal at the behavioral level differs from the other studies in that self-focused reappraisal was used instead of situation-focused reappraisal (Rive et al. 2015). Regarding the explicit ER strategy of maintaining emotions (Gruber et al. 2013a), euthymic patients with BD-I showed reduced maintenance of negative emotions. No impairments were found for positive emotions. Phases of extensively elevated positive mood (= mania) are one core characteristic of BD. The results imply that patients with BD experience such phases because negative emotions that otherwise suppress positive emotions are maintained deficiently. In contrast to patients with BD, patients with UD were as able as HC in maintaining negative emotions (Gruber et al. 2013a, b). By explaining elevated mood in BD by a deficit in maintaining negative emotions, the authors thus provide an interesting etiological explanation for manic phases in patients with BD that distinguishes BD from other affective disorders. Further research is needed to provide a solution for inconsistencies that arise from this approach. For example, it does not explain depressive episodes in BD or that BD patients rate positive emotions less positively (Kanske et al. 2015). Further research with patients in different mood states could help resolve these inconsistencies.

In sum, the reviewed studies descriptively suggest differences in the effectiveness of different explicit ER strategies for euthymic patients. While the results indicate that (situation-focused) reappraisal may be an effective strategy for euthymic patients, due to increased cognitive effort during distraction in patients with BD, distraction seems less effective. On the other hand, studies systematically comparing distraction and reappraisal in euthymic patients did not find significant differences in both strategies' effectiveness (Kanske et al. 2015; Lois et al. 2017). Given further research efforts in this field, future studies may use meta-analytical methods to clarify differences in both strategies in euthymic patients.

***Neural deviations in euthymic patients during explicit emotion regulation***

Regarding neural measures, structural and functional aberrations in euthymic patients with BD were revealed (Caseras et al. 2015). During distraction, this group exhibited hyperactivity in DLPFC, amygdala, and nucleus accumbens. Interestingly, these findings differ between patients with BD-I and patients with BD-II. While the BD-I group exhibited hyperactivity in the areas mentioned above during distraction from happiness, the BD-II group exhibited the most pronounced aberrations during distraction from fear. Unlike BD-I patients, BD-II patients also exhibited increased inverse functional connectivity between DLPFC and amygdala during the distraction from fear. This finding is particularly interesting, combined with the behavioral findings of BD-II patients. Behaviorally, patients with BD-II showed no differences in the distraction of fear distractors compared to HC, which suggests that the strengthened connection between DLPFC and amygdala may be a compensatory mechanism that prevents behavioral losses.

Another study did not find any significant differences between euthymic BD patients and HC on the neural level (Kanske et al. 2015). However, again taking into account findings of hyperactivity in the right parietal cortex of patients with BD-I during distraction with an arithmetic task, a different picture emerges (Kanske et al. 2013). The right parietal cortex is associated with arithmetic tasks (Park et al. 2013). In line with the behavioral results, both studies suggest that BD patients can distract from emotions, but only by investing more resources in the distraction task.

Regarding reappraisal, hyperactivity in the amygdala of euthymic patients indicates impairments in ER (Corbalán et al. 2015; Kanske et al. 2015). Further, the reviewed studies revealed aberrations in frontal areas' functional connectivity and the amygdala (Kanske et al. 2015; Townsend et al. 2013; Zhang et al. 2018). However, the results are ambiguous as to which frontal areas are involved. Aberrant connectivity to the amygdala was found for the VLPFC, occipital gyrus, right posterior cingulate, right middle frontal gyrus (Townsend et al. 2013), DLFPC (Zhang et al. 2018), OFC, and ventral ACC (Kanske et al. 2015). While VLPFC and DLPFC were previously associated with explicit ER, the OFC and ventral ACC was more likely to be associated with implicit ER (Etkin et al. 2015; Phillips et al. 2008). Of particular interest here is the aberrant activity in the ventral ACC. Given that the ventral ACC and rACC together build a subsystem of the rACC (Etkin et al. 2011), as described above, aberrant activity in the rACC of euthymic patients is evidence for the scar hypothesis, which claims that the experience of affective episodes leads to permanent changes in patients with affective disorder. An interesting pending question is whether changes in activity in the ventral ACC predict the likelihood of recurrence.

#### *Discrepancies between behavioral and neural measures in euthymic patients*

A remarkable result of the studies investigating distraction in euthymic patients is the discrepancy between behavioral and neural results. While especially the studies that investigated situation-focused reappraisal did not find any significant behavioral differences between euthymic BD patients and HC (Corbalán et al. 2015; Gruber et al. 2014; Kanske et al. 2015; Kjærstad et al. 2016; Townsend et al. 2013; Zhang et al. 2018), neural aberrations in the amygdala, frontal areas, as well as in the functional connectivity between these areas were found. Regarding distraction, the studies reviewed suggest that euthymic patients with BD can successfully distract themselves from emotions, but this ability is associated with increased connectivity between areas associated with cognitive control and the amygdala (Caseras et al. 2015).

One possible explanation for the discrepancy is that it may be a statistical artifact resulting from underpowered study designs. (see the Limitations section of this article). An alternative explanation may be that neural aberrations represent compensatory mechanisms that prevent impairments on the behavioral level (Kjærstad et al. 2016). Considering that models of the neural basis of ER assume that frontal areas associated with cognitive control act to regulate striatal areas of emotion reactivity, this explanation also seems plausible. Aberrations were found in frontal areas and the connectivity between frontal and striatal areas. Further indications of a compensatory mechanism can be inferred from studies in which euthymic patients showed increased recruitment of areas associated with the distraction task but did not differ significantly from HC in terms of perceived emotions (Kanske et al. 2013, 2015). Further plausibility for the compensation hypothesis arises from the fact that most euthymic patients examined in the reviewed studies were on medication and/or psychotherapeutic treatment.

Given that medication and psychotherapy have compensatory effects on symptoms of mental disorders, it seems plausible if compensatory mechanisms are also reflected in brain activity. In any case, the interpretation of neural changes in euthymic patients must consider the effects of medication and psychotherapy. The next section outlines the implications of the findings for psychotherapy and trainability in more detail.

#### Implications

The studies that examined explicit ER in patients with BD showed aberrations in areas associated with explicit ER (e.g., DLPFC and VLPFC) and areas associated with implicit ER (e.g., OFC and ACC). These findings are also consistent with the model of Phillips et al. (2008); it assumes a partially joint route of explicit and implicit ER. This joint route is particularly interesting in light of studies showing that patients with BD exhibit deficits in using effective implicit ER in their daily lives. If activating the explicit route also activates the implicit route, this has important implications for trainability. Frequent (co-) activation of the implicit route when using explicit ER might also lead to implicit ER improvements. Since explicit ER can be trained in a controlled manner, it could also improve implicit ER.

Indeed, previous studies reveal evidence for the trainability of ER (Schweizer et al. 2013). Training with an emotional working memory paradigm affects neural activity in areas associated with explicit emotion regulation (like the DLPFC and VLPFC) and areas more associated with implicit emotion regulation (like the OFC and ACC) as well as the connectivity between them.

Another approach to improving ER in BD patients is to train patients to use ER strategies that are most effective for them, as studies have shown the importance of choosing an appropriate ER strategy for successful ER (Sheppes et al. 2014). This point is particularly relevant in light of the reviewed studies that have directly compared different ER strategies. On the one hand, these studies can show whether and how BD patients can fall back on successful ER strategies and, on the other hand, whether there are deficits that still need to be addressed. Given that it is relatively spared in BD, distraction may be a resource that BD patients can exploit, while they may not benefit from applying reappraisal. On the other hand, patients could benefit from more frequent reappraisal use in the long run because repeated use could act like training and lead to a more successful application. The frequently found aberrations in fronto-limbic connectivity during reappraisal in BD may indicate precisely this potential for improvement. Moreover, as healthy individuals at risk for BD show similar fronto-limbic abnormalities, training reappraisal may also function as a preventive intervention.

In summary, our review suggests the following conclusions. First, individuals at risk for BD exhibit neural aberrations, which may be a specific marker to distinguish the risk of BD from the risk of unipolar depression. Secondly, individuals at risk for BD and euthymic patients may compensate for ER deficits by enhanced recruitment of structures related to cognitive control and/or relevant for the distraction task. Our review found that both distraction and reappraisal are effective strategies for BD patients and individuals at risk for BD to regulate their emotions.

#### Limitations

The present review aimed to apply a strict definition of explicit ER to describe specific neural and behavioral aberrations in explicit ER in individuals at risk for BD, patients with a current affective episode, and euthymic patients. We further classified the reviewed studies based on the ER strategy investigated (i.e., reappraisal, distraction, and maintenance). These classifications entail limitations because, regarding specific samples in combination with specific ER strategies, only a few studies are available. Further, it should be noted that not all ER strategies are equally represented in research. Most studies investigated reappraisal, followed by distraction, and last, maintenance. Similarly, in terms of mood state, most studies investigated euthymic patients. Only two studies investigated patients with an affective episode.

Although these classifications lead to less robust conclusions due to the small number of studies in each class, they have the advantage of allowing a more fine-grained description of the variations in ER of individuals with or at risk for BD.

Furthermore, the conclusions on explicit ER as a marker for BD are subject to limitations. On the one hand, the reviewed studies show that altered explicit ER is present in risk groups, primarily evidenced by altered neural processing; on the other hand, it is unclear how specific these alterations are in differentiating them from other disorders with alterations in emotion regulation. While we addressed the differences between patients with BD and unipolar depression in discussing the results, we did not include other disorders in which ER disorders are present (e.g., borderline personality disorder and schizophrenia). This selection is due to the lack of studies comparing these groups. In particular, it should be emphasized here that the known markers according to which risk groups can be determined cannot themselves specifically distinguish between different affective disorders. For example, the first-degree relatives of BD patients who constitute the risk group in some of the reviewed studies show not only an increased risk of developing BD themselves but also an increased vulnerability to other disorders (Rasic et al. 2014). Longitudinal studies are needed that allow classification into specific risk groups after the onset of the disorder and assess explicit ER before the onset.

Many of the reviewed studies reported null findings, making it difficult to reach a conclusive estimate of intact or impaired ER in individuals with BD or at risk for BD. On the one hand, this is due to the theoretical conception of frequentist significance tests, and on the other hand, many neuroscientific studies are underpowered (Poldrack 2017). Reporting statistical power in frequentist statistics or a switch to bayesian hypothesis tests with planned precision would allow a more precise interpretation of the results (Kruschke and Liddell 2018). All of the reviewed studies used frequentist significance tests. Most of them did not report statistical power that would allow more accurate handling of any null results. Accordingly, caution is advised in our synthesis and interpretation of the findings. In future research, meta-analytic approaches may draw more accurate conclusions.

Another difficulty concerning the interpretation of the present studies arises from the medication of the samples studied. Only a single study, which examined patients with BD, investigated a medication-free patient sample. Although studying medicated samples can provide important insights, it is essential for causal research of BD to increasingly control for medication. Similar concerns apply to research on patients in euthymic mood state. On the one hand, research with remitted patients provides essential insights, particularly concerning the consequences of affective episodes. On the other hand, it reveals little about the causes of BD, as any differences between remitted patients and HC may result from medication, psychotherapy, or change in life circumstances related to the disorder. Without adequately accounting for these factors, it remains difficult to separate them in interpretation.

In recent research, different response styles of emotion regulation have been increasingly studied (Nolen-Hoeksema 2004). The term response styles describe the individual tendency to react to emotions in a certain way (e.g., a tendency to ruminate). Since this tendency is rather implicit, it is outside the scope of the present review. This exclusion is a possible limitation of the present review, as the explicit regulation of different response styles could represent an interesting interaction between explicit and implicit ER. On the other hand, this would contradict the strict definition of explicit ER that we based the review on and further complicate the already difficult distinction between explicit and implicit ER at the neural level. For this reason, we decided against including research on response styles.

#### Acknowledgements

None.

#### Authors' contributions

PK provided the conception of the review, PM did the literature research, KF and MK classified, interpreted, and discussed the results of the literature research. MB and PK supervised the work on the manuscript. MK wrote the manuscript. All authors read and approved the final manuscript.

**Author details**
[1] Clinical Psychology and Behavioral Neuroscience, Faculty of Psychology, Technische Universität Dresden, Chemnitzer Str. 46, 01187 Dresden, Germany.
[2] Department of Psychiatry and Psychotherapy, Medical Faculty, University Hospital Carl Gustav Carus, Technische Universität Dresden, Dresden, Germany.
[3] Max Planck Institute for Human Cognitive and Brain Sciences, Leipzig, Germany.

**References**

Ajaya Y, Peckham AD, Johnson SL. Emotion regulation and mania risk: Differential responses to implicit and explicit cues to regulate. J Behav Ther Exp Psychiatry. 2016;50:283–8. https://doi.org/10.1016/j.jbtep.2015.10.004.

Aldao A, Nolen-Hoeksema S, Schweizer S. Emotion-regulation strategies across psychopathology: a meta-analytic review. Clin Psychol Rev. 2010;30(2):217–37. https://doi.org/10.1016/j.cpr.2009.11.004.

Almeida JRC, Phillips ML. Distinguishing between unipolar depression and bipolar depression: current and future clinical and neuroimaging perspectives. Biol Psychiat. 2013;73(2):111–8.

American Psychiatric Association. (2013). *Diagnostic and statistical manual of mental disorders: DSM-5* (5th ed.). American Psychiatric Association.

Bauer M, Glenn T, Alda M, Bauer R, Grof P, Marsh W, Monteith S, Munoz R, Rasgon N, Sagduyu K, Whybrow PC. Trajectories of adherence to mood stabilizers in patients with bipolar disorder. Int J Bipolar Disord. 2019;7(1):19.

Becerra R, Cruise K, Murray G, Bassett D, Harms C, Allan A, Hood S. Emotion regulation in bipolar disorder: Are emotion regulation abilities less compromised in euthymic bipolar disorder than unipolar depressive or anxiety disorders? Open J Psychiatry. 2013;03(04):1–7. https://doi.org/10.4236/ojpsych.2013.34A001.

Braunstein LM, Gross JJ, Ochsner KN. Explicit and implicit emotion regulation: A multi-level framework. Social Cogn Affect Neurosci. 2017;12(10):1545–57. https://doi.org/10.1093/scan/nsx096.

Bürger C, Redlich R, Grotegerd D, Meinert S, Dohm K, Schneider I, Zaremba D, Förster K, Alferink J, Bölte J, Heindel W, Kugel H, Arolt V, Dannlowski U. Differential abnormal pattern of anterior cingulate gyrus activation in unipolar and bipolar depression: an fmri and pattern classification approach. Neuropsychopharmacology. 2017;42(7):1399–408. https://doi.org/10.1038/npp.2017.36.

Canli T, Sivers H, Thomason ME, Whitfield-Gabrieli S, Gabrieli JDE, Gotlib IH. Brain activation to emotional words in depressed vs healthy subjects. NeuroReport. 2004;15(17):2585–8. https://doi.org/10.1097/00001756-200412030-00005.

Caseras X, Murphy K, Lawrence NS, Fuentes-Claramonte P, Watts J, Jones DK, Phillips ML. Emotion regulation deficits in euthymic bipolar I versus bipolar II disorder: a functional and diffusion-tensor imaging study. Bipolar Disord. 2015;17(5):461–70. https://doi.org/10.1111/bdi.12292.

Corbalán F, Beaulieu S, Armony JL. Emotion regulation in bipolar disorder type I: an fMRI study. Psychol Med. 2015;45(12):2521–31. https://doi.org/10.1017/S0033291715000434.

Craddock N, Sklar P. Genetics of bipolar disorder. Lancet. 2013;381(9878):1654–62. https://doi.org/10.1016/S0140-6736(13)60855-7.

Denny BT, Ochsner KN. Behavioral effects of longitudinal training in cognitive reappraisal. Emotion. 2014;14(2):425–33. https://doi.org/10.1037/a0035276.

Dodd A, Lockwood E, Mansell W, Palmier-Claus J. Emotion regulation strategies in bipolar disorder: A systematic and critical review. J Affect Disord. 2019;246:262–84. https://doi.org/10.1016/j.jad.2018.12.026.

Eckblad M, Chapman LJ. Development and validation of a scale for hypomanic personality. J Abnorm Psychol. 1986;95(3):214–22. https://doi.org/10.1037//0021-843X.95.3.214.

Elliott R, Ogilvie A, Rubinsztein JS, Calderon G, Dolan RJ, Sahakian BJ. Abnormal ventral frontal response during performance of an affective go/no go task in patients with mania. Biol Psychiat. 2004;55(12):1163–70. https://doi.org/10.1016/j.biopsych.2004.03.007.

Etkin A, Egner T, Peraza DM, Kandel ER, Hirsch J. Resolving emotional conflict: a role for the rostral anterior cingulate cortex in modulating activity in the amygdala. Neuron. 2006;51(6):871–82. https://doi.org/10.1016/j.neuron.2006.07.029

Etkin A, Egner T, Kalisch R. Emotional processing in anterior cingulate and medial prefrontal cortex. Trends Cogn Sci. 2011;15(2):85–93. https://doi.org/10.1016/j.tics.2010.11.004.

Green MJ, Lino BJ, Hwang E-J, Sparks A, James C, Mitchell PB. Cognitive regulation of emotion in bipolar I disorder and unaffected biological relatives. Acta Psychiatr Scand. 2011;124(4):307–16. https://doi.org/10.1111/j.1600-0447.2011.01718.x.

Gross JJ. Antecedent- and response-focused emotion regulation: Divergent consequences for experience, expression, and physiology. J Pers Soc Psychol. 1998a;74(1):224–37.

Gross JJ. The Emerging Field of Emotion Regulation: An Integrative Review. Rev Gen Psychol. 1998b;2(3):271–99. https://doi.org/10.1037/1089-2680.2.3.271.

Gross JJ. Handbook of Emotion Regulation, Second Edition (2nd ed.). Guilford Publications. 2013. http://gbv.eblib.com/patron/FullRecord.aspx?p=1578364

Gross JJ. The Extended Process Model of Emotion Regulation: Elaborations, Applications, and Future Directions. Psychol Inq. 2015;26(1):130–7. https://doi.org/10.1080/1047840X.2015.989751.

Grotegerd D, Suslow T, Bauer J, Ohrmann P, Arolt V, Stuhrmann A, Heindel W, Kugel H, Dannlowski U. Discriminating unipolar and bipolar depression by means of fMRI and pattern classification: a pilot study. Eur Arch Psychiatry Clin Neurosci. 2013;263(2):119–31.

Gruber J. Can Feeling Too Good Be Bad? Curr Dir Psychol Sci. 2011;20(4):217–21. https://doi.org/10.1177/0963721411414632.

Gruber J, Harvey AG, Gross JJ. When trying is not enough: Emotion regulation and the effort-success gap in bipolar disorder. Emotion. 2012;12(5):997–1003. https://doi.org/10.1037/a0026822.

Gruber J, Purcell AL, Perna MJ. Letting go of the bad: deficit in maintaining negative, but not positive, emotion in bipolar disorder. Emotion. 2013a;13(1):168–75. https://doi.org/10.1037/a0029381.

Gruber J, Kogan A, Mennin D, Murray G. Real-world emotion? An experience-sampling approach to emotion experience and regulation in bipolar I disorder. J Abnorm Psychol. 2013b;122(4):971–83. https://doi.org/10.1037/a0034425.

Gruber J, Hay AC, Gross JJ. Rethinking emotion: Cognitive reappraisal is an effective positive and negative emotion regulation strategy in bipolar disorder. Emotion. 2014;14(2):388–96. https://doi.org/10.1037/a0035249.

Gyurak A, Gross JJ, Etkin A. Explicit and implicit emotion regulation: a dual-process framework. Cogn Emot. 2011;25(3):400–12. https://doi.org/10.1080/02699931.2010.544160.

Heissler J, Kanske P, Schönfelder S, Wessa M. Inefficiency of emotion regulation as vulnerability marker for bipolar disorder: evidence from healthy individuals with hypomanic personality. J Affect Disord. 2014;152–154:83–90. https://doi.org/10.1016/j.jad.2013.05.001.

Izard CE. Facial expressions and the regulation of emotions. J Pers Soc Psychol. 1990;58(3):487–98. https://doi.org/10.1037/0022-3514.58.3.487.

Johnson SL, Carver CS, Joormann J, Cuccaro M. A genetic analysis of the validity of the Hypomanic Personality Scale. Bipolar Disord. 2015;17(3):331–9. https://doi.org/10.1111/bdi.12251.

Kanske P, Heissler J, Schönfelder S, Wessa M. Neural correlates of emotion regulation deficits in remitted depression: The influence of regulation strategy, habitual regulation use, and emotional valence. Neuroimage. 2012;61(3):686–93. https://doi.org/10.1016/j.neuroimage.2012.03.089.

Kanske P, Heissler J, Schönfelder S, Forneck J, Wessa M. Neural correlates of emotional distractibility in bipolar disorder patients, unaffected relatives, and individuals with hypomanic personality. Am J Psychiatry. 2013;170(12):1487–96. https://doi.org/10.1176/appi.ajp.2013.12081044.

Kanske P, Schönfelder S, Forneck J, Wessa M. Impaired regulation of emotion: Neural correlates of reappraisal and distraction in bipolar disorder and unaffected relatives. Transl Psychiatry. 2015;5:e497. https://doi.org/10.1038/tp.2014.137.

Khoury B, Lecomte T. Emotion regulation and schizophrenia. Int J Cogn Ther. 2012;5(1):67–76.

Kjærstad HL, Vinberg M, Goldin PR, Køster N, Støttrup MMD, Knorr U, Kessing LV, Miskowiak KW. Impaired down-regulation of negative emotion in self-referent social situations in bipolar disorder: a pilot study of a novel experimental paradigm. Psychiatry Res. 2016;238:318–25. https://doi.org/10.1016/j.psychres.2016.02.047

Kohn N, Eickhoff SB, Scheller M, Laird AR, Fox PT, Habel U. Neural network of cognitive emotion regulation—an ALE meta-analysis and MACM analysis. Neuroimage. 2014;87:345–55.

Koole SL. The psychology of emotion regulation: an integrative review. Cogn Emot. 2009;23(1):4–41. https://doi.org/10.1080/02699930802619031.

Kruschke JK, Liddell TM. The Bayesian new statistics: hypothesis testing, estimation, meta-analysis, and power analysis from a Bayesian perspective. Psychon Bull Rev. 2018;25(1):178–206.

Kwapil TR, Miller MB, Zinser MC, Chapman LJ, Chapman J, Eckblad M. A longitudinal study of high scorers on the Hypomanic Personality Scale. J Abnorm Psychol. 2000;109(2):222–6. https://doi.org/10.1037//0021-843X.109.2.222.

Ladouceur CD, Diwadkar VA, White R, Bass J, Birmaher B, Axelson DA, Phillips ML. Fronto-limbic function in unaffected offspring at familial risk for bipolar disorder during an emotional working memory paradigm. Dev Cogn Neurosci. 2013;5:185–96. https://doi.org/10.1016/j.dcn.2013.03.004.

Larkin GR, Cartensen LL. Divergent trajectories in the aging mind: changes in working memory for affective versus visual information with age. Psychol Aging. 2005;20(4):542–53. https://doi.org/10.1037/0882-7974.20.4.542.

Lawrence NS, Williams AM, Surguladze S, Giampietro V, Brammer MJ, Andrew C, FrangouEckerPhillips SCML. Subcortical and ventral prefrontal cortical neural responses to facial expressions distinguish patients with bipolar disorder and major depression. Biol Psychiat. 2004;55(6):578–87.

Lois G, Gerchen MF, Kirsch P, Kanske P, Schönfelder S, Wessa M. Large-scale network functional interactions during distraction and reappraisal in remitted bipolar and unipolar patients. Bipolar Disord. 2017;19(6):487–95. https://doi.org/10.1111/bdi.12512.

Malhi GS, Morris G, Hamilton A, Outhred T, Mannie Z. Is "early intervention" in bipolar disorder what it claims to be? Bipolar Disord. 2017;19(8):627–36. https://doi.org/10.1111/bdi.12576.

Mauss IB, Cook CL, Cheng JYJ, Gross JJ. Individual differences in cognitive reappraisal: experiential and physiological responses to an anger provocation. Int J Psychophysiol. 2007;66(2):116–24. https://doi.org/10.1016/j.ijpsycho.2007.03.017.

Mercer L, Becerra R. A unique emotional processing profile of euthymic bipolar disorder? A critical review. J Affect Disord. 2013;146(3):295–309. https://doi.org/10.1016/j.jad.2012.10.030.

Mikels JA, Reuter-Lorenz PA, Beyer JA, Fredrickson BL. Emotion and working memory: evidence for domain-specific processes for affective maintenance. Emotion. 2008;8(2):256–66. https://doi.org/10.1037/1528-3542.8.2.256.

Morris RW, Sparks A, Mitchell PB, Weickert CS, Green MJ. Lack of cortico-limbic coupling in bipolar disorder and schizophrenia during emotion regulation. Transl Psychiatry. 2012;2:e90. https://doi.org/10.1038/tp.2012.16.

Nolen-Hoeksema S. The response styles theory. In: Papageorgiou C, Wells A, editors. Depressive rumination: Nature, theory and treatment. Chichester: Wiley; 2004. p. 107–23.

Ochsner KN, Gross JJ. The cognitive control of emotion. Trends Cogn Sci. 2005;9(5):242–9. https://doi.org/10.1016/j.tics.2005.03.010.

Ochsner KN, Gross JJ. The neural bases of emotion and emotion regulation: A valuation perspective. In: Gross JJ, editor. Handbook of emotion regulation. 2nd ed. New York: Guilford; 2014. p. 23–42.

Ochsner KN, Ray RD, Cooper JC, Robertson ER, Chopra S, Gabrieli JDE, Gross JJ. For better or for worse: Neural systems supporting the cognitive down- and up-regulation of negative emotion. Neuroimage. 2004;23(2):483–99. https://doi.org/10.1016/j.neuroimage.2004.06.030.

Park J, Park DC, Polk TA. Parietal functional connectivity in numerical cognition. Cerebral Cortex. 2013 ;23(9):2127–2135.

Phillips ML. Understanding the neurobiology of emotion perception: Implications for psychiatry. The British Journal of Psychiatry : The Journal of Mental Science. 2003;182:190–2. https://doi.org/10.1192/bjp.182.3.190.

Phillips ML, Kupfer DJ. Bipolar disorder diagnosis: challenges and future directions. Lancet. 2013;381(9878):1663–71.

Phillips ML, Ladouceur CD, Drevets WC. A neural model of voluntary and automatic emotion regulation: Implications for understanding the pathophysiology and neurodevelopment of bipolar disorder. Mol Psychiatry. 2008;13(9):833–57. https://doi.org/10.1038/mp.2008.65.

Pilhatsch M, Glenn T, Rasgon N, Alda M, Sagduyu K, Grof P, Munoz R, Marsh W, Monteith S, Severus E, Bauer R, Ritter P, Whybrow PC, Bauer M. Regularity of self-reported daily dosage of mood stabilizers and antipsychotics in patients with bipolar disorder. Int J Bipolar Disord. 2018;6(1):10. https://doi.org/10.1186/s40345-018-0118-8.

Poldrack RA, Baker CI, Durnez J, Gorgolewski KJ, Matthews PM, Munafò MR, Yarkoni T. Scanning the horizon: towards transparent and reproducible neuroimaging research. Nat Rev Neurosci. 2017;18(2):115.

Rasic D, Hajek T, Alda M, Uher R. Risk of mental illness in offspring of parents with schizophrenia, bipolar disorder, and major depressive disorder: a meta-analysis of family high-risk studies. Schizophr Bull. 2014;40(1):28–38. https://doi.org/10.1093/schbul/sbt114.

Redlich R, Almeida JJR, Grotegerd D, Opel N, Kugel H, Heindel W, Arolt V, Phillips ML, Dannlowski U. Brain morphometric biomarkers distinguishing unipolar and bipolar depression. A voxel-based morphometry-pattern classification approach. JAMA Psychiatry. 2014;71(11):1222–30. https://doi.org/10.1001/jamapsychiatry.2014.1100.

Repple J, Meinert S, Grotegerd D, Kugel H, Redlich R, Dohm K, Zaremba D, Opel N, Buerger C, Förster K, Nick T, Arolt V, Heindel W, Deppe M, Dannlowski U. A voxel-based diffusion tensor imaging study in unipolar and bipolar depression. Bipolar Disord. 2017;19(1):23–31. https://doi.org/10.1111/bdi.12465.

Rive MM, van Rooijen G, Veltman DJ, Phillips ML, Schene AH, Ruhé HG. Neural correlates of dysfunctional emotion regulation in major depressive disorder. A systematic review of neuroimaging studies. Neurosci Biobehav Rev. 2013;37(10):2529–53.

Rive MM, Mocking RJT, Koeter MWJ, van Wingen G, de Wit SJ, van den Heuvel OA, Veltman DJ, Ruhé HG, Schene AH. State-dependent differences in emotion regulation between unmedicated bipolar disorder and major depressive disorder. JAMA Psychiat. 2015;72(7):687–96. https://doi.org/10.1001/jamapsychiatry.2015.0161.

Rohde P, Lewinsohn PM, Seeley JR. Are people changed by the experience of having an episode of depression? A further test of the scar hypothesis. J Abnorm Psychol. 1990;99(3):264–71. https://doi.org/10.1037/0021-843X.99.3.264.

Rosen HR, Rich BA. Neurocognitive correlates of emotional stimulus processing in pediatric bipolar disorder: A review. Postgrad Med. 2010;122(4):94–104. https://doi.org/10.3810/pgm.2010.07.2177.

Schweizer S, Grahn J, Hampshire A, Mobbs D, Dalgleish T. Training the emotional brain: Improving affective control through emotional working memory training. J Neurosci. 2013;33(12):5301–11. https://doi.org/10.1523/JNEUROSCI.2593-12.2013.

Sheppes G, Scheibe S, Suri G, Radu P, Blechert J, Gross JJ. Emotion regulation choice: a conceptual framework and supporting evidence. J Exp Psychol Gen. 2014;143(1):163–81. https://doi.org/10.1037/a0030831.

Simsek F, Oguz K, Kitis O, Akan ST, Kempton MJ, Gonul AS. Neural activation during cognitive reappraisal in girls at high risk for depression. Prog Neuropsychopharmacol Biol Psychiatry. 2017;77:49–56. https://doi.org/10.1016/j.pnpbp.2017.03.022.

Surguladze SA, Marshall N, Schulze K, Hall MH, Walshe M, Bramon E, McDonald C. Exaggerated neural response to emotional faces in patients with bipolar disorder and their first-degree relatives. Neuroimage. 2010;53(1):58–64.

Tang W, Jbabdi S, Zhu Z, Cottaar M, Grisot G, Lehman JF, Yendiki A, Haber SN. A connectional hub in the rostral anterior cingulate cortex links areas of emotion and cognitive control. Elife. 2019. https://doi.org/10.7554/eLife.43761.

Townsend JD, Altshuler LL. Emotion processing and regulation in bipolar disorder: A review. Bipolar Disord. 2012;14(4):326–39. https://doi.org/10.1111/j.1399-5618.2012.01021.x.

Townsend JD, Torrisi SJ, Lieberman MD, Sugar CA, Bookheimer SY, Altshuler LL. Frontal-amygdala connectivity alterations during emotion downregulation in bipolar I disorder. Biol Psychiat. 2013;73(2):127–35. https://doi.org/10.1016/j.biopsych.2012.06.030.

Tugade MM, Fredrickson BL. Regulation of Positive Emotions: Emotion Regulation Strategies that Promote Resilience. J Happiness Stud. 2007;8(3):311–33. https://doi.org/10.1007/s10902-006-9015-4.

van Dillen LF, Heslenfeld DJ, Koole SL. Tuning down the emotional brain: an fMRI study of the effects of cognitive load on the processing of affective images. Neuroimage. 2009;45(4):1212–9. https://doi.org/10.1016/j.neuroimage.2009.01.016.

Walsh MA, DeGeorge DP, Barrantes-Vidal N, Kwapil TR. A 3-Year Longitudinal Study of Risk for Bipolar Spectrum Psychopathology. J Abnorm Psychol. 2015;124(3):486–97. https://doi.org/10.1037/abn0000045.

Wessa M, Linke J. Emotional processing in bipolar disorder: Behavioural and neuroimaging findings. Int Rev Psychiatry. 2009;21(4):357–67. https://doi.org/10.1080/09540260902962156.

Wessa M, Houenou J, Paillère-Martinot M-L, Berthoz S, Artiges E, Leboyer M, Martinot J-L. Fronto-striatal overactivation in euthymic bipolar patients during an emotional go/nogo task. Am J Psychiatry. 2007;164(4):638–46. https://doi.org/10.1176/ajp.2007.164.4.638.

Wessa M, Heissler J, Schönfelder S, Kanske P. Goal-directed behavior under emotional distraction is preserved by enhanced task-specific activation. Social Cogn Affect Neurosci. 2013;8(3):305–12. https://doi.org/10.1093/scan/nsr098.

Wessa M, Kanske P, Linke J. Bipolar disorder: a neural network perspective on a disorder of emotion and motivation. Restor Neurol Neurosci. 2014;32(1):51–62. https://doi.org/10.3233/RNN-139007.

Willroth EC, Hilimire MR. Differential effects of self- and situation-focused reappraisal. Emotion. 2016;16(4):468–74. https://doi.org/10.1037/emo0000139.

Zhang L, Opmeer EM, van der Meer L, Aleman A, Ćurčić-Blake B, Ruhé HG. Altered frontal-amygdala effective connectivity during effortful emotion regulation in bipolar disorder. Bipolar Disord. 2018;20(4):349–58. https://doi.org/10.1111/bdi.12611.

# 7

# The futility of long-term predictions in bipolar disorder: mood fluctuations are the result of deterministic chaotic processes

Abigail Ortiz[1,2*], Kamil Bradler[3], Maxine Mowete[4], Stephane MacLean[5], Julie Garnham[6], Claire Slaney[6], Benoit H. Mulsant[1,2] and Martin Alda[7,8]

**Abstract**

**Background:** Understanding the underlying architecture of mood regulation in bipolar disorder (BD) is important, as we are starting to conceptualize BD as a more complex disorder than one of recurring manic or depressive episodes. Nonlinear techniques are employed to understand and model the behavior of complex systems. Our aim was to assess the underlying nonlinear properties that account for mood and energy fluctuations in patients with BD; and to compare whether these processes were different in healthy controls (HC) and unaffected first-degree relatives (FDR). We used three different nonlinear techniques: Lyapunov exponent, detrended fluctuation analysis and fractal dimension to assess the underlying behavior of mood and energy fluctuations in all groups; and subsequently to assess whether these arise from different processes in each of these groups.

**Results:** There was a positive, short-term autocorrelation for both mood and energy series in all three groups. In the mood series, the largest Lyapunov exponent was found in HC (1.84), compared to BD (1.63) and FDR (1.71) groups [$F(2, 87) = 8.42$, $p < 0.005$]. A post-hoc Tukey test showed that Lyapunov exponent in HC was significantly higher than both the BD ($p = 0.003$) and FDR groups ($p = 0.03$). Similarly, in the energy series, the largest Lyapunov exponent was found in HC (1.85), compared to BD (1.76) and FDR (1.67) [$F(2, 87) = 11.02$; $p < 0.005$]. There were no significant differences between groups for the detrended fluctuation analysis or fractal dimension.

**Conclusions:** The underlying nature of mood variability is in keeping with that of a chaotic system, which means that fluctuations are generated by deterministic nonlinear process(es) in HC, BD, and FDR. The value of this complex modeling lies in analyzing the nature of the processes involved in mood regulation. It also suggests that the window for episode prediction in BD will be inevitably short.

**Keywords:** Bipolar disorder, Mood fluctuations, Nonlinear analyses, Episode prediction, Unaffected first-degree relatives

## Background

Bipolar disorder (BD) is a mood disorder characterized by (hypo)manic, mixed, or depressive episodes, interspersed with low amplitude mood fluctuations or, at times, with subsyndromal mood symptoms. Understanding how mood is regulated is important in BD, as we are only starting to conceptualize it as a more complex disorder than simply one of recurring manic and depressive episodes.

Mood regulation is a complex and poorly understood process, which can be conceived as a "buffer" system that allows flexible responses to changing conditions (Ortiz and Alda 2018). All complex systems, including mood, are continuously subject to stochastic variations in external conditions. From a dynamic point of view,

*Correspondence: abigail.ortiz@utoronto.ca
[1] Department of Psychiatry, University of Toronto, Toronto, ON, Canada
Full list of author information is available at the end of the article

the properties that enable the system to adapt to these stochastic variations are considered "complex". These properties include: (i) nonlinearity, i.e., systems do not respond in a way that is proportional to the amount they are stimulated; (ii) the lack of a single or characteristic scale, i.e., fractal organization; and (iii) emergent properties, i.e., properties that emerge from the whole but were not present in the parts. Nonlinearity, however, does not imply a lack of underlying structure; on the contrary, nonlinear systems have organized, discoverable principles. The challenge is that these principles are difficult to uncover by conventional analyses and require nonlinear methods for their study.

Nonlinear methods offer new tools to quantify, model, and predict the behavior of complex systems (Ehlers 1995; Pincus 2001). Time-series analysis is a type of nonlinear method employed to study a collection of observations made sequentially in time (Chatfield 2016). Its special feature is that successive observations are not independent, and that the analysis must take into account the time order of the observations. Using time-series analysis, we have recently described higher regularity—a "pathologically stable" or organized mood in patients with BD (Ortiz et al. 2015) and their unaffected first-degree relatives (FDR) (Ortiz et al. 2019). Other authors have also described that mood in patients with BD is a process that becomes more organized over a longer time scale, as opposed to processes in healthy controls (Gottschalk et al. 1995; Bayani et al. 2017; Bonsall et al. 2012).

Although this increased degree of organization of mood in BD may seem paradoxical, these data fit an increasingly apparent pattern in Biology, where aging (Goldberger et al. 2002a, b), cardiovascular diseases (Jelinek et al. 2013; Olde Rikkert et al. 2016; Peng et al. 1995a), metabolic diseases (Wu et al. 2013; Gomolka et al. 2018), and psychiatric diseases (Cowdry et al. 1991; Golier et al. 2001; Katerndahl et al. 2007; Pincus et al. 2008) are marked by increasing degrees of organization. In other words, these systems are less flexible and able to cope with the demands of a constantly changing environment. These observations have led to hypothesize that mood variability might be better described in terms of chaotic dynamics (Bonsall et al. 2012; Bonsall et al. 2015; Huber et al. 1999, 2000).

In this paper, we aim to further characterize the nonlinear dynamics of mood and energy regulation in time-series data from 90 participants (30 healthy controls (HC), 30 euthymic patients with BD, and 30 unaffected FDR) using nonlinear methods. While our research shares a foundation with our previous work using paper-based time-series analysis to compare mood regulation in HC, unaffected FDR, and euthymic patients with BD, in this study we analyzed mood and energy series using three nonlinear indicators (Lyapunov exponent, detended fluctuation analysis, and fractal dimension), with the aim of understanding whether mood fluctuations stem from different processes in each of these groups.

## Material and methods

### Participant recruitment

As per our previous papers (Ortiz et al. 2015, 2019), we obtained data from 90 participants: 30 HC, 30 euthymic patients with BD, and 30 unaffected FDR. Euthymia was operationalized as at least 3 months of a Young Mania Rating Scale (YMRS) score $\leq 5$ (Young et al. 1978) and a Hamilton Depression Rating Scale (HDRS) score $\leq 7$ (Hamilton 1960). All participants were interviewed by the same investigator (AO), using the Schedule for Affective Disorders and Schizophrenia-Lifetime version (SADS-L) (Endicott and Spitzer 1978); diagnosis was confirmed in a blind fashion in consensus meetings with the research team. The investigation was carried out in accordance with the latest version of the Declaration of Helsinki. The study design was approved by the local ethical committee and written informed consent of participants was obtained after the nature of the procedures had been fully explained.

### Measurements

We used paper-based visual analog scales (VAS) to measure mood, energy, anxiety, and sleep. The scale ranges from '1' to '9', with '5' being 'their usual'. Participants provided measurements on these variables over a three-month period, twice each day. The first rating was completed 1 h after waking up, and the second rating 1 h before bedtime. For incomplete data in the VAS scale (2 days in a row), we used interpolation methods; if more than 2 days were missing consecutively (usually at the end of the study), the rest of the data were removed from the calculations.

### Analytical consideration for nonlinear analyses

1. Time-series analyses

   The analyses performed relies on three assumptions:

   (i) The character of the collected data: the data-points *Si* (for $i = \{1, 2, 9\}$), represent an interval scale. This means that we consider the data not only to be a totally ordered set *{Si}* ($S_i < S_{i+1}$ for all measured quantities) but also that the differences between *i* and *j* ($i \neq j$) do have a specific meaning. This is a strong assumption, given that the underlying process(es) we try to shed light on need not be proportional to the measurement scale and most likely are logarithmic, as seen in other human phenomena (Varshney and Sun 2013).

(ii) The validity of a model to which we try to fit the data. The collected data are noisy, and the resolution in both the domain and range of the time series is low. We were cautious not to overfit the data by using simple models (i.e., first-order departure from a completely random process (white noise) or the autoregressive process AR (Ortiz and Alda 2018).

(iii) Finally, given the character of the data, we cannot verify the requirement of strict stationarity, but we may relax this notion and ask the time series to satisfy *weak* stationarity. That is, we require only the first two moments (mean and variance) to be time invariant. The requirement of at least weak stationarity is crucial for time-series analysis. For a complete description of the analyses, please see (Ortiz et al. 2015).

In summary, we assumed that the difference between intervals in the scale has a specific meaning and that the time series are weak non-stationary. We were cautious not to overfit the data by using simple models.

2. Lyapunov exponent (LE)
   LE is a quantitative measurement of a parameter's sensitive dependence on initial conditions, which provides a quantitative indication of the chaotic level of a system. In medicine, LE has been used to analyze heart rate variability (Hu et al. 2009 and EEG signals (Hu et al. 2009; Hu et al. 2010). LE defines the average rate of divergence or convergence of two neighboring trajectories in the state-space (Nayak et al. 2018). Positive LE values indicate that the phase space trajectories are diverging (i.e., the closely located points in the initial state are quickly separating from each other in the $i$ direction), and the system is losing its predictability, exhibiting chaotic behavior. Conversely, a negative LE represents the average rate of the convergence of the phase space trajectories. Additional file 1 describes specific analytical considerations for LE.
3. Detendred fluctuation analysis (DFA)
   DFA is used to measure long range dependence in a time-series (Peng et al. 1994, 1995b). A parameter referred as "Hurst exponent" ($H$) describes the correlation properties of the dataset; it quantifies the relative tendency of a time series cluster in a direction over time. A value $H$ in the range 0.5–1, indicates a time series with positive autocorrelation, which means that a high value in the series will probably be followed by another high value. A value in the range of 0–0.5 indicates a time-series with long-term switching between high and low values in adjacent pairs, which means that a single high value will be probably followed by a low value and that the value after that will tend to be high, with this tendency to switch between values lasting a long time into the future. Additional file 1 describes specific analytical considerations for DFA.
4. Fractal dimension ($D$)
   $D$ is a ratio providing a statistical index of complexity, and a highly sensitive measure for detecting hidden information contained in physiological time series (Raghavendra and Dutt 2010). There are many methods used to calculate $D$, but the most accurate estimate is achieved by Higuchi's method. Higuchi's fractal dimension originates from chaos theory and for almost 30 years it has been successfully applied as a complexity measure of artificial or physiological signals, including EEG and EKG (Gomolka et al. 2018; Skinner et al. 1992; Kesic and Spasic 2016; Ma et al. 2018). Values associated with natural phenomena are estimated to be between 1 and 2 (Higuchi 1988). A value of 1 corresponds to a regular time-series; while for Gaussian-type noise, it might attain higher values; i.e., 1.5 for Brownian, 1.8 for pink noise, and 2.0 for white noise (Gomolka et al. 2018). For information on the calculation of $D$, please refer to Additional file 1.

### Statistical analyses

After all nonlinear parameters had been calculated, we conducted analyses of variance for each of them (LE, DFA, and $D$) to determine whether there were any differences between the three groups in mood or energy series. All analyses were performed using MATLAB ®.

## Results

### Demographic and clinical characteristics of the sample

Ninety participants were included in the analyses: 30 HC, 30 euthymic BD and 30 FDR. In the BD subgroup, 76.6% were BD type I and all patients were on long-term pharmacotherapy (see Table 1). With proportions of participants completing >84 days of consecutive entries of 96% in the HC group, 93.3% in the BD group, and 86.6% in the FDR groups, we analyzed 14,980 datapoints (5200 in the HC group, 4970 in the BD group and 4810 in the FDR group). Please refer to our original paper for the complete description of the sample and distribution of individual measures (Ortiz et al. 2019).

**Table 1** Pharmacotherapy (patients with BD, N = 30)

| Medication | % of patients |
|---|---|
| Mood stabilizers | 90 |
| Lithium carbonate | 50 |
| Lamotrigine | 20 |
| Valproic acid | 13.3 |
| Carbamazepine | 6.7 |
| None | 10 |
| Combination treatment with antidepressants | 30 |
| SSRI | 3.3 |
| SNRI | 3.3 |
| MAOI | 13.3 |
| Other | 10 |
| None | 70 |
| Combination treatment with antipsychotics | 50 |
| First-generation | 6.7 |
| Second-generation | 43.3 |
| None | 50 |
| Other treatments | 43.2 |
| Sleep-inductors/benzodiazepines | 16.6 |
| Thyroid supplementation | 20 |
| Tryptophan | 3.3 |
| Atomoxetine | 3.3 |
| None | 56.8 |

MAOI: monoamine oxidase inhibitor; SNRI: serotonin–norepinephrine reuptake inhibitor; SSRI: selective serotonin reuptake inhibitor

***Lyapunov exponent (LE)***

Table 2 describes LE for all groups, for both mood and energy series. For the mood series, the largest LE was found in HC (1.84), compared to BD (1.63) and FDR (1.71). An ANOVA yielded a statistically significant difference between groups (F (2, 87) = 8.42, p < 0.005), with a post-hoc Tukey test showing that LE was significantly higher in HC than in the BD (p = 0.003) and FDR groups (p = 0.03). Similarly, for the energy series, HC showed a LE of 1.85, compared to 1.76 for BD and 1.61 for FDR (F (2, 87) = 11.02; p < 0.005), with a post-hoc Tukey test showing that LE was significantly higher in HC group compared to FDR group (p < 0.001), but not the BD group (p = 0.1).

***Detrended fluctuation analysis (DFA)***

Table 2 describes the Hurst (*H*) exponent for all groups, for both mood and energy series. There were no statistically significant differences between groups for either mood or energy series (p > 0.5).

***Fractal dimension (D)***

Table 2 describes *D* for all groups, for both mood and energy series. There were no statistically significant differences between groups for either mood or energy series (p > 0.05).

## Discussion

The underlying nature of mood variability is in keeping with that of a chaotic system, rather than noise, which means that fluctuations are generated by deterministic nonlinear process(es) in HC, BD, and FDR participants. The three different techniques used in these analyses have all demonstrated that chaotic behavior can originate from deterministic systems that have simple mathematical descriptions (Klonowski 2007).

Our main findings include a positive, short-term, autocorrelation in the time-series for mood and energy series in all groups; with a more chaotic pattern in the time-series for mood in HC, than in BD or FDR participants, which is in keeping with our previous results.

The limitations of this analysis include using one-dimensional time-series, as these may not not sufficient to reconstruct the complex dynamics of mood regulation. However, despite the 'low resolution' of the visual analog scale employed, this is a measure that has been validated in mood disorders and it meets the assumptions needed to validate the analysis employed. Moreover, using nonlinear methods allowed us to detect hidden information in physiological time-series, which

**Table 2** Nonlinear coefficients for mood and energy series

| Coefficient | Series | HC (mean ± SD) | BD (mean ± SD) | FDR (mean ± SD) | Statistic |
|---|---|---|---|---|---|
| LE | Mood | 1.84 | 1.63 | 1.71 | F(2, 87) = 8.42; p < 0.005 |
| | Energy | 1.85 | 1.76 | 1.61 | F(2, 87) = 11.02; p < 0.005 |
| DFA | Mood | 0.53 ± 0.03 | 0.50 ± 0.01 | 0.52 ± 0.03 | F(2, 87) = 0.14, p = 0.86 |
| | Energy | 0.54 ± 0.04 | 0.54 ± 0.04 | 0.53 ± 0.03 | F(2, 87) = 0.02; p = 0.97 |
| Fractal Dimension | Mood | 1.54 ± 0.11 | 1.51 ± 0.05 | 1.52 ± 0.04 | F(2, 87) = 1.48, p = 0.2 |
| | Energy | 1.42 ± 0.12 | 1.41 ± 0.05 | 1.41 ± 0.06 | F(2, 87) = 0.18, p = 0.8 |

LE: Lyapunov exponent; DFA: Detrended fluctuation analysis; HC: Healthy controls; BD: bipolar disorder; FDR: Unaffected first-degree relatives supports conceptualizing mood variability as an inherent nonlinear process.

LE showed differences between the three groups: for both mood and energy series, LE was higher in HC than in BD and FDR participants, which is indicative of a more chaotic pattern. As mentioned above, LE is a nonlinear parameter that quantifies the sensitivity to initial conditions. The existence of a positive exponent for almost all initial conditions in a bounded dynamic system is a widely used definition of deterministic chaos (Zhong et al. 2007; Gao et al. 2007). Positive values (as shown in all groups) mean that two trajectories starting very close together will rapidly diverge from each other, and thereafter have totally different futures. The practical implication is that long-term prediction becomes impossible in such a system, because small uncertainties are quickly amplified. This is relevant when it comes to calculating the window of episode prediction: a positive LE indicates the futility of trying to predict the detailed long-term behavior of a chaotic system. However, short-term prediction may be feasible in BD, as: (i) mood can be considered as a short-term memory process (Ortiz et al. 2015); (ii) our previous studies using machine-learning models for episode prediction have shown the last 4 days as preferred over other windows of prediction (Ortiz et al. 2018).

For DFA, our results show that all three groups have *H* values close to 0.5, which is indicative of a positive autocorrelation in their time series; i.e., a high value in the series will probably be followed by another high value. This result is consistent with our prior finding of an ARIMA (1,1,0) model, that conceptualizes mood as a short-term memory process (Ortiz et al. 2015) and with prior studies that also described a lag of 1 day in mood fluctuations (Gottschalk et al. 1995; Werf et al. 2006). This process could explain the daily fluctuations (perturbations or "micro-recoveries") in mood seen in all groups. This behavior will likely be different in untreated patients, patients with mood symptoms but not a primary mood disorder (e.g., borderline personality disorder) or in patients with BD experiencing an acute episode.

Lastly, in the fractal dimension analysis, all three groups have *D* values close to 1.5, which is in keeping with the values in time-series associated with natural phenomena. As a highly sensitive measure for detecting hidden information contained in physiological time series, our results show, as expected, an underlying complexity in mood variability in the three groups.

Overall, these findings suggest that a more chaotic pattern is present in healthy systems; whereas compromised systems show a more rigid pattern, not as flexible or resilient to adjust to the demands of a changing environment. Resilience is defined as the capacity to tolerate disturbance without collapsing (Clements and Ozgul 2018). Efforts to understand resilience in humans are relatively advanced in Geriatrics (Olde Rikkert et al. 2016; Lagro et al. 2012) and Cardiology (Quail et al. 2015). The breakdown of resilience proposed only recently as a characteristic of mood disorders (Ortiz and Alda 2018; Golier et al. 2001; Cochran et al. 2018; Scheffer et al. 2018; Kossakowski et al. 2019; Leemput et al. 2014). As resilience approaches zero, a critical transition can be triggered even by a minor event (Scheffer et al. 2001, 2009; Nelson et al. 2017; Nes et al. 2016; O'Regan and Burton 2018). In other words, slower recovery from small perturbations is an indicator that the system is in a fragile state and that a tipping point might be near (Nelson et al. 2017).

Our findings have several clinical implications. First, it is important to recognize that mood variability is an important characteristic of healthy systems, and we can inform clinicians and patients about the importance of these 'low amplitude' mood fluctuations. Patients do not need to feel 'flat' to be stable. Second, we should recognize the role of other physiological factors, such as sleep, in increasing the ability of the system to recover from small perturbations. Cognitive strategies could also be important tools to help decrease co-morbid anxiety or substance use disorders, which can easily be "the tipping point" for a system that is already fragile. By increasing the system's resilience, it would be more prone to small, but not critical transitions (e.g., minor life events would lead to adjustment disorder symptoms, rather than a depressive episode).

Other future clinical applications from our findings include the use of time-series analysis to assess mood variability in difficult diagnostic cases (e.g., borderline personality disorder versus bipolar disorder). Finally, nonlinear techniques can be used to model clinical trajectories and forecast the onset of depressive, manic, or mixed episodes, keeping in mind that these will be necessarily short-term forecasts.

## Conclusions

Mood fluctuations are generated by deterministic chaotic process(es) in healthy controls, patients with BD and their unaffected first-degree relatives. Mood regulation is a short-term memory process, which implies that it is autocorrelated in the short term (e.g., mood today will be correlated with mood tomorrow, but not farther than that). This has clinical implications when predicting mood episodes in BD: due to the underlying nature of mood fluctuations, only short-term forecasts are possible.

With the uptake in passive sensing and smartphone data to improve clinical care in BD (Ortiz et al. 2021), including predicting episodes of illness, we need to be aware that mood is regulated by a system sensitive to initial conditions. This means that two trajectories starting very close together will rapidly diverge from each other, and thereafter have completely different futures. The practical implication is that long-term prediction becomes impossible in a system like this, in which small uncertainties are quickly amplified. In other words, it is futile trying to predict the detailed long-term behavior of a chaotic system. Instead, we should focus on demonstrating the feasibility and clinical impact of short-term prediction in BD.

In closing, living systems are complex and operate far from equilibrium. Mood disorders, like any other clinical disorder, should be conceptualized as the result of a loss of complexity, rather than the loss of regularity.

## Supplementary Information

**Additional file 1.** Analytical considerations and calculations for LE, DFA and *D*.

**Acknowledgements**
Not applicable.

**Authors' contributions**
AO and MA designed the study. JG, CS and SM collected clinical data and entered it in the database. MM conducted the analyses and KB supervised nonlinear calculations. AO and BHM wrote the manuscript. All authors read and approved the final manuscript and provided critical comments.

**Author details**
[1]Department of Psychiatry, University of Toronto, Toronto, ON, Canada. [2]Centre for Addiction & Mental Health, CAMH 100 Stokes St., Rm 4229, Toronto, ON M6J 1H4, Canada. [3]ORCA Quantum Computing, Toronto, ON, Canada. [4]Department of Electrical Engineering, University of Ottawa, Ottawa, ON, Canada. [5]Institute for Mental Health Research, The Royal Ottawa Hospital, Ottawa, ON, Canada. [6]Nova Scotia Health Authority, Halifax, NS, Canada. [7]Department of Psychiatry, Dalhousie University, Halifax, NS, Canada. [8]National Institute of Mental Health, Klecany, Czech Republic.

**References**

Bayani A, Hadaeghi F, Jafari S, Murray G. Critical slowing down as an early warning of transitions in episodes of bipolar disorder: a simulation study based on a computational model of circadian activity rhythms. Chronobiol Int. 2017;34(2):235–45.

Bonsall MB, Wallace-Hadrill SM, Geddes JR, Goodwin GM, Holmes EA. Nonlinear time-series approaches in characterizing mood stability and mood instability in bipolar disorder. Proc Biol Sci. 2012;279(1730):916–24.

Bonsall MB, Geddes JR, Goodwin GM, Holmes EA. Bipolar disorder dynamics: affective instabilities, relaxation oscillations and noise. J R Soc Interface. 2015;12(112):20150670.

Chatfield C. The analysis of time series: an introduction. Boca Raton: CRC Press; 2016.

Clements CF, Ozgul A. Indicators of transitions in biological systems. Ecol Lett. 2018;21(6):905–19.

Cochran AL, Schultz A, McInnis MG, Forger DB. Testing frameworks for personalizing bipolar disorder. Transl Psychiatry. 2018;8(1):36.

Cowdry RW, Gardner DL, O'Leary KM, Leibenluft E, Rubinow DR. Mood variability: a study of four groups. Am J Psychiatry. 1991;148(11):1505–11.

Doyle TLA, Dugan EL, Humphries B, Newton RU. Discriminating between elderly and young using a fractal dimension analysis of centre of pressure. Int J Med Sci. 2004;1(1):11–20.

Ehlers CL. Chaos and complexity. Can it help us to understand mood and behavior? Arch General Psychiatry. 1995;52(11):960–4.

Endicott J, Spitzer RL. A diagnostic interview: the schedule for affective disorders and schizophrenia. Arch Gen Psychiatry. 1978;35(7):837–44.

Gao J, Gao Y, Tung WW, Hu J. Multiscale analysis of complex time series: integration of chaos and random fractal theory. Hoboken: Wiley; 2007.

Goldberger AL, Amaral LA, Hausdorff JM, Ivanov P, Peng CK, Stanley HE. Fractal dynamics in physiology: alterations with disease and aging. Proc Natl Acad Sci USA. 2002a;99(Suppl 1):2466–72.

Goldberger AL, Peng CK, Lipsitz LA. What is physiologic complexity and how does it change with aging and disease? Neurobiol Aging. 2002b;23(1):23–6.

Golier JA, Yehuda R, Schmeidler J, Siever LJ. Variability and severity of depression and anxiety in post traumatic stress disorder and major depressive disorder. Depress Anxiety. 2001;13(2):97–100.

Gomez C, Mediavilla A, Hornero R, Abasolo D, Fernandez A. Use of the Higuchi's fractal dimension for the analysis of MEG recordings from Alzheimer's disease patients. Med Eng Phys. 2009;31(3):306–13.

Gomolka RS, Kampusch S, Kaniusas E, Thurk F, Szeles JC, Klonowski W. Higuchi fractal dimension of heart rate variability during percutaneous auricular vagus nerve stimulation in healthy and diabetic subjects. Front Physiol. 2018;9:1162.

Gottschalk A, Bauer MS, Whybrow PC. Evidence of chaotic mood variation in bipolar disorder. Arch Gen Psychiatry. 1995;52(11):947–59.

Hamilton M. A rating scale for depression. J Neurol Neurosurg Psychiatry. 1960;23:56–62.

Higuchi T. Approach to an irregular time series on the basis of the fractal theory. Physica D. 1988;31(2):277–83.

Hu K, Ivanov PC, Chen Z, Carpena P, Stanley HE. Effect of trends on detrended fluctuation analysis. Phys Rev E Stat Nonlin Soft Matter Phys. 2001;64(1 Pt 1):011114.

Hu J, Gao J, Tung WW. Characterizing heart rate variability by scale-dependent Lyapunov exponent. Chaos. 2009;19(2):028506.

Hu J, Gao J, Tung WW, Cao Y. Multiscale analysis of heart rate variability: a comparison of different complexity measures. Ann Biomed Eng. 2010;38(3):854–64.

Huber MT, Braun HA, Krieg JC. Consequences of deterministic and random dynamics for the course of affective disorders. Biol Psychiatry. 1999;46(2):256–62.

Huber MT, Braun HA, Krieg JC. Effects of noise on different disease states of recurrent affective disorders. Biol Psychiatry. 2000;47(7):634–42.

Jelinek HF, Md Imam H, Al-Aubaidy H, Khandoker AH. Association of cardiovascular risk using non-linear heart rate variability measures with the framingham risk score in a rural population. Front Physiol. 2013;4:186.

Katerndahl D, Ferrer R, Best R, Wang CP. Dynamic patterns in mood among newly diagnosed patients with major depressive episode or panic disorder and normal controls. Prim Care Companion J Clin Psychiatry. 2007;9(3):183–7.

Katz MJ. Fractals and the analysis of waveforms. Comput Biol Med. 1988;18(3):145–56.

Kesic S, Spasic SZ. Application of Higuchi's fractal dimension from basic to clinical neurophysiology: a review. Comput Methods Programs Biomed. 2016;133:55–70.

Klonowski W. From conformons to human brains: an informal overview of nonlinear dynamics and its applications in biomedicine. Nonlinear Biomed Phys. 2007;1(1):5.

Kossakowski JJ, Gordijn MCM, Riese H, Waldorp LJ. Applying a dynamical systems model and network theory to major depressive disorder. Front Psychol. 2019;10:1762.

Lagro J, Laurenssen NC, Schalk BW, Schoon Y, Claassen JA, Olde Rikkert MG. Diastolic blood pressure drop after standing as a clinical sign for increased mortality in older falls clinic patients. J Hypertens. 2012;30(6):1195–202.

Ma Y, Shi W, Peng CK, Yang AC. Nonlinear dynamical analysis of sleep electroencephalography using fractal and entropy approaches. Sleep Med Rev. 2018;37:85–93.

Nayak SK, Bit A, Dey A, Mohapatra B, Pal K. A review on the nonlinear dynamical system analysis of electrocardiogram signal. J Healthc Eng. 2018;2018:6920420.
Nelson B, McGorry PD, Wichers M, Wigman JTW, Hartmann JA. Moving from static to dynamic models of the onset of mental disorder: a review. JAMA Psychiat. 2017;74(5):528–34.
Olde Rikkert MG, Dakos V, Buchman TG, Boer R, Glass L, Cramer AO, et al. Slowing down of recovery as generic risk marker for acute severity transitions in chronic diseases. Crit Care Med. 2016;44(3):601–6.
O'Regan SM, Burton DL. How stochasticity influences leading indicators of critical transitions. Bull Math Biol. 2018;80(6):1630–54.
Ortiz A, Alda M. The perils of being too stable: mood regulation in bipolar disorder. J Psychiatry Neurosci. 2018;43(6):363–5.
Ortiz A, Bradler K, Garnham J, Slaney C, Alda M. Nonlinear dynamics of mood regulation in bipolar disorder. Bipolar Disord. 2015;17(2):139–49.
Ortiz A, Bradler K, Hintze A. Episode forecasting in bipolar disorder: is energy better than mood? Bipolar Disord. 2018;20(5):470–6.
Ortiz A, Bradler K, Garnham J, Slaney C, MacLean S, Alda M. Corrigendum to nonlinear dynamics of mood regulation in unaffected first-degree relatives of bipolar disorder patients [Journal of Affective disorders 243 (2019) 274–279]. J Affect Disord. 2019;245:16.
Ortiz A, Maslej MM, Husain I, Daskalakis J, Mulsant BH. Apps and gaps in bipolar disorder: a systematic review on electronic monitoring for episode prediction. J Affect Disord. 2021;295:1190–200.
Peng CK, Buldyrev SV, Havlin S, Simons M, Stanley HE, Goldberger AL. Mosaic organization of DNA nucleotides. Phys Rev E. 1994;49(2):1685–9.
Peng CK, Havlin S, Stanley HE, Goldberger AL. Quantification of scaling exponents and crossover phenomena in nonstationary heartbeat time series. Chaos. 1995a;5(1):82–7.
Peng CK, Havlin S, Hausdorff JM, Mietus JE, Stanley HE, Goldberger AL. Fractal mechanisms and heart rate dynamics Long-range correlations and their breakdown with disease. J Electrocardiol. 1995b;28:59–65.
Pincus S. Assessing serial irregularity and its implications for health. Ann N Y Acad Sci. 2001;954:245–67.
Pincus SM, Schmidt PJ, Palladino-Negro P, Rubinow DR. Differentiation of women with premenstrual dysphoric disorder, recurrent brief depression, and healthy controls by daily mood rating dynamics. J Psychiatr Res. 2008;42(5):337–47.
Quail T, Shrier A, Glass L. Predicting the onset of period-doubling bifurcations in noisy cardiac systems. Proc Natl Acad Sci USA. 2015;112(30):9358–63.
Raghavendra BS, Dutt DN. Signal characterization using fractal dimension. Fractals. 2010;18(3):287–92.
Rosenstein MT, Collins JJ, De Luca CJ. A practical method for calculating largest Lyapunov exponents from small data sets. Physica D. 1993;65(1):117–34.
Scheffer M, Carpenter S, Foley JA, Folke C, Walker B. Catastrophic shifts in ecosystems. Nature. 2001;413(6856):591–6.
Scheffer M, Bascompte J, Brock WA, Brovkin V, Carpenter SR, Dakos V, et al. Early-warning signals for critical transitions. Nature. 2009;461(7260):53–9.
Scheffer M, Bolhuis JE, Borsboom D, Buchman TG, Gijzel SMW, Goulson D, et al. Quantifying resilience of humans and other animals. Proc Natl Acad Sci USA. 2018;115(47):11883–90.
Skinner JE, Molnar M, Vybiral T, Mitra M. Application of chaos theory to biology and medicine. Integr Physiol Behav Sci. 1992;27(1):39–53.
van de Leemput IA, Wichers M, Cramer AO, Borsboom D, Tuerlinckx F, Kuppens P, et al. Critical slowing down as early warning for the onset and termination of depression. Proc Natl Acad Sci USA. 2014;111(1):87–92.
van der Werf SY, Kaptein KI, de Jonge P, Spijker J, de Graaf R, Korf J. Major depressive episodes and random mood. Arch Gen Psychiatry. 2006;63(5):509–18.
van Nes EH, Arani BMS, Staal A, van der Bolt B, Flores BM, Bathiany S, et al. What do you mean, "tipping point"? Trends Ecol Evol. 2016;31(12):902–4.
Varshney LR, Sun JZ. Why do we perceive logarithmically? Significance. 2013;10(1):28–31.
Wu HT, Liu CC, Lo MT, Hsu PC, Liu AB, Chang KY, et al. Multiscale cross-approximate entropy analysis as a measure of complexity among the aged and diabetic. Comput Math Methods in Med. 2013;2013:324325.
Young RC, Biggs JT, Ziegler VE, Meyer DA. A rating scale for mania: reliability, validity and sensitivity. Br J Psychiatry. 1978;133:429–35.
Zhong Y, Jan KM, Ju KH, Chon KH. Representation of time-varying nonlinear systems with time-varying principal dynamic modes. IEEE Trans Biomed Eng. 2007;54(11):1983–92.

# Combination of dextromethorphan and memantine in treating bipolar spectrum disorder: a 12-week double-blind randomized clinical trial

Sheng-Yu Lee[1,2,3,4], Tzu-Yun Wang[4], Shiou-Lan Chen[5], Yun-Hsuan Chang[6], Po-See Chen[4], San-Yuan Huang[7], Nian-Sheng Tzeng[7], Liang-Jen Wang[8], I-Hui Lee[4], Kao-Ching Chen[4], Yen-Kuang Yang[4], Jau-Shyong Hong[9] and Ru-Band Lu[4,10,11*]

**Abstract**

**Background:** The aim of this study is to determine whether adding combination of agents with anti-inflammatory and neurotrophic effects is more efficacious than mood stabilizer alone in improving clinical symptoms, plasma brain-derived neurotrophic factor (BDNF), cytokine levels, and metabolic profiles in patients with bipolar spectrum disorder.

**Methods:** In a randomized, double-blind, controlled 12-week clinical trial, patients with moderate mood symptoms (HDRS ≥ 18 or YMRS ≥ 14) were recruited. The patients were randomly assigned to a group while still undergoing regular valproate (VPA) treatments: VPA + dextromethorphan (DM) (30 mg/day) + memantine (MM) (5 mg/day) (DM30 + MM5) (n = 66), VPA + DM (30 mg/day) (DM30) (n = 69), VPA + MM (5 mg/day) (MM5) (n = 66), or VPA + Placebo (Placebo) (n = 69). Symptom severity, immunological parameters [plasma tumor necrosis factor (TNF)-α and C-reactive protein (CRP)] and plasma brain-derived neurotrophic factor (BDNF) were regularly examined. Metabolic profiles [cholesterol, triglycerides, glycosylated hemoglobin (HbA1C), fasting serum glucose, body mass index (BMI)] were measured at baseline and at 2, 8, and 12 weeks.

**Results:** Depression scores were significantly ($P = 0.03$) decreases and BDNF levels significantly ($P = 0.04$) increased in the DM30 + MM5 group than in the Placebo group. However, neither depressive scores nor BDNF levels were significantly different between the DM30, MM5, and Placebo groups. Changes in certain plasma cytokine and BDNF levels were significantly correlated with metabolic parameters.

**Conclusion:** We concluded that add-on DM30 + MM5 was significantly more effective than placebo for clinical symptoms and plasma BDNF levels. Additional studies with larger samples and mechanistic studies are necessary to confirm our findings.

*Trial registration* NCT03039842 (https://register.clinicaltrials.gov/). Trial date was from 1 Jan 2013 to 31 December 2016 in National Cheng Kung University Hospital. Registered 28 February 1 2017-Retrospectively registered, https://clinicaltrials.gov/ct2/show/NCT03039842?term=NCT03039842&rank=1.

**Keywords:** Bipolar spectrum disorder, Bipolar II disorder, Dextromethorphan, Memantine, Cytokines, BDNF

*Correspondence: rblu@mail.ncku.edu.tw
[4] Department of Psychiatry, National Cheng Kung University Hospital, College of Medicine, National Cheng Kung University, 138 Sheng-Li Road, Tainan 70428, Taiwan
Full list of author information is available at the end of the article

## Background

Bipolar II disorder (BD-II) is a subtype of bipolar disorder (BD) characterized as recurrent episodes of depression and hypomania. BD-II is frequently misdiagnosed in clinical settings because the diagnosis is frequently made based on recollections of past hypomania while patients present with symptoms of depression (Mosolov et al. 2014). A consequence of the frequent misdiagnosis or delayed diagnosis of BD-II is ineffective treatment (Drancourt et al. 2013): Patients with BD-II are at a greater risk of suicide, a prolonged clinical course, more mood episodes, more major and minor depressive episodes, and shorter interepisode intervals, than are patients with BD-I (Karanti et al. 2019).

Neurodegeneration and inflammation are considered the pathogenesis of BD (Berk et al. 2011; Drevets 2000; Peng et al. 2005). Brain-derived neurotrophic factor (BDNF) is important for the development and survival of monoamine neurons (Cotman and Berchtold 2002). Several lines of evidence suggest the involvement of BDNF in the pathogenesis of mood disorders and the mechanism of action of mood stabilizing medication, which indicates probable neurotrophic and neuronal dysfunction in patients with BD (Duman 2002; Mora et al. 2019). Two meta-analyses reported significantly lower-than-normal-range serum BDNF levels in patients with BD during episodes of mania and depression, but not different from controls during euthymic state (Fernandes et al. 2015; Munkholm et al. 2016). Level of BDNF increased after patients were treated for mood episode (Tunca et al. 2014). Plasma BDNF levels might also be associated with the degree of neurodegeneration in BD (de Oliveira et al. 2009). Because BDNF can cross the blood–brain barrier (Karege et al. 2005), BDNF levels in the brain and plasma might undergo similar changes during maturation and aging in vivo (Cirulli et al. 2009). Therefore, plasma BDNF levels might reflect BDNF levels in the human brain (Pan et al. 1998; Klein et al. 2011). In addition, peripheral BDNF has been proposed as a candidate biomarker of mood states and disease progression for BD (Fernandes et al. 2011).

Increasing evidence suggests that abnormal cytokine-mediated inflammatory responses might be another pathogenesis of BD (Goldstein et al. 2009; Rosenblat et al. 2016). Strakowski et al. (2000) proposed that subcortical structural abnormalities in the striatum, amygdala, and prefrontal cortex might lead to neuroinflammation and then contribute to the progression of brain atrophy and exacerbation of the symptoms of BD. Meta-analyses have also reported higher-than-normal levels of the proinflammatory cytokine tumor necrosis factor (TNF)-α and of C-reactive protein (CRP) during acute manic and depressive episodes; both substances decreased after treatment (Fernandes et al. 2016; Goldsmith et al. 2016). Cytokines have also been proposed as diagnostic and staging biomarkers for BD (Goldstein et al. 2015; Jacoby et al. 2016).

Patients with BD appear to have a higher prevalence rate of metabolic syndrome than does the general population (Vancampfort et al. 2013). In BD, obesity has been associated with greater illness severity and cognitive dysfunction, and even suicide attempts (Goldstein et al. 2011; Yim et al. 2012). One main link between metabolic disturbance and BD was postulated as inflammation (Yamagata et al. 2017). Manipulating central and peripheral BDNF levels modified metabolic dysfunction in an animal study (Lyons et al. 1999). BDNF was also suggested to play a crucial role in the pathophysiology of obesity and metabolic syndrome in neurodegenerative disorder such as depression (Motamedi et al. 2017) because low plasma levels of BDNF were reported in patients with metabolic syndrome (Chaldakov et al. 2004). Therefore, the relationship between metabolic abnormality and BD might be a consequence of aberrant inflammatory and neural networks. It is of interest to investigate the correlation between cytokines and BDNF with the metabolic profile in BD.

Although the treatment guidelines for BD are well established (Yatham et al. 2018), many patients remain symptomatic while on mood stabilizers (Rybakowski 2013). It is possible that current mood stabilizers might not prevent ongoing inflammation and neurodegeneration. Therefore, adding agents with anti-inflammatory and neurotrophic effects to current therapy for BD might provide more effective therapy. Both low-dose DM and MM have anti-inflammatory and neurotrophic effects.

DM is an antitussive drug used for more than 50 years (Turchan-Cholewo et al. 2009). DM is a *N*-methyl-D-aspartate (NMDA) receptor antagonist which was reported to be useful at a high dose (480 mg/day) to reduce methadone tolerance in opioid-dependent patients (Cornish et al. 2002). DM also protects monoaminergic neurons against inflammation-mediated degeneration (Liu and Hong 2003) and endotoxicity (Liu and Hong 2003; Zhang et al. 2004; Zhang et al. 2005). Apart from its being an NMDA receptor, DM and its metabolite may stimulate sigma-1 receptor, inhibit serotonin reuptake, and block L-type calcium channel mediating anti-inflammation, anti-convulsive, anti-parkinsonian, anti-ischemic, antioxidant, and alleviation of pseudobulbar effects (Chen 2011; Shin et al. 2011). Above evidence suggests that DM offers promising neuroprotective and anti-inflammatory benefits in neurodegenerative disorders such as are BD. Memantine is a noncompetitive NMDA receptor antagonist. It is also an alternative mechanism: anti-inflammatory effect that downregulates the activity of microglia and upregulates astroglia-released of neurotrophic factors (Wu et al. 2009).

In one of our prior randomized clinical trials, we added low-dose DM (30 mg or 60 mg) or placebo to the pharmacological therapy of BD patients for 12 weeks (Chen et al. 2014); in another, we added low-dose MM (5 mg/day) or placebo (Lee et al. 2013). Although there was no significant improvement in clinical symptoms, the add-on agents reduced the levels of inflammatory markers and increased the levels of plasma BDNF. We then wondered whether the combination effect of DM and MM, both which provide anti-inflammatory and neurotrophic effects, might benefit patients with BD-II more than adding only one of them.

Therefore, we conducted a double-blind, placebo-controlled study of add-on low-dose DM (30 mg) (DM30), MM (5 mg/day) (MM5), DM30+MM5, or placebo to evaluate their efficacy as augmenting agents in treating BD-II. The outcome measures included clinical severity, levels of cytokine and plasma BDNF expression, and metabolic profiles. In addition, we investigated the correlation between changes in plasma cytokines and BDNF with mood symptoms and metabolic indices over the 12-week pharmacological intervention.

## Methods

The Institutional Review Board for the Protection of Human Subjects at National Cheng Kung University Hospital reviewed and approved the research protocol. All participants were given a detailed description of the study before they signed written informed consent forms.

Patients with BP-II were recruited from outpatient and inpatient settings. All patients were initially evaluated by an attending psychiatrist, once diagnosed with BP-II, they then received a structural interview conducted by a clinical psychologist to confirm the Diagnostic and Statistical Manual of Mental Disorders, fourth edition (DSM-IV) diagnoses, using the Chinese Version of the Modified Schedule of Affective Disorder and Schizophrenia-Life Time (SADS-L) (Endicott and Spitzer 1978), which has good inter-rater reliability (Huang et al. 2004). Patients with other mood and psychotic disorders, borderline personality disorder, drug dependence, or cognitive disorders other than BD-II were excluded. Patients who had taken DM or MM within 1 week before the first dose of the double-blind medication were also excluded. In addition, due to safety reasons, women of childbearing potential not using adequate contraception, pregnant or nursing females, and those who have clinically significant medical condition (i.e. cardiac, hepatic and renal disease) were excluded.

Although DSM-IV-TR criteria require a minimum of 4 days of hypomania, current epidemiologic data suggest that 2 days is more prevalent in community samples; therefore, we used the 2-day minimum for hypomania in the diagnosis of BD-II. However, because some patients may not fulfill criteria of BD-II according to the DSM-IV-TR criteria, it is better to refer our study group as "bipolar spectrum patients" to avoid misleading.

### Study design

After they had been initially screened, the patients were randomly assigned to add-on DM30 group (30 mg/day), the add-on MM5 group (5 mg/day), the add-on DM30+MM5 group, or to the add-on Placebo group for 12 weeks, during which they were also given open-label VPA treatment [500 mg and 1000 mg daily (50–100 μg/ml in plasma)], which had begun when they joined the study. All patients were prescribed with VPA treatment when they agreed to join the study. It will than take about 1 week for the patients to pass initial screen and undergo randomization for add-on experimental drugs. Therefore, the patients usually receive VPA about 1 week before they were given the experimental drugs. We hired a third party local pharmacological company to prepare the trial medication and perform randomization. They had constructed a combined capsule of either DM30, MM5 or DM30+MM5 and placebo. The randomization method was block randomization. The add-on medication was delivered by research assistant to the patients after doctor visit. Both the clinician and the research assistants were blind to the add-on therapy throughout the trial. Clinical psychologists with good inter-rater reliability managed the rating of symptoms during each visits in the follow-up duration. Symptom severity was assessed at baseline, and treatment responses were measured on day 7 of weeks 1, 2, 4, 8, and 12. The severity of mood symptoms was assessed using the Hamilton Depression Rating Scale (HDRS) and the Young Mania Rating Scale (YMRS). Only patients with moderate mood symptoms (HDRS $\geq$ 18 or YMRS $\geq$ 14) were recruited. Concomitant benzodiazepine medication (lorazepam < 8 mg) was used for nighttime sedation, and to treat agitation and insomnia during the study. Up to 20 mg/daily of fluoxetine was permitted for associated depressive symptoms. Risperidone (1–6 mg/day) were allowed for agitation.

Ten milliliters of whole blood was withdrawn from the antecubital vein of each patient when clinical severity was assessed, at baseline, and on day 7 of weeks 1, 2, 4, 8, and 12. Plasma, which was isolated from the whole blood after it had been centrifuged at 3000*g* for 15 min at 4 °C, was immediately stored at − 80 °C. Cytokine levels were quantified using an antibody pair assay system (Flexia; BioSource Intl., Camarillo, CA). Sample processing and data analysis were done according to the manufacturer's instructions. The immunological parameters plasma TNF-α and CRP and plasma BDNF were analyzed.

**Statistical analysis**

The demographic and clinical characteristics of the patients, their baseline YMRS and HDRS scores, and their baseline cytokine levels were compared between groups using one-way analysis of variance (ANOVA) for continuous variables, and $\chi^2$ tests for categorical variables. Data are mean ± standard deviation (SD). Both CRP and TNF-α levels were distributed erratically and showed a significant level of positive skew (Table 1). Arithmetic transformations were used to produce approximately normal distributions for further analysis; log $(x+1)$ was used for cytokine levels.

The intent to-treat (ITT) analysis set included all patients who had taken at least one dose of a study drug, and had undergone one baseline assessment and at least one post-baseline assessment. All outcome variables—HDRS, YMRS, cytokine levels, plasma BDNF levels, and metabolic parameters—in the ITT set were analyzed. Missing data were filled in using the last observation carried forward (LOCF) method.

The overall within-group changes of each outcome over the 12 weeks were analyzed using paired-sample *t*-tests. To compare the difference in outcomes of add-on medication (DM30, MM5, and DM30 + MM5) versus placebo, the generalized estimating equation (GEE) was used. We ran 10 models with each outcome as a dependent variable. In each model, add-on medication (DM30, MM5, and DM30 + MM5 vs. Placebo), treatment duration, treatment given × treatment duration, gender, and age were included as independent variables. The covariance structure used was the autoregressive (AR (Mosolov et al. 2014)) model. The placebo group was the reference group. The interaction term of treatment given × treatment duration was regarded as the effect of add-on DM30, MM5, and DM30 + MM5. To analyze correlations between cytokines, BDNF, and metabolic profiles, GEE analysis was also used. Plasma cytokines and BDNF were set as independent variables and metabolic profile components were set as dependent variables; The analyses were controlled for time effects (treatment period from baseline to week 12), gender and age, and clinical severity. By setting clinical outcomes (HDRS and YMRS) to remission (HDRS $\leq 7$ and YMRS $< 8$), response (change of HAMD or YMRS $\geq 50\%$) and non-response/remission (Tohen et al. 2009), survival analysis was conducted according to the above defined categorical data and time to response or to remission. The response and remission rate was estimated using the Kaplan–Meier product-limit estimate method, and survival curves were compared using the Cox regression. SPSS 22.0 for Windows was used for all statistical computations. Significance was set at $P < 0.05$.

## Results

The timeframe for inclusion was from 1 Jan 2013 to 31 December 2016. We initially screened 312 patients: 32 were excluded because they did not meet the inclusion criteria and 10 because they refused to participate. We then randomly assigned 270 BD-II patients to the DM30 (n = 69), MM5 (n = 66), DM30 + MM5 (n = 66),

**Table 1 Characteristics of the BD-II patients in different treatment groups at baseline**

| Treatment groups | DM30 (n = 69) | MM5 (n = 66) | DM30 + MM5 (n = 66) | Placebo (n = 69) | F or $\chi^2$ | *P*-value |
|---|---|---|---|---|---|---|
| Age (years) | 36.3 ± 13.3 | 37.4 ± 14.0 | 35.7 ± 13.2 | 35.2 ± 13.8 | 0.32 | 0.81 |
| Gender (M/F) | 34/35 | 27/39 | 22/44 | 34/35 | 4.83 | 0.19 |
| Age at onset (years) | 15.4 ± 5.0 | 14.8 ± 5.0 | 14.9 ± 4.3 | 13.6 ± 2.8 | 1.79 | 0.15 |
| HDRS | 15.3 ± 4.2 | 15.8 ± 4.2 | 15.9 ± 3.8 | 15.2 ± 3.7 | 0.51 | 0.68 |
| YMRS | 13.1 ± 3.2 | 13.5 ± 2.9 | 13.5 ± 3.4 | 13.6 ± 2.8 | 0.34 | 0.80 |
| TNF-α (pg/ml) | 1.7 ± 1.3 | 2.1 ± 1.8 | 1.8 ± 1.3 | 1.9 ± 1.6 | 0.88 | 0.45 |
| CRP (ng/ml) | 1658.4 ± 1346.6 | 1635.4 ± 1237.1 | 1814.5 ± 1489.6 | 1878.0.5 ± 1525.0 | 0.47 | 0.70 |
| BDNF (ng/ml) | 12.6 ± 7.3 | 12.6 ± 6.9 | 12.1 ± 6.3 | 14.0 ± 6.6 | 0.90 | 0.44 |
| TC (mg/dl) | 179.8 ± 44.9 | 172.5 ± 29.9 | 182.0 ± 39.9 | 180.9 ± 39.8 | 0.71 | 0.50 |
| HDL-C (mg/dl) | 55.9 ± 15.2 | 57.5 ± 16.6 | 59.4 ± 12.7 | 55.0 ± 17.9 | 1.00 | 0.40 |
| LDL-C (mg/dl) | 117.4 ± 33.4 | 109.0 ± 28.0 | 117.5 ± 36.5 | 114.2 ± 31.4 | 0.97 | 0.41 |
| Triglycerides (mg/dl) | 106.0 ± 68.5 | 94.6 ± 51.2 | 91.8 ± 44.1 | 119.6 ± 86.4 | 1.84 | 0.14 |
| FBS (mg/dl) | 96.1 ± 37.7 | 88.8 ± 9.6 | 88.2 ± 13.7 | 92.7 ± 22.5 | 1.60 | 0.19 |

All data are mean ± SD unless otherwise stipulated

*SD* standard deviation, *HDRS* 17-item Hamilton Depression Rating Scale, *YMRS* Young Mania Rating Scale, *TNF-α* tumor necrosis factor α, *CRP* C-reactive protein, *BDNF* brain-derived neurotrophic factor, *TC* total cholesterol, *HDL-C* high-density lipoprotein-cholesterol, *LDL-C* low-density lipoprotein-cholesterol, *DM30* dextromethorphan (30 mg/day), *MM5* memantine (5 mg/day), *DM30 + MM5* dextromethorphan (30 mg/day) combined with memantine (5 mg/day), *FBS* fasting blood sugar and Placebo (n = 69) groups for 12 weeks. One hundred thirty-six (50.4%) of the 270 patients completed the double-blind phase, and 134 (49.6%) dropped out (Fig. 1): MM5 group: dizziness = 1, refusal of follow-up = 35; DM30: refusal of follow-up = 30; DM30 + MM5: refusal of follow-up = 26; Placebo: refusal of follow-up = 42. Throughout the trial, only one patient in the MM5 group reported dizziness and dropped out from the trial on week 2.

Patient demographic and clinical characteristics, HDRS and YMRS scores, cytokine and BDNF levels, and metabolic profiles of the patients were similar at baseline in the 4 treatment groups at baseline (Table 1). After 12 weeks of treatment, mean within-group changes in clinical severity (HDRS and YMRS scores) were significant in all treatment groups (Table 2). CRP levels were significantly lower in the DM30 + MM5 group, and BDNF levels were significantly higher in the DM30 and DM30 + MM5 groups. Total cholesterol and low density lipoprotein-cholesterol (LDL-C) levels were significantly lower in the Placebo group.

GEE analysis showed a significant change in the HDRS score in the DM30 + MM5 group compared with that in the Placebo group ($P = 0.03$) (Table 3; Fig. 2a); a trend of difference in the change in the YMRS score in the DM30 + MM5 group compared with that in the Placebo group was also noted, though not significant. BDNF levels were significantly higher in the DM30 + MM5 group than in the Placebo group ($P = 0.04$) (Fig. 2b).

The change in plasma BDNF level was significantly correlated with the changes in total cholesterol ($P = 0.04$) levels. The change in CRP level was significantly correlated with the change in YMRS scores ($P = 0.03$) and high-density lipoprotein-cholesterol (HDL-C) ($P = < 0.001$) and triglyceride levels ($P \leq 0.001$). The change in TNF-α level was also significantly associated with change in HDL-C ($P = 0.01$) and triglyceride levels ($P = 0.001$) (Table 4). As categorical analysis, we found no significance in the four treatment groups in either response nor remission rate (Table 5, Fig. 3). The frequency of concomitant use of medication are: fluoxetinen (7.8%), lorazepam (89.4%) and risperdone (80.8%). We further analyzed the difference in addition of fluoxetine, benzodiazepine, or risperdone in responders and non-responders. The addition of fluoxetine (P = 0.95), benzodiazepines (P = 0.53) or risperidone (P = 0.77) was not significantly different in those who improved and those who did not improve.

The data that support the findings of this study are available from the corresponding author upon reasonable request.

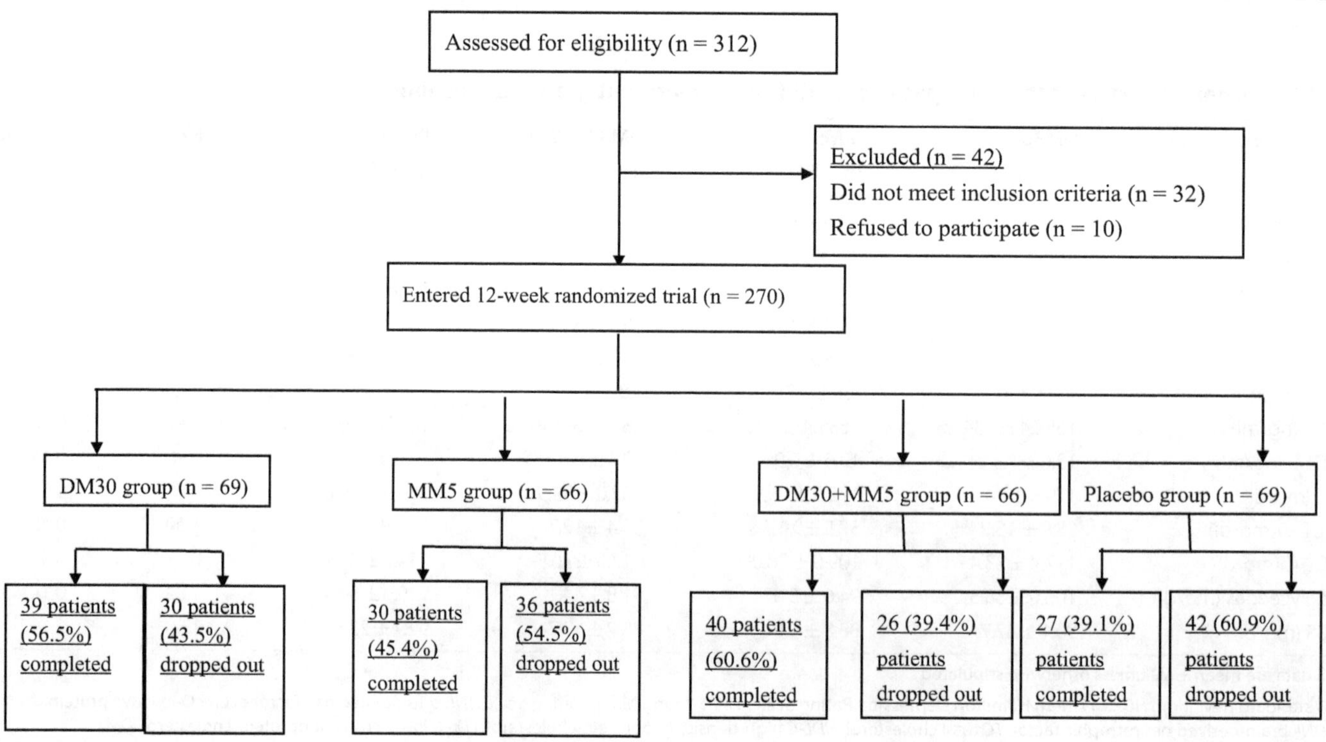


**Fig. 1** CONSORT diagram

**Table 2 Within-group changes (baseline minus endpoint) in clinical characteristics of the BD-II patients in different treatment groups after 12 weeks of follow-up**

| Treatment groups | DM30 | | MM5 | | DM30 + MM5 | | Placebo | |
|---|---|---|---|---|---|---|---|---|
| Change | Mean ± SD | *P*-value | Mean ± SD | *P*-value | Mean ± SD | *P*-value | Mean ± SD | *P*-value |
| Primary outcomes | | | | | | | | |
| HDRS | 6.4 ± 4.7 | < 0.001** | 6.3 ± 4.9 | < 0.001** | 6.6 ± 4.6 | < 0.001** | 5.0 ± 4.1 | < 0.001** |
| YMRS | 4.7 ± 3.4 | < 0.001** | 4.6 ± 3.9 | < 0.001** | 4.9 ± 4.0 | < 0.001** | 3.6 ± 4.1 | < 0.001** |
| Cytokines and BDNF | | | | | | | | |
| TNF-α (pg/ml) | 0.1 ± 2.5 | 0.76 | 0.3 ± 1.8 | 0.09 | 0.3 ± 1.4 | 0.16 | − 0.2 ± 1.6 | 0.87 |
| CRP (ng/ml) | 10.9 ± 1290.3 | 0.20 | − 12.6 ± 1269.4 | 0.98 | 371.3 ± 1157.9 | 0.005** | 20.9 ± 978.8 | 0.17 |
| BDNF (ng/ml) | − 2.3 ± 8.3 | 0.035* | 0.3 ± 7.6 | 0.75 | − 2.2 ± 8.2 | 0.044* | 0.09 ± 8.9 | 0.94 |
| Metabolic parameters | | | | | | | | |
| TC (mg/dl) | − 0.1 ± 28.7 | 0.98 | 0.5 ± 24.5 | 0.90 | 0.6 ± 28.6 | 0.89 | 8.3 ± 24.6 | 0.034* |
| HDL-C (mg/dl) | 1.6 ± 10.2 | 0.28 | 2.4 ± 8.7 | 0.10 | − 10.7 ± 82.4 | 0.41 | 1.3 ± 7.2 | 0.26 |
| LDL-C (mg/dl) | − 0.9 ± 23.1 | 0.79 | 2.6 ± 22.0 | 0.48 | 4.6 ± 24.4 | 0.23 | 7.7 ± 21.9 | 0.034* |
| Triglycerides (mg/dl) | − 11.6 ± 168.4 | 0.68 | − 10.7 ± 38.7 | 0.17 | − 2.5 ± 44.3 | 0.73 | − 14.0 ± 57.0 | 0.20 |
| FBS (mg/dl) | 9.0 ± 38.1 | 0.10 | − 3.3 ± 22.6 | 0.33 | 2.8 ± 9.9 | 0.06 | 2.0 ± 14.2 | 0.34 |

The difference between baseline and endpoint after 12 weeks of follow-up analyzed using a paired sample *t*-test

*SD* standard deviation, *HDRS* 17-item Hamilton Depression Rating Scale, *YMRS* Young Mania Rating Scale, *TNF-α* tumor necrosis factor α, *CRP* C-reactive protein, *BDNF* brain-derived neurotrophic factor, *TC* total cholesterol, *HDL-C* high-density lipoprotein-cholesterol, *LDL-C* low-density lipoprotein-cholesterol, *DM30* dextromethorphan (30 mg/day), *MM5* memantine (5 mg/day), *DM30+MM5* dextromethorphan (30 mg/day) combined with memantine (5 mg/day), *FBS* fasting blood sugar

*$P<0.05$; **$P<0.01$

## Discussion

Our most important finding was that add-on DM30 + MM5 was significantly more effective than was placebo for improving HDRS scores (depressive symptoms) and raising plasma BDNF levels. However, the treatment effects of add-on DM30 only and of add-on MM5 only were not significantly different from those of placebo. We also found a significant correlation between changes in cytokine and BDNF levels and in metabolic profiles. However, changes in plasma BDNF levels and HDRS scores were not correlated. Our study provides the first evidence that combination of low-dose DM and MM attenuated symptoms of depression in patients with BD-II.

The treatment effects of DM and MM alone on depressive symptoms remains inconsistent. A recent meta-analysis (Kishi et al. 2017) reported that MM alone had no therapeutic effect on major depressive disorder or BD. We previously reported (Wu et al. 2009; Lee et al. 2014) that low-dose MM (5 mg), though had no significant effect on depressive symptoms in BD-II, showed anti-inflammatory and neurotrophic effects. Lauterbach (2016), however, reported that high-dose (60 mg bid) DM had an antidepressant effect in treatment-refractory depression, and Kelly and Lieberman (2014) said that DM (20 mg) + quinidine (10 mg) once or twice a day attenuated BD-II depression. Others have reported that DM protected monoaminergic neurons against inflammation-mediated degeneration (Liu and Hong 2003) and endotoxicity (Liu and Hong 2003; Zhang et al. 2004; Zhang et al. 2005). We reported (Chen et al. 2014) that low-dose (60 mg/day) add-on DM was not more effective than placebo in treating BD, however, we found that DM significantly raised plasma BDNF levels in BD patients after 12 weeks of treatment. No previous studies reported the therapeutic effect of DM + MM in depressive symptoms. From our past study, we propose that the possible mechanism of the therapeutic efficacy of add-on low-dose DM + MM may be related to anti-inflammation and neurotrophic effects. However, since we found no correlation between HDRS and BDNF nor other cytokines, this hypothesis requires additional investigations.

We found no significant changes in metabolic parameters between the add-on treatment groups and the Placebo group. Such changes are affected by various factors—diet, exercise, daily activities, smoking, and underlying body composition—all of which were difficult to control for in the current study because most of our participants were outpatients. It would be ideal if we could control their daily caloric intake and consumption in future studies. Furthermore, we did not find significantly lower TNF-α or CRP levels in the treatment groups than in the Placebo group. We previously reported (Lee et al. 2014), in an independent sample of 214 participants, that MM (5 mg) alone might significantly decrease plasma

**Table 3 Difference in outcomes of add-on medication (DM30, MM5, and DM30 + MM5) versus Placebo in BD-II patients**

| | B | Wald $\chi^2$ | *P*-value |
|---|---|---|---|
| HDRS[a] | | | |
| DM30 | − 1.38 | 3.36 | 0.07 |
| MM5 | − 1.33 | 2.96 | 0.09 |
| DM30 + MM5 | − 1.60 | 4.61 | 0.03* |
| YMRS[a] | | | |
| DM30 | − 1.00 | 2.44 | 0.12 |
| MM5 | − 0.98 | 2.07 | 0.15 |
| DM30 + MM5 | − 1.32 | 3.68 | 0.06 |
| TNF-α[b] | | | |
| DM30 | − 0.04 | 0.14 | 0.71 |
| MM5 | − 0.15 | 2.00 | 0.16 |
| DM30 + MM5 | − 0.07 | 0.68 | 0.41 |
| CRP[b] | | | |
| DM30 | 0.05 | 0.40 | 0.53 |
| MM5 | 0.09 | 1.18 | 0.28 |
| DM30 + MM5 | − 0.05 | 0.41 | 0.52 |
| BDNF[b] | | | |
| DM30 | 2.94 | 2.97 | 0.09 |
| MM5 | 0.02 | < 0.001 | 0.99 |
| DM30 + MM5 | 3.44 | 4.23 | 0.04* |
| TC[b] | | | |
| DM30 | 6.95 | 1.60 | 0.21 |
| MM5 | 3.14 | 0.38 | 0.54 |
| DM30 + MM5 | 4.37 | 0.60 | 0.44 |
| HDL-C[b] | | | |
| DM30 | 0.79 | 0.11 | 0.74 |
| MM5 | − 0.07 | 0.001 | 0.98 |
| DM30 + MM5 | 14.45 | 1.04 | 0.31 |
| LDL-C[b] | | | |
| DM30 | 8.80 | 3.35 | 0.07 |
| MM5 | 4.45 | 0.80 | 0.37 |
| DM30 + MM5 | 3.21 | 0.38 | 0.54 |
| Triglycerides[b] | | | |
| DM30 | 28.08 | 0.94 | 0.33 |
| MM5 | 8.81 | 0.29 | 0.59 |
| DM30 + MM5 | 11.69 | 0.52 | 0.47 |
| FBS[b] | | | |
| DM30 | − 5.33 | 0.90 | 0.34 |
| MM5 | 7.63 | 2.82 | 0.09 |
| DM30 + MM5 | − 0.31 | 0.02 | 0.90 |

*B* standardized coefficient, *HDRS* 17-item Hamilton Depression Rating Scale, *YMRS* Young Mania Rating Scale, *TNF-α* tumor necrosis factor α, *CRP* C-reactive protein, *BDNF* brain-derived neurotrophic factor, *TC* total cholesterol, *HDL-C* high-density lipoprotein-cholesterol, *LDL-C* low-density lipoprotein-cholesterol, *DM30* dextromethorphan (30 mg/day), *MM5* memantine (5 mg/day), *DM30 + MM5* dextromethorphan (30 mg/day) combined with memantine (5 mg/day), *FBS* fasting blood sugar

*$P < 0.05$

[a] Using the Placebo group as a reference group, controlling for age, gender, and treatment duration. The data shown are the interaction term, treatment group, and treatment duration

[b] Using the Placebo group as a reference group, controlling for age, gender, treatment duration, HDRS, and YMRS. The data shown are the interaction term, treatment group, and treatment duration

TNF-α levels compared with placebo. Our current negative finding might be attributable to a smaller sample.

We also found a significant association between changes in plasma BDNF levels and changes in total cholesterol (TC) levels; changes in CRP levels and changes in YMRS scores; changes in CRP levels and changes in HDL-C and triglyceride levels; and changes in TNF-α levels and changes in HDL-C and triglyceride levels. These findings mostly agree with our previous findings in an independent sample (Lee et al. 2013, 2015). We concluded then that the correlation between metabolic disturbance, clinical severity, and inflammatory aberrations might support the hypothesis that inflammation is the common underlying pathogenesis for the frequently comorbidity of BD and metabolic disturbances. In addition, because peripheral CRP levels might indicate central inflammation in the brain, Zhu et al. (2006) reported that the inflammation might decrease neurotrophic support and lead to brain dysfunction. By demonstrating concurrent increase in plasma BDNF, it is possible that the elevated plasma BDNF level observed is a compensatory response to the process of inflammation and metabolic disturbance. Our hypothesis is supported by Noren Hooten et al. (2015), who suggested that BDNF might attenuate the inflammatory stress related to high levels of CRP. The correlation between BDNF and CRP with metabolic parameters in BD requires additional investigation.

Our study has some limitations. First, we sampled only peripheral BDNF and cytokines instead of central nervous system samples because the former samples were easier to obtain. In addition, it has been suggested that changes in central BDNF and cytokine secretion might be partly reflected by the changes in peripheral levels (Pan et al. 1998; Pan and Kastin 1999). We did not explore other factors, such as smoking, diet, health supplements, or weight, all of which can affect the correlation between metabolic profiles and proinflammatory factors. Second, our study sample is small. The difference in main reduction in HDRS between the four treatment group is small. Therefore, our result should be interpreted with caution for the effect of the combination group may not have clinical superiority or significance. Studies with larger samples are needed to confirm our findings. Furthermore, it is possible that other medication permitted in the study obscured the mood stabilizing effect of the add-on medication. We did not take a ceiling effect into consideration when planning the study; however, it does appear that the patients recruited were not severely depressed. In future studies, to avoid a ceiling effect, it will be important to include patients with more severe symptoms of depression. Although we tried to limit concomitant treatment medication to only three

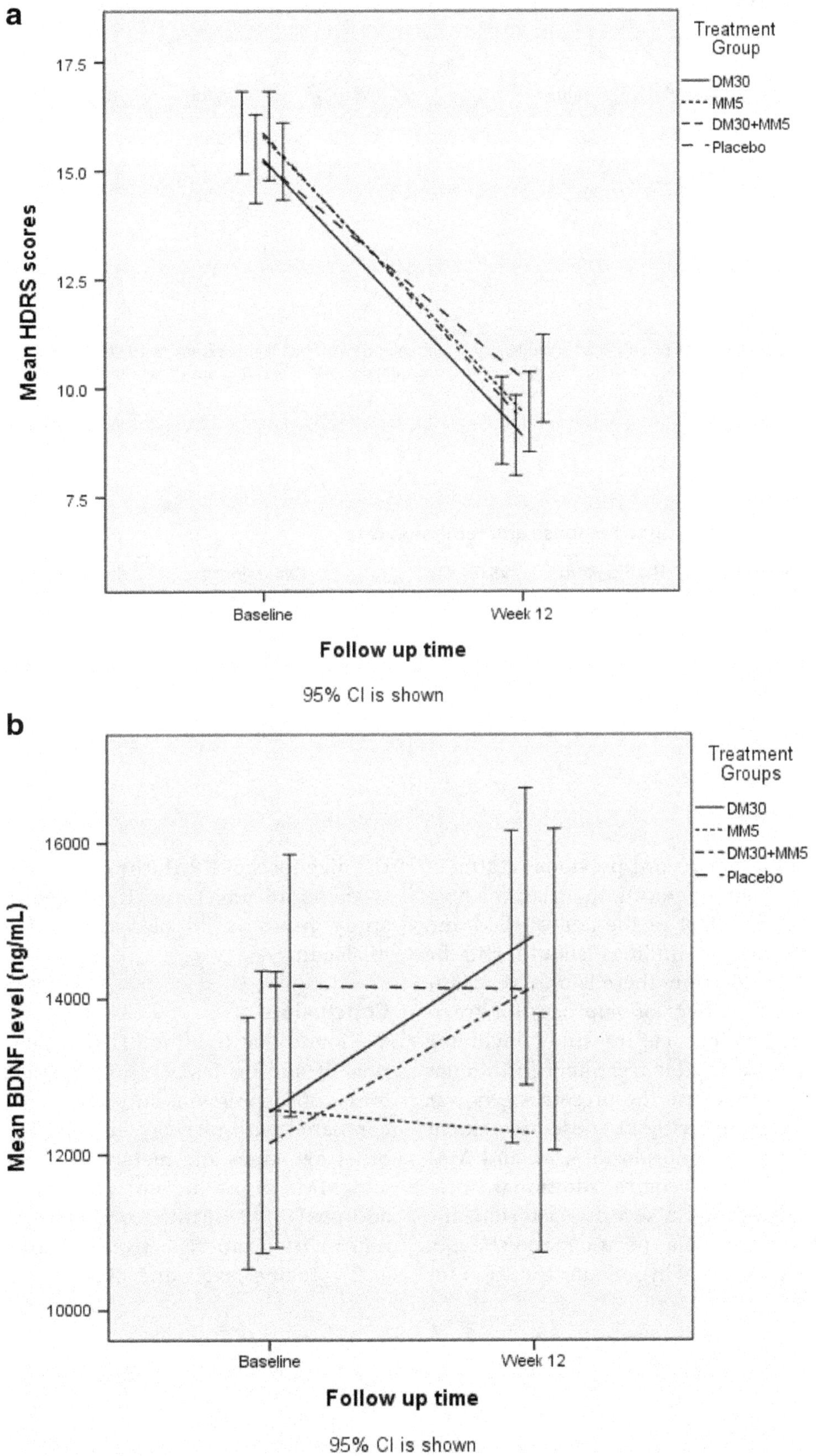


**Fig. 2** **a** Difference in symptoms of depression in BD-II patients taking add-on DM30, MM5, and DM30+MM5 versus placebo. **b** Difference in plasma BDNF levels in BD-II patients taking add-on DM30, MM5, and DM30+MM5 versus placebo

**Table 4 Correlation between TNF-α, CRP, and BDNF with clinical symptoms and metabolic parameters**

| | TNF-α | | | CRP | | | BDNF | | |
|---|---|---|---|---|---|---|---|---|---|
| | B | Wald $\chi^2$ | *P*-value | B | Wald $\chi^2$ | *P*-value | B | Wald $\chi^2$ | *P*-value |
| HDRS | 0.45 | 1.07 | 0.30 | 0.22 | 0.62 | 0.43 | 0.11 | 1.94 | 0.16 |
| YMRS | 0.20 | 0.32 | 0.57 | 0.72 | 4.82 | 0.03* | − 0.01 | 0.30 | 0.58 |
| TC | − 1.83 | 0.28 | 0.60 | 1.98 | 0.32 | 0.58 | 0.52 | 4.20 | 0.04* |
| HDL-C | − 5.34 | 6.24 | 0.01* | − 11.61 | 24.82 | < 0.001** | 0.02 | 0.02 | 0.89 |
| LDL-C | − 1.91 | 0.41 | 0.53 | 5.51 | 3.19 | 0.07 | 0.38 | 2.69 | 0.10 |
| Triglycerides | 22.78 | 10.67 | 0.001** | 34.58 | 22.38 | < 0.001** | 0.97 | 3.46 | 0.06 |
| FBS | − 6.37 | 1.30 | 0.26 | 0.73 | 0.13 | 0.72 | 0.27 | 3.41 | 0.07 |

*TNF-α* tumor necrosis factor α, *CRP* C-reactive protein, *BDNF* brain-derived neurotrophic factor, *B* standardized coefficient, *HDRS* 17-item Hamilton Depression Rating Scale, *YMRS* Young Mania Rating Scale, *TC* total cholesterol, *HDL-C* high-density lipoprotein-cholesterol, *LDL-C* low-density lipoprotein-cholesterol, *FBS* fasting blood sugar

**P* < 0.05; ***P* < 0.01

**Table 5 Survival analysis according to response and remission rate**

| | Response rate N/total N (%) | Hazard Ratio | 95.0% CI | P | Remission rate N/total N (%) | Hazard Ratio | 95.0% CI | P |
|---|---|---|---|---|---|---|---|---|
| DM30 | 44/69 (63.7%) | 0.92 | 0.59–1.43 | 0.70 | 18/69 (26.1%) | 0.78 | 0.40–1.52 | 0.46 |
| MM5 | 34/66 (51.5%) | 0.73 | 0.46–1.18 | 0.20 | 12/66 (18.2%) | 0.56 | 0.27–1.18 | 0.13 |
| DM30 + MM5 | 39/66 (59.1%) | 0.82 | 0.51–1.29 | 0.39 | 19/66 (28.8%) | 0.86 | 0.44–1.65 | 0.64 |
| Placebo | 39/69 (56.5%) | 1 (ref) | | | 17/69 (24.6%) | 1 (ref) | | |

drugs, however, we did not record previous treatment the patients were on before entering the trial; the possible anti-inflammatory effect of the add-on DM and MM interpreted from our findings should still be taken with caution. In addition, there is only very limited data supporting the effect of valproate for treatment of bipolar depression. Future study including the use of lamotrigine, a reliable treatment for bipolar depression, is needed. Because the present study was a fixed-dose comparison without dose-assessment trials, the definitive effects of add-on DM and MM and their clinical efficacy require additional studies. Finally, although we had a severity criterion, the patients recruited were not in a specific mood state, in addition, we utilized the 2-day hypomanic duration for the diagnosis of BP-II, the generalizability of our result is therefore uncertain. It will be better to refer our study group as "bipolar spectrum patients" to avoid misleading.

## Conclusion

We found that treating BD-II patients with a combination of add-on DM30 + MM5 might attenuate symptoms of depression and raise plasma BDNF levels compared with placebo, but that it had little effect on other cytokines and metabolic profiles. Add-on DM30 and MM5 alone did not have the same effect as did add-on DM30 + MM5 combined. We also found significant associations between changes in plasma BDNF and cytokine levels and changes in certain metabolic

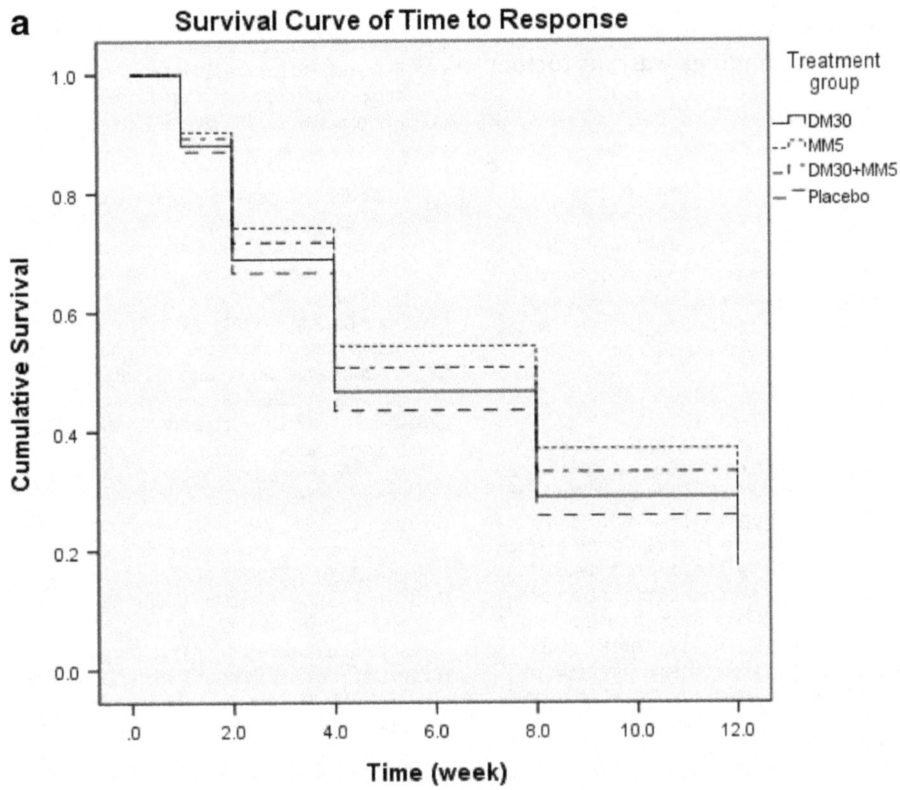


**b** Survival curve of time to remission

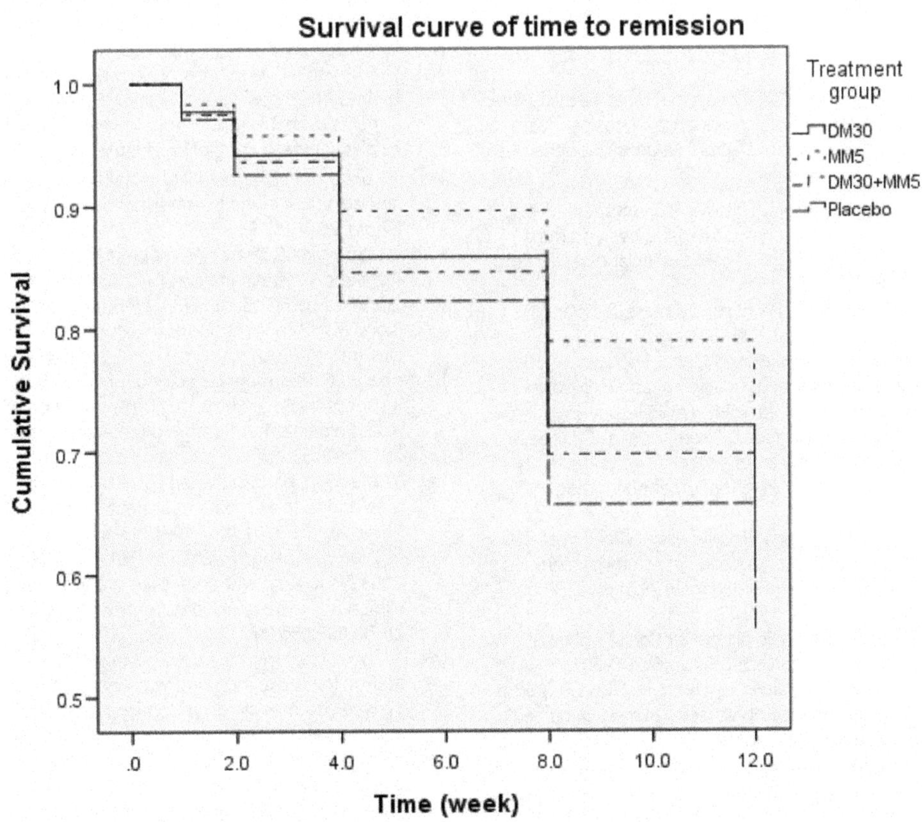


**Fig. 3** **a** Survival curve of time to response in BD-II patients taking add-on DM30, MM5, and DM30 + MM5 versus placebo. **b** Survival curve of time to response in BD-II patients taking add-on DM30, MM5, and DM30 + MM5 versus placebo

parameters, which suggested that inflammation might be the common pathogenesis between metabolic disturbance and BD. Our positive findings warrant further studies with larger samples.

**Acknowledgements**
We thank Dr. Shih-Hsien Lin for his statistical advice.

**Authors' contributions**
RBL and JSH conceived and planned the trial. SYL, TYW, PSC, SYH, NST, IHL, KCC, YKY and RBL managed participant recruitment. SYL wrote the first draft. SYL, TYW, SLC, YHC and LJW managed the lab work and statistics. RBL and JSH supervised this work and edited the manuscript. All authors reviewed the manuscript. All authors read and approved the final manuscript.

**Author details**
[1] Department of Psychiatry, Kaohsiung Veterans General Hospital, Kaohsiung, Taiwan. [2] Department of Psychiatry, School of Medicine, College of Medicine, Kaohsiung Medical University, Kaohsiung, Taiwan. [3] Department of Psychiatry, College of Medicine, National Yang-Ming University, Taipei, Taiwan. [4] Department of Psychiatry, National Cheng Kung University Hospital, College of Medicine, National Cheng Kung University, 138 Sheng-Li Road, Tainan 70428, Taiwan. [5] Department of Neurology, School of Medicine, Kaohsiung Medical University, Kaohsiung, Taiwan. [6] Department of Psychology, College of Medical and Health Science, Asia University, Taichung, Taiwan. [7] Department of Psychiatry, Tri-Service General Hospital, National Defense Medical Center, Taipei, Taiwan. [8] Department of Child and Adolescent Psychiatry, Kaohsiung Chang Gung Memorial Hospital and Chang Gung University College of Medicine, Kaohsiung, Taiwan. [9] Laboratory of Toxicology and Pharmacology, NIH/NIEHS, Research Triangle Park, Durham, NC, USA. [10] Yanjiao Furen Hospital, Hebei, China. [11] Addiction Research Center, National Cheng Kung University, Tainan, Taiwan.

**References**

Berk M, Kapczinski F, Andreazza AC, Dean OM, Giorlando F, Maes M, et al. Pathways underlying neuroprogression in bipolar disorder: focus on inflammation, oxidative stress and neurotrophic factors. Neurosci Biobehav Rev. 2011;35(3):804–17.

Chaldakov GN, Fiore M, Stankulov IS, Manni L, Hristova MG, Antonelli A, et al. Neurotrophin presence in human coronary atherosclerosis and metabolic syndrome: a role for NGF and BDNF in cardiovascular disease? Prog Brain Res. 2004;146:279–89.

Chen JJ. Pharmacologic safety concerns in Parkinson's disease: facts and insights. Int J Neurosci. 2011;121(Suppl 2):45–52.

Chen SL, Lee SY, Chang YH, Chen PS, Lee IH, Wang TY, et al. Therapeutic effects of add-on low-dose dextromethorphan plus valproic acid in bipolar disorder. Eur Neuropsychopharmacol. 2014;24(11):1753–9.

Cirulli F, Francia N, Branchi I, Antonucci MT, Aloe L, Suomi SJ, et al. Changes in plasma levels of BDNF and NGF reveal a gender-selective vulnerability to early adversity in rhesus macaques. Psychoneuroendocrinology. 2009;34(2):172–80.

Cornish JW, Herman BH, Ehrman RN, Robbins SJ, Childress AR, Bead V, et al. A randomized, double-blind, placebo-controlled safety study of high-dose dextromethorphan in methadone-maintained male inpatients. Drug Alcohol Depend. 2002;67(2):177–83.

Cotman CW, Berchtold NC. Exercise: a behavioral intervention to enhance brain health and plasticity. Trends Neurosci. 2002;25(6):295–301.

de Oliveira GS, Cereser KM, Fernandes BS, Kauer-Sant'Anna M, Fries GR, Stertz L, et al. Decreased brain-derived neurotrophic factor in medicated and drug free bipolar patients. J Psychiatr Res. 2009;43(14):1171–4.

Drancourt N, Etain B, Lajnef M, Henry C, Raust A, Cochet B, et al. Duration of untreated bipolar disorder: missed opportunities on the long road to optimal treatment. Acta Psychiatr Scand. 2013;127(2):136–44.

Drevets WC. Neuroimaging studies of mood disorders. Biol Psychiatry. 2000;48(8):813–29.

Duman RS. Synaptic plasticity and mood disorders. Mol Psychiatry. 2002;7(Suppl 1):S29–34.

Endicott J, Spitzer RL. A diagnostic interview: the schedule for affective disorders and schizophrenia. Arch Gen Psychiatry. 1978;35(7):837–44.

Fernandes BS, Gama CS, Cereser KM, Yatham LN, Fries GR, Colpo G, et al. Brain-derived neurotrophic factor as a state-marker of mood episodes in bipolar disorders: a systematic review and meta-regression analysis. J Psychiatr Res. 2011;45(8):995–1004.

Fernandes BS, Molendijk ML, Kohler CA, Soares JC, Leite CM, Machado-Vieira R, et al. Peripheral brain-derived neurotrophic factor (BDNF) as a biomarker in bipolar disorder: a meta-analysis of 52 studies. BMC Med. 2015;13:289.

Fernandes BS, Steiner J, Molendijk ML, Dodd S, Nardin P, Goncalves CA, et al. C-reactive protein concentrations across the mood spectrum in bipolar disorder: a systematic review and meta-analysis. Lancet Psychiatry. 2016;3(12):1147–56.

Goldsmith DR, Rapaport MH, Miller BJ. A meta-analysis of blood cytokine network alterations in psychiatric patients: comparisons between schizophrenia, bipolar disorder and depression. Mol Psychiatry. 2016;21(12):1696–709.

Goldstein BI, Kemp DE, Soczynska JK, McIntyre RS. Inflammation and the phenomenology, pathophysiology, comorbidity, and treatment of bipolar disorder: a systematic review of the literature. J Clin Psychiatry. 2009;70(8):1078–90.

Goldstein BI, Liu SM, Zivkovic N, Schaffer A, Chien LC, Blanco C. The burden of obesity among adults with bipolar disorder in the United States. Bipolar Disord. 2011;13(4):387–95.

Goldstein BI, Lotrich F, Axelson DA, Gill MK, Hower H, Goldstein TR, et al. Inflammatory markers among adolescents and young adults with bipolar spectrum disorders. J Clin Psychiatry. 2015;76(11):1556–63.

Huang SY, Lin WW, Ko HC, Lee JF, Wang TJ, Chou YH, et al. Possible interaction of alcohol dehydrogenase and aldehyde dehydrogenase genes with the dopamine D2 receptor gene in anxiety-depressive alcohol dependence. Alcohol Clin Exp Res. 2004;28(3):374–84.

Jacoby AS, Munkholm K, Vinberg M, Pedersen BK, Kessing LV. Cytokines, brain-derived neurotrophic factor and C-reactive protein in bipolar I disorder—results from a prospective study. J Affect Disord. 2016;197:167–74.

Karanti A, Kardell M, Joas E, Runeson B, Pålsson E, Landén M. Characteristics of bipolar I and II disorder: a study of 8766 individuals. Bipolar Disord. 2019. https://doi.org/10.1111/bdi.12867.

Karege F, Bondolfi G, Gervasoni N, Schwald M, Aubry JM, Bertschy G. Low brain-derived neurotrophic factor (BDNF) levels in serum of depressed patients probably results from lowered platelet BDNF release unrelated to platelet reactivity. Biol Psychiatry. 2005;57(9):1068–72.

Kelly TF, Lieberman DZ. The utility of the combination of dextromethorphan and quinidine in the treatment of bipolar II and bipolar NOS. J Affect Disord. 2014;167:333–5.

Kishi T, Matsunaga S, Iwata N. A meta-analysis of memantine for depression. J Alzheimers Dis. 2017;57(1):113–21.

Klein AB, Williamson R, Santini MA, Clemmensen C, Ettrup A, Rios M, et al. Blood BDNF concentrations reflect brain-tissue BDNF levels across species. Int J Neuropsychopharmacol. 2011;14(3):347–53.

Lauterbach EC. Treatment resistant depression with loss of antidepressant response: rapid-acting antidepressant action of dextromethorphan, a possible treatment bridging molecule. Psychopharmacol Bull. 2016;46(2):53–8.

Lee SY, Chen SL, Chang YH, Chen PS, Huang SY, Tzeng NS, et al. Add-on memantine to valproate treatment increased HDL-C in bipolar II disorder. J Psychiatr Res. 2013a;47(10):1343–8.

Lee SY, Chen SL, Chang YH, Chen PS, Huang SY, Tzeng NS, et al. Inflammation's association with metabolic profiles before and after a twelve-week clinical trial in drug-naive patients with bipolar II disorder. PLoS ONE. 2013b;8(6):e66847.

Lee SY, Chen SL, Chang YH, Chen PS, Huang SY, Tzeng NS, et al. The effects of add-on low-dose memantine on cytokine levels in bipolar II depression: a 12-week double-blind, randomized controlled trial. J Clin Psychopharmacol. 2014;34(3):337–43.

Lee SY, Chen SL, Chang YH, Chen PS, Huang SY, Tzeng NS, et al. Correlation of plasma brain-derived neurotrophic factor and metabolic profiles in drug-naive patients with bipolar II disorder after a twelve-week pharmacological intervention. Acta Psychiatr Scand. 2015;131(2):120–8.

Liu B, Hong JS. Primary rat mesencephalic neuron-glia, neuron-enriched, microglia-enriched, and astroglia-enriched cultures. Methods Mol Med. 2003;79:387–95.

Lyons WE, Mamounas LA, Ricaurte GA, Coppola V, Reid SW, Bora SH, et al. Brain-derived neurotrophic factor-deficient mice develop aggressiveness and hyperphagia in conjunction with brain serotonergic abnormalities. Proc Natl Acad Sci USA. 1999;96(26):15239–44.

Mora E, Portella MJ, Pinol-Ripoll G, Lopez R, Cuadras D, Forcada I, et al. High BDNF serum levels are associated to good cognitive functioning in bipolar disorder. Eur Psychiatry. 2019;60:97–107.

Mosolov S, Ushkalova A, Kostukova E, Shafarenko A, Alfimov P, Kostyukova A, et al. Bipolar II disorder in patients with a current diagnosis of recurrent depression. Bipolar Disord. 2014;16(4):389–99.

Motamedi S, Karimi I, Jafari F. The interrelationship of metabolic syndrome and neurodegenerative diseases with focus on brain-derived neurotrophic factor (BDNF): kill two birds with one stone. Metab Brain Dis. 2017;32(3):651–65.

Munkholm K, Vinberg M, Kessing LV. Peripheral blood brain-derived neurotrophic factor in bipolar disorder: a comprehensive systematic review and meta-analysis. Mol Psychiatry. 2016;21(2):216–28.

Noren Hooten N, Ejiogu N, Zonderman AB, Evans MK. Protective effects of BDNF against C-reactive protein-induced inflammation in women. Mediat Inflamm. 2015;2015:516783.

Pan W, Kastin AJ. Penetration of neurotrophins and cytokines across the blood–brain/blood–spinal cord barrier. Adv Drug Deliv Rev. 1999;36(2–3):291–8.

Pan W, Banks WA, Fasold MB, Bluth J, Kastin AJ. Transport of brain-derived neurotrophic factor across the blood–brain barrier. Neuropharmacology. 1998;37(12):1553–61.

Peng GS, Li G, Tzeng NS, Chen PS, Chuang DM, Hsu YD, et al. Valproate pretreatment protects dopaminergic neurons from LPS-induced neurotoxicity in rat primary midbrain cultures: role of microglia. Brain Res Mol Brain Res. 2005;134(1):162–9.

Rosenblat JD, Kakar R, Berk M, Kessing LV, Vinberg M, Baune BT, et al. Anti-inflammatory agents in the treatment of bipolar depression: a systematic review and meta-analysis. Bipolar Disord. 2016;18(2):89–101.

Rybakowski JK. Genetic influences on response to mood stabilizers in bipolar disorder: current status of knowledge. CNS Drugs. 2013;27(3):165–73.

Shin EJ, Bach JH, Lee SY, Kim JM, Lee J, Hong JS, et al. Neuropsychotoxic and neuroprotective potentials of dextromethorphan and its analogs. J Pharmacol Sci. 2011;116(2):137–48.

Strakowski SM, DelBello MP, Adler C, Cecil DM, Sax KW. Neuroimaging in bipolar disorder. Bipolar Disord. 2000;2(3 Pt 1):148–64.

Tohen M, Frank E, Bowden CL, Colom F, Ghaemi SN, Yatham LN, Malhi GS, Calabrese JR, Nolen WA, Vieta E, Kapczinski F, Goodwin GM, Suppes T, Sachs GS, Chengappa KR, Grunze H, Mitchell PB, Kanba S, Berk M. The International Society for Bipolar Disorders (ISBD) Task Force report on the nomenclature of course and outcome in bipolar disorders. Bipolar Disord. 2009;11(5):453–73.

Tunca Z, Ozerdem A, Ceylan D, Yalcin Y, Can G, Resmi H, et al. Alterations in BDNF (brain derived neurotrophic factor) and GDNF (glial cell line-derived neurotrophic factor) serum levels in bipolar disorder: the role of lithium. J Affect Disord. 2014;166:193–200.

Turchan-Cholewo J, Dimayuga FO, Gupta S, Keller JN, Knapp PE, Hauser KF, et al. Morphine and HIV-Tat increase microglial-free radical production and oxidative stress: possible role in cytokine regulation. J Neurochem. 2009;108(1):202–15.

Vancampfort D, Vansteelandt K, Correll CU, Mitchell AJ, De Herdt A, Sienaert P, et al. Metabolic syndrome and metabolic abnormalities in bipolar disorder: a meta-analysis of prevalence rates and moderators. Am J Psychiatry. 2013;170(3):265–74.

Wu HM, Tzeng NS, Qian L, Wei SJ, Hu X, Chen SH, et al. Novel neuroprotective mechanisms of memantine: increase in neurotrophic factor release from astroglia and anti-inflammation by preventing microglial activation. Neuropsychopharmacology. 2009;34(10):2344–57.

Yamagata AS, Mansur RB, Rizzo LB, Rosenstock T, McIntyre RS, Brietzke E. Selfish brain and selfish immune system interplay: a theoretical framework for metabolic comorbidities of mood disorders. Neurosci Biobehav Rev. 2017;72:43–9.

Yatham LN, Kennedy SH, Parikh SV, Schaffer A, Bond DJ, Frey BN, et al. Canadian Network for Mood and Anxiety Treatments (CANMAT) and International Society for Bipolar Disorders (ISBD) 2018 guidelines for the management of patients with bipolar disorder. Bipolar Disord. 2018;20(2):97–170.

Yim CY, Soczynska JK, Kennedy SH, Woldeyohannes HO, Brietzke E, McIntyre RS. The effect of overweight/obesity on cognitive function in euthymic individuals with bipolar disorder. Eur Psychiatry. 2012;27(3):223–8.

Zhang W, Wang T, Qin L, Gao HM, Wilson B, Ali SF, et al. Neuroprotective effect of dextromethorphan in the MPTP Parkinson's disease model: role of NADPH oxidase. FASEB J. 2004;18(3):589–91.

Zhang W, Qin L, Wang T, Wei SJ, Gao HM, Liu J, et al. 3-hydroxymorphinan is neurotrophic to dopaminergic neurons and is also neuroprotective against LPS-induced neurotoxicity. FASEB J. 2005;19(3):395–7.

Zhu CB, Blakely RD, Hewlett WA. The proinflammatory cytokines interleukin-1beta and tumor necrosis factor-alpha activate serotonin transporters. Neuropsychopharmacology. 2006;31(10):2121–31.

9

# Socio-demographic and clinical predictors of outcome to long-term treatment with lithium in bipolar disorders: A systematic review of the contemporary literature and recommendations from the ISBD/IGSLI Task Force on treatment with lithium

Diane Grillault Laroche[1,2], Bruno Etain[1,2,3,4*], Emanuel Severus[5], Jan Scott[3,4,6], Frank Bellivier[1,2,3] and On behalf of the ISBD-IGSLI Joint Task Force on Lithium Treatment

**Abstract**

**Objective:** To identify possible socio-demographic and clinical factors associated with Good Outcome (GO) as compared with Poor Outcome (PO) in adult patients diagnosed with Bipolar Disorder (BD) who received long-term treatment with lithium.

**Methods:** A comprehensive search of major electronic databases was performed to identify relevant studies that included adults patients (18 years or older) with a diagnosis of BD and reported sociodemographic and/or clinical variables associated with treatment response and/or with illness outcome during long-term treatment to lithium (>=6 months). The quality of the studies was scored using the Quality Assessment Tool for Observational Cohort and Cross-Sectional Studies from the National Institute of Health.

**Results:** Following review, 34 publications (from 31 independent datasets) were eligible for inclusion in this review. Most of them (n=25) used a retrospective design. Only 11 studies were graded as good or borderline good quality. Forty-three potential predictors of outcome to lithium were identified. Four factors were associated with PO to lithium: alcohol use disorder; personality disorders; higher lifetime number of hospital admissions and rapid cycling pattern. Two factors were associated with GO in patients treated with lithium: good social support and episodic evolution of BD. However, when the synthesis of findings was limited to the highest (good or borderline good) quality studies (11 studies), only higher lifetime number of hospitalization admissions remained associated with PO to lithium and no associations remained for GO to lithium.

**Conclusion:** Despite decades of research on lithium and its clinical use, besides lifetime number of hospital admissions, no factor being consistently associated with GO or PO to lithium was identified. Hence, there remains a substantial gap in our understanding of predictors of outcome of lithium treatment indicating there is a need of high quality research on large representative samples.

*Correspondence: bruno.etain@inserm.fr
[2] AP-HP, DMU Neurosciences, GH Saint-Louis – Lariboisière – F. Widal, Hôpital Fernand Widal, Département de Psychiatrie et de Médecine Addictologique, Paris, France
Full list of author information is available at the end of the article

**Keywords:** Bipolar disorder, Lithium, Response, Prediction, Mania, Depression, Treatment, Psychiatry, Clinical markers, Predictors

## Background

Bipolar disorder (BD) is a highly prevalent psychiatric disorder. With the combination of an early age of onset (peak 15–25 years) and a recurrent course, it is one of the most burdensome disorders worldwide, being ranked 4th in terms of DALYs (disability-adjusted life-year) for all medical conditions in individuals aged less than 25 years, and 6th in working age adults (Gore et al. 2011; Collins et al. 2011). BD is a leading cause of increased premature all-cause mortality including not only suicide, but also medical conditions and, compared with the general population, the estimated decrease in life expectancy is about 10 years (Kessing et al. 2015).

Mood stabilizers are the mainstay of prophylaxis for BD and lithium (Li) is the most frequently recommended first-line treatment in Clinical Practice Guidelines (CPG) (e.g. the National Institute for Health and Clinical Excellence (NICE) 2020 (https://www.nice.org.uk/guidance/cg185); the British Association for Psychopharmacology (BAP) (Goodwin et al. 2016); the Canadian Network for Mood and Anxiety Treatments (CANMAT) (Yatham et al. 2018), Royal Australian and New Zealand College of Psychiatrists (Malhi et al. 2018)). Furthermore, a network meta-analysis comparing the efficacy and tolerability of several classes of mood stabilizers concluded that a particular advantage of Li is that it prevents mood episode relapses and recurrences of all polarities (Miura et al. 2014). Despite evidence of efficacy and support for the use of Li in CPG recommendations, prescribing of Li has plateaued (Kessing 2019) and in many countries patients' and clinicians' preference for Li is lower than expected (Tondo et al. 2019). Indeed, antidepressants, despite not recommended as monotherapy or first line use, remain a widely used therapy (Kessing et al. 2016) and other agents such as atypical antipsychotics have been aggressively marketed as alternatives. Another reason for this apparent ambivalence is that a substantial proportion of individuals (probably between 30 and 60%) do not achieve a good outcome with Li prophylaxis in day-to-day clinical settings (Scott et al. 2018). Furthermore, predictors of poor outcome are poorly understood or there is limited evidence supporting their validity. As such, patients are often faced with a 'trial and error' approach that requires their commitment to take Li for about several months in order to determine the magnitude of their individual response. Unsurprisingly, this scenario, plus the narrow therapeutic window (requiring plasma monitoring), is associated with high attrition rates and suboptimal exposure to Li treatment, e.g. due to fluctuating adherence, in individuals with BD.

To avoid lengthy and ineffective treatment trials in individuals with a low likelihood of benefit from Li, a number of studies aimed to identify socio-demographic and clinical predictors of good prophylactic response to lithium. Some reviews and meta-analyses have been undertaken to try to summarize findings from a broad range of individual studies (Severus et al. 2014; Kessing et al. 2018). However, both approaches have encountered problems. For example, reviews published in the last 15 years have rarely followed current guidelines on systematic reviews and/or the reported findings show significant inconsistencies across the reviews (Tighe et al. 2011; Rybakowski 2014; Kleindienst et al. 2005; Montlahuc et al. 2019). Likewise, the use of meta-analytic approaches that try to quantify the relative importance of potential predictors of good or poor response to Li are undermined by the fact that many of the original studies are of low quality and so there are significant differences in the estimated importance (and valency of effect) of many factors. For instance, a recent meta-analysis by Hui and colleagues (Hui et al. 2019) identified six predictors of good response (Manic Depressive Interval (MDI) sequence, absence of rapid cycling, absence of psychotic symptoms, family history of BD, shorter duration of illness prior to the start of lithium, and later age of onset). However, findings of large and significant associations between these identified factors and good response (e.g. MDI sequence had an odds ratio of about 4.3) were undermined by the fact that < 10% of the 71 publications included in the systematic review and meta-analysis were rated as good quality. For example, in the case of MDI sequence–one of the core features of the classical manic-depressive clinical profile associated with lithium response by Mogens Schou and others in 1970's (Schou 1982)–five of the six studies included in the pooled analysis were rated as poor quality which highlights the need to be very cautious in interpreting the relevance of this potential predictor. Indeed, several guidelines suggest that it is inappropriate to undertake meta-analyses under these circumstances or that the use of this approach requires justification (Thompson et Pocock 1991; NIH Quality Assurance Guidelines 2019). On the other hand, in case of MDI sequence, the sixth study in the afore mentioned meta-analysis (Hui et al. 2019), which was considered of fair quality (Maj et al. 1989), also showed that MDI sequence, compared to DMI sequence, was associated with good outcome to lithium treatment.

From a methodological point of view, to be able to truly identify clinical or socio-demographic predictors of outcome to prophylactic treatment with optimal lithium levels a 3-arm randomized placebo- and "active comparator"- controlled study design would be needed—to differentiate between predictors of "treatment versus no treatment" and "treatment with lithium versus treatment with another approved drug". However we are not aware that any such study has been conducted. Therefore, for this review, we decided that it is more prudent to use the wording "predictors of outcome to long-term treatment with lithium" instead of "predictors of response to long-term treatment with lithium" when it comes to interpret the results of the vast majority of the studies conducted so far.

Given the above, the International Society of BD (ISBD) Task Force on the treatment with Lithium concluded that a gap in the knowledge-base about Li response still remained. Further, it was agreed that this gap might best be addressed by a qualitative review (i.e. design and quality of available studies) that adhered to established guidelines on systematic reviews and that employed a protocol that had been subjected to peer-review (via a recognized international body) and was published (to allow external scrutiny). It was agreed that the review would focus on contemporary publications and that eligibility criteria for inclusion would stipulate the need for any study to provide clear documentation of the procedure for diagnosing BD and for defining Li response, etc. The key aims of the review were:

(a) To identify socio-demographic and clinical factors that are associated with good outcome as compared with poor outcome to Li prophylaxis in adults with BD;
(b) to determine if the list of putative predictors remained robust when considering number of studies identifying each specific factor, study quality (good versus fair/poor) and design (prospective versus retrospective).

Due to the known weaknesses in the literature, quantitative analyses were disregarded pre-hoc, but instead a range of qualitative techniques were utilized to assess the above concepts.

## Methods

### Protocol

The protocol for the systematic review was lodged with the international prospective register of systematic reviews in July 2019 (PROSPERO: CRD42019141329) and we adhered to the Preferred Reporting Items for Systematic Reviews and Meta-Analyses (PRISMA) and Meta-Analysis Of Observational Studies in Epidemiology (MOOSE) guidelines (Liberati et al. 2009; Moher et al. 2015). A PRISMA flowchart is provided in Fig. 1 and a PRISMA checklist is provided in the Additional file 1: (Appendix 1).

### Search strategy

A systematic strategy was employed to search for studies relevant to the review. We employed search terms referring to socio-demographic and clinical variables that may predict response to or can be associated with outcome during long-term exposure to Li in adults with a presentation that met diagnostic criteria for BD. For example, terms such as lithium OR prophylactic lithium AND bipolar dis* AND predict* OR respons* OR remission OR Retrospective Assessment of Response to Lithium Scale OR Alda scale OR treatment outcome OR non-response OR relapse OR remission OR recurrence were cross-referenced with terms identifying observational, retrospective, prospective, cohort, case control, epidemiological and/or database studies, and randomized or non-randomized trials. Searches were repeated using the terms affective psychosis or manic depression related terms (mani*, manic depress*, hypomani*) instead of bipolar dis* and using terms that ensured we focused on adult-pattern disorders (i.e. excluding paediatric/juvenile BD). Also, we incorporated selected search terms used in previous systematic reviews of lithium response and prediction of outcomes for individuals (e.g. Li blood level, etc.).

Electronic databases (MedLINE, PubMed, Cochrane Library, Web of Sciences, EMBASE, and Google Scholar) were searched for the last 30 years (from July 1st 1989 until July 31st, 2019). This time frame was chosen to ensure we focused on more recent research and studies that primarily employed diagnostic criteria for BD that show greater consistency across current classification systems (DSM-IIIR onwards and/or equivalent iterations of ICD). Alerts were set up until December 2019 for the electronic databases so that researchers were notified of new publications up to and including the submission date for this review (e.g. manuscripts listed as Epub ahead of print). A handsearch of primary and secondary publication reference lists was conducted to identify further studies.

### Selection Criteria

Publications were eligible for screening if they were written in English and reported data from peer-reviewed studies in samples that comprised of adults (minimum age 18 years) who met internationally recognized diagnostic criteria for BD (DSM-IIIR and later, ICD9 and later, RDC) and that reported sociodemographic and/or clinical variables associated with treatment response

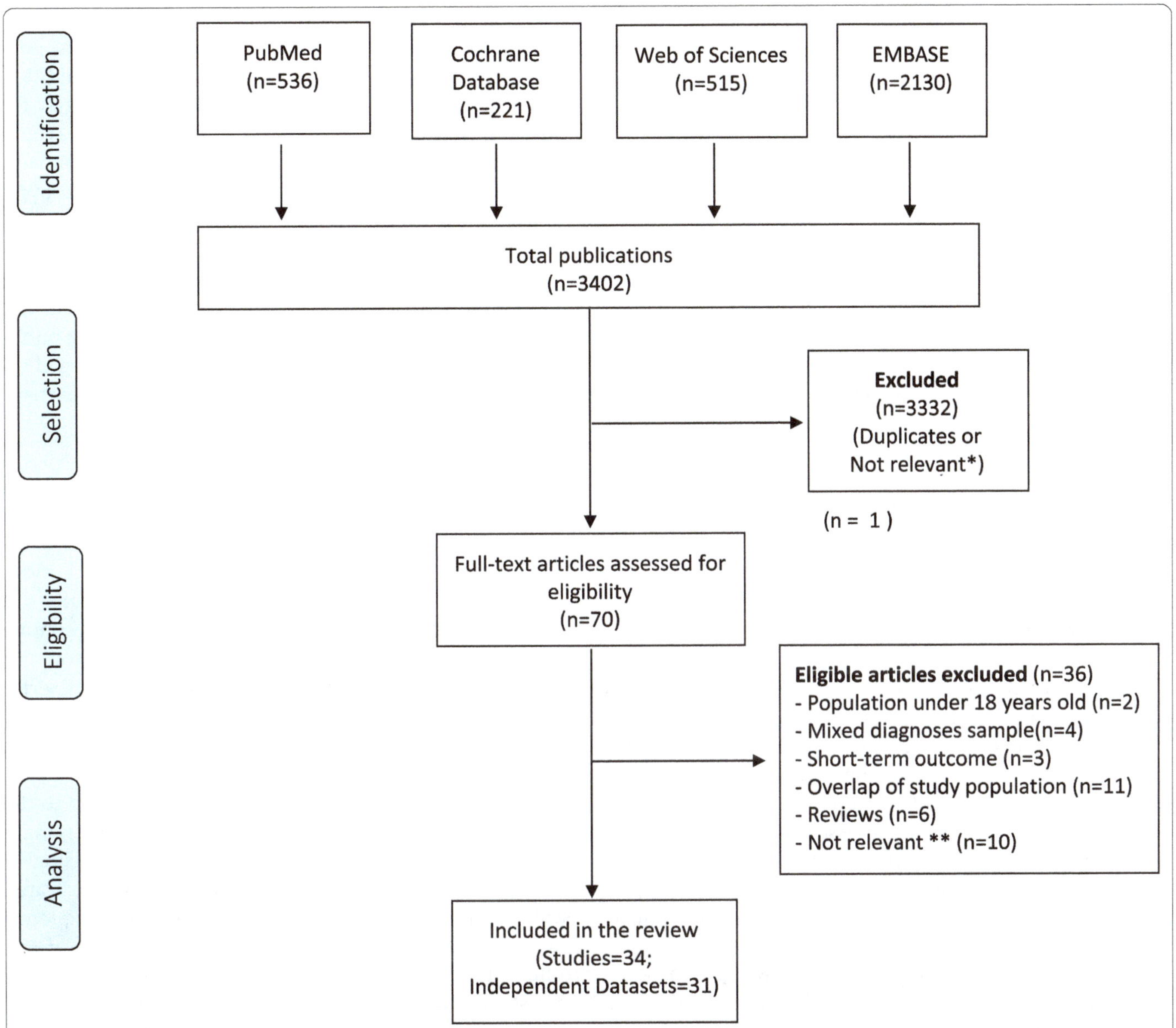


**Fig. 1** Flow-chart of articles included in the systematic qualitative analysis. (*) not relevant: keywords met selection criteria, but publication did not represent a study of outcome with Lithium. (**) not relevant: studies failed to meet inclusion criteria regarding predictors or met ≥ 1 exclusion criterion e.g. comparison of outcome to Li versus other mood stabilizers

and/or with illness outcome during long-term exposure to Li. Lithium could be used alone, in combination with other psychotropics and/or co-prescribed with another mood stabilizer.

### Eligibility

We selected only those articles reporting sociodemographic and/or clinical factors associated with good outcome to Li treatment compared with poor outcome to Li treatment in adults with a presentation of BD that met internationally recognized diagnostic criteria according to the Diagnostic and Statistical Manual (DSM IIIR or later), the International Statistical Classification of Diseases and Related Health Problems (ICD-9 or later; World Health Organization, 1978; ibid 1992), or the Research Diagnostic Criteria (RDC) (Spitzer et al. 1978). To be included in the systematic review, publications had to fulfill the following eligibility criteria:

### Inclusion criteria

(i) the article clearly indicated that Li was prescribed as a long-term, continuation, maintenance or prophylactic treatment (if the publication did not use any of these descriptors, it could be included if the reported mean duration of Li treatment was at least 6 months),

(ii) 'outcome' was defined as any outcome in terms of mood episodes or illness course or activity, but did not include outcomes that were related only to the anti-suicidal properties of lithium,

(iii) raw data about potential socio-demographic or clinical predictors of Li response (measured as a categorical or continuous variable) or of outcomes associated with exposure to Li (e.g. social functioning) were reported,

(iv) findings were reported separately regarding good outcome or poor outcome to Li (where Li was prescribed as a single or combined treatment),

(v) studies where a subsample of the study population met the eligibility criteria could be included in the review provided relevant data were available for that subsample or could be obtained from the authors.

**Exclusion criteria**

(i) comparative studies that only reported predictors of outcome to Li versus predictors of outcome to other mood stabilizers (unless the publication separately reported factors specifically associated with good versus poor outcome to Li),

(ii) studies of samples that were wholly or partly comprised of children or adolescents and/or of mixed diagnoses such as BD with unipolar disorder and/or schizo-affective disorders (unless the analyses were stratified according to age groups or to diagnosis, and findings reported separately),

(iii) studies that only reported outcomes for Li treatment in BD samples with an acute manic or depressive episode,

(iv) studies that reported only on putative biomarkers of good or poor outcome to lithium treatment (such as genetic or brain imaging research) without data on socio-demographic or clinical variables associated with good or poor outcome to lithium,

(v) studies where the sample comprised only of a 'special population' or subgroup (e.g. seasonal affective or post-partum disorders, or BD in individuals with learning difficulties or with a particular medical disorder such as thyroid disease),

(vi) review articles or non-data based publications.

A priori, we agreed upon a strategy for determining study eligibility when several publications arose from the same database or when publications included overlapping samples. The consensus was that later publications were eligible for inclusion if they included novel findings e.g. a later follow-up had revealed additional possible predictors of outcome to Li treatment (in addition to the initial report). If data were reported separately for repeated follow-ups of the same sample, then we would prioritize findings from the most recent publication with the longest follow-up. If the publications reported overlapping samples, then we would prioritize findings from the largest sample size.

Data publications that included the key search terms in the title, abstract, or index term fields were screened, and full text articles obtained as appropriate. Duplicate publications were removed and uncertainties regarding eligibility of individual articles were reconciled by consensus (by DGL, BE, and checked independently by JS).

**Data extraction**

Data were extracted from studies meeting selection criteria and key information was entered into an Excel file proforma (by DGL and BE; then checked independently by FB). This recorded key study details e.g. authors, study location, design (cross-sectional; cohort; retrospective; prospective), and year of publication and noted whether the publication was included in a series of publications by the same research group of investigators and/or whether the study arose from a project being undertaken by a larger network or consortium, etc. Also, the proforma collated specific information related to the review topic, namely sampling frame (sample size, diagnostic assessment procedure); method for assessing Li response (e.g. clinical judgement, self- or observer-rated scale, change in social functioning or episode frequency etc.); duration of observation period and timing of any follow-up assessments (if appropriate). We noted any statistical measures of association between potential predictors and response status (e.g. correlations, odds ratios, etc....), the magnitude of any associations, and whether the analyses were uni- or multi-variate, were adjusted for covariates (e.g. sex), and/or if they examined confounders, etc. If summary statistics were not reported, the researchers requested raw data from the original authors.

**Quality assurance (QA) assessment**

Quality of included studies was assessed independently by three raters (JS, DGL and BE) using the 14-item Quality Assessment Tool for Observational Cohort and Cross-Sectional Studies (available at https://www.nhlbi.nih.gov/health-topics/study-quality-assessment-tools). Assessors reviewed and critically appraised each publication and differences in their independent ratings were resolved by consensus. The final ratings provided a total score (range 0–14) and a quality grading (good, fair or poor).

### Qualitative synthesis of findings

Findings were summarized from all eligible studies and we generated a list of socio-demographic and clinical variables that were reported in at least two studies undertaken in independent datasets. Each study was then assessed separately and any factor associated with a good outcome to Li was labelled as GO (Good Outcome), whilst those associated with poor outcome were labelled as PO (Poor Outcome). If the analysis of a factor in an individual study showed no statistical association with GO or PO, it was labelled as UA (uncertain association with Li response status). By the term 'outcome', we refer to the primary outcome that has been defined in each study (for examples: score at the Alda scale for retrospective studies if this scale was used, morbidity index before/after lithium initiation for other retrospective studies, time to relapse or presence of a relapse during follow-up for prospective studies, among different types of response assessment).

We then estimated the percentage of studies in which a factor was classified as GO, UA, or PO (i.e. number of studies in which factor was classified/total number of studies measuring that factor). The relative proportions of studies identifying a given factor respectively as GO, UA and PO were then plotted for all factors in a '100% stacked column' chart. Three schematic diagrams were produced, one included all relevant studies regardless of QA assessment, the second selected studies graded as good quality only and the third selected only prospective studies. For the second and third schematic diagrams, we applied the same threshold for inclusion of a factor as used for the first schematic, namely that it was measured in at least two studies.

Lastly, we assessed concordance regarding the valence of any putative predictors by assessing the level of agreement (regarding factors associated with GO, PO or UA) according to study quality grading (categorized as Good versus Fair or Poor (combined into one category)) or study design (categorized as Retrospective versus Prospective). We considered that a factor gave concordant results when it was associated with the same type of response (GO, PO or UR) in more than 50% of independent studies. We then calculated the proportion of concordance: number of 'concordant factors' divided by the number of factors being studied.

## Results

### Selected articles

The initial literature search identified 3402 articles, of which 70 met criteria for full text review (see flow-chart in Fig. 1). Following review, 34 publications derived from 31 independent datasets were eligible for inclusion in the systematic review.

### Population and study design

Key characteristics of the methodology, design and samples from the included studies are presented in Additional file 2: Table S3. Location of publication varied widely, but 13 of the 34 studies were undertaken in Europe (38%). The median sample size was 112 but again varied widely (n = 21 to 4714, total sample size = 12.602), while seven studies (20%) included < 50 individuals. About 20% of studies included only individuals with a diagnosis of BD-I, whilst eleven of the studies did not specify the distribution of BD subtypes. The prevalence of females ranged from 29 to 79%, although the majority of samples included more females than males.

Twenty-five studies used a retrospective design; of these 11 studies assessed Li response using the Alda scale (Kapur et al. 2019; Saito et al. 2017; Etain et al. 2016; Sportiche et al. 2017; Scott et al. 2017; Silva et al. 2016; Rybakowski et al. 2013; Garnham et al. 2007; Grof et al. 2002; Martinsson et al. 2013; Guloksuz et al. 2012), whilst two community cohort studies used change in illness activity (e.g. readmission rates) (Kessing et al. 2011; Kessing et al. 2014). The 14 other retrospective studies employed a variety of assessments of outcome of prophylaxis ranging from number of relapses over a given time period through to change in Clinical Global Improvement (CGI) or Global Assessment Scale (GAS) scores (Shan et al. 2016; Tharoor et al. 2013; Rybakowski et al. 2009; Ozyildirim et al. 2010; Masui et al. 2008; Rybakowski et al. 2007; Washizuka et al. 2003; Tondo et al. 2001; Yazici et al. 1999; O'Connell et al. 1991; Okuma 1993). Nine studies were categorized as prospective, of which eight reported only prospective outcomes of Li treatment such as change in number of BD episodes by polarity, overall change in illness burden before/after lithium initiation for example (Post et al. 2016; Cakir et al. 2016; Kato et al. 2000; Gasperini et al. 1993; Maj et al. 1998; Degenhardt et al. 2012; Denicoff et al. 1997; Stefos et al. 1996; Kusalic et al. 1998), whilst one study reported both retrospective and prospective outcome assessments (Kulhara et al. 1999). As described in Additional file 2: Table S3, 16 studies did not report serum lithium levels while 18 studies did.

### Quality assessment of eligible studies

The median quality rating score was 7/14. However, quality gradings revealed that, whilst 11 studies (33% - n = 9.981) were graded as good or borderline good quality, 10 studies (30% - n = 2.621) were graded as poor or borderline poor (see Additional file 3: Table S1). There were recurring design and methodological weaknesses that could bias reported study findings including e.g. reliance on small and/or convenience samples, case

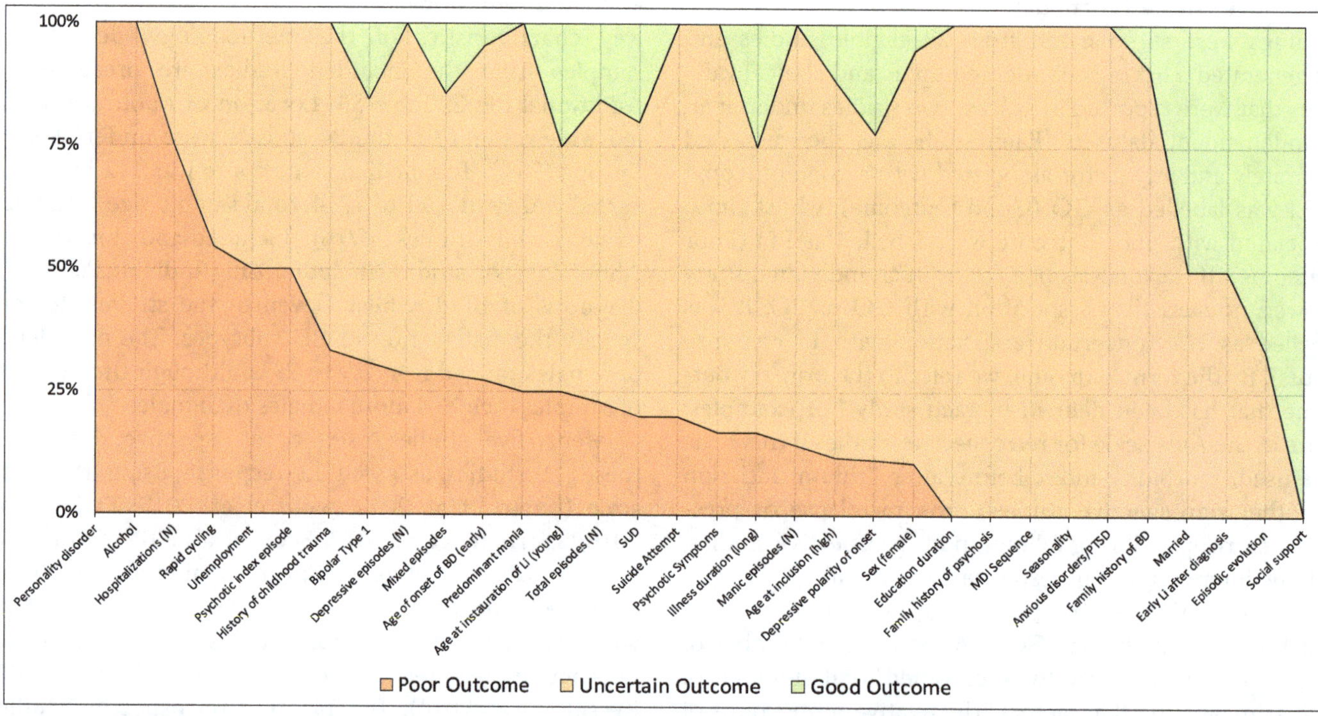


X axis displays the factors being studied in association with the outcome to Lithium. Y axis display the percentage of studies showing an association with Poor Outcome (red), Uncertain Outcome (orange) and Good Outcome (green) to lithium

**Fig. 2** Diagram graph of all potential predictors being studied in at least 2 studies

note assessment of outcome to Li treatment by a single, unblinded investigator (without corroboration or review by another rater), failure to systematically assess putative predictors using reliable and valid tools (e.g. reliance on patient reports to assess family history of BD).

#### Putative predictors of outcome to lithium treatment

Although a total of 43 potential predictors of outcome to Li were reported at least in one study, only 32 of these factors were eligible for the review (for a detailed summary of factors, see Additional file 4: Table S2). The three most frequently examined factors were: age at onset of BD (n = 22 studies), gender (n = 19) and current age/age at study inclusion (n = 17). Six other factors were examined in > 30% studies: psychotic symptoms, illness duration of BD, BD subtype, family history of BD, rapid cycling and lifetime number of mood episodes.

As shown in Fig. 2, six factors were reported to be associated with either PO or GO status. Factors associated with PO were: comorbid alcohol use disorder (reported in 2 out of 2 studies); comorbid personality disorders (2/2 studies); higher lifetime number of hospitalizations (PO = 6/8; UA = 2/8 studies); and rapid cycling pattern (PO = 6/11; UA = 5/11 studies). Two factors were associated with GO: good social support (2/2 studies) and episodic (i.e. sequence of mood episodes being separated by clear periods of euthymia) evolution of illness (GO = 2/3; UA = 1/3 studies).

The other 26 factors (i.e. 81% of all factors examined) repeatedly failed to show any statistically significant positive or negative association with Li treatment (and were mainly classified as UA). Among these, five factors were classified as UA in all the eligible studies in which the factor was examined: seasonality (2/2 studies), MDI sequence (3/3 studies), time in education (5/5 studies), family history of psychosis (2/2 studies), and presence of any anxiety disorders (including PTSD) (4/4 studies).

When the synthesis of findings was limited to the highest (good or borderline good) quality studies (11 studies; 9 independent datasets), only higher lifetime number of hospitalizations remained associated with PO and no associations were maintained for GO (see Fig. 3). When the descriptive analysis was restricted to only good quality studies, some variables being associating to PO or GO were lost (personality disorders, alcohol misuse, social support, episodic evolution and rapid cycling). This was mainly due to an insufficient number of (good quality) studies reporting these variables (personality disorders, alcohol misuse, social support, episodic evolution). For rapid cycling, it was observed that 2 of 5 good quality studies reported an association with PO, while 4 of 6 studies (fair to poor quality) reported such an association. This observation makes it possible that for rapid cycling, the quality of the studies may impact on the reports of the potential associations to PO.

As shown in Fig. 4, when the synthesis of findings was limited to prospective studies (n = 9), we noted that rapid cycling and number of hospitalizations were associated with PO, but no associations were maintained for GO.

Regarding concordance, we found that the level of agreement between studies regarding the predictive utility of a factor (and the valence of the association) was lower in higher quality studies (concordance rates: Higher versus Lower Quality = 65% versus 85%) and in prospective studies (concordance rates: Retrospective versus Prospective Design = 92% versus 86%).

## Discussion

After decades of research into clinical predictors of response to Li prophylaxis in BD, our disappointing findings highlight the lack of consistency across individual studies. The conclusions of this systematic review can be deduced simply by examining the dwindling number of factors associated with GO and PO status when we focus on higher quality studies or prospective designs (Figs. 1, 2 and 3). One of the most obvious conclusions is that, despite many decades of research, there remains a substantial gap in our understanding of predictors of outcome of lithium treatment indicating there is a need of high quality research on large representative samples. We do not underestimate the difficulties faced by researchers in this field and recognize the impossibility of perfect studies and the complexity of undertaking very high quality projects on this topic. However, a key message from this review is that this remains an unanswered question. The other obvious point is that there is a potential problem in undertaking further qualitative or quantitative reviews as they are all faced with the difficulties of deriving reliable and valid conclusions regarding predictors when synthesizing findings from the existing literature. This is perhaps best illustrated by the fact that higher quality or prospective studies (theoretically more reliable and/or valid) show a somewhat lower concordance (i.e. less agreement) regarding the best predictors than lower quality or retrospective studies. It is also noteworthy that meta-analyses cannot solve this conundrum, as a lack of high quality studies (compared to the number of fair/poor quality studies) is a recognized contra-indication to use that strategy or an indication to being cautious in the application of any findings in such circumstances.

Regarding specific outputs of this review, we highlight that 26 out of 32 putative predictors (selected on the basis that they were examined in at least two studies from independent datasets) failed to show any significant association with either GO or PO status. Further, the six factors identified as associated with either GO (n = 2) or PO (n = 4) did not manifest a robust association with Li response when the synthesis of data focused on studies selected for their higher quality (good or borderline fair/good) or optimal design (prospective follow-up). Interestingly, the two factors identified as being associated with GO in all the studies in which they were examined (good social support and episodic evolution of illness) were only assessed on five occasions in total and were the factors most likely to be lost from the list of predictors when studies were stratified by quality or design—partly because there were no high quality studies available assessing, for example,"good social support". The majority of the variables associated with PO were no more robust, with the exception of higher number of prior hospitalizations and the mainly consistent evidence of poor outcome in those with rapid cycling BD in prospective studies.

Overall, the most relevant clinical implication of this review is that clinicians might have marginally more confidence in stating which factors are associated with poor outcome to Li prophylaxis, but very little certainty about the factors that are associated with good outcome. As higher lifetime number of hospitalizations consistently predicted poor outcome in the overall analyses, in the highest quality studies and in the prospective studies, another clinical implication from the review might be that lithium should be offered early in the course of bipolar disorder as also concluded in the study by Kessing et al. 2014 specifically investigating this issue. Whilst this is disappointing at one level, the clinical translation of the findings, especially if this trend continues in future studies and high quality systematic reviews, is that psychiatrists may eventually be able to avoid asking some individuals with BD to participate in a lengthy trial of Li when the clinical history reveals the presence of the factors most robustly associated with poor outcome (as they are unlikely to show any significant health gain). Unfortunately, we are still far away from being confident about this assertion, and it may well be that poor outcome associated with higher lifetime number of hospitalizations may have nothing to do with lithium in particular but may simply be a marker for poor general outcome (to psychopharmacological treatment) in patients with bipolar disorders. This is suggested by a randomized controlled study comparing lithium and lamotrigine (Licht et al. 2010). In this study the number of previous episodes (and rapid cycling), independently of treatment, was associated with poor outcome, which also has been found by others (Perlis et al. 2006).

Several factors that even meta-analytic studies have suggested may be associated with good outcome lacked a clear signal for predicting Li response in this review. Indeed, when the current review is compared with the most recent meta-analysis (Hui et al. 2019), the only findings in common are the association of poor outcome with rapid cycling BD or number of prior hospitalizations (but the strength of the reported associations was reversed between these two reviews). In part, this may be due to differences in inclusion and exclusion criteria as, for example, there was no overlap in the studies selected regarding the predictor "MDI sequence" between this review and the recent meta-analysis (Hui et al. 2019). In addition very few of the studies (e.g. Etain et al. 2017; Scott et al. 2017) selected for this review as well as the recent meta-analysis (Hui et al. 2019) studied the possibility of interdependence/interaction between predictors. Moreover, several of the included studies (n = 16) did not report lithium plasma levels in the studied samples, nor comparisons of lithium plasma level by outcome status (n = 11). Among the 7 remaining studies, the subdivision of lithium concentrations, associated with the various outcomes, was so inconsistent that this fact alone made it impossible to include lithium concentrations as a predictive factor in our systematic review. However, lithium serum levels in a range above a lower threshold around 0.45/0.60 and up to 0.80/1.00 mmol/L have been associated with superior efficacy compared to lower lithium serum levels in the maintenance treatment of bipolar disorders (Nolen et al. 2019). All of this presents a dilemma for clinicians seeking answers from the literature. Do they follow the evidence from a meta-analysis that the authors themselves report to be sub-optimal, or do they ignore even the weak signal regarding outcome prediction to lithium treatment because a rigorous review failed to find sufficient support for the factor in question? At this point of time, it seems prudent to suggest clinicians, when there are no contraindications, to offer a trial of lithium prophylaxis as the gold standard maintenance treatment in bipolar disorders to all of their patients with theses disorders, irrespective of the presence or absence of predictors potentially associated with good or poor outcome to long-term treatment with lithium.

## Perspectives and recommendations

The search for clinical predictors of response to Li remains inconclusive and unconvincing. There has been a trend for reviews and meta-analyses of existing studies, but many of these are flawed (e.g. low quality or fail to employ reliable assessments or multivariate analyses). It is perhaps more important to encourage high quality large scale studies, rather than undertaking further

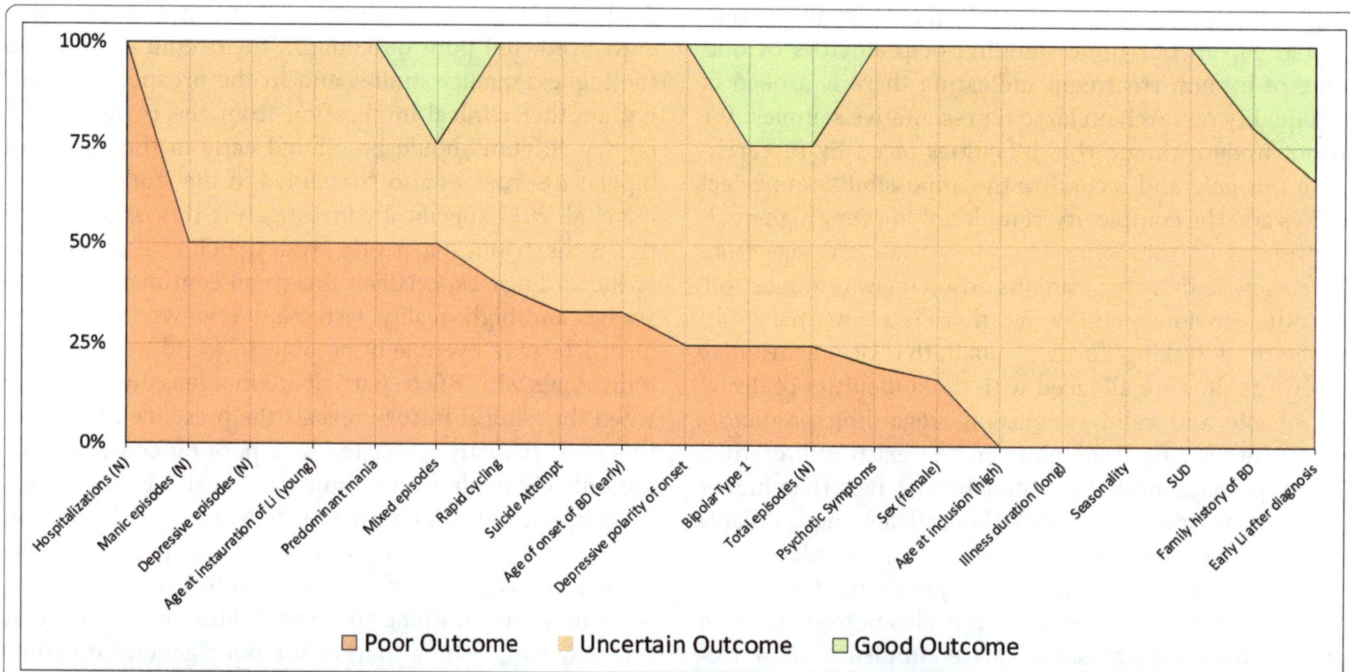


X axis displays the factors being studied in association with the outcome to Lithium. Y axis display the percentage of studies showing an association with Poor Outcome (red), Uncertain Outcome (orange) and Good Outcome (green) to lithium

**Fig. 3** Diagram graph of all potential predictors being studied in at least 2 studies, only in good or borderline good quality studies

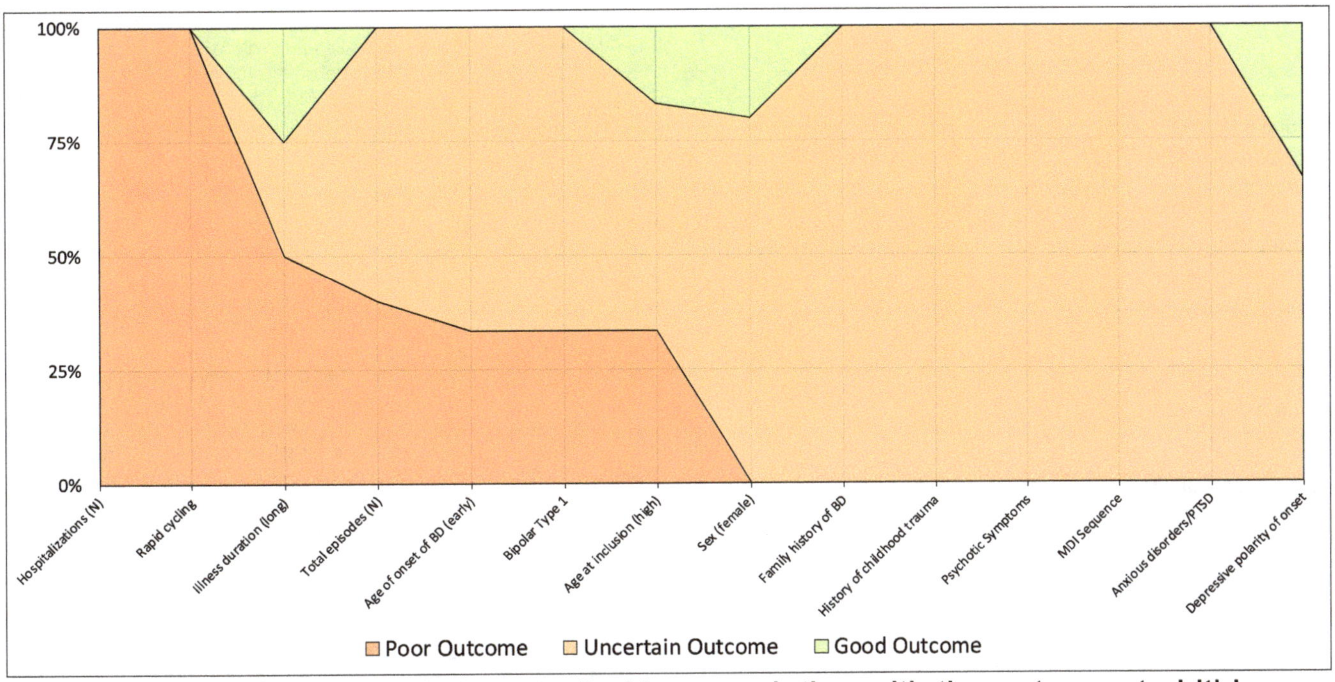


X axis displays the factors being studied in association with the outcome to Lithium. Y axis display the percentage of studies showing an association with Poor Outcome (red), Uncertain Outcome (orange) and Good Outcome (green) to lithium

**Fig. 4** Diagram graph of all potential predictors being studied in at least 2 studies, only in prospective studies

reviews or pooled analyses. Despite the longevity of use of Li in clinical practice, more research is required of clinically representative samples (with adequate statistical power) that employ modern analytic techniques and consider co-associations between putative predictors, including serum lithium levels, to identify individual demographic or clinical factors associated with GO or PO or specific combinations of factors or key variables underlying Li response (Passos et al. 2019; Nunes et al. 2020).

A comprehensive, reliable and valid clinical assessment needs to be incorporated into any future studies since some potential predictors of good/poor outcome to Li remain understudied (familial response to Li, alcohol use disorder, personality disorders, etc.), and/or are poorly operationalized (MDI sequence, childhood maltreatment, etc.) (Scott et al. 2018).

Although there is increasing research on potential biomarkers or biosignatures of Li response (e.g. RLiNK, https://rlink.eu.com/ in which most authors are involved, other on-going longitudinal studies or registry-based studies), they are likely to be used as well as, rather than instead of clinical factors (if any) (Hui et al. 2019; Scott et al. 2019), so an integrated science approach including rigorous clinical phenotyping remains a cornerstone of any biological or genetic research in this field (Scott et al. 2018).

## Conclusions

This systematic review of publications from the last three decades of research in the field of predictors of Li response failed to identify predictors of outcome to Li prophylaxis, except lifetime number of hospitalizations, that remained robust when the synthesis of findings was restricted to higher quality or prospective studies. Hence, it is suggested from the review that lithium should be offered early in the course of BD. It emerged that several factors are under-researched (including some potentially associated with GO such as good social support) and/or are worthy of further investigation (such as early initiation of Li and axis II disorders and alcohol use disorders). However, we conclude that the current clinical approach, i.e. a trial of Li undertaken on a case by case basis, is still required. This is because a careful examination of the design and quality of available studies identified sufficient methodological concerns to suggest that earlier reviews and meta-analyses might have significant drawbacks. Also, further systematic reviews or meta-analyses are not easy to justify until new high quality studies in large clinically representative samples are available.

## Supplementary information

**Additional file 1:** PRISMA checklist.

**Additional file 2: Table S3.** Characterization of selected studies (n=34) and the clinical predictors of outcome to long-term treatment with lithium.

**Additional file 3: Table S1.** Summary of Quality Assessment gradings for studies meeting eligibility criteria for the systematic review.

**Additional file 4: Table S2.** Number factors investigated in >= 2 from independent datasets.

**Acknowledgements**
Not applicable.

**Authors' contributions**
Conception and design: DGL, BE, JS, FB. Data analyses and interpretation: DGL, BE, JS, FB. Drafted the manuscript: DGL, BE, JS, FB. Critically revised the manuscript: DGL, BE, ES, JS, FB. Final approval: DGL, BE, ES, JS, FB. Agrees to be accountable for all aspect of work ensuring integrity and accuracy: DGL, BE, ES, JS, FB. All authors read and approved the final manuscript.

**Members of the ISBD/IGSLI task force on the treatment with lithium who critically revised the article**
M Bauer (University Hospital Carl Gustav Carus, TU Dresden, Dresden, Germany); M. Berk (Deakin University, Geelong, Australia); A.F. Carvalho (Centre for Addiction & Mental Health (CAMH), University of Toronto, Toronto, Canada); K.N. Fountoulakis (Aristotle University of Thessaloniki, Thessaloniki, Greece); P. Grof (Mood Disorders Center of Ottawa, University of Toronto, Canada); L.V. Kessing (Psychiatric Center Copenhagen, Copenhagen, Denmark); U. Lewitzka (Klinik und Poliklinik für Psychiatrie und Psychotherapie, Universitätsklinikum Carl Gustav Carus, Dresden, Germany); R.W. Licht (Aalborg University Hospital, Psychiatry, and Department of Clinical Medicine, Aalborg University, Aalborg, Denmark); B. Müller-Oerlinghausen (Drug Commission of the German Medical Association, Berlin, Germany); R.E. Nielsen (Aalborg University Hospital, Psychiatry, and Department of Clinical Medicine, Aalborg University, Aalborg, Denmark); W.A. Nolen (Department of Psychiatry, University Medical Center Groningen, University of Groningen, Groningen, the Netherlands); I. Pacchiarotti (Bipolar Disorder Program, Hospital Clinic, University of Barcelona, IDIBAPS, CIBERSAM, Barcelona, Spain); J.K. Rybakowski (Poznan University of Medical Sciences, Poznan, Poland); C. Simhandl (Medical Faculty, Bipolar Center, Sigmund Freud Private University, Wiener Neustadt, Austria); T. Suppes (Department of Psychiatry & Behavioral Sciences, Stanford University School of Medicine, Palo Alto, USA); E. Vieta (Bipolar Disorder Program, Hospital Clinic, University of Barcelona, IDIBAPS, CIBERSAM, Barcelona, Spain); A.H. Young (Department of Psychological Medicine, Institute of Psychiatry, Psychology and Neuroscience, King's College London, London, UK); C. Zarate (National Institute of Mental Health (NIMH), Bethesda, Maryland, USA).

**Author details**
[1] INSERM U1144 – Optimisation Thérapeutique en Neuropsychopharmacologie, Université de Paris Descartes, Paris, France. [2] AP-HP, DMU Neurosciences, GH Saint-Louis – Lariboisière – F. Widal, Hôpital Fernand Widal, Département de Psychiatrie et de Médecine Addictologique, Paris, France. [3] Faculté de Médecine, Université de Paris, Paris, France. [4] Centre for Affective Disorders, Institute of Psychiatry, Psychology and Neurosciences, London, UK. [5] Department of Psychiatry and Psychotherapy, University Hospital Carl Gustav Carus, TU Dresden, Dresden, Germany. [6] Academic Psychiatry, Institute of Neuroscience, Newcastle University, Newcastle, UK.

**References**
Cakir S, Tasdelen Durak R, Ozyildirim I, Ince E, Sar V. Childhood trauma and treatment outcome in bipolar disorder. J Trauma Dissociation. 2016;17(4):397–409. https://doi.org/10.1080/15299732.2015.1132489.

Collins PY, Patel V, Joestl SS, March D, Insel TR, Daar AS. Scientific Advisory Board and the Executive Committee of the Grand Challenges on Global Mental Health, et al. Grand challenges in global mental health. Nature. 2011;475(7354):27–30. https://doi.org/10.1038/475027a.

Degenhardt EK, Gatz JL, Jacob J, Tohen M. Predictors of relapse or recurrence in bipolar I disorder. J Affect Disord. 2012;136(3):733–9. https://doi.org/10.1016/j.jad.2011.09.051.

Denicoff KD, Smith-Jackson EE, Disney ER, Ali SO, Leverich GS, Post RM. Comparative prophylactic efficacy of lithium, carbamazepine, and the combination in bipolar disorder. J Clin Psychiatr. 1997;58(11):470–8. https://doi.org/10.4088/jcp.v58n1102.

Etain B, Lajnef M, Brichant-Petitjean C, Geoffroy PA, Henry C, Gard S, Kahn JP, Leboyer M, Young AH, Bellivier F. Childhood trauma and mixed episodes are associated with poor response to lithium in bipolar disorders. Acta Psychiatr Scand. 2017;135(4):319–27. https://doi.org/10.1111/acps.12684.

Garnham J, Munro A, Slaney C, Macdougall M, Passmore M, Duffy A, O'Donovan C, Teehan A, Alda M. Prophylactic treatment response in bipolar disorder: results of a naturalistic observation study. J Affect Disord. 2007;104(1–3):185–90. https://doi.org/10.1016/j.jad.2007.03.003.

Gasperini M, Scherillo P, Manfredonia MG, Franchini L, Smeraldi E. A study of relapses in subjects with mood disorder on lithium treatment ». Eur Neuropsychopharmacol. 1993;3(2):103–10.

Goodwin GM, Haddad PM, Ferrier IN, Aronson JK, Barnes TRH, Cipriani A, Coghill DR, et al. Evidence-based guidelines for treating bipolar disorder: revised third edition Recommendations from the British Association for Psychopharmacology. J Psychopharmacol. 2016;30(6):495–553. https://doi.org/10.1177/0269881116636545.

Gore FM, Bloem PJN, Patton GC, Ferguson J, Joseph V, Coffey C, Sawyer SM, Mathers CD. Global burden of disease in young people aged 10-24 years: a systematic analysis. Lancet. 2011;377(9783):2093–102. https://doi.org/10.1016/S0140-6736(11)60512-6.

Grof P, Duffy A, Cavazzoni P, Grof E, Garnham J, MacDougall M, O'Donovan C, Alda M. Is response to prophylactic lithium a familial trait? J Clin Psychiatr. 2002;63(10):942–7.

Guloksuz S, Altinbas K, Aktas Cetin E, Kenis G, Bilgic Gazioglu S, Deniz G, Timucin Oral E, van Os J. Evidence for an association between Tumor Necrosis Factor-alpha levels and lithium response. J Affect Disord. 2012;143(1–3):148–52. https://doi.org/10.1016/j.jad.2012.04.044.

Hui TP, Kandola A, Shen L, Lewis G, Osborn DPJ, Geddes JR, Hayes JF. A systematic review and meta-analysis of clinical predictors of lithium response in bipolar disorder. Acta Psychiatr Scand. 2019;140(2):94–115. https://doi.org/10.1111/acps.13062.

Kapur V, Nadella RK, Sathur Raghuraman B, Saraf G, Mishra S, Srinivasmurthy N, Jain S, Del Zompo M, Viswanath B. Clinical factors associated with lithium treatment response in bipolar disorder patients from India. Asian J Psychiatr. 2019;39:165–8. https://doi.org/10.1016/j.ajp.2018.04.006.

Kato T, Inubushi T, Kato N. Prediction of lithium response by 31P-MRS in bipolar disorder. The International Journal of Neuropsychopharmacology. 2000;3(1):83–5. https://doi.org/10.1017/S1461145799001674.

Kessing LV, Vradi E, Andersen PK. Nationwide and population-based prescription patterns in bipolar disorder. Bipolar Disord. 2016;18(2):174–82.

Kessing LV. Lithium as the drug of choice for maintenance treatment in bipolar disorder. Acta Psychiatr Scand. 2019;140(2):91–3. https://doi.org/10.1111/acps.13070.

Kessing LV, Bauer M, Nolen WA, Severus E, Goodwin GM, Geddes J. Effectiveness of maintenance therapy of lithium vs other mood stabilizers in monotherapy and in combinations: a systematic review of evidence from observational studies. Bipolar Disord. 2018;20(5):419–31. https://doi.org/10.1111/bdi.12623.

Kessing LV, Hellmund G, Andersen PK. Predictors of excellent response to lithium: results from a nationwide register-based study. Int Clin Psychopharmacol. 2011;26(6):323–8. https://doi.org/10.1097/YIC.0b013e32834a5cd0.

Kessing LV, Vradi E, Andersen PK. Starting lithium prophylaxis early v late in bipolar disorder. Br J Psychiatr. 2014;205(3):214–20. https://doi.org/10.1192/bjp.bp.113.142802.

Kessing LV, Vradi E, Andersen PK. Life expectancy in bipolar disorder. Bipolar Disord. 2015;17(5):543–8. https://doi.org/10.1111/bdi.12296.

Kleindienst N, Engel R, Greil W. Which clinical factors predict response to prophylactic lithium? A systematic review for bipolar disorders. Bipolar Disord. 2005;7(5):404–17. https://doi.org/10.1111/j.1399-5618.2005.00244.x

Kulhara P, Basu D, Mattoo SK, Sharan P, Chopra R. Lithium prophylaxis of recurrent bipolar affective disorder: long-term outcome and its psychosocial correlates. J Affect Disord. 1999;54(1–2):87–96.

Kusalic M, Engelsmann F. Predictors of lithium treatment responsiveness in bipolar patients. A two-year prospective study. Neuropsychobiology. 1998;37(3):146–9. https://doi.org/10.1159/000026497.

Liberati A, Altman DG, Tetzlaff J, Mulrow C, Gøtzsche PC, Ioannidis JPA, Clarke M, Devereaux PJ, Kleijnen J, Moher D. The PRISMA statement for reporting systematic reviews and meta-analyses of studies that evaluate healthcare interventions: explanation and elaboration. BMJ. 2009;339:b2700. https://doi.org/10.1136/bmj.b2700.

Licht RW, Nielsen JN, Gram LF, Vestergaard P, Bendz H. Lamotrigine versus lithium as maintenance treatment in bipolar I disorder: an open, randomized effectiveness study mimicking clinical practice The 6th trial of the Danish University Antidepressant Group (DUAG-6). Bipolar Disord. 2010;12(5):483–93.

Maj M, Pirozzi R, Magliano L, Bartoli L. Long-term outcome of lithium prophylaxis in bipolar disorder: a 5-year prospective study of 402 patients at a lithium clinic. Journal Psychiatr. 1998;155(1):30–5. https://doi.org/10.1176/ajp.155.1.30.

Maj M, Pirozzi R, Starace F. Previous pattern of course of the illness as a predictor of response to lithium prophylaxis in bipolar patients. J Affect Disord. 1989;17(3):237–41.

Malhi GS, Outhred T, Morris G, Boyce PM, Bryant R, Fitzgerald PB, Hopwood MJ, et al. Royal Australian and New Zealand college of psychiatrists clinical practice guidelines for mood disorders: bipolar disorder summary. Medical J Australia. 2018;208(5):219–25.

Martinsson L, Wei Y, Xu D, Melas PA, Mathé AA, Schalling M, Lavebratt C, Backlund L. Long-term lithium treatment in bipolar disorder is associated with longer leukocyte telomeres. Translational Psychiatr. 2013;21(3):e261. https://doi.org/10.1038/tp.2013.37.

Masui T, Hashimoto R, Kusumi I, Suzuki K, Tanaka T, Nakagawa S, Suzuki T, et al. A possible association between missense polymorphism of the breakpoint cluster region gene and lithium prophylaxis in bipolar disorder. Prog Neuropsychopharmacol Biol Psychiatry. 2008;32(1):204–8. https://doi.org/10.1016/j.pnpbp.2007.08.010.

Miura T, Noma H, Furukawa TA, Mitsuyasu H, Tanaka S, Stockton S, Salanti G, et al. Comparative efficacy and tolerability of pharmacological treatments in the maintenance treatment of bipolar disorder: a systematic review and network meta-analysis. Lancet Psychiatr. 2014;1(5):351–9. https://doi.org/10.1016/S2215-0366(14)70314-1.

Moher D, Shamseer L, Clarke M, Ghersi D, Liberati A, Petticrew M, Shekelle P, Stewart LA, PRISMA-P Group. Preferred reporting items for systematic review and meta-analysis protocols (PRISMA-P) 2015 Statement. Syst Rev. 2015;4:1. https://doi.org/10.1186/2046-4053-4-1.

Montlahuc C, Curis E, Grillault Laroche D, Bagoe G, Etain B, Bellivier F, Chevret S. Response to lithium in patients with bipolar disorder: what are psychiatrists' experiences and practices compared to literature review? Pharmacopsychiatry. 2019;52(2):70–7. https://doi.org/10.1055/s-0044-100521.

NIH Quality Assurance Guidelines. Study quality assessment tools, National Heart, Lung, and Blood Institute (NHLBI). 2019. https://www.nhlbi.nih.gov/health-topics/study-quality-assessment-tools.

Nolen WA, Licht RW, Young AH, Malhi GS, Tohen M, Vieta E, Kupka RW, Zarate C, Nielsen RE, Baldessarini RJ, Severus E. ISBD/IGSLI Task Force on the treatment with lithium What is the optimal serum level for lithium in the maintenance treatment of bipolar disorder? A systematic review and recommendations from the ISBD/IGSLI Task Force on treatment with lithium Version 2. Bipolar Disord. 2019;21(5):394–409. https://doi.org/10.1111/bdi.12805.

Nunes A, Ardau R, Berghöfer A, Bocchetta A, Chillotti C, Deiana V, et al. Prediction of lithium response using clinical data. Acta Psychiatr Scand. 2020;141(2):131–41.

O'Connell RA, Mayo JA, Flatow L, Cuthbertson B, O'Brien BE. Outcome of bipolar disorder on long-term treatment with lithium. Br J Psychiatr. 1991;159:123–9. https://doi.org/10.1192/bjp.159.1.123.

Okuma T. Effects of carbamazepine and lithium on affective disorders. Neuropsychobiology. 1993;27(3):138–45. https://doi.org/10.1159/000118969.

Ozyildirim I, Cakir S, Yazici O. Impact of psychotic features on morbidity and course of illness in patients with bipolar disorder. European Psychiatry. 2010;25(1):47–51. https://doi.org/10.1016/j.eurpsy.2009.08.004.

Passos IC, Ballester PL, Barros RC, Librenza-Garcia D, Mwangi B, Birmaher B, et al. Machine learning and big data analytics in bipolar disorder: a position paper from the International Society for Bipolar Disorders Big Data Task Force. Bipolar Disord. 2019;21(7):582–94.

Perlis RH, Ostacher MJ, Patel JK, Marangell LB, Zhang H, Wisniewski SR, et al. Predictors of recurrence in bipolar disorder: primary outcomes from the Systematic Treatment Enhancement Program for Bipolar Disorder (STEP-BD). Am J Psychiatry. 2006;163(2):217–24.

Post RM, Leverich GS, Kupka R, Keck PE, McElroy SL, Altshuler LL, Frye MA, et al. Clinical correlates of sustained response to individual drugs used in naturalistic treatment of patients with bipolar disorder. Compr Psychiatry. 2016;66:146–56. https://doi.org/10.1016/j.comppsych.2016.01.009.

Rybakowski JK. Factors Associated with Lithium Efficacy in Bipolar Disorder ». Harvard Rev Psychiatr. 2014;22(6):353–7. https://doi.org/10.1097/HRP.0000000000000006.

Rybakowski JK, Dembinska D, Kliwicki S, Akiskal KK, Akiskal HH. TEMPS-A and long-term lithium response: positive correlation with hyperthymic temperament. J Affect Disord. 2013;145(2):187–9. https://doi.org/10.1016/j.jad.2012.07.028.

Rybakowski JK, Permoda-Osip A, Borkowska A. Response to prophylactic lithium in bipolar disorder may be associated with a preservation of executive cognitive functions. Eur Neuropsychopharmacol. 2009;19(11):791–5. https://doi.org/10.1016/j.euroneuro.2009.06.002.

Rybakowski JK, Suwalska A, Skibinska M, DmitrzakWeglarz M, Leszczynska-Rodziewicz A, Hauser J. Response to lithium prophylaxis: interaction between serotonin transporter and BDNF Genes American Journal of Medical Genetics Part B. Neuropsychiatric Genetics. 2007;144B(6):820–3. https://doi.org/10.1002/ajmg.b.30420.

Saito S, Fujii K, Ozeki Y, Ohmori K, Honda G, Mori H, Kato K, et al. Cognitive function, treatment response to lithium, and social functioning in Japanese patients with bipolar disorder. Bipolar Disord. 2017;19(7):552–62. https://doi.org/10.1111/bdi.12521.

Schou M. Trends in lithium treatment and research during the last decade. Pharmacopsychiatria. 1982;15(4):128–30.

Scott J, Etain B, Bellivier F. Can an integrated science approach to precision medicine research improve lithium treatment in bipolar disorders? Frontiers Psychiatr. 2018;9:360. https://doi.org/10.3389/fpsyt.2018.00360.

Scott J, Geoffroy PA, Sportiche S, Brichant-PetitJean C, Gard S, Kahn JP, Azorin JM, Henry C, Etain B, Bellivier F. Cross-validation of clinical characteristics and treatment patterns associated with phenotypes for lithium response defined by the Alda scale. J Affect Disord. 2017;208:62–7. https://doi.org/10.1016/j.jad.2016.08.069.

Scott J, Hidalgo-Mazzei D, Strawbridge R, Young AH, Resche-Rigon M, Etain B, Andreassen OA, et al. Prospective cohort study of early biosignatures of response to lithium in bipolar I disorders: overview of the H2020-funded R-LiNK initiative. Int J Bipolar Disord. 2019;7(1):20. https://doi.org/10.1186/s40345-019-0156-x.

Severus E, Taylor MJ, Sauer C, Pfennig A, Ritter P, Bauer M, Geddes JR. Lithium for prevention of mood episodes in bipolar disorders: systematic review and meta-analysis. Int J Bipolar Disord. 2014;2:15. https://doi.org/10.1186/s40345-014-0015-8.

Shan GW, Makmor-Bakry M, Omar MS. Long term use of lithium and factors associated with treatment response among patients with bipolar disorder. Psychiatria Danubina. 2016;28(2):146–53.

Silva, LF, Cunha Loureiro J, Raposo Franco SC, de Lima Santos M, Secolin R, Lopes-Cendes I, de Rosalmeida Dantas C, et al. 2016. Assessing treatment response to prophylactic lithium use in patients with bipolar disorder. Jornal Brasileiro de Psiquiatria.2016;65 (1):9-16. https://doi.org/10.1590/0047-2085000000097.

Sportiche S, Geoffroy PA, Brichant-Petitjean C, Gard S, Khan JP, Azorin JM, Henry C, et al. Clinical factors associated with lithium response in bipolar disorders. Australian New Zealand J Psychiatr. 2017;51(5):524–30. https://doi.org/10.1177/0004867416664794.

Stefos G, Bauwens F, Staner L, Pardoen D, Mendlewicz J. Psychosocial predictors of major affective recurrences in bipolar disorder: a 4-year longitudinal study of patients on prophylactic treatment. Acta Psychiatr Scand. 1996;93(6):420–6. https://doi.org/10.1111/j.1600-0447.1996.tb10672.x.

Tharoor H, Kotambail A, Jain S, Sharma PSVN, Satyamoorthy K. Study of the association of serotonin transporter triallelic 5-HTTLPR and STin2 VNTR polymorphisms with lithium prophylaxis response in bipolar disorder. Psychiatr Genet. 2013;23(2):77–81. https://doi.org/10.1097/YPG.0b013e32835d6fad.

Thompson SG, Pocock SJ. Can meta-analyses be trusted? Lancet. 1991;338(8775):1127–30. https://doi.org/10.1016/0140-6736(91)91975-z.

Tighe SK, Mahon B, Potash JB. Predictors of lithium response in bipolar disorder. Therapeutic AdvChronic Dis. 2011;2(3):209–26. https://doi.org/10.1177/2040622311399173.

Tondo L, Baldessarini RJ, Floris G. Long-term clinical effectiveness of lithium maintenance treatment in types I and II bipolar disorders ». Br J Psychiatr. 2001;178(Suppl 41):S184–90.

Tondo L, Alda M, Bauer M, Bergink V, Grof P, Hajek T, Lewitka U, et al. Clinical use of lithium salts: guide for users and prescribers. Int J Bipolar Disord. 2019;7(1):16. https://doi.org/10.1186/s40345-019-0151-2.

Washizuka S, Ikeda A, Kato N, Kato T. Possible relationship between mitochondrial DNA polymorphisms and lithium response in bipolar disorder. Int J Neuropsychopharmacol. 2003;6(4):421–4. https://doi.org/10.1017/S1461145703003778.

Yatham LN, Kennedy SH, Parikh SV, Schaffer A, Bond DJ, Frey BN, Sharma V, et al. Canadian Network for Mood and Anxiety Treatments (CANMAT) and International Society for Bipolar Disorders (ISBD) 2018 Guidelines for the Management of Patients with Bipolar Disorder. Bipolar Disord. 2018;20(2):97–170. https://doi.org/10.1111/bdi.12609.

Yazici O, Kora K, Uçok A, Tunali D, Turan N. Predictors of lithium prophylaxis in bipolar patients. J Affect Disord. 1999;55(2–3):133–42.

# 10

# Affective lability as a prospective predictor of subsequent bipolar disorder diagnosis

Rosie H. Taylor[1], Andrea Ulrichsen[1], Allan H. Young[1,2] and Rebecca Strawbridge[1*]

**Abstract**

**Objectives:** The early pathogenesis and precursors of Bipolar Disorder (BD) are poorly understood. There is some cross-sectional and retrospective evidence of affective lability as a predictor of BD, but this is subject to recall biases. The present review synthesises the prospective evidence examining affective lability and the subsequent development of BD at follow-up.

**Methods:** The authors performed a systematic search of PubMed, PsycInfo and Embase (1960–June 2020) and conducted hand searches to identify studies assessing affective lability (according to a conceptually-inclusive definition) at baseline assessment in individuals without a BD diagnosis, and a longitudinal follow-up assessment of bipolar (spectrum) disorders. Results are reported according to the PRISMA guidelines, and the synthesis without meta-analysis (SWiM) reporting guidelines were used to strengthen the narrative synthesis. The Newcastle–Ottawa Scale was used to assess risk of bias (ROB).

**Results:** 11 articles describing 10 studies were included. Being identified as having affective lability at baseline was associated with an increased rate of bipolar diagnoses at follow-up; this association was statistically significant in six of eight studies assessing BD type I/II at follow-up and in all four studies assessing for bipolar spectrum disorder (BSD) criteria. Most studies received a 'fair' or 'poor' ROB grade.

**Conclusions:** Despite a paucity of studies, an overall association between prospectively-identified affective lability and a later diagnosis of BD or BSD is apparent with relative consistency between studies. This association and further longitudinal studies could inform future clinical screening of those who may be at risk of BD, with the potential to improve diagnostic accuracy and facilitate early intervention.

**Keywords:** Bipolar disorder, Systematic review, Affective lability, Mood instability, Prospective, Predictor, Risk-factor, Bipolar spectrum

## Background

The chronic nature and disabling impacts of bipolar disorders (BD) are well recorded and addressed in translational research, (American Psychiatric Association 2013; Merikangas et al. 2007) but diagnosis remains delayed (for many individuals, by a decade after symptom onset) and these delays precede poorer outcomes and additional illness burdens (Lloyd et al. 2011). The distinct gaps in understanding how to predict and/or prevent BD (Woo et al. 2015) mean that there is little to offer people prior to receipt of a diagnosis. These challenges could be attenuated with the use of predictive clinical features describing bipolar signatures (Woo et al. 2015).

Newly emerging prodromal features of BD include dysregulated sleep, mood, and energy, including irritability

*Correspondence: Becci.strawbridge@kcl.ac.uk
[1] Department of Psychological Medicine, Institute of Psychiatry, Psychology and Neuroscience, King's College London, London SE5 8AF, UK
Full list of author information is available at the end of the article

(Correll et al. 2007; Skjelstad et al. 2010) (Trait) dysregulation of affect as a whole is also putatively associated with subsequent diagnosis of BD (Correll et al. 2007; Lish et al. 1994). Diverse terminology is used to describe various measures broadly assessing dysregulated affect, with examples including 'mood lability', 'cyclothymic temperament', 'affective instability' and 'mood swings' (Correll et al. 2007; Faedda et al. 1995; Miklowitz and Chang 2008; Rucklidge 2008). In this review, we use the term 'affective lability' to inclusively refer to these variable measures of extreme and alternating moods. The term affective lability is purposefully broad and is used by the present paper to encompass fluctuations of mood and emotional state, in addition to arousal/activation. A commonality between these aforementioned measures of fluctuating affect is its consideration as a *trait* construct. The nature of BD as an illness where individuals, by definition, experience switches in affect renders it plausible that (trait) fluctuating affect could be a durable preceding characteristic of people who subsequently develop BD. Affective lability will be conceptualised broadly in the present review as a 'predictor' or 'precursor' of BD without determination of a strict developmental timeline.

The relationship between affective lability and BDs which fall just outside of DSM type I/II, conceptualised as not otherwise specified (NOS), also referred to as bipolar spectrum disorders (BSD), is also worthy of review. As well as being increasingly recognised in diagnostic manuals, clinical assessment tools are also validated accordingly for BSDs (e.g. SADS) (Akiskal 1996; Angst 2013). There is further evidence of BSDs being common illnesses to BD-I and BD-II (Angst 2013) and of BSDs being used to predict diagnostic conversion to BD (Woo et al. 2015). Therefore, the present review will not limit definitions of bipolarity or BSDs.

There is also some evidence that affective lability may influence and predict the clinical course, features, and outcomes of BD or BSD after diagnosis. For example, cyclothymic temperament in BD patients has a significant impact on longitudinal functional outcomes such as impairments to home-management, social life, and leisure activities (Nilsson et al. 2012). The present review intends to consider and clarify these emerging associations.

The present review is novel in its synthesis of the existing literature incorporating an inclusive definition of affective lability and consequent inclusivity of assessment tools. Previous research and reviews assessing the relationship between affective lability and BDs have used retrospective and cross-sectional study designs (Correll et al. 2007; Egeland et al. 2000; Özgürdal et al. 2009; Leopold et al. 2012). Because these are susceptible to recall bias, the present review will only review prospective studies which used longitudinal study designs (Howes et al. 2011).

### Objectives

The primary aim of this systematic review is to establish whether people without BD, prospectively identified as having affective lability, are more likely to meet criteria for BSD/BD at a follow-up timepoint than those without affective lability at baseline. To our knowledge, this has not yet been subject to systematic review. As a secondary objective, the present review will also include and synthesise any further measures of diagnostic subtypes in BD patients whose affective lability was prospectively identified.

## Materials and methods

### Protocol and registration

The present review adheres to the preferred reporting items for systematic reviews and meta-analyses (PRISMA) statement (Moher et al. 2009). A protocol was pre-registered to the international prospective register of systematic reviews (PROSPERO 2020, registration CRD42020183945).

Initially the review registration specified that BD diagnoses should follow DSM or ICD-10 conceptualisation. Shortly after the protocol publication, and before the search had been run, it was decided that the broader BSDs have sufficient evidence of potential use in future clinical practice to be considered and reported. Results for DSM BD and BSD have been differentiated in this review. No other changes were made to the methodology after protocol registration.

### Eligibility criteria

Studies were eligible for inclusion if (i) the study design was longitudinal; (ii) human participants of any age were assessed; (iii) affective lability was measured prospectively (i.e. baseline measurement in participants not currently meeting criteria for bipolar (spectrum) disorder); (iv) a measure of affective lability, as deemed to be assessing fluctuations in mood or affect, was assessed at baseline; (vi) BD or BSD was assessed at a follow-up timepoint. Reasons for exclusion included participants having a diagnosis of borderline personality disorder (BPD) or BD at intake.

### Search strategy

Key search terms were entered into the following electronic databases: PubMed, PsycInfo and EMBASE (all dates from inception to June 2020). The search comprised the following terms: (bipolar* or psychiatric or affective disorder* or mood disorder* or psychopathology) and (mood instability or mood shift* or moodiness or cyclothymic temperament or mood lability or mood swing* or TEMPS or temperament*) and (prospective or longitud* or follow up). All generated studies were limited to those with a title and abstract available in the English language.

Two reviewers (RHT and AU) independently screened the titles and abstracts of all retrieved articles using Rayyan open-source review management software (Ouzzani et al. 2016). Reviewers were not blinded to the objectives of the review. Each article was formally screened against eligibility criteria by these two reviewers. The reviewers discussed all conflicts in study selections and a consensus was reached with the support of a third reviewer (RS). Reviewers had access to the same articles but were blinded to one another's selections during the screening process. This process was repeated for the full-text screening of all articles selected as being potentially eligible. Reference lists of eligible papers were manually handsearched to identify further articles for screening.

### Data extraction

Reviewer RHT extracted relevant study details such as citation details, recruitment methods, sample size, follow-up duration, proportional rates of BD diagnoses, and affective lability assessment tools. Information regarding participants' characteristics, measures, and study design were also extracted for both baseline and follow-up. Any available measure of association used to assess the relationship between affective lability and BD conversion was examined. The accuracy of data extraction was checked by a second reviewer (AU). Any disagreements were discussed in conjunction with a third reviewer (RS).

### Risk of bias assessments

The quality of all selected articles was assessed independently by RHT and AU using the Newcastle Ottawa scale (NOS) grading system for longitudinal studies in systematic reviews using a 'star grade system' before consensus was reached by examination of a third reviewer (RS) (Wells et al. 2012). Two reviewers (RHT, RS) were involved in establishing the assessment criterion specifications from the NOS scale, specific to this review topic, a priori. Any individual article could be awarded between zero and nine stars. As recommended in quality improvement reviews, seven stars or more is deemed a 'good' study, five or six stars is deemed 'fair', and less than five stars is deemed 'poor' (for more detail regarding criteria for ROB ratings, see Additional file 1) (McPheeters et al. 2012). ROB assessments were used to guide the narrative synthesis in the present review, with more emphasis given to studies with higher star-graded quality ratings.

### Analysis

Due to the heterogeneity of populations studied, measures and study designs employed, a quantitative meta-analysis was not considered appropriate. Findings and methodology across the selected articles are presented and analysed using tables and a narrative synthesis. To strengthen the narrative synthesis of results, the present review has used the synthesis without meta-analysis (SWiM) reporting guidelines for systematic reviews (Campbell et al. 2020).

## Results

### Study selection

As demonstrated in the PRISMA flowchart (Fig. 1), the systematic search generated 2280 records. Deduplication removed 936 and 8 further articles were identified through handsearches. 1267 studies were excluded on the basis of their abstract and titles not fulfilling eligibility criteria e.g. due to clearly not having a prospective study design, assessment of bipolarity or affective lability. The resulting 85 full texts were reviewed, with 74 being excluded, most commonly for not having an assessment of affective lability. During the screening process, authors of all conference abstracts were contacted to glean potentially relevant grey literature. No eligible studies were identified through this process. 11 articles were deemed eligible for inclusion and synthesis. The reference lists of these selected manuscripts were hand checked to identify any remaining studies by reviewer RHT; none were identified. One study was reported in two articles (DeGeorge et al. 2014; Sperry et al. 2020). These employed distinct measures, both of which fell under the present review's inclusive conceptualisation of affective lability.

### Study characteristics

The baseline study characteristics for all included studies are presented in Table 1. All studies employed an assessment for BD at intake.

From the 10 included studies, a range of cohorts were assessed. 5 studies recruited non-clinical cohorts (DeGeorge et al. 2014; Sperry et al. 2020; Hafeman et al. 2017; Angst et al. 2003; Egeland et al. 2012). However, each of these non-clinical cohorts had been screened for a factor that put them at risk, such as having a family history of BD. The other 5 studies assessed clinical cohorts, 4 with participants who had MDD (with or without psychotic features) and 1 recruiting a mix of individuals with MDD, anxiety or substance use disorders (Ratheesh et al. 2015). Recruitment methods varied and included using inpatients (Tohen et al. 2012; Salvatore et al. 2013; Kochman et al. 2005), outpatients, hospital records and advertising (Hafeman et al. 2017; Angst et al. 2003; Ratheesh

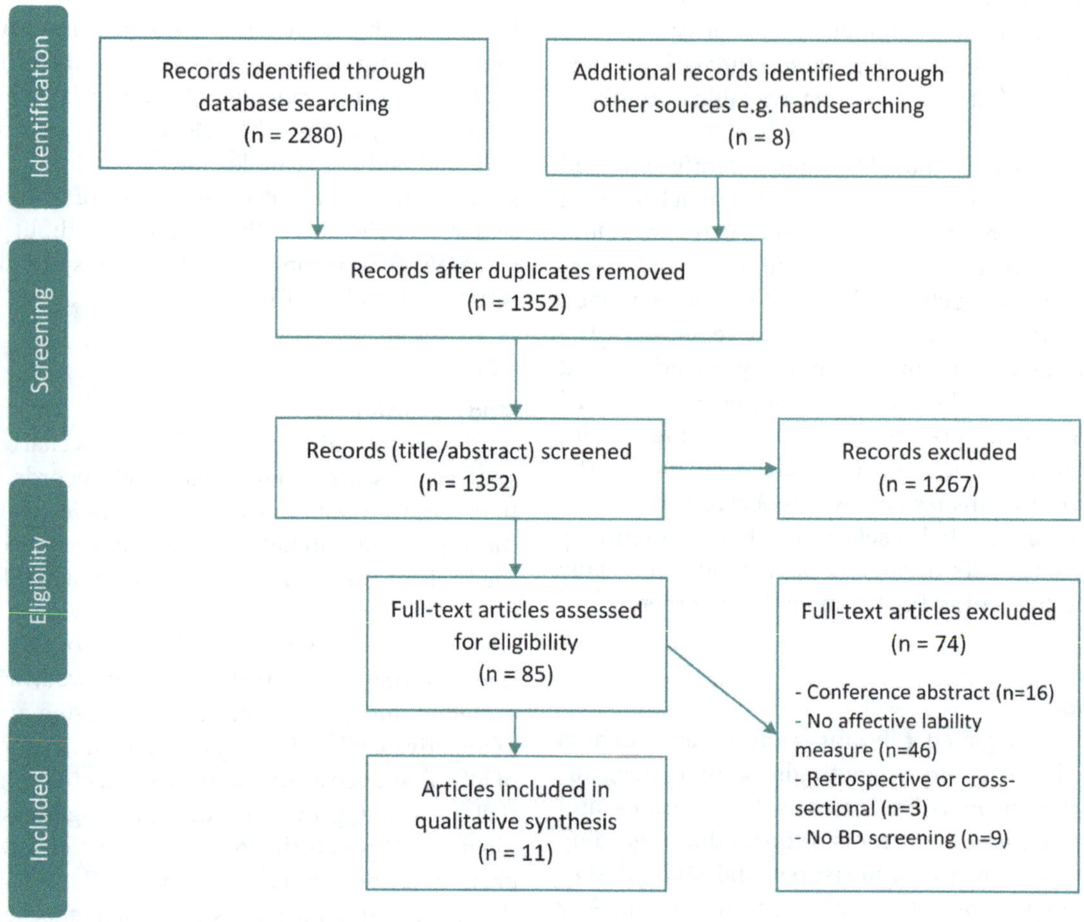


**Fig. 1** PRISMA flow diagram of the study selection process. Study flow diagram showing the Preferred Reporting Items for Systematic Reviews and Meta-Analyses. BD = bipolar disorder

et al. 2015; Gan et al. 2011), sub-populations from larger studies (Egeland et al. 2012; Akiskal et al. 1995) and psychology students (DeGeorge et al. 2014; Sperry et al. 2020).

A wide range of tools were employed to assess affective lability. Three studies (DeGeorge et al. 2014; Ratheesh et al. 2015; Kochman et al. 2005) used validated versions of the Temperament Evaluation of Memphis, Pisa, Paris and San Diego Auto-questionnaire (TEMPS-A) (Akiskal and Akiskal 2005; Vázquez and Akiskal 2005). Terminology used to describe unstable and alternating moods varied. The term 'mood lability' was used by three studies, employing different assessment tools (see Table 1). Other terminology used included 'diurnal variation in mood' (n = 1), 'cyclothymic temperament' (n = 1), 'emotional and vegetative lability' (n = 1) 'affective lability' (n = 1), 'affective or psychomotor instability' (n = 1), 'cyclothymic/irritable temperament' (n = 1), 'cyclothymic-hypersensitive temperament' (n = 1), and 'emotional instability' (n = 1).

Study characteristics at follow-up are reported in Table 2. Most studies followed up a participant pool of more than 100 participants (n = 7). Follow-up durations ranged from 1 year (Ratheesh et al. 2015; Gan et al. 2011) to 16 years (Egeland et al. 2012). Diagnoses of BD or BSD were provided by clinicians (n = 6) or trained interviewers (n = 4) and the number of conversions to BSD/BD ranged from four (Sperry et al. 2020; Ratheesh et al. 2015) to 86 (Angst et al. 2003) individuals. The proportion of the sample who converted ranged from 4% (Sperry et al. 2020; Egeland et al. 2012) to 43% (Kochman et al. 2005). Diagnostic tools also varied, as presented in Table 2.

### Primary outcome

As presented in Table 2, six studies reported a statistically significant association between prospectively-identified affective lability and a later diagnosis of BD as defined by the DSM (Hafeman et al. 2017; Angst et al. 2003; Tohen et al. 2012; Salvatore et al. 2013; Gan et al. 2011; Akiskal et al. 1995). One small study of 70 participants with a mixture of diagnoses at baseline (depression, anxiety,

**Table 1** Study and participant characteristics at baseline

| Article | Location | Clinical Status | Age | N | Sex | Recruitment Method | Affective Lability measure | Affective Lability assessment tool | Ascertainment of affective lability |
|---|---|---|---|---|---|---|---|---|---|
| Akiskal et al. 1995 | US | MDD | 17+ | NR | NR | Sub-population from larger depression study | Mood Lability | GZTS (emotional stability) + MMPI (neuroticism) combined | Self-report |
| Angst et al. 2003 | Switzer-land | Non-clinical | Range = 19–20 Mean = 20 | 591 | F = 51% | Community cohort study | Emotional & vegetative lability | SCI-90-R | Self-report |
| DeGeorge et al. 2014* | US | At-risk, clinical, non-clinical | Mean = 20 SD = 2 | 123 | F = 69% | Introductory Psychology course | Cyclothymic/irritable temperament | TEMPS-A | Self-report |
| Sperry et al. 2020* | | | | 101 | | | Emotion dynamics (positive & negative affect) | ESM for PA and NA | |
| Egeland et al. 2012 | US | At-risk offspring & non-clinical | Most < 14 | 221 | F = 51% | Sub-population from larger study (CARE) | Mood Lability | Interview developed by expert panel | Clinician |
| Gan et al. 2011 | China | MDD | NR | 344 | F = 62% | Hospital archive records, outpatient clinical records | Diurnal variation in mood | Clinical assessments | Self-report |
| Hafeman et al., 2017 | US | Non-clinical BD offspring | Range = 6–18 Mean = 12 SD = 4 | 480 | NR | Advertisement, research studies, outpatient clinics | Affective Lability | CALS | Self-report |
| Kochman et al. 2005 | France | MDD | Mean = 13 SD = 3 | 109 | NR | Child inpatient admissions | Cyclothymic-hypersensitive temperament | Adapted TEMPS-A cyclothymic scale | Self-report |
| Ratheesh et al. 2015 | Australia | MDD, anxiety, SUD, ADD | Range = 15–25 Mean = 20 SD = 3 | 70 | F = 85% | At-risk youth seeking mental health support | Cyclothymic temperament | TEMPS-A | Self-report |
| Salvatore et al. 2013 | Italy, US | MDDP | Range = 10–82 Mean = 35 SD = 16 | 500 | F = 45% | Psychiatric inpatients | Affective or psychomotor instability | AMDP and BSABS | Trained evaluator assessments |
| Tohen et al. 2012 | US | MDDP | Range = 18–72 Mean = 36 SD = 15 | 56 | F = 50% | Inpatient unit | Mood lability | AMDP + BABS | Research assistant |

*US* United states, *MDD* major depressive disorder, *NR* not reported, *GZTS* Guilford-Zimmerman Temperament Survey, *MMPI-N* The Minnesota Multiphasic Personality Inventory, for Neuroticism, *F* female, *M* male, *SCI-90-R* Symptom Checklist-90-R, *SD* standard deviation, *TEMPS-A* Temperament Evaluation of Memphis, Pisa, Paris and San Diego Auto-questionnaire, *ESM* experience sampling method, *PA* positive affect, *NA* negative affect, *CARE* prospective Children and Adolescent Research Evaluation study, *SCID* Structured clinical interview for the Diagnostic and Statistical Manual of Mental Disorders, *BD* bipolar disorder, *CALS* Children's Affective Lability Scale, *SUD* substance use disorder, *ADD* attention deficit disorder, *MDDP* MDD with psychosis, *AMDP* Manual for the Assessment and Documentation of Psychopathology, *BSABS/BABS* Bonn Scale for the Assessment of Basic Symptoms

* Sperry et al. 2020 and DeGeorge et al. 2014 are two papers from the same study. Although analyses were conducted for participants without BD at baseline, participant sex and age averages were not provided for the subgroup considered in this review (we report averages from the total sample, which are expected to be comparable)

**Table 2** Study characteristics and findings at follow-up

| Article | FU n | % lost at FU | FU duration (years) | Diagnostic Tool | Diagnostic assessor | Diagnosed with BD n (%) | Rates of BD type | Affective lability/ BD association |
|---|---|---|---|---|---|---|---|---|
| Akiskal et al. 1995 | 559 | NR | 11 | SADS (DSM / RDC) | Clinician | 70 (13) | 22 BD-I, 48 BD-II | BD-II $X^2=19.92$+ + + (specificity = 86%, sensitivity = 42%) |
| Angst et al. 2003 | 591 | NR | 15 | DSM-IV criteria | Clinician | 86 (15) | 41 BD-II, 45 BSD | BD-II+ + BSD OR = 3.4, 95% CI [1.7, 6.6]+ + |
| DeGeorge et al. 2014* | 112 | 23% | 3.1 (SD = 0.5, range 1.7—4.8) | SCID | Advanced grad (81%), psychologist + undergrad (19%) | 13 (14) | BSD and BD BSD | BSD OR = 2.99+ BD OR = .532, CI [.08–3.45] |
| Sperry et al. 2020* | 108 | 22% | | | | 4 (4) | | PA: OR = 1.91, 95% CI [1.14, 3.18]+ NA: OR = 1.54, 95% CI [1.00, 2.38]+ |
| Egeland et al. 2012 | 221 | NR | 16 | Adapted K-SADS, clinical records | Clinician | 9 (4) | All BD-I | Mood lability more present in BD at risk sample than controls (p = 0.063) |
| Gan et al. 2011 | 268 | 22% | 1 | SCID-I | Psychiatrist | 27 (24) | 2 BD-I, 25 BD-II | OR = 0.487+ |
| Hafeman et al. 2017 | 412 | 14% | Mean = 8.34 | K-SADS (DSM-IV) | Trained interviewers + psychiatrist review | 44/299 at-risk (15) | 15 BD-I/II, 29 BSD | $X^2=4.00$+ |
| Kochman et al. 2005 | 80 | 27% | 2–4 (27 months, SD = 9 months) | K-SADS | Investigator | 35 (43) | All BSD | Prior instability in 64% of BSD; BSD vs non-BSD difference+ + + |
| Ratheesh et al. 2015 | 52 | 26% | 1 | LIFE | Unspecified | 4 (8) | 3 BD-II, 1 BD-NOS | SES = 0.27 (p = 0.13), 95% CI [0.00,0.59] |
| Salvatore et al. 2013 | 107 | 79% | Mean = 4 | SCID | Blinded investigator | 20 (19) | 10 BD-I, 10 BD-NOS | RR = 1.45+ |
| Tohen et al. 2012 | 49 | 13% | 4 | SCID | Blinded experienced raters | 14 (33) | BD-I or BD-NOS | $X^2=4.85$+ |

*FU* follow-up, *n* number of, *BD* bipolar disorder, *BPSD* bipolar spectrum disorder, *DSM* Diagnostic and Statistical Manual of Mental Disorders, *NR* not reported, *SADS* The Schedule for Affective Disorders and Schizophrenia, *RDC* the Research Diagnostic Criteria, *BPI* Bipolar Disorder Type 1, *BPII* bipolar disorder type 2, *DSM-IV* the fifth edition of the Diagnostic and Statistical Manual of Mental Disorders, *BSD* bipolar spectrum disorders, *OR* Odds ratio, *CI* Confidence intervals, *SD* standard deviation, *SCID* Structured Clinical Interviews for DSM, *PA* positive affect, *NA* negative affect, *K-SADS* Kiddie Schedule for Affective Disorders and Schizophrenia, *SCID-I* Structured Clinical Interview for the fifth edition of the Diagnostic and Statistical Manual of Mental Disorders for Axis I Disorders, *LIFE* The Longitudinal Interval Follow-up Evaluation for DSM IV, *BD-NOS* Bipolar disorder not otherwise specified, *SES* standardised effect size. *RR* Risk Ratio

* Sperry et al. 2020 and DeGeorge et al. 2014 are two papers from the same study. In both papers '% lost at FU' and 'FU duration' are reported for the participant pool including some participants with initial BD diagnoses (we report averages from the total sample, which are expected to be comparable)

+p < 0.05, + +p < 0.01, + + +p < 0.001

substance use disorder and attention deficit disorder) did not find a statistically significant association with BD (p = 0.13) although only 4 conversions to BD were recorded (Ratheesh et al. 2015). The other (Egeland et al. 2012) reported that mood lability tended to be more frequent in those at-risk for BD than controls who were not at risk but also had a low conversion rate to BD (n = 9) and as such did not undertake statistical analyses for this comparison.

Four articles reported findings for the analyses of BSD, with all identifying statistically significant relationships with this diagnosis (DeGeorge et al. 2014; Sperry et al. 2020; Angst et al. 2003; Kochman et al. 2005). Two articles reporting results for prospectively identified BSD were drawn from the same study, with each paper independently reporting distinct findings with different measures of affective lability (DeGeorge et al. 2014; Sperry et al. 2020).

Therefore, across all studies, nine of 11 articles reported a statistically significant relationship with BD/BSD.

### Secondary outcomes

As a secondary objective, we planned to explore any further BD-related clinical associations with prospectively identified affective lability. In our review protocol, the examples considered were symptom severity, episode frequency or BD diagnostic subtype pending data availability. The former two examples were not synthesisable given limited reporting and heterogeneity of included studies, however we were able to examine the type of BD diagnosis. Only one study reported on the independent statistical analyses of BD-I and BD-II, finding a significant association for the latter but not the former (Akiskal et al. 1995).

No studies only assessed BD-I. Statistically significant associations were identified where: all developed BD-I or Bipolar Disorder Not Otherwise Specified (BD-NOS), (Tohen et al. 2012) there was an even split between BD-I and BD-NOS, (Salvatore et al. 2013) a preponderance of BD participants met criteria for BD-II, (Gan et al. 2011) a preponderance met criteria for BD-NOS, (Hafeman et al. 2017) and where only BSD was considered (Sperry et al. 2020; Kochman et al. 2005). The only non-significant associations were in studies with very low conversion rates to any BD type (Egeland et al. 2012; Ratheesh et al. 2015).

### Risk of bias

Quality assessments were carried out for all 11 eligible articles and presented in Table 3. Most studies' ROB was deemed 'fair' (n = 6). The highest star grading which classified as 'good' (7 stars) was given to only one study (Hafeman et al. 2017). A star grade of six ('fair'), was also given to only one study (Akiskal et al. 1995). Both studies found a significant relationship between prospectively identified affective lability and later diagnoses of BD. Five studies received a star grading of five ('fair'), of which four reported significant associations (Angst et al. 2003; Tohen et al. 2012; Salvatore et al. 2013; Gan et al. 2011) and the other reported having too low a conversion rate to undertake statistical analyses (Egeland et al. 2012). Four studies received a star grading of three and were and were therefore deemed 'poor', of which three identified significant associations (DeGeorge et al. 2014; Sperry et al. 2020; Kochman et al. 2005) and one did not but had a very low bipolar conversion rate (Ratheesh et al. 2015). No studies recruited cohorts which can be deemed representative of the average person without BD in the community. However, all studies screened for psychopathology at baseline (n = 11).

## Discussion

This systematic review set out to determine whether prospectively identified affective lability in cohorts without BD was associated with subsequent diagnoses of bipolar (spectrum) disorders. All selected and synthesised studies are prospective, making them less susceptible to recall bias. Studies are further strengthened by their use of validated diagnostic BD assessments at both baseline and follow-up.

The present systematic review revealed a reasonably consistent, positive association between prospectively identified affective lability and follow-up BD diagnoses, with 9 out of 11 studies finding a significant association with BD/BSD. For DSM-defined BD, significant associations were identified in 6/8 studies, with the remaining two having extremely small BD sample sizes, which precluded statistical analyses (Egeland et al. 2012) or led to a non-significant association (Ratheesh et al. 2015). The strength of this result is limited by the fact that most ROB assessments were 'fair'. If anything, the relationship between prospectively identified affective lability and follow-up diagnoses of broader BSD diagnoses appears stronger, being identified in all four studies examining this (DeGeorge et al. 2014; Sperry et al. 2020; Angst et al. 2003; Kochman et al. 2005). However, 1/4 studies received a 'fair' ROB rating, and all others received 'poor', weakening the strength of this result.

Whether affective lability differentially predicts one type of bipolar illness from another is unclear. Proportional rates of various BD diagnoses were identified and have been reported in Table 2. Only one study reported on the independent statistical analyses of BD-I and BD-II, finding a significant association for the latter but not the former (Akiskal et al. 1995). This corresponds to cross-sectional findings which associate temperamental instability with BD-II disorder more so than BD-I (Akiskal et al. 2003). Despite this, there is not enough relevant data in the present review to draw firm conclusions. Furthermore, although this study received one of the highest ROB assessments in the present review, this grading was only classed as 'fair'. This finding may also not be specific to bipolar disorders, and affective lability may commonly be a risk factor for developing other mood or personality diagnoses, something that was not in scope of the current review but clearly deserving of future evidence synthesis.

The secondary objective of this review also sought to explore any further clinical implications of prospectively identified affective lability (such as, for example, the experience of rapid cycling, mixed affective episodes, preponderance of mania or depression, or comorbid anxiety). These are all putative correlates of affective lability

**Table 3** Risk of bias assessment of included studies

| ROB scale and accepted criteria | Akiskal et al. 1995 | Angst et al. 2003 | Egeland et al. 2012 | Gan et al. 2011 | Hafeman et al. 2017 | Ratheesh et al. 2015 | Salvatore et al. 2013 | Tohen et al. 2012 | DeGeorge et al. 2014 | Kochman et al. 2005 | Sperry et al. 2020 |
|---|---|---|---|---|---|---|---|---|---|---|---|
| Selection | | | | | | | | | | | |
| Exposed cohort is representative of the average person without BD | – | – | – | – | – | – | – | – | – | – | – |
| Non-exposed cohort is drawn from the same community as the exposed cohort | * | * | * | * | * | * | * | * | * | * | * |
| Exposure ascertained through secure record or structured interview | – | – | * | * | – | – | * | * | – | – | – |
| Demonstration that outcome of interest was not present at start of study | * | * | * | * | * | * | * | * | * | * | * |
| Comparability | | | | | | | | | | | |
| Study controls for family history of BD or additional factor | ** | * | – | – | ** | – | * | – | – | – | – |
| Outcome | | | | | | | | | | | |
| Assessment of outcome uses structured clinical assessment or record linkage | * | * | * | * | * | * | * | * | * | * | * |
| Follow-up long enough for outcome to occur (5 + years)? | * | * | * | – | * | – | – | – | – | – | – |
| Adequacy of follow up of cohorts (> 80% follow up or description provided of those lost) | – | – | – | * | * | – | – | * | – | – | – |
| Total (max = 9) | 6 | 5 | 5 | 5 | 7 | 3 | 5 | 5 | 3 | 3 | 3 |

Risk of bias (ROB) assessment for all included studies, using the Newcastle–Ottawa Scale for cohort studies. The criteria employed for ROB ratings are described in text and Additional file 1

* Method accepted. – Method not accepted

but no further clinical outcome measures were examinable in the current review.

There were several limitations of the present review. The first is that only 10 studies, with 11 sets of analyses, were included for review. This is likely attributable due to methodological and logistical challenges of undertaking long-term longitudinal studies. The quality and risk of bias of studies is also a limiting factor, with most included studies rated as 'poor' (n=7) or 'fair' (n=4). Only one study was 'good'.

Although the reviewed measures of affective lability are deemed relatively consistent, conclusions could have been stronger if the field used a consistent, well-validated measure across all studies. ROB assessments were also graded down by low follow-up rates. Participant loss to follow-up rates is a reasonable and common limitation of long-term studies, participants who developed mental health difficulties might have been more likely to discontinue the study and represents a potential confounding factor. Low conversion rates to BD limit the strength of analyses. Diagnostic rates were likely to have been even lower had the studies not selected at-risk cohorts. However, all studies selected their samples in this way, limiting how easily the results can be generalised to the general population.

Many studies did not follow up participants for longer than two to three years. Many participants might have developed BD after this timeframe and the analyses would not represent these participants. Although these factors collectively graded most ROB assessments down, low gradings do not necessarily reflect low quality studies. Further, many studies did not assess for affective lability as a primary objective. It is therefore not surprising that this was not carefully controlled for or measured in a structured interview. The possibility of publication bias affecting these associations also cannot be disregarded.

Other methodological differences between the studies should be considered as our findings combined samples of different ages (baseline age ranging from pre-adolescence to adults) and with different types of risk factors (e.g. synthesising those with familial risk and clinical populations). However, the consistency of the associations reported in spite of these variabilities supports its potential as a valid risk factor.

The identification of stable risk factors such as affective lability, is critical to developing accurate at-risk predictive models that have the potential to consequentially improve illness detection, intervention and ultimately prognosis. Recently developed instruments for the early detection of BD include the BAR-criteria, BPSS, EPIbipolar and SIBARS (Leopold et al. 2012; Bechdolf et al. 2012; Correll et al. 2014; Fusar-Poli et al. 2018). Existing measures of bipolarity, such as the bipolarity index, also hold potential as tools for identification of those who are at-risk (Aiken et al. 2015). There is some preliminary evidence distinguishing mood lability as a precursor specific to BD when compared to schizophrenia (Correll et al. 2007). These distinctions require further clarification (Howes et al. 2011).

Clinical implications of predictive models may include minimising delays to diagnosis and improved early intervention; (Hafeman et al. 2017) BD patients respond better to medication if they receive it earlier in their illness course (Beesdo et al. 2009; Swann et al. 1999). It has even been suggested that comprehensive and reliable predictive models could also contribute to preventing the development of a full disorder (Skjelstad et al. 2010). Predictive models can help to advance this new field of research by improving the identification of appropriate non-clinical cohorts for research. For these reasons, researchers have argued that clinically applicable predictive assessment tools have the potential to transform the treatment, clinical outcomes, and illness progression of BD (Skjelstad et al. 2010; Malhi et al. 2014). However, it is important to emphasise that clinical implementation of these risk-prediction tools is challenging e.g. ethically in informing individuals that they are at-risk for BD, the potential for premature treatment initiation, identifying false positive cases, eliciting self-stigmatization. Thus, care and consideration is required not only in relation to the sensitivity and specificity of such a tool (to maximise true positive and minimise false positive cases) but also how its implementation would be managed in terms of supporting the wellbeing of individuals with being informed they are at risk, particularly relating to stigma and intervention.

There are specific cohorts who could particularly benefit from improved clinical screening bolstered by an understanding of precursor features. This will be critical for those who face BD, schizophrenia, BPD, or MDD misdiagnoses. For example, many of those with BD can initially experience years of depressive episodes without the occurrence of mania or hypomania (Bowden 2001). This can lead to a lack of treatment or being misdiagnosed with MDD. Patients can consequently receive inappropriate treatment which may exacerbate bipolar symptoms. Crucially, for those whose BD begins with depressive episodes, more severe long-term clinical outcomes, such as higher rates of suicide, have been reported (Correll et al. 2007; Baldessarini et al. 2014).

Further research into predictive features could improve the identification and treatment of BD-II. Although there is not enough research for the present review to draw conclusions regarding BD subtypes, hypomanic episodes do not always result in hospitalisation and can easily be missed, making the diagnosis of BD-II particularly challenging. This could contribute to the relatively high rates of suicide attempts and completed suicides that occur in affected patients (Rihmer and Pestality 1999). Similarly, precursor features could distinguish the pathogenesis of treatment-resistant depression from DSM-defined MDD, with potential to bring to light a broader spectrum of illness and unacknowledged features of bipolarity.

## Conclusions

The present review has found that prominently, longitudinal studies demonstrate a significant association between prospectively identified affective lability in cohorts without BD and subsequent diagnoses of BD or BSD. This pattern was observed across 9 of the 10 studies reviewed. Future studies should aim to establish this pattern using larger sample sizes, in samples which are more representative of the general population and use longer follow-up durations. Whether affective lability leads to a particular type of bipolar illness and/or trajectory should also be determined, particularly since the present review employed an inclusive approach to bipolar diagnoses. More broadly, affective lability should be further explored using well-validated measures, in combination with a range of other possible precursors in order to develop clinical predictive models and contribute to early intervention efforts, accurate diagnosis, and improved outcomes for those with BD.

## Supplementary Information

**Additional file 1**: The Newcastle Ottawa scale (NOS) grading system tailored criteria.

**Acknowledgements**

The authors would like to extend their thanks to other members of the Centre for Affective Disorders and the MSc Affective Disorders course leaders for their inspiration, collaboration and support, particularly Dr Nefize Yalin whose input was instrumental to the conceptualisation of this project.

**Authors' contributions**

RS conceived the project. RHT, AHY and RS drafted the protocol. RHT conducted the searches. RHT and AU screened articles for inclusion and extracted data from included studies. RS and AHY provided supervision and facilitated consensus on any discrepancies between the two main review authors. RHT with input from all other authors completed the results and wrote the first draft of the manuscript. All authors have read and approved the final manuscript.

**Author details**

[1]Department of Psychological Medicine, Institute of Psychiatry, Psychology and Neuroscience, King's College London, London SE5 8AF, UK. [2]South London & Maudsley NHS Foundation Trust, Maudsley Hospital, London, UK.

**References**

Aiken CB, Weisler RH, Sachs GS. The bipolarity index: a clinician-rated measure of diagnostic confidence. J Affect Disord. 2015;177:59–64.

Akiskal HS. The prevalent clinical spectrum of bipolar disorders: beyond DSM-IV. J Clin Psychopharmacol. 1996;16(2):4S.

Akiskal KK, Akiskal HS. The theoretical underpinnings of affective temperaments: implications for evolutionary foundations of bipolar disorder and human nature. J Affect Disord. 2005;85(1):231–9.

Akiskal HS, Maser JD, Zeller PJ, Endicott J, Coryell W, Keller M, et al. Switching from 'unipolar' to bipolar II: an 11-year prospective study of clinical and temperamental predictors in 559 patients. Arch Gen Psychiatry. 1995;52(2):114–23.

Akiskal HS, Hantouche EG, Allilaire JF. Bipolar II with and without cyclothymic temperament: "dark" and "sunny" expressions of soft bipolarity. J Affect Disord. 2003;73(1):49–57.

Angst J. Problems in the current concepts and definitions of bipolar disorders. World Psychiatry. 2013;10(3):191.

Angst J, Gamma A, Endrass J. Risk factors for the bipolar and depression spectra. Acta Psychiatr Scand. 2003;108(s418):15–9.

American Psychiatric Association. Diagnostic and Statistical Manual of Mental Disorders (DSM-5®). American Psychiatric Pub; 2013.

Baldessarini RJ, Tondo L, Visioli C. First-episode types in bipolar disorder: predictive associations with later illness. Acta Psychiatr Scand. 2014;129(5):383–92.

Baldessarini RJ, Salvatore P, Khalsa H-MK, Tohen M. Dissimilar morbidity following initial mania versus mixed-states in type-I bipolar disorder. J Affect Disord. 2010;126(1):299–302.

Bechdolf A, Ratheesh A, Wood S, Tecic T, Conus P, Nelson B, et al. Rationale and first results of developing at-risk (Prodromal) criteria for bipolar disorder. Curr Pharm Des. 2012;18(4):358–75.

Beesdo K, Knappe S, Pine DS. Anxiety and anxiety disorders in children and adolescents: developmental issues and implications for DSM-V. Psychiatr Clin North Am. 2009;32(3):483–524.

Bowden CL. Strategies to reduce misdiagnosis of bipolar depression. Psychiatr Serv. 2001;52(1):51–5.

Campbell M, McKenzie JE, Sowden A, Katikireddi SV, Brennan SE, Ellis S, et al. Synthesis without meta-analysis (SWiM) in systematic reviews: reporting guideline. BMJ. 2020;16(368):l6890.

Correll CU, Penzner JB, Frederickson AM, Richter JJ, Auther AM, Smith CW, et al. Differentiation in the preonset phases of schizophrenia and mood disorders: evidence in support of a bipolar mania prodrome. Schizophr Bull. 2007;33(3):703–14.

Correll CU, Olvet DM, Auther AM, Hauser M, Kishimoto T, Carrión RE, et al. The bipolar prodrome symptom interview and scale-prospective (BPSS-P): description and validation in a psychiatric sample and healthy controls. Bipolar Disord. 2014;16(5):505–22.

DeGeorge DP, Walsh MA, Barrantes-Vidal N, Kwapil TR. A three-year longitudinal study of affective temperaments and risk for psychopathology. J Affect Disord. 2014;164:94–100.

Egeland JA, Hostetter AM, Pauls DL, Sussex JN. Prodromal symptoms before onset of manic-depressive disorder suggested by first hospital admission histories. J Am Acad Child Adolesc Psychiatry. 2000;39(10):1245–52.

Egeland JA, Endicott J, Hostetter AM, Allen CR, Pauls DL, Shaw JA. A 16-year prospective study of prodromal features prior to BPI onset in well amish children. J Affect Disord. 2012;142(1):186–92.

Faedda L, Baldessarini RJ, Suppes T, Tondo L, Becker I, Lipschitz DS. Pediatric-onset bipolar disorder: a neglected clinical and public health problem gianni. Harv Rev Psychiatry. 1995;3(4):171–95.

Fusar-Poli P, De Micheli A, Rocchetti M, Cappucciati M, Ramella-Cravaro V, Rutigliano G, et al. Semistructured interview for bipolar at risk states (SIBARS). Psychiatry Res. 2018;1(264):302–9.

Gan Z, Diao F, Wei Q, Wu X, Cheng M, Guan N, et al. A predictive model for diagnosing bipolar disorder based on the clinical characteristics of major depressive episodes in Chinese population. J Affect Disord. 2011;134(1):119–25.

Hafeman DM, Merranko J, Goldstein TR, Axelson D, Goldstein BI, Monk K, et al. Assessment of a person-level risk calculator to predict new-onset bipolar spectrum disorder in youth at familial risk. JAMA Psychiat. 2017;74(8):841–7.

Howes OD, Lim S, Theologos G, Yung AR, Goodwin GM, McGuire P. A comprehensive review and model of putative prodromal features of bipolar affective disorder. Psychol Med. 2011;41(8):1567–77.

Kochman FJ, Hantouche EG, Ferrari P, Lancrenon S, Bayart D, Akiskal HS. Cyclothymic temperament as a prospective predictor of bipolarity and suicidality in children and adolescents with major depressive disorder. J Affect Disord. 2005;85(1):181–9.

Leopold K, Ritter P, Correll CU, Marx C, Özgürdal S, Juckel G, et al. Risk constellations prior to the development of bipolar disorders: rationale of a new risk assessment tool. J Affect Disord. 2012;136(3):1000–10.

Lish JD, Dime-Meenan S, Whybrow PC, Price RA, Hirschfeld RMA. The National Depressive and Manic-depressive Association (DMDA) survey of bipolar members. J Affect Disord. 1994;31(4):281–94.

Lloyd LC, Giaroli G, Taylor D, Tracy DK. Bipolar depression: clinically missed, pharmacologically mismanaged. Ther Adv Psychopharmacol. 2011;1(5):153–62.

Malhi GS, Bargh DM, Coulston CM, Das P, Berk M. Predicting bipolar disorder on the basis of phenomenology: implications for prevention and early intervention. Bipolar Disord. 2014;16(5):455–70.

McPheeters ML, Kripalani S, Peterson NB, Idowu RT, Jerome RN, Potter SA, et al. Closing the quality gap: revisiting the state of the science (vol. 3: quality improvement interventions to address health disparities). Evid Rep Technol Assess. 2012;208.3:1–475.

Merikangas KR, Akiskal HS, Angst J, et al. Lifetime and 12-month prevalence of bipolar spectrum disorder in the National Comorbidity Survey replication. Arch Gen Psychiatry. 2007;64(5):543–52.

Miklowitz DJ, Chang KD. Prevention of bipolar disorder in at-risk children: theoretical assumptions and empirical foundations. Dev Psychopathol. 2008;20(3):881–97.

Moher D, Liberati A, Tetzlaff J, Altman DG, Group TP. Preferred reporting items for systematic reviews and meta-analyses: the PRISMA statement. PLOS Med. 2009;6(7):e1000097.

Nilsson KK, Straarup KN, Jørgensen CR, Licht RW. Affective temperaments' relation to functional impairment and affective recurrences in bipolar disorder patients. J Affect Disord. 2012;138(3):332–6.

Ouzzani M, Hammady H, Fedorowicz Z, Elmagarmid A. Rayyan—a web and mobile app for systematic reviews. Syst Rev. 2016;5(1):210.

Özgürdal S, van Haren E, Hauser M, Ströhle A, Bauer M, Assion H-J, et al. Early mood swings as symptoms of the bipolar prodrome: preliminary results of a retrospective analysis. Psychopathology. 2009;42(5):337–42.

Ratheesh A, Cotton SM, Betts JK, Chanen A, Nelson B, Davey CG, et al. Prospective progression from high-prevalence disorders to bipolar disorder: exploring characteristics of pre-illness stages. J Affect Disord. 2015;183:45–8.

Rihmer Z, Pestality P. Bipolar II disorder and suicidal behavior. Psychiatr Clin North Am. 1999;22(3):667–73.

Rucklidge JJ. Retrospective parent report of psychiatric histories: do checklists reveal specific prodromal indicators for postpubertal-onset pediatric bipolar disorder? Bipolar Disord. 2008;10(1):56–66.

Salvatore P, Baldessarini RJ, Khalsa H-MK, Amore M, Vittorio CD, Ferraro G, et al. Predicting diagnostic change among patients diagnosed with first-episode *DSM-IV-TR* major depressive disorder with psychotic features. J Clin Psychiatry. 2013;74(7):723–31.

Skjelstad DV, Malt UF, Holte A. Symptoms and signs of the initial prodrome of bipolar disorder: a systematic review. J Affect Disord. 2010;126(1):1–13.

Sperry SH, Walsh MA, Kwapil TR. Emotion dynamics concurrently and prospectively predict mood psychopathology. J Affect Disord. 2020;261:67–75.

Swann AC, Bowden CL, Calabrese JR, Dilsaver SC, Morris DD. Differential effect of number of previous episodes of affective disorder on response to lithium or divalproex in acute mania. Am J Psychiatry. 1999;156(8):1264–6.

Tohen M, Khalsa H-MK, Salvatore P, Vieta E, Ravichandran C, Baldessarini RJ. Two-year outcomes in first-episode psychotic depression: the McLean–Harvard first-episode project. J Affect Disord. 2012;136(1):1–8.

Vázquez GH, Akiskal H. The temperament evaluation of the Memphis, Pisa, Paris, and San Diego autoquestionnaire, Argentine version (TEMPS-A Buenos Aires). Vertex. 2005;16(60):89–94.

Wells G, Shea B, O'Connell D, Robertson J, Peterson J, Losos M, et al. The Newcastle-Ottawa Scale (NOS) for Assessing the Quality of Nonrandomized Studies in Meta- Analysis. 2012.

Woo YS, Shim IH, Wang H-R, Song HR, Jun T-Y, Bahk W-M. A diagnosis of bipolar spectrum disorder predicts diagnostic conversion from unipolar depression to bipolar disorder: A 5-year retrospective study. J Affect Disord. 2015;174:83–8.

11

# Early detection of bipolar disorders and treatment recommendations for help-seeking adolescents and young adults: Findings of the Early Detection and Intervention Center Dresden

Julia Martini[1], Karolina Leopold[1,2], Steffi Pfeiffer[1], Christina Berndt[1], Anne Boehme[1], Veit Roessner[3], Paolo Fusar-Poli[4,5], Allan H. Young[6], Christoph U. Correll[7,8,9], Michael Bauer[1] and Andrea Pfennig[1*]

**Abstract**

**Background:** Early identification and intervention of individuals with risk factors for or subtle prodromal symptoms of bipolar disorders (BD) may improve the illness course and prevent adverse long-term consequences.

**Methods:** We examined sociodemographic, clinical and psychopathological characteristics of help-seeking adolescents and young adults who consulted the Early Detection and Intervention Center Dresden at the University of Dresden (Germany) and presented with or without pre-defined at-risk criteria for BD. The standardized diagnostic procedure for all help-seeking youth included a comprehensive psychiatric history and a structured clinical interview. When BD at-risk state was suspected, early detection instruments (EPI*bipolar*, BPSS-FP) were applied. Treatment recommendations were formulated in multi-professional case conferences.

**Results:** Out of 890 help-seeking persons between 05/2009 and 04/2018, 582 (65%) completed the diagnostic process. Of these, 24 (4%) had manifest BD and 125 (21%) fulfilled at-risk BD criteria (age = 23.9 ± 0.6 years, female = 62%). Of the pre-defined main risk factors, family history for BD was reported in 22% of the at-risk persons, (hypo-)mania risk state in 44%, and increasing cyclothymic mood swings with increased activity in 48%. The most common secondary risk factors were decreased psychosocial functioning (78%), lifetime diagnosis of depressive disorder (67%) and specific sleep/circadian rhythm disturbances (59%). Substance use was very common in subjects at-risk for BD (cannabis = 50%, alcohol = 33%) and highest in patients with BD (cannabis = 75%, alcohol = 40%). Psychiatric treatment history, including psychopharmacological therapy, was similar between the groups, while treatment recommendations differed, with more advice for psychotherapy and antidepressants in the at-risk group with a lifetime diagnosis of depression and more advice for specialized BD treatment including mood stabilizers in patients with BD.

**Conclusion:** This analysis on the phenomenology of different BD at-risk stages suggests that early detection of individuals presenting with suggested risk factors for the development of BD is feasible in help-seeking young people.

*Correspondence: andrea.pfennig@uniklinikum-dresden.de
[1] Department of Psychiatry and Psychotherapy, Carl Gustav Carus University Hospital, Technische Universität Dresden, Fetscherstraße 74, 01307 Dresden, Germany
Full list of author information is available at the end of the article

Future research should further develop/test stage-specific prevention and early targeted intervention approaches that were described in a naturalistic setting.

## Background

Bipolar disorders (BD) are severe mental disorders that are associated with an early onset and substantial psychosocial impairment (Carlson et al. 2000; Perlis et al. 2004). According to the World Health Organization Global Burden of Disease Study, BD rank within the top 10 causes of disability among all medical conditions worldwide, and about 3 million people suffer from BD in the European Union (Vos et al. 2012; Wittchen et al. 2011).

First signs of emerging BD frequently occur in early adolescence, and manifestation of the full disorder (at least one depressive and one (hypo-)manic/mixed episode) typically occurs in late adolescence or early adulthood (Carlson et al. 2000). Early onset BD is associated with greater rates of comorbid disorders (e.g., substance abuse), more recurrences, shorter periods of euthymia and a greater likelihood of suicide attempts (Perlis et al. 2004). Diagnosis of a first episode and adequate treatment are often delayed (up to ten years) (Baldessarini et al. 2003; Pfennig et al. 2011). Reasons for delayed diagnosis and treatment include: i) the natural development of the disease with depressive episodes as the first manifestation in about half of the patients (frequently leading to a diagnosis of unipolar depression), ii) non-specific symptoms in early stages that are not classified as bipolar symptomatology, iii) suboptimal health care access and provision, and iv) fear of stigmatization by affected subjects (Leopold et al. 2012; Faedda et al. 2019). Treatment delay is associated with an impaired age-appropriate development, worse social adjustment and functional outcome, more hospitalizations, higher comorbidity rates, elevated risk of suicide, and reduced response to mood stabilizing drug treatment (Chen and Dilsaver 1996; Goldberg and Ernst 2002; Kessing et al. 2014; Matza et al. 2005; Miller et al. 2014; Post et al. 2010). Thus, early recognition of at-risk persons and early BD and primary interventions before the onset of the disorder and at early stages of BD are promising avenues for improving outcomes of the disorder (Collins et al. 2011; Forsman et al. 2014, 2015) in line with clinical staging models (Berk et al. 2017). Prevention of BD can target asymptomatic subgroups of individuals with risk factors for BD (selective prevention) or individuals with subthreshold symptoms that do not meet diagnostic BD criteria (indicated prevention, Fusar-Poli et al. 2019). For example, due to its high heritability (Craddock and Sklar 2009), a positive family history for BD is one of the major criteria for selective prevention of BD (Duffy et al. 2010, 2014; Mendlewicz and Rainer 1977; Smoller and Finn 2003). However, since many patients with BD do not have a positive family history, efforts are being made to develop clinical at-risk criteria so as to improve

Prevention of BD (Axelson et al. 2015; Bechdolf et al. 2010; Brietzke et al. 2012; Correll and Olvet et al. 2014; Duffy et al. 2017; Faedda et al. 2014; Hafeman et al. 2016; Howes et al. 2010; Hunt et al. 2016; Leopold et al. 2012; Luby and Navsaria 2010; van Meter et al. 2016; Singh 2015; Skjelstad et al. 2010). In a systematic literature review, Rios and colleagues postulated a clinical staging model and determined stage I as a symptomatic period that can last up to years preceding the first manifest manic episode/BD. The first manifest manic episode/ BD itself was defined as stage II (Rios et al. 2015). Early symptoms include (sub-)syndromal major depressive disorder/changes in mood/affective liability, fearfulness/ anxiety, sleep disturbances, anger/irritability, and functional impairment (Bechdolf et al. 2010; Leopold et al. 2012; Correll and Hauser et al. 2014; van Meter et al. 2016; Faedda et al. 2019). Furthermore, longitudinal studies suggest a progression of psychopathology over time (Duffy et al. 2017; Hafeman et al. 2016), with symptoms usually becoming more specific and more similar to those of manifest BD (Axelson et al. 2015; van Meter et al. 2016; Pfennig et al. 2017; Tohen et al. 2003).

Based on this knowledge and clinical staging models, some semistructured instruments have been developed to identify young people at clinical risk for BD and to allow indicated prevention (i) the Early Phase Inventory for bipolar disorders (EPI*bipolar*, Leopold et al. 2012); (ii) the Bipolar Prodrome Symptom Scale (BPSS-FP, Correll and Olvet et al. 2014); (iii) Bipolar at-risk (BAR) criteria, Bechdolf et al. 2012/ the Semistructured Interview for Bipolar At Risk States, SIBARS, Fusar-Poli et al. 2018). Cross-sectional studies revealed promising results on the internal reliability and consistency of these instruments (Correll and Olvet et al. 2014; Bechdolf et al. 2012). Emerging longitudinal studies reported a transition risk to BD of 14% at 1-year (Bechdolf et al. 2014) and 23% at 2-years (Fusar-Poli et al. 2018), and adequate prognostic accuracy for conversion to BD (0.7 at 18 months, Fusar-Poli et al. 2018). Research is ongoing to validate the findings in larger cohorts.

Following early and appropriate detection, prevention of illness progression becomes crucial. Therefore, increasing research efforts are being targeted towards the development and evaluation of early selective and indicated interventions (McNamara et al. 2012). Choosing the appropriate intervention requires careful balancing risks and benefits in a shared decision process. Preliminary clinical category models and treatment guidance have been formulated based on emerging evidence and clinical expertise (Berk et al. 2007; Kapczinski et al. 2009; Leopold and Pfeiffer et al. 2013; Leopold and Pfennig et al. 2013; Chia et al. 2019). The basic proposed approach encompasses psychoeducation, counselling on illicit drug use, improvement of sleep quality and stable social rhythms, and further mental health strategies on preserving the young person's ability to meet age-appropriate developmental tasks (Berk et al. 2007; Kapczinski et al. 2009; Leopold and Pfeiffer et al. 2013). Additionally, psychotherapy is an early intervention strategy, since (i) early symptoms (such as mood swings, disruptions of diurnal rhythm/ sleep disturbances) may be especially responsive to psychotherapy, (ii) it has an exceptionally favorable benefit/risk ratio, and (iii) is usually more acceptable to young patients compared to pharmacotherapy. Family focused psychotherapy tailored to the needs of the young at-risk subjects was associated with reduction of depressive symptoms, increase of psychosocial functioning and a longer time in remission (Miklowitz et al. 2013). Additionally, first data from small, open and uncontrolled studies show that Interpersonal and social rhythm therapy (IPSRT, Goldstein et al. 2014) led to better sleep, and Mindfulness-based cognitive therapy (MBCT, (Cotton et al. 2016; Strawn et al. 2016) to better emotion regulation and less anxiety. However, IPSRT plus informed referral were not significantly better compared to informed referral only in a succeeding small study (Goldstein et al. 2018). Recently published first data from early tailored cognitive behavioral group therapy applied to at-risk subjects show a reduction of affective symptoms and better psychosocial functioning after up to six month. However, there was no significant difference compared to the unstructured control group treatment (Leopold et al. 2020).

Evidence on pharmacological interventions in persons at-risk for BD is scarce (Chang et al. 2003; DelBello et al. 2007; Findling et al. 2007; Geller et al. 1998). Pharmacological treatment approaches with mood stabilizers (lithium and divalproex) for treatment of at-risk patients have only been investigated in small-sample studies not showing effectivity over placebo (Findling et al. 2007; Geller et al. 1998). In a larger sample aripiprazole ($n = 30$) was significantly better over 12 weeks in improving manic symptomatology and global clinical illness severity compared to placebo ($n = 29$, Findling et al. 2017).

Thus far, treatment guidelines do not contain specific recommendations on interventions of patients at-risk for BD (DGBS and DGPPN 2019), and no consistent recommendations for early stage disorder, except with respect to the indications for maintenance medication treatments (Chia et al. 2019). Additionally, clinical practice is poorly examined. Initiatives for the early detection of BD have been started to clarify whether early detection of at-risk stages for the development of BD is possible and which early intervention strategies may be most appropriate (Pfennig et al. 2012; Faedda et al. 2019).

Taken together, evidence for a progression of BD across early at-risk states is growing, and it is hypothesized that symptoms become more specific and similar to those of manifest BD over time (Axelson et al. 2015; Duffy et al. 2017; Hafeman et al. 2016; van Meter et al. 2016; Pfennig et al. 2017). However, clinical at-risk stages for BD are poorly examined regarding clinical characteristics/phenomenology, attendant symptoms and comorbid psychiatric disorders. Moreover, detail on the psychiatric and psychotherapeutic care offered to persons at risk for BD is largely missing. Clinical data from Early Detection and Intervention Center are useful to gain insight into clinical characteristics, care and treatment histories as well as treatments recommended and provided in early stages of developing BD. Based on clinical data of young people seen during the first nine years of the Early Detection and Intervention Center at the university hospital in Dresden, this analysis aimed to thoroughly describe different clinical at-risk constellations for BD with regard to individual risk factors and (comorbid) psychiatric disorders. Moreover, treatment history as well as treatment recommendations by the service were examined.

## Methods

### Design

This analysis was conducted in accordance to the REporting of studies Conducted using Observational Routinely-collected health Data (RECORD) statement (Benchimol et al. 2015). All data were collected as part of the service routine process. The analysis was in accordance to the APA ethical standards (American Psychiatric Association 2003) and the Declaration of Helsinki (World Medical Association 1964) and approved by the Ethics Committee of the Medical Faculty of the Technische Universität Dresden (EK290082014). All participants provided informed consent.

### Study population and setting

The analysis comprised sociodemographic, clinical and psychopathological characteristics as well as previous treatment experiences of help-seeking adolescents and young adults that consulted the Early Detection and Intervention Center at the university hospital Dresden, Germany, from May 2009 to April 2018. In addition, treatment recommendations given by the service specialists after multi-professional case conferences discussed with the clients in the shared decision process were analyzed.

### Proceeding at the Early Detection and Intervention Center Dresden

The Early Detection and Intervention Center Dresden was established in 2008 for help-seeking young people aged 15 to 35 years. It is open to clients with a broad symptomatology and/or need for counselling, and employs staff specifically trained in the early detection and treatment of BD (https://www.ddfruehdran.de/). Being a secondary care service, individuals can consult the service directly or via referral by psychologists, psychiatrists, primary care physicians or counselling services. Patients are assessed by clinical psychologists and/or psychiatrists in a comprehensive standardized, stepped diagnostic procedure, including early recognition instruments, if indicated. Diagnostic information is evaluated in multi-professional case conferences by experienced, specialized service staff members. Treatment decisions are based on the best available evidence. The content of the particular treatment recommendations does not follow a specific protocol but is given naturalistically based on the clinical experience of the service clinical experts, published evidence and clinical guideline recommendations as appropriate (Leopold et al. 2014). Recommendations might cover pharmacotherapy, psychotherapy, sociotherapy and other (e.g. additional specialized diagnostics) and can be administered in an outpatient, day care or inpatient setting, both at our university hospital and other hospitals or resident clinicians and psychotherapists. Clients and staff engage in a shared-decision process to agree upon the option most appropriate for the client at that point in time. In case patients already fulfill the diagnostic criteria for manifest BD, specific treatment is offered at the in- and outpatient facilities of the department of psychiatry at the same institution.

### Study measures, follow-up and clinical outcomes

At the initial contact, sociodemographic characteristics and reasons for visiting the service are assessed. If a diagnostic procedure is offered after the initial case conference, a comprehensive structured history is taken, including information about family history of psychiatric disorders and past treatment (incl. history of in- or outpatient (child-)psychiatric treatment, psychotherapy, pharmacotherapy with antidepressants, mood stabilizer and/or antipsychotics). History of substance use includes frequency of use of nicotine, alcohol, cannabis, amphetamines, hallucinogens, and cocaine (never, once, sporadically, frequently).

After obtaining a detailed psychiatric history and assessment of psychopathology, the German version of Structured Clinical Interview for DSM-IV Axis I disorders (SCID-I, First and Spitzer et al. 1997) is conducted by a different staff member that blinded to the results of the initial diagnostic interview to prevent premature assumptions and to ensure the patient is evaluated by two staff members (four-eye-principle). The SCID-I is a semi-structured clinical interview administered by trained psychiatrists/ psychologists and designed to yield psychiatric diagnoses consistent with DSM-IV/DSM-IV-TR (American Psychiatric Association 2007) diagnostic criteria. The duration of administration ranges from 30 to 120 min. The SCID-I possesses very good psychometric properties (First and Spitzer et al. 1997). To reach a good reliability regular rater trainings should be provided (Gorgens 2018). The reach a good validity the interview should be applied according to the LEAD procedure including longitudinal assessment performed by expert diagnosticians using all data that are available about the subject (Spitzer 1983). As part of the quality assurance of our Early Detection and Intervention Center we regularly train our diagnosticians and conduct all diagnostics according to the LEAD procedure.

When the development or manifestation of a personality disorder is suggested in the diagnostic process, the German version of Structured Clinical Interview for DSM-IV Axis II personality disorders (First and Gibbon et al. 1997) is applied.

Subjects with any suggestion of an at-risk state for BD, such as mood swings, and/or positive family history for affective or schizoaffective disorders, are additionally assessed with the following two instruments:

The Early Phase Inventory for Bipolar Disorders (EPI-*bipolar*, Leopold et al. 2012) is a semi-structured interview comprising the categories disturbances in sleep and circadian rhythm, mood swings and affective lability, fearfulness and anxiety, psychosocial functioning, course of illness, former or current behavioral problems, and/or attention-deficit/hyperactivity disorder (ADHD) and substance use. Specific sleep and circadian rhythm disturbances were pre-defined and included for instance a high variability in sleeping times without external causation, phases of feeling fresh despite substantially less sleep than usual and having substantial problems with time zone changes. Specific features of the first depressive episode in disease history were pre-defined and included for instance substantial suicidal behavior, hypersomnia and hyperphagia. Additional data from history taking, including family history and data from the Bipolar Prodrome Symptom Scale-Full Prospective (BPSS-FP) completes the information. The BPSS-FP (Correll and Olvet et al. 2014) is a semi-structured interview with sections rating subthreshold (hypo-)manic, depressive and general symptoms. Patients fulfilling at least moderate severity in two or more (hypo-)mania items (attention and increased psychomotor activity are counted as one symptom) meet operationally defined criteria for a (hypo-)mania risk state. The BPSS-FP Mania scale has good to excellent psychometric properties in terms of internal consistency (Cronbachs α: 0.87) and interrater-reliability (intraclass correlation coefficient, ICC: 0.934) and satisfying scores for convergent validity (e.g. with the Young Mania Rating Scale) (Correll and Olvet et al. 2014).

Pre-defined *main* risk factors within EPI*bipolar* assessed within the above mentioned semi-structured interviews are I) a family history of BD, II) increasing cyclothymic mood swings with increased activity, and III) a (hypo-)mania risk state (at least moderate severity score in at least two (hypo-)mania items, taken from the BPSS-FP). *Secondary* risk factors are assigned to clusters A and B, that is: A1) specific sleep and circadian rhythm disturbances, A2) increasing cyclothymic mood swings without increased activity, A3) depressive episodes with specific features, B1) family history of schizophrenia, schizoaffective disorder or major depression, B2) lifetime diagnosis of depressive disorder, B3) lifetime diagnosis of ADHD, B4) decreased psychosocial functioning (work/school, social life, family or global), B5) episodic course of illness psychopathology, B6) increasing and periodic substance use of alcohol and/or cannabis. The EPI*bipolar* at-risk status was defined as presenting with (a) at least one secondary risk factor of each cluster (A & B), (b) at least one main risk factor and at least one secondary risk factor, or (c) at least two main risk factors. The EPI*bipolar* at-risk status was used in the analysis in order to generate baseline data for validation of the interview developed at our research group. It has been designed in cooperation with Dr. Correll to complement the BPSS-FP and capture very early signs of developing BD.

### Statistical analysis

All data were sampled in the project database of the Early Detection and Intervention Center Dresden (employing ACCESS). Routinely, data quality and completeness were checked; before analysis, data were cleaned. The software-package IBM SPSS Statistics Version 25 was used to compute descriptive statistics. Chi$^2$-tests and t-tests were applied to test whether clinical and sociodemographic characteristics of subjects not at-risk/no manifest mania/BD (N = 433) vs. at-risk for or manifest mania/BD (N = 149) differed.

For the subsequent analyses, the following groups of patients were defined according to the considered predefined risk factors for BD:

- Group 1 (AR): EPI*bipolar* at-risk status, no lifetime depression (SCID-I), mania risk state (BPSS-FP)
- Group 2 (AR + LD): EPI*bipolar* at-risk status plus lifetime depression (SCID-I), mania risk state (BPSS-FP)
- Group 3 [AR + (H)MR]: EPI*bipolar* at risk status plus (hypo-)mania risk state (BPSS-FP), with or without lifetime depression (SCID-I)
- Group 4 (M/BD): manifest mania/BD (SCID-I).

In addition to the calculation of pairwise group comparison (with Bonferroni correction) we also analyzed planned contrasts representing assumed increases in risk for BD using Chi$^2$-tests and t-tests.

Two-sided statistical significance was evaluated at the 5% level for all analyses. We additionally report results that failed to reach significance as a trend (10% level).

## Results

### Patient sample

Altogether, 890 help-seeking adolescents and young adults were seen at the Early Detection and Intervention Center Dresden between May 2009 and April 2018. About a quarter of all contacts (N = 220, 25%) did not enter the full diagnostic process after the initial contact. Reasons were that clients (1) did not describe symptoms that would meet the diagnostic criteria for a psychiatric disorder or at-risk states (e.g., symptoms could be explained as heartsickness or grief, N = 29, 3%), (2) were already in adequate treatment (N = 11, 1%), (3) had to be referred to a more specific service right away (e.g. trauma care service, addiction counselling) (N = 175, 20%), or (4) presented with the necessity of immediate crisis intervention/ in-patient treatment (N = 5, 1%). Another 88 persons (10%) left the diagnostic process prematurely (e.g. did not show up to further appointments despite several offers).

Overall, 582 (65%) patients completed the diagnostic procedure of the service and were included into the following analyses. The flow chart is presented in Fig. 1.

There were no significant differences regarding age and sex between subjects who did not enter the diagnostic process after the initial contact (N = 220; age: M = 25.0, SD = 10.2; female: N = 110, 50%), subjects who left the diagnostic process prematurely (N = 88; age: M = 25.2, SD = 8.3, female: N = 35, 40%), and subjects who completed the full diagnostic procedure (N = 582; age: M = 24.7, SD = 6.0, female: N = 279, 48%).

### Comparison of those with and without risk of BD

Table 1 presents sociodemographic and clinical characteristics of help-seeking adolescents and young adults who completed the diagnostic process (N = 582). Overall,

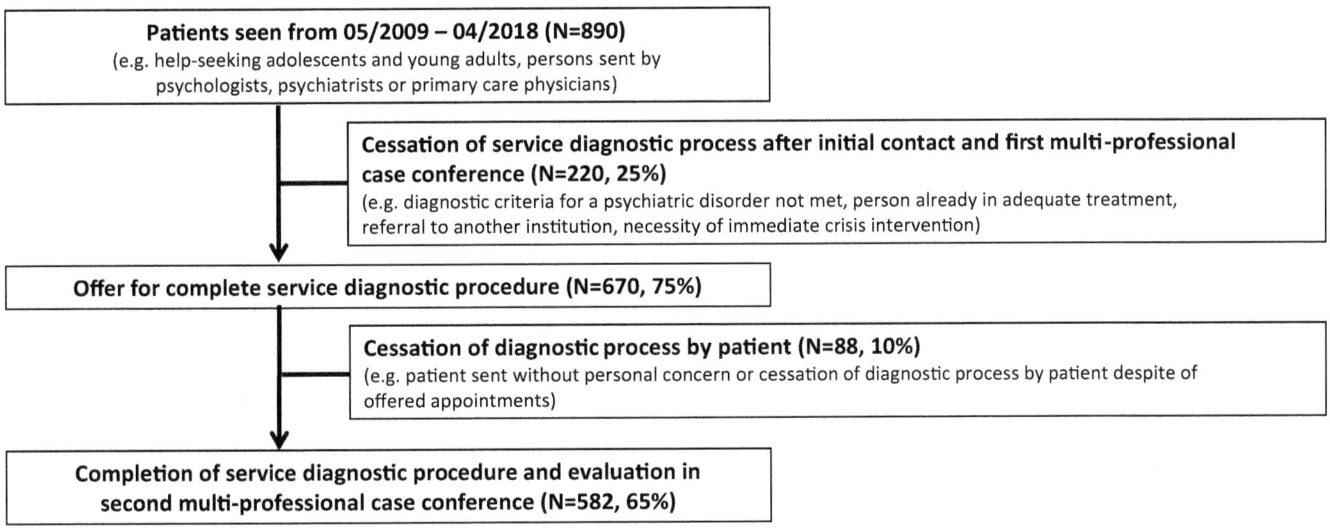


**Fig. 1** Subject flow chart

149 patients met any of the pre-defined risk factors for BD (N = 125, 21% of those with complete diagnostics) or received a diagnosis of manifest mania/ BD (N = 24, 4%).

Patients at-risk for BD or with manifest mania/BD were of an equivalent age profile but more likely to be female (57% vs. 45%, p = 0.011). The educational profiles (representing the highest degree achieved) were somewhat different between the groups. Patients at-risk for BD or with manifest mania/BD reported significantly more frequent substance use (especially nicotine, alcohol, cannabis, and hallucinogens). They indicated significantly more often a preceding or comorbid mental disorder (especially recurrent depressive disorder, misuse of alcohol, eating disorder, and/or ADHD/ hyperkinetic disorder). Twice as many reported a history of (child-)psychiatric treatment (16% vs 8%, p = 0.005) and 44% vs. 34% (p = 0.031) had received outpatient treatment within adult psychiatry/ psychotherapy.

Figure 2 presents the rates and distribution of the pre-defined risk factors for BD according to EPI*bipolar* in at-risk patients (N = 125). Regarding the pre-defined *main* risk factors, 22% of at-risk patients presented with a family history of BD (first degree relative), 44% a (hypo-) mania risk state and 48% increasing cyclothymic mood swings with increased activity. From the *secondary* risk factors, decreased psychosocial functioning was the most frequent (78%), followed by lifetime diagnosis of depressive disorder (67%) and specific sleep and circadian rhythm disturbances (59%).

For the subsequent analyses, four groups of patients were defined as mentioned in the methods section according to the considered pre-defined risk factors for BD: AR (N = 21), AR + LD (N = 49), AR + (H)MR (N = 55), and M/BD (N = 24).

Table 2 presents sociodemographic and clinical characteristics of patients of the above-defined groups. Patients with manifest mania or BD (M/BD) were less often female compared to at-risk subjects (significantly compared to AR + LD, p = 0.036) and compared to the all subjects at-risk (p = 0.039). Substance use was common in all four groups with increasing frequency along the risk groups from AR to AR + (H)MR. Patients with mania/BD indicated more frequent cannabis and cocaine use compared to all at-risk subjects (cannabis by trend: p = 0.056, cocaine: p = 0.041). Manifest mental disorders were very common in all four groups, most frequently alcohol- or cannabis- related disorders, depression, anxiety and related disorders, and ADHD. The frequency of fulfilling at least two diagnoses apart from BD was increasing along the risk groups (AR 19%, AR + LD 49%, AR + (H)MR 47%).

Table 3 presents the treatment history patients reported and treatment recommendations given by the service after the diagnostic process. There was no significant difference with regard to history of (child-)psychiatric treatment/ psychotherapy and history of drug treatment in the four groups. In all groups pretreatment with antidepressants was relatively common (14%-46%), whereas pretreatment with mood stabilizers was rare (< 5%). Planned contrasts revealed that patients with M/ BD indicated more often a history of inpatient treatment (by trend: p = 0.077) as well as antidepressant (p = 0.017) and antipsychotic (p = 0.012) medication compared all at-risk persons.

**Table 1** Sociodemographic and clinical characteristics of help-seeking adolescents and young adults completing the diagnostic process with vs without BD at-risk/manifest BD status (N = 582)

| | Not at-risk for and no manifest mania/ Bipolar Disorder (N = 433) | | At-risk for or manifest mania/ Bipolar Disorder (N = 149) | | Group differences | P-value |
|---|---|---|---|---|---|---|
| | M | SD | M | SD | t | |
| Age | 24.9 | 6.4 | 24.1 | 4.6 | 1.336 | 0.182 |
| | N | % | N | % | Chi² | |
| Sex | | | | | | |
| Female | 194 | 44.9 | 85 | 57.0 | **6.541** | **0.011** |
| Education | | | | | | |
| Studies not finished (yet) | 41 | 10.9 | 9 | 7.1 | **13.663** | **0.008** |
| 9th or 10th grade | 142 | 37.8 | 37 | 29.4 | | |
| a-level | 141 | 37.5 | 70 | 55.6 | | |
| University level | 41 | 10.9 | 9 | 7.1 | | |
| No educational degree | 11 | 2.9 | 1 | 0.8 | | |
| First contact to the health care system for present symptoms | | | | | | |
| General practitioner or specialist physician | 99 | 37.1 | 42 | 45.2 | 3.607 | 0.307 |
| Counselling center | 46 | 17.2 | 17 | 18.3 | | |
| Early Recognition Center | 117 | 43.8 | 31 | 33.3 | | |
| Other | 5 | 1.9 | 3 | 3.2 | | |
| Substance use | | | | | | |
| Nicotine use[a] | 138 | 35.6 | 64 | 45.4 | **4.228** | **0.040** |
| Alcohol[a] | 95 | 24.7 | 49 | 34.8 | **5.271** | **0.022** |
| Cannabis use[a] | 145 | 37.6 | 78 | 55.3 | **13.33** | **<0.001** |
| Amphetamine use[b] | 48 | 12.4 | 23 | 16.3 | 1.332 | 0.249 |
| Hallucinogen use[b] | 24 | 6.2 | 18 | 12.8 | **6.038** | **0.014** |
| Cocaine use[b] | 21 | 5.4 | 12 | 8.5 | 1.697 | 0.193 |
| Diagnoses according to DSM-IV (current or lifetime) | | | | | | |
| Mental/behavioral dis. due to psychoactive substance use (F1x.x) | 49 | 11.3 | 26 | 17.4 | *3.715* | *0.054* |
| Mental/behavioral dis. due to use of alcohol (F10.x) | 20 | 4.6 | 20 | 13.4 | **13.424** | **<0.001** |
| Mental/behavioral dis. due to use of cannabis (F12.x) | 20 | 4.6 | 12 | 8.1 | 2.517 | 0.113 |
| Mood (Affective) Disorders (3x.x) | 175 | 40.4 | 108 | 72.5 | **45.632** | **<0.001** |
| Manic episode/Bipolar affective disorder (wo Hypomania) (F30.x-F31.x) | 0 | 0.0 | 24 | 16.1 | **72.745** | **<0.001** |
| Depressive episode (F32.x) | 80 | 18.5 | 27 | 18.1 | 0.009 | 0.923 |
| Recurrent depressive disorder (F33.x) | 79 | 18.2 | 51 | 34.2 | **16.325** | **<0.001** |
| Persistent mood (affective) disorders (F34.x) | 25 | 5.8 | 6 | 4.0 | 0.671 | 0.413 |
| Neurotic, stress-related and somatoform disorders (F4x.x) | 136 | 31.4 | 42 | 28.2 | 0.542 | 0.462 |
| Phobic anxiety disorders and other anxiety disorders (F40.x-F41.x) | 99 | 22.9 | 31 | 20.8 | 0.271 | 0.603 |
| Obsessive–compulsive disorder (F42.x) | 16 | 3.7 | 6 | 4.0 | 0.034 | 0.855 |
| Reaction to severe stress, adjustment disorder (F43.x) | 23 | 5.3 | 8 | 5.4 | 0001 | 0.979 |
| Eating disorders (F50x) | 8 | 1.8 | 10 | 6.7 | **8.750** | **0.003** |
| Specific, mixed & other personality disorders (F60.x-F61.x) | 18 | 4.2 | 9 | 6.0 | 0.889 | 0.346 |
| ADHD/ hyperkinetic disorder[c](F90.x) | 13 | 3.0 | 15 | 10.1 | **12.082** | **0.001** |
| Comorbidity of above mentioned diagnoses | | | | | | |
| 0 | 147 | 33.9 | 22 | 14.8 | **34.884** | **<0.001** |
| 1 | 194 | 44.8 | 62 | 41.6 | | |
| 2+ | 92 | 21.2 | 65 | 43.6 | | |
| History of child psychiatric treatment | 35 | 8.1 | 24 | 16.1 | **7.835** | **0.005** |

**Table 1** (continued)

| | Not at-risk for and no manifest mania/ Bipolar Disorder (N=433) | | At-risk for or manifest mania/ Bipolar Disorder (N=149) | | Group differences | P-value |
|---|---|---|---|---|---|---|
| | M | SD | M | SD | t | |
| Outpatient | 20 | 4.6 | 11 | 7.4 | 1.679 | 0.195 |
| Inpatient | 19 | 4.4 | 18 | 12.1 | **11.019** | **0.001** |
| History of psychiatric treatment/ psychotherapy | 197 | 45.5 | 79 | 53.0 | 2.517 | 0.113 |
| Outpatient | 149 | 34.4 | 66 | 44.3 | **4.649** | **0.031** |
| Inpatient | 96 | 22.2 | 35 | 23.5 | 0.111 | 0.739 |
| History of medication treatment | | | | | | |
| Antidepressant | 91 | 21.0 | 39 | 26.2 | 1.700 | 0.192 |
| Mood stabilizer | 4 | 0.9 | 4 | 2.7 | 2.535 | 0.111 |
| Antipsychotic | 60 | 13.9 | 12 | 8.1 | *3.444* | *0.063* |

*N* number, % percentage, *M* mean, *SD* standard deviation, *Chi*²Chi-square, t t-test, *p* p-value,

[a] never, once, sporadically vs. frequently; [b]never, once vs.sporadically, frequently; [c]including anamnestic information;

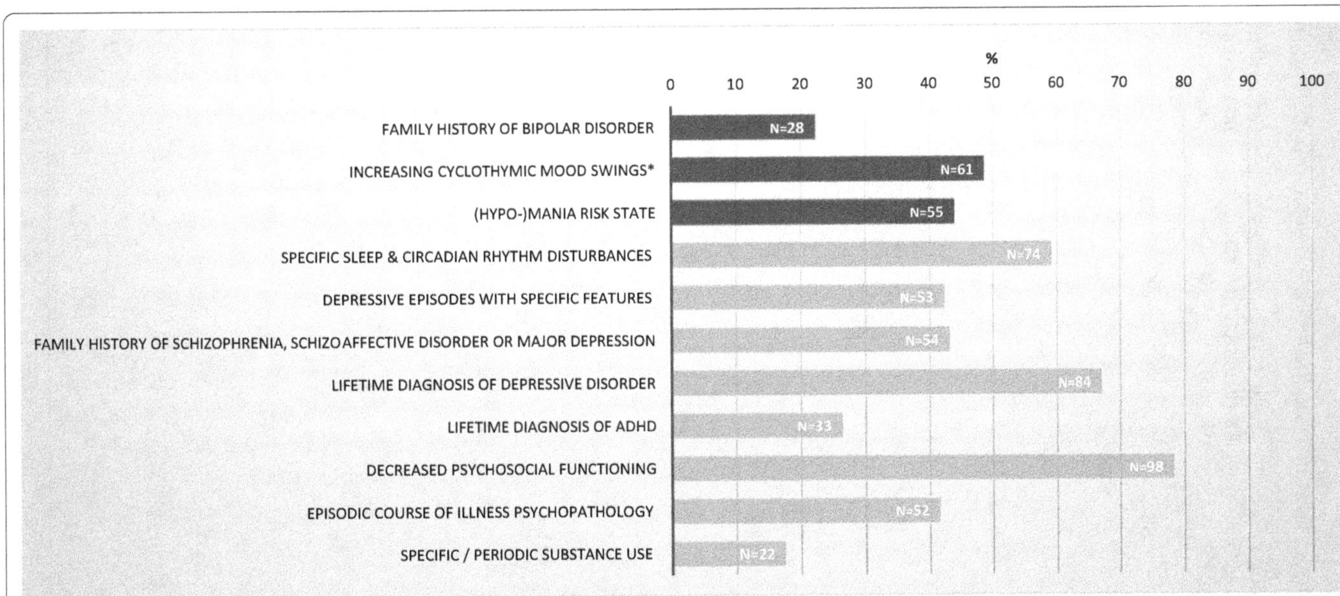


Legend: pre-defined main risk factors in dark.

*with and without increased activity; ADHD: attention-deficit/hyperactivity disorder

**Fig. 2** Distribution of a priori defined risk-factors for Bipolar Disorders according to EPI*bipolar* and BPSS (N=125)

Patients of the four groups received differential treatment recommendations by the service. In subjects of the AR+LD group significantly more frequently outpatient psychotherapy (74%), outpatient psychiatric treatment (43%) and medication with antidepressant drugs (35%) was recommended compared to the other groups. Every second person diagnosed with manifest M/BD (50%) was referred to the in-house outpatients' department with specialization on BD treatment. The remaining persons with manifest mania/BD were offered inpatient treatment (17%) or psychotherapeutic/psychiatric outpatient treatment (38%).

**Table 2** Sociodemographic and clinical characteristics for subjects in the four pre-defined groups (three BD at-risk and one manifest mania/BD) (N=149)

| | Group 1 AR (N=21) | | Group 2 AR+LD (N=49) | | Group 3 AR+(H)MR (N=55) | | Group 4 M/BD (N=24) | | Group differences with Bonferroni correction (significant results, only)[d] | p-value | Group differences for planned contrasts representing increasing risk for BD (significant results, only)[d] | p-value |
|---|---|---|---|---|---|---|---|---|---|---|---|---|
| | M | SD | M | SD | M | SD | M | SD | | | | |
| Age | 23.7 | 4.8 | 24.5 | 5.1 | 23.4 | 4.0 | 25.6 | 4.5 | | | | |
| | N | % | N | % | N | % | N | % | | | | |
| Sex | | | | | | | | | | | | |
| Female | 12 | 57.1 | 33 | 67.3 | 32 | 58.2 | 8 | 33.3 | G2 vs G4: $Chi^2=7.570$ | 0.036 | G1+G2+G3 vs G4: $Chi^2=6.565$ | 0.039 |
| Substance use | | | | | | | | | | | | |
| Nicotine use[a] | 9 | 42.9 | 21 | 44.7 | 22 | 41.5 | 12 | 60.0 | | | | |
| Alcohol[a] | 4 | 19.0 | 16 | 34.0 | 21 | 39.6 | 8 | 40.0 | | | | |
| Cannabis use[a] | 11 | 52.4 | 22 | 46.8 | 30 | 56.6 | 15 | 75.0 | | | *G1+G2+G3 vs G4:* $Chi^2=3.652$ | *0.056* |
| Amphetamine use[b] | 4 | 19.0 | 5 | 10.6 | 9 | 17.0 | 5 | 25.0 | | | | |
| Hallucinogen use[b] | 3 | 14.3 | 6 | 12.8 | 6 | 11.3 | 3 | 15.0 | | | | |
| Cocaine use[b] | 1 | 4.8 | 2 | 4.3 | 5 | 9.4 | 4 | 20.0 | | | G1+G2+G3 vs G4: $Chi^2=3.951$ | 0.041 |
| Diagnoses according to DSM-IV (current or lifetime)[#] | | | | | | | | | | | | |
| Mental/behavioral dis. due to psychoactive substance use (F1x.x) | 2 | 9.5 | 11 | 22.4 | 9 | 16.4 | 4 | 16.7 | | | | |
| Mental/behavioral dis. due to use of alcohol (F10.x) | 1 | 4.8 | 9 | 18.4 | 7 | 12.7 | 3 | 12.5 | | | | |
| Mental/behavioral dis. due to use of cannabis (F12.x) | 2 | 9.5 | 4 | 8.2 | 3 | 5.5 | 3 | 12.5 | | | | |
| Mood (Affective) Disorders (3x.x) | 0 | 0.0 | 49 | 100.0 | 35 | 63.6 | 24 | 100.0 | n.a | | n.a | |
| Manic episode/Bipolar affective disorder (wo Hypomania) (F30.x-F31.x) | 0 | 0.0 | 0 | 0.0 | 0 | 0.0 | 24 | 100.0 | n.a | | n.a | |
| Depressive Episode (F32.x) | 0 | 0.0 | 20 | 40.8 | 7 | 12.7 | 0 | 0.0 | n.a | | n.a | |
| Recurrent depressive disorder (F33.x) | 0 | 0.0 | 24 | 49.0 | 27 | 49.1 | 0 | 0.0 | n.a | | n.a | |
| Persistent mood (affective) disorders (F34.x) | 0 | 0.0 | 5 | 10.2 | 1 | 1.8 | 0 | 0.0 | n.a | | n.a | |
| Neurotic, stress-related and somatoform disorders (F4x.x) | 7 | 33.3 | 10 | 20.4 | 17 | 30.9 | 8 | 33.3 | | | | |
| Phobic anxiety disorders and other anxiety disorders (F40.x-F41.x) | 4 | 19.0 | 6 | 12.2 | 15 | 27.3 | 6 | 25.0 | | | *G1+G2vsG3+G4:* $Chi^2=3.406$ | *0.065* |
| Eating disorders (F50x) | 1 | 4.8 | 3 | 6.1 | 5 | 9.1 | 1 | 4.2 | | | | |

**Table 2** (continued)

| | Group 1 AR (N=21) | | Group 2 AR+LD (N=49) | | Group 3 AR+(H)MR (N=55) | | Group 4 M/BD (N=24) | | Group differences with Bonferroni correction (significant results, only)[d] | p-value | Group differences for planned contrasts representing increasing risk for BD (significant results, only)[d] | p-value |
|---|---|---|---|---|---|---|---|---|---|---|---|---|
| | M | SD | M | SD | M | SD | M | SD | | | | |
| Specific, mixed and other personality disorders (F60.x-F61.x) | 3 | 14.3 | 3 | 6.1 | 3 | 5.5 | 0 | 0.0 | | | *G1vsG2+G3+G4: $Chi^2=2.928$* | *0.087* |
| ADHD/ hyperkinetic disorder (F90.x)[c] | 1 | 4.8 | 4 | 8.2 | 7 | 12.7 | 3 | 12.5 | | | | |
| Comorbidity of above mentioned diagnoses 0 | 11 | 52.4 | 0 | 0.0 | 11 | 20.0 | 0 | 0.0 | G1 vs G2: $Chi^2=30.632$<br>*G1 vs G3: $Chi^2=8.655$*<br>G1 vs G4: $Chi^2=16.720$<br>G2 vs G3: $Chi^2=11.913$ | $p<0.001$<br>*$p=0.078$*<br>$p<0.001$<br>$p=0.018$ | G1vsG2+G3+G4: $Chi^2=27.810$<br>*G1+G2+G3vsG4: $Chi^2=5.340$* | $p<0.001$<br>*$p=0.069$* |
| 1 | 6 | 28.6 | 25 | 51.0 | 18 | 32.7 | 13 | 54.2 | | | | |
| 2+ | 4 | 19.0 | 24 | 49.0 | 26 | 47.3 | 11 | 45.8 | | | | |

*N* number, % percentage, *M* mean, *SD*: standard deviation, *$Chi^2$*: Chi-square, p: p-value, *n.a.* not applicable, *AR* at-risk for bipolar disorder, *LD*: lifetime depression, *(h)MR* (Hypo-)Mania Risk State, *M/BD* Manifest Mania/ Bipolar Disorder, *G1* group 1, *G2* group 2, *G3* group 3, *G4* group 4.

[a] never, once, sporadically vs. frequently; [b]never, once vs. sporadically; [c] including anamnestic information; [d]For reason of clarity we decided to present significant results only.

Statistics for non-significant results are available on request to inform future meta-analyses,

**Table 3** Treatment history and treatment recommendation of the service for subjects in the four pre-defined groups (three BD at-risk and one manifest mania/BD) (N = 149)

| | Group 1 AR (N = 21) | | Group 2 AR + LD (N = 49) | | Group 3 AR + (H)MR (N = 55) | | Group 4 M/BD (N = 24) | | Group differences with Bonferroni correction (significant results, only)[a] | p-value | Group differences for planned contrasts representing increasing risk for BD (significant results, only)[a] | p-value |
|---|---|---|---|---|---|---|---|---|---|---|---|---|
| | N | % | N | % | N | % | N | % | | | | |
| History of child psychiatric treatment | 3 | 14.3 | 6 | 12.2 | 11 | 20.0 | 4 | 16.7 | | | | |
| Outpatient | 2 | 9.5 | 2 | 4.1 | 4 | 7.3 | 3 | 12.5 | | | | |
| Inpatient | 2 | 9.5 | 5 | 10.2 | 9 | 16.4 | 2 | 8.3 | | | | |
| History of psychiatric treatment/ psychotherapy | 10 | 47.6 | 25 | 51.0 | 29 | 52.7 | 15 | 62.5 | | | | |
| Outpatient | 8 | 38.1 | 22 | 44.9 | 24 | 43.6 | 12 | 50.0 | | | | |
| Inpatient | 4 | 19.0 | 9 | 18.4 | 13 | 23.6 | 9 | 37.5 | | | *G1 + G2 + G3 vs G4: $Chi^2$ = 3.124* | *0.077* |
| History of medication treatment | | | | | | | | | | | | |
| Antidepressant | 3 | 14.3 | 13 | 26.5 | 12 | 21.8 | 11 | 45.8 | | | G1 + G2 + G3 vs G4: $Chi^2$ = 5.722 | 0.017 |
| Mood stabilizer | 1 | 4.8 | 1 | 2.0 | 1 | 1.8 | 1 | 4.2 | | | | |
| Antipsychotic | 2 | 9.5 | 2 | 4.1 | 3 | 5.5 | 5 | 20.8 | | | G1 + G2 + G3 vs G4: $Chi^2$ = 6.310 | 0.012 |
| Treatment recommendation of service | | | | | | | | | | | | |
| Psychotherapy (outpatient) | 9 | 42.9 | 36 | 73.5 | 24 | 43.6 | 9 | 37.5 | *G1 vs G2: $Chi^2$ = 6.000*<br>G2 vs G3: $Chi^2$ = 9.499<br>G2 vs G4: $Chi^2$ = 8.815 | *0.084*<br>0.012<br>0.018 | G2 + G3 vs G3 + G4: $Chi^2$ = 7.541 | 0.024 |
| Psychiatrist (outpatient) | 2 | 9.5 | 21 | 42.9 | 10 | 18.2 | 9 | 37.5 | G1 vs G2: $Chi^2$ = 7.404<br>G2 vs G3: $Chi^2$ = 7.541 | 0.042<br>0.036 | | |
| Psychiatric institutional outpatients' department (PIA) | 1 | 4.8 | 8 | 16.3 | 10 | 18.2 | 12 | 50.0 | G1 vs G4: $Chi^2$ = 11.157<br>G2 vs G4: $Chi^2$ = 9.183<br>G3 vs G4: $Chi^2$ = 8.419 | 0.006<br>0.012<br>0.024 | *G1 vs G2 + G3 + G4: $Chi^2$ = 3.819*<br>G1 + G2 vs G3 + G4: $Chi^2$ = 5.062<br>G1 + G2 + G3 vs G4: $Chi^2$ = 14.799 | *0.051*<br>0.024<br>< 0.001 |
| Inpatient treatment | 2 | 9.5 | 9 | 18.4 | 10 | 18.2 | 4 | 16.7 | | | | |
| Recommended medication of service | | | | | | | | | | | | |
| Antidepressant | 0 | 0.0 | 17 | 34.7 | 4 | 7.3 | 1 | 4.2 | G1 vs G2: $Chi^2$ = 9.623<br>G2 vs G3: $Chi^2$ = 12.091<br>G2 vs G4: $Chi^2$ = 8.081 | 0.012<br>0.006<br>0.024 | G1 vs.G2 + G3 + G4: $Chi^2$ = 4.235<br>G1 + G2vsG3 + G4: $Chi^2$ = 9.509 | 0.040<br>0.002 |
| Mood stabilizer | 0 | 0.0 | 3 | 6.1 | 5 | 9.1 | 9 | 37.5 | G1 vs G2: $Chi^2$ = 9.844<br>G2 vs G4: $Chi^2$ = 11.547<br>G3 vs G4: $Chi^2$ = 9.249 | 0.012<br>0.006<br>0.012 | *G1 vs G2 + G3 + G4: Chi2 = 3.148*<br>G1 + G2 vs G3 + G4: $Chi^2$ = 6.629<br>G1 + G2 + G3 vs G4: $Chi^2$ = 19.267 | *0.076*<br>0.010<br>< 0.001 |
| Antipsychotic | 2 | 9.5 | 0 | 0.0 | 3 | 5.5 | 1 | 4.2 | | | | |

*N* number, % percentage, *M* mean, *SD* standard deviation, *$Chi^2$* Chi-square, *t* t-test, *p* p-value, *n.a.* not applicable, *AR* at-risk for bipolar disorder, *LD* lifetime depression, *(h)MR* (Hypo-)Mania Risk State, *M/BD* Manifest Mania/ Bipolar Disorder, G1: group 1, G2: group 2, G3: group 3, G4: group 4.

[a] For reason of clarity we decided to present significant results only.

Statistics for non-significant results are available on request to inform future meta-analyses

Moodwstabilizers were recommended with increasing frequency from the AR to the M/BD group (0%, 6%, 9% and 38%).

## Discussion

This analysis examined sociodemographic, clinical and psychopathological characteristics as well as treatment histories of help-seeking persons who were seen at the Early Detection and Intervention Center Dresden from 2009 to 2018. Based on the characteristics, differential at-risk groups for BD were compared and treatment recommendations analyzed. The at-risk sample of our cohort is distinct from offspring samples of BD patients who were focused on in risk research so far (Canadian offspring study, Duffy et al. 2010; Pittsburgh Bipolar Offspring Study, BIOS, Birmaher et al. 2010; Dutch Bipolar Offspring Cohort Study, Wals et al. 2001 and Preisig et al. 2016).

The main findings of the analysis are:

- About one in five young help-seeking clients that completed the diagnostic process met the at-risk definition for bipolar disorders.
- Of the pre-defined main risk factors, increasing cyclothymic mood swings with increased activity was present in about half of the at-risk patients, a (hypo-) mania risk state in about forty percent, a positive family history in only about one in five. Decreased psychosocial functioning (about four in five), lifetime depression (two thirds) and specific sleep and rhythm disturbances (about 60%) were the most frequent secondary risk factors.
- Manifest diagnoses apart from BD were present in the majority of at-risk patients with increasing frequency of at least two diagnoses along the risk groups. Substance use was very common in at-risk patients and highest in patients diagnosed with manifest mania/BD, with use of cannabis in up to three quarters and alcohol in up to 40%.
- Treatment history was rather similar across groups.
- Regarding treatment recommendations, psychotherapy was frequently recommended in subjects at-risk for BD with a lifetime depression. Specialized treatment, including mood stabilizers, was recommended most frequently in manifest mania/BD patients.

Given a lifetime prevalence of BD of about 3%, a substantial amount of persons (one in five) met the at-risk definition for BD in this help-seeking sample of adolescents and young adults. Data to relate this frequency to are rare. For instance, in the Orygen Youth Health study 11% (N=59/559) of the clients fulfilled BAR criteria and did not meet the exclusion criteria (including an (un) treated hypomania, a psychotic episode or current/past mood stabilizer treatment, Bechdolf et al. 2014). Reasons for the higher frequency compared to the Australian help-seeking sample might be that we included patients older than 25 years and did not exclude those with a history of mood stabilizer treatment. Moreover, the EPI-*bipolar* risk assessment interview used in our study includes more potential risk symptoms for BD.

About 22% of at-risk patients indicated a history of BD in a first degree relative. Whether or not at-risk patients will develop BD is being evaluated as part of our ongoing follow-up analyses. Studies in offspring cohorts reported that 9–22% of children of BD patients developed BD-spectrum disorders (Faedda et al. 2019). In our sample about four out of five help-seeking youth at potential risk did not report a positive family history. This renders the assessment and integration of psychopathological and other clinical information into the early detection process vital, as merely the monitoring of offspring will not detect all people at-risk for BD. Early detection and intervention services that are able to offer low-threshold and comprehensive diagnostic procedures to help-seeking young people, as "Dresden early on", could undertake this challenge.

Data is scarce regarding the prevalence of individual at-risk symptoms for the development of BD in help-seeking patients. A recent meta-analysis including 11 studies of differential cohorts revealed that the most common symptoms before the first mood episode were too much energy (68%), diminished ability to think, (63%), indecisiveness (62%), pressured speech (60%), talkativeness (60%), elated mood (58%), academic or work difficulties (56%), insomnia (54%, coded separately from decreased need for sleep), depressed mood (53%), and over-productive/goal-directed behavior (50%) (van Meter et al. 2016). The findings are in part overlapping with our data with respect to e.g. subthreshold hypomanic symptoms and depression. Additionally, sleep disturbances were seen in equal frequency and academic or work difficulties in more than half of our at-risk patients, too. We also observed an overlap with psychosis risk syndromes, e.g. regarding depressive symptoms and those related to anxiety (Fusar-Poli et al. 2020).

The finding of substance use in a high proportion of at-risk patients and in patients diagnosed with manifest mania/BD (with cannabis and alcohol being the most frequent substances) is in line with published evidence (Brietzke et al. 2012; Goldstein et al. 2013; Leopold et al. 2012; van Meter et al. 2016). Results are indicative of an early onset of substance misuse or substance use disorders in persons who later manifest BD (Beesdo-Baum et al. 2015). Patients with substance use disorders usually show low utilization of mental health care services

(Mack et al. 2014). The Early Detection and Intervention Center Dresden with its low-threshold service seems to be an early opportunity to reach individuals at-risk for BD who present with unfavorable substance use habits. Drug counselling was recommended by our service in all identified cases and was part of the recommended psychotherapy. Overall, the frequency of substance use in subjects was higher compared to those published in 2008 for a German help-seeking sample of the Early Recognition and Intervention Center Cologne (Germany) (4–5%) (Schultze-Lutter et al. 2008). This difference might be partially due to varying diagnostic procedures (with differences in the detail of screening) and clinical foci of the two institutions (e.g. the service in Cologne is specialized in the early recognition of psychosis whereas that in Dresden has a somewhat broader outreach) and due to a change in overall substance use rates in Germany during this period. In the above mentioned recent meta-analysis regarding psychosis risk syndromes, 27% of young people at risk for psychosis were cannabis users, a lower proportion compared to our risk-sample. It has to be kept in mind when comparing our rates of substance use to that in other samples that our clientele to a great extend did not present for drug use issues as there are local low-threshold community drug counselling services available that are highly responsive to that issues.

Treatment histories were rather similar in help-seeking persons with and without risk for BD. Interestingly, 50% of subjects who fulfilled any of the pre-defined at-risk factors for BD or even satisfied the diagnostic criteria for manifest BD reported a history of psychiatric treatment, including psychotherapy. However, the increased risk for BD was rarely recognized by the previous care provider and only few patients were referred to the Early Detection and Intervention Center Dresden to evaluate the suspected diagnosis of BD or subthreshold symptomatology. This finding can be partially explained by the fact that emerging BD often is characterized by heterogeneous and non-specific symptomatology (Leopold and Pfennig et al. 2013; Lambert et al. 2016; Hauser and Correll 2013). However, early recognition of BD is very important as persons at-risk for BD or manifest BD/mania often suffer from symptoms such as sleep/circadian rhythm disturbances and functional impairment (60% and 80% of those persons in our sample). Additionally, antidepressant monotherapy was rather frequent in our at-risk subjects. This treatment approach should have been accompanied by close clinical monitoring because of its potential to generate or accelerate (hypo)manic symptomatology (DGBS and DGPPN 2019).

Psychiatric comorbidity in BD is often associated with a more severe course, poorer treatment adherence, and worse outcomes related to suicide and other complications. Additionally, it requires consideration when prescribing drugs (DGBS and DGPPN 2019). In line with previous evidence (Krishnan 2005), patients at-risk for BD or with manifest BD had significantly elevated rates of mental or behavioral disorders due to the (mis-)use of alcohol, recurrent depressive disorder, eating disorders and/or ADHD/hyperkinetic disorder. However, it is often unclear whether a co-occurring disorder is truly comorbid, a precursor of the disorder, a consequence of treatment, or a combination of those options (Faedda et al. 2019). Of the aforementioned comorbidities, that of eating disorders and BD seems the most underestimated in research and clinical service. There is recent evidence for higher rates of binge eating disorder and bulimia nervosa in BD (McElroy et al. 2016; Thiebaut et al. 2019). However, little is known about the timing of symptom onset, the individual trajectories of the disorders when co-occurring and the interaction of symptoms (Thiebaut et al. 2019). Data from a qualitative study suggest that in some patients symptoms of the eating disorder preceded the onset of BD (McAulay et al. 2021). Clinicians have to evaluate and monitor patients with BD and at-risk for BD for the presence and the development of any comorbid psychiatric condition to ensure appropriate interventions while avoiding potential iatrogenic complications. Moreover, clinicians should consider underlying or developing BD when evaluating individuals with other psychiatric diagnoses that often coexist with BD (not just unipolar depression). Anticonvulsants and other mood stabilizers may be especially helpful in treating BD patients with significant comorbidity (Krishnan 2005).

At the Early Detection and Intervention Center Dresden, no pre-defined treatment algorithm was followed and treatment recommendations were reached in a decision making process based on the clinical need, best available evidence and clinical expertise. Psychotherapy was recommended for the majority of subjects at-risk for BD, especially for patients who also met criteria for depression. Psychotherapy seems to be more acceptable to young patients at-risk compared to pharmacologic treatments (Rios et al. 2015). Preliminary studies of various psychotherapies, including psychoeducation strategies tailored specifically for BD in adolescents and young adults show promising results (Pavuluri et al. 2005; Pfennig et al. 2017) and should be considered when developing or revising evidence-based treatment guidelines for the early stages of BD.

Our results show that drug recommendation differed across the four at-risk BD groups. In at-risk youth with depression and no (hypo-)mania risk state (AR+LD), more frequently antidepressants were recommended. When a (hypo-)mania risk was present (AR+(H)MR), monotherapy with antidepressants was discouraged and mood stabilizers were recommended, the latter with the highest percentage in case of manifest mania/BD. These pharmacological recommendations are in line with current guideline recommendations. They reflect the favorable risk to benefit ratio of antidepressants compared to mood stabilizers in case of young people at risk for BD without (hypo-)mania risk state and the higher risk of instability and switch of antidepressant monotherapy when (hypo-)manic symptomatology becomes more present (DGBS and DGPPN 2019; Leopold and Pfennig et al. 2013).

Limitations: Although this analysis summarizes the experience of nine years work at the Early Detection and Intervention Center Dresden and provides clues for a better description and understanding of various risk constellations for BD, the following limitations have to be noticed: (1) data were collected in a clinical routine setting over a period of nine years. Within this period, progression regarding treatment recommendations and increasing clinical experiences of the service staff have to be considered. (2) Early detection instruments were not fully validated yet and psychometric properties need further examination (Correll and Olvet et al. 2014; Leopold et al. 2012). (3) Recall bias and inaccuracies regarding e.g. former treatment cannot be ruled out. Information on preceding mental disorders and treatment history can be biased or incomplete, since it was assessed retrospectively. However, illness history information is very important since preceding psychopathology is associated with the course of disease, and pretreatment experiences might be relevant for further health care utilization and treatment adherence (Duffy et al. 2017; Hafeman et al. 2016). (4) Another concern pertains to the phenotypic heterogeneity of at-risk states of BD. Due to the episodic character, the fluctuation of symptom severity and variations of functional impairment, early stages of BD are more complex and more difficult to identify than that of psychotic disorders (Brietzke et al. 2012; Duffy et al. 2017; Kafali et al. 2019; Rios et al. 2015; Hauser and Correll 2013). Non-specific symptoms may lead to false positive cases, and the typical overlap with potential preceding disorders and comorbidities further hampers adequate staging (Axelson et al. 2015; Duffy et al. 2017; Geller et al. 2002). However, help-seeking behavior and impairing symptomatology confirm the need of early diagnosis and individual treatment. (5) Thus far, this analysis only includes baseline data, a follow-up survey is underway to investigate long-term outcomes. (6) Finally, our findings stem from a sample of help-seeking adolescents and young adults. Results might not be generalizable to adolescents and young adults in general or to persons who decide not to engage in counselling, diagnostics or treatment.

## Conclusion

Despite the limitations inherent to the naturalistic research design and its descriptive character, in view of implications of the results for the long-term trajectory of the illness course this study clearly indicates the necessity of more research on stage-specific interventions, especially for the early phases of BD. A better understanding of the risk factors for BD and a clearer picture of the phenomenology of emerging BD offer hope for early identification and prevention (Pavuluri et al. 2005). Early detection and intervention of BD require detailed prospective examination in further studies, focusing on phenomenology of different at-risk states and examination of adequate, stage-specific treatment (Rios et al. 2015). Especially during early stages of BD, it is hoped that these research efforts will help provide data that guide clinicians towards tailored interventions with greater effectiveness in preventing or, at least, postponing the conversion to manifest BD. Clinical follow-up data could promote further development of evidence-based treatment approaches in early stages of BD (Berk et al. 2007; Kapczinski et al. 2009; Leopold and Pfeiffer et al. 2013). Studies on the feasibility, efficacy and cost-effectiveness of clinical approved interventions could be a next step (McGorry et al. 2006).

### Abbreviations

ADHD: Attention-deficit/hyperactivity disorder; APA: American Psychiatric Association; AR: EPI*bipolar* at-risk status; BAR criteria: Bipolar at-risk criteria; BD: Bipolar Disorder; BPSS-FP: Bipolar Prodrome Symptom Scale-Prospective; DSM-IV: Diagnostic and Statistical Manual of mental Disorders, 4th Edition; DSM-IV-TR: Diagnostic and Statistical Manual of mental Disorders, 4th Edition, Text revision; EPI*bipolar*: Early Phase Inventory for Bipolar Disorders; (H)MR: (Hypo-)mania risk state (BPSS-FP); ICC: Intraclass correlation coefficient; IBM SPSS: Software package Statistical Package for the Social Sciences (SPSS) produced by International Business Machines Corporation (IBM); LD: Lifetime depression (SCID-I); M/BD: Manifest mania/ BD (SCID-I); SCID-I: Structured Clinical Interview for DSM-IV Axis I disorders; SIBARS: Semistructured Interview for Bipolar At Risk States.

### Acknowledgements

Professor Young's independent research funded by the National Institute for Health Research (NIHR) Biomedical Research Centre at South London and Maudsley NHS Foundation Trust and King's College London. The views expressed are those of the authors and not necessarily those of the NHS, the NIHR, or the Department of Health. We thank Dr. Philipp Ritter from the Department of Psychiatry and Psychotherapy, Carl Gustav Carus University Hospital, Technische Universität Dresden for commenting the manuscript and language editing.

### Authors' contributions

JM conceptualized and designed the analyses, carried out the statistical analyses and the interpretation of the data, drafted the initial manuscript and approved the final manuscript as submitted. AP and KLdesigned the data collection instruments, established "Dresden early on", collected data for the study, critically reviewed the manuscript and approved the final manuscript as submitted. MB established "Dresden early on" together with AP and KL, collected data for the study, critically reviewed the manuscript and approved the final manuscript as submitted. S. Pfeiffer is responsible for data management, was involved in the statistical analyses critically reviewed the manuscript and approved the final manuscript as submitted. AY, PFP, CC and AB critically reviewed the manuscript and approved the final manuscript as submitted. All authors read and approved the final manuscript.

#### Competing interests

AP has received speakers honoraria and travel support from Janssen and Lundbeck. KL has been an advisor to and received speakers honoraria and travel support from Janssen, Lundbeck, Otsuka and Recordati. She received grant support from Janssen and Otsuka. JM, AY has received speakers honoraria and travel support from Janssen and Lundbeck, Sunovion, COMPASS and Livanova. CC has been a consultant and/or advisor to or have received honoraria from: Acadia, Alkermes, Allergan, Angelini, Axsome, Gedeon Richter, Gerson Lehrman Group, Indivior, IntraCellular Therapies, Janssen/J&J, Karuna, LB Pharma, Lundbeck, MedAvante-ProPhase, MedInCell, Medscape, Merck, Mylan, Neurocrine, Noven, Otsuka, Pfizer, Recordati, Rovi, Servier, Sumitomo Dainippon, Sunovion, Supernus, Takeda, and Teva. He provided expert testimony for Janssen and Otsuka. He served on a Data Safety Monitoring Board for Lundbeck, Rovi, Supernus, and Teva. He has received grant support from Janssen and Takeda. He is also a stock option holder of LB Pharma. AB, SP, MB state to have no conflict of interest.

#### Author details

[1]Department of Psychiatry and Psychotherapy, Carl Gustav Carus University Hospital, Technische Universität Dresden, Fetscherstraße 74, 01307 Dresden, Germany. [2]Department of Psychiatry, Psychotherapy and Psychosomatics, Vivantes Klinikum Am Urban, Berlin, Germany. [3]Department of Child- and Adolescent Psychiatry and Psychotherapy, Carl Gustav Carus University Hospital, Technische Universität Dresden, Dresden, Germany. [4]Early Psychosis: Intervention and Clinical-Detection (EPIC) Lab, Institute of Psychiatry, Psychology and Neuroscience, King's College London, London, UK. [5]Department of Brain and Behavioral Sciences, University of Pavia, Pavia, Italy. [6]Department of Psychological Medicine, Institute of Psychiatry, Psychology and Neuroscience, King's College London & South London and Maudsley NHS Foundation Trust, Bethlem Royal Hospital, London, UK. [7]Department of Child- and Adolescent Psychiatry and Psychotherapy, Charité Universitätsmedizin, Berlin, Germany. [8]Department of Psychiatry, The Zucker Hillside Hospital, Northwell Health, Glen Oaks, NY, USA. [9]Donald and Barbara Zucker School of Medicine At Hofstra/Northwell, Department of Psychiatry and Molecular Medicine, Hempstead, NY, USA.

#### References

American Psychiatric Association. Ethical principles of psychologists and code of conduct. 2003. https://www.apa.org/ethics/code/ethics-code-2017.pdf. Accessed 15 Aug 2019.

American Psychiatric Association. Diagnostic and statistical manual of mental disorders: DSM-IV-TR. 4th ed. Arlington, VA: American Psychiatric Assoc; 2007.

Axelson D, Goldstein B, Goldstein T, Monk K, Yu H, Hickey MB, et al. Diagnostic precursors to bipolar disorder in offspring of parents with bipolar disorder: a longitudinal study. Am J Psychiatry. 2015;172(7):638–46. https://doi.org/10.1176/appi.ajp.2014.14010035.

Baldessarini RJ, Tondo L, Hennen J. Treatment-latency and previous episodes: Relationships to pretreatment morbidity and response to maintenance treatment in bipolar I and II disorders. Bipolar Disord. 2003;5(3):169–79.

Bechdolf A, Nelson B, Cotton SM, Chanen A, Thompson A, Kettle J, et al. A preliminary evaluation of the validity of at-risk criteria for bipolar disorders in help-seeking adolescents and young adults. J Affect Disord. 2010;127(1–3):316–20. https://doi.org/10.1016/j.jad.2010.06.016.

Bechdolf A, Ratheesh A, Wood SJ, Tecic T, Conus P, Nelson B, et al. Rationale and first results of developing at-risk (prodromal) criteria for bipolar disorder. Curr Pharm Des. 2012;18(4):358–75.

Bechdolf A, Ratheesh A, Cotton SM, Nelson B, Chanen AM, Betts J, et al. The predictive validity of bipolar at-risk (prodromal) criteria in help-seeking adolescents and young adults: A prospective study. Bipolar Disord. 2014;16(5):493–504. https://doi.org/10.1111/bdi.12205.

Beesdo-Baum K, Knappe S, Asselmann E, Zimmermann P, Brückl T, Höfler M, et al. The "Early Developmental Stages of Psychopathology (EDSP) study": a 20-year review of methods and findings. Soc Psychiatry Psychiatr Epidemiol. 2015;50(6):851–66. https://doi.org/10.1007/s00127-015-1062-x

Benchimol EI, Smeeth L, Guttmann A, Harron K, Moher D, Petersen I, et al. The REporting of studies Conducted using Observational Routinely-collected health Data (RECORD) statement. PLoS Med. 2015;12(10):e1001885. https://doi.org/10.1371/journal.pmed.1001885.

Berk M, Conus P, Lucas N, Hallam K, Malhi GS, Dodd S, et al. Setting the stage: From prodrome to treatment resistance in bipolar disorder. Bipolar Disord. 2007;9(7):671–8.

Berk M, Post R, Ratheesh A, Gliddon E, Singh A, Vieta E, et al. Staging in bipolar disorder: from theoretical framework to clinical utility. World Psychiatry. 2017;16(3):236–44. https://doi.org/10.1002/wps.20441.

Birmaher B, Axelson D, Goldstein B, Monk K, Kalas C, Obreja M, et al. Psychiatric disorders in preschool offspring of parents with bipolar disorder: the Pittsburgh Bipolar Offspring Study (BIOS). Am J Psychiatry. 2010;167(3):321–30. https://doi.org/10.1176/appi.ajp.2009.09070977.

Brietzke E, Mansur RB, Soczynska JK, Kapczinski F, Bressan RA, McIntyre RS. Towards a multifactorial approach for prediction of bipolar disorder in at risk populations. J Affect Disord. 2012;140(1):82–91. https://doi.org/10.1016/j.jad.2012.02.016.

Carlson GA, Bromet EJ, Sievers S. Phenomenology and outcome of subjects with early- and adult-onset psychotic mania. Am J Psychiatry. 2000;157(2):213–9. https://doi.org/10.1176/appi.ajp.157.2.213.

Chang KD, Dienes K, Blasey C, Adleman N, Ketter T, Steiner H. Divalproex monotherapy in the treatment of bipolar offspring with mood and behavioral disorders and at least mild affective symptoms. J Clin Psychiatry. 2003;64(8):936–42.

Chen YW, Dilsaver SC. Lifetime rates of suicide attempts among subjects with bipolar and unipolar disorders relative to subjects with other Axis I disorders. Biol Psychiatry. 1996;39(10):896–9. https://doi.org/10.1016/0006-3223(95)00295-2.

Chia MF, Cotton S, Filia K, Phelan M, Conus P, Jauhar S, et al. Early intervention for bipolar disorder - Do current treatment guidelines provide recommendations for the early stages of the disorder? J Affect Disord. 2019;257:669–77. https://doi.org/10.1016/j.jad.2019.07.062.

Collins PY, Patel V, Joestl SS, March D, Insel TR, Daar AS, et al. Grand challenges in global mental health. Nature. 2011;475(7354):27–30. https://doi.org/10.1038/475027a.

Correll CU, Olvet DM, Auther AM, Hauser M, Kishimoto T, Carrion RE, et al. The bipolar prodrome symptom interview and scale-prospective (BPSS-P): Description and validation in a psychiatric sample and healthy controls. Bipolar Disord. 2014a;16(5):505–22. https://doi.org/10.1111/bdi.12209.

Correll CU, Hauser M, Penzner JB, Auther AM, Kafantaris V, Saito E, et al. Type and duration of subsyndromal symptoms in youth with bipolar I disorder prior to their first manic episode. Bipolar Disord. 2014b;16(5):478–92. https://doi.org/10.1111/bdi.12194.

Cotton S, Luberto CM, Sears RW, Strawn JR, Stahl L, Wasson RS, et al. Mindfulness-based cognitive therapy for youth with anxiety disorders at risk for bipolar disorder: A pilot trial. Early Interv Psychiatry. 2016;10(5):426–34. https://doi.org/10.1111/eip.12216.

Craddock N, Sklar P. Genetics of bipolar disorder: Successful start to a long journey. Trends Genet. 2009;25(2):99–105. https://doi.org/10.1016/j.tig.2008.12.002.

DelBello MP, Adler CM, Whitsel RM, Stanford KE, Strakowski SM. A 12-week single-blind trial of quetiapine for the treatment of mood symptoms in adolescents at high risk for developing bipolar I disorder. J Clin Psychiatry. 2007;68(5):789–95.

DGBS, DGPPN. S3-Leitlinie zur Diagnostik und Therapie Bipolarer Störungen: Langversion 2.0 Update vom Februar 2019; 2019.

Duffy A, Alda M, Hajek T, Sherry SB, Grof P. Early stages in the development of bipolar disorder. J Affect Disord. 2010;121(1–2):127–35. https://doi.org/10.1016/j.jad.2009.05.022.

Duffy A, Horrocks J, Doucette S, Keown-Stoneman C, McCloskey S, Grof P. The developmental trajectory of bipolar disorder. Br J Psychiatry. 2014;204(2):122–8. https://doi.org/10.1192/bjp.bp.113.126706.

Duffy A, Vandeleur C, Heffer N, Preisig M. The clinical trajectory of emerging bipolar disorder among the high-risk offspring of bipolar parents: current understanding and future considerations. Int J Bipolar Disord. 2017;5(1):37. https://doi.org/10.1186/s40345-017-0106-4.

Faedda GL, Serra G, Marangoni C, Salvatore P, Sani G, Vazquez GH, et al. Clinical risk factors for bipolar disorders: A systematic review of prospective studies. J Affect Disord. 2014;168:314–21. https://doi.org/10.1016/j.jad.2014.07.013.

Faedda GL, Baldessarini RJ, Marangoni C, Bechdolf A, Berk M, Birmaher B, et al. An International Society of bipolar disorders task force report: Precursors and prodromes of bipolar disorder. Bipolar Disord. 2019;21(8):720–40. https://doi.org/10.1111/bdi.12831.

Findling RL, Frazier TW, Youngstrom EA, McNamara NK, Stansbrey RJ, Gracious BL, et al. Double-blind, placebo-controlled trial of divalproex monotherapy in the treatment of symptomatic youth at high risk for developing bipolar disorder. J Clin Psychiatry. 2007;68(5):781–8.

Findling RL, Youngstrom EA, Rowles BM, Deyling E, Lingler J, Stansbrey RJ, et al. A double-blind and placebo-controlled trial of Aripiprazole in symptomatic youths at genetic high risk for bipolar disorder. J Child Adolesc Psychopharmacol. 2017;27(10):864–74. https://doi.org/10.1089/cap.2016.0160.

First MB, Spitzer RL, Gibbon M, Williams JBW. Structured Clinical Interview for DSM-IV Axis I Disorders (SCID I). New York: State Psychiatric Institute; 1997a.

First MB, Gibbon M, Spitzer RL, Williams JBW, Benjamin LS. Structured Clinical Interview for DSM-IV Axis II Personality Disorders, (SCID-II). Washington, DC: American Psychiatric Press; 1997b.

Forsman AK, Ventus DBJ, van der Feltz-Cornelis CM, Wahlbeck K. Public mental health research in Europe: A systematic mapping for the ROAMER project. Eur J Public Health. 2014;24(6):955–60. https://doi.org/10.1093/eurpub/cku055.

Forsman AK, Wahlbeck K, Aarø LE, Alonso J, Barry MM, Brunn M, et al. Research priorities for public mental health in Europe: Recommendations of the ROAMER project. Eur J Public Health. 2015;25(2):249–54. https://doi.org/10.1093/eurpub/cku232.

Fusar-Poli P, De MA, Rocchetti M, Cappucciati M, Ramella-Cravaro V, Rutigliano G, et al. Semistructured interview for bipolar at risk states (SIBARS). Psychiatry Res. 2018;264:302–9. https://doi.org/10.1016/j.psychres.2018.03.074.

Fusar-Poli P, Bauer M, Borgwardt S, Bechdolf A, Correll CU, Do KQ, et al. European college of neuropsychopharmacology network on the prevention of mental disorders and mental health promotion (ECNP PMD-MHP). Eur Neuropsychopharmacol. 2019;29(12):1301–11. https://doi.org/10.1016/j.euroneuro.2019.09.006.

Fusar-Poli P, de Pablo GS, Correll CU, Meyer-Lindenberg A, Millan MJ, Borgwardt S, et al. Prevention of psychosis: advances in detection, prognosis, and intervention. JAMA Psychiat. 2020;77(7):755–65. https://doi.org/10.1001/jamapsychiatry.2019.4779.

Geller B, Cooper TB, Zimerman B, Frazier J, Williams M, Heath J, Warner K. Lithium for prepubertal depressed children with family history predictors of future bipolarity: A double-blind, placebo-controlled study. J Affect Disord. 1998;51(2):165–75.

Geller B, Zimerman B, Williams M, DelBello MP, Frazier J, Beringer L. Phenomenology of prepubertal and early adolescent bipolar disorder: examples of elated mood, grandiose behaviors, decreased need for sleep, racing thoughts and hypersexuality. J Child Adolesc Psychopharmacol. 2002;12(1):3–9. https://doi.org/10.1089/10445460252943524.

Goldberg JF, Ernst CL. Features associated with the delayed initiation of mood stabilizers at illness onset in bipolar disorder. J Clin Psychiatry. 2002;63(11):985–91.

Goldstein BI, Strober M, Axelson D, Goldstein TR, Gill MK, Hower H, et al. Predictors of first-onset substance use disorders during the prospective course of bipolar spectrum disorders in adolescents. J Am Acad Child Adolesc Psychiatry. 2013;52(10):1026–37. https://doi.org/10.1016/j.jaac.2013.07.009.

Goldstein TR, Fersch-Podrat R, Axelson DA, Gilbert A, Hlastala SA, Birmaher B, Frank E. Early intervention for adolescents at high risk for the development of bipolar disorder: pilot study of Interpersonal and Social Rhythm Therapy (IPSRT). Psychotherapy (chic). 2014;51(1):180–9. https://doi.org/10.1037/a0034396.

Goldstein TR, Merranko J, Krantz M, Garcia M, Franzen P, Levenson J, et al. Early intervention for adolescents at-risk for bipolar disorder: A pilot randomized trial of Interpersonal and Social Rhythm Therapy (IPSRT). J Affect Disord. 2018;235:348–56. https://doi.org/10.1016/j.jad.2018.04.049

Gorgens KA. Structured Clinical Interview for DSM-IV (SCID-I/SCID-II). In: Kreutzer et al. (eds.) Encyclopedia of Clinical Neuropsychology. Springer International Publishing AG; 2018.

Hafeman DM, Merranko J, Axelson D, Goldstein BI, Goldstein T, Monk K, et al. Toward the Definition of a Bipolar Prodrome: Dimensional Predictors of Bipolar Spectrum Disorders in At-Risk Youths. Am J Psychiatry. 2016;173(7):695–704. https://doi.org/10.1176/appi.ajp.2015.15040414.

Hauser M, Correll CU. The significance of at-risk or prodromal symptoms for bipolar I disorder in children and adolescents. Can J Psychiatry. 2013;58(1):22–31.

Howes OD, Lim S, Theologos G, Yung AR, Goodwin GM, McGuire P. A comprehensive review and model of putative prodromal features of bipolar affective disorder. Psychological Medicine. 2010;FirstView:1–11.

Hunt J, Schwarz CM, Nye P, Frazier E. Is there a bipolar prodrome among children and adolescents? Curr Psychiatry Rep. 2016;18(4):35. https://doi.org/10.1007/s11920-016-0676-3.

Kafali HY, Bildik T, Bora E, Yuncu Z, Erermis HS. Distinguishing prodromal stage of bipolar disorder and early onset schizophrenia spectrum disorders during adolescence. Psychiatry Res. 2019;275:315–25. https://doi.org/10.1016/j.psychres.2019.03.051.

Kapczinski F, Dias VV, Kauer-Sant'Anna M, Frey BN, Grassi-Oliveira R, Colom F, Berk M. Clinical implications of a staging model for bipolar disorders. Expert Rev Neurother. 2009;9(7):957–66. https://doi.org/10.1586/ern.09.31.

Kessing LV, Vradi E, Andersen PK. Starting lithium prophylaxis early versus late in bipolar disorder. Br J Psychiatry. 2014;205(3):214–20. https://doi.org/10.1192/bjp.bp.113.142802.

Krishnan KRR. Psychiatric and medical comorbidities of bipolar disorder. Psychosom Med. 2005;67(1):1–8. https://doi.org/10.1097/01.psy.0000151489.36347.18.

Lambert M, Niehaus V, Correll C. Pharmacotherapy in children and adolescents at clinical-high risk for psychosis and bipolar disorder. Pharmacopsychiatry. 2016;49(6):229–44. https://doi.org/10.1055/s-0042-116668.

Leopold K, Ritter P, Correll CU, Marx C, Ozgurdal S, Juckel G, et al. Risk constellations prior to the development of bipolar disorders: Rationale of a new risk assessment tool. J Affect Disord. 2012;136(3):1000–10. https://doi.org/10.1016/j.jad.2011.06.043.

Leopold K, Pfeiffer S, Correll CU, Bauer M, Pfennig A. Early recognition centers for mental disorders - A complementary supply in the German health system. Psychiatr Prax. 2013a. https://doi.org/10.1055/s-0032-1332972.

Leopold K, Pfennig A, Severus E, Bauer M. Prevention of bipolar disorders. Nervenarzt. 2013b;84(11):1310–5. https://doi.org/10.1007/s00115-013-3834-4.

Leopold K, Ratzer S, Correll CU, Rottmann-Wolf M, Pfeiffer S, Ritter P, et al. Characteristics, symptomatology and naturalistic treatment in individuals at-risk for bipolar disorders: Baseline results in the first 180 help-seeking individuals assessed at the Dresden high-risk project. J Affect Disord. 2014;152–154:427–33. https://doi.org/10.1016/j.jad.2013.10.009.

Leopold K, Bauer M, Bechdolf A, Correll CU, Holtmann M, Juckel G, et al. Efficacy of cognitive-behavioral group therapy in patients at risk for serious mental illness presenting with subthreshold bipolar symptoms: Results from a prespecified interim analysis of a multicenter, randomized, controlled study. Bipolar Disord. 2020. https://doi.org/10.1111/bdi.12894.

Luby JL, Navsaria N. Pediatric bipolar disorder: evidence for prodromal states and early markers. J Child Psychol Psychiatry. 2010;51(4):459–71. https://doi.org/10.1111/j.1469-7610.2010.02210.x.

Mack S, Jacobi F, Gerschler A, Strehle J, Höfler M, Busch MA, et al. Self-reported utilization of mental health services in the adult German population–evidence for unmet needs? Results of the DEGS1-Mental Health Module (DEGS1-MH). Int J Methods Psychiatr Res. 2014;23(3):289–303. https://doi.org/10.1002/mpr.1438.

Matza LS, Rajagopalan KS, Thompson CL, de Lissovoy G. Misdiagnosed patients with bipolar disorder: Comorbidities, treatment patterns, and direct treatment costs. J Clin Psychiatry. 2005;66(11):1432–40.

McAulay C, Dawson L, Mond J, Outhred T, Touyz S. "The food matches the mood": experiences of eating disorders in bipolar disorder. Qual Health Res. 2021;31(1):100–12. https://doi.org/10.1177/1049732320956267.

McElroy SL, Crow S, Blom TJ, Biernacka JM, Winham SJ, Geske J, et al. Prevalence and correlates of DSM-5 eating disorders in patients with bipolar disorder. J Affect Disord. 2016;191:216–21. https://doi.org/10.1016/j.jad.2015.11.010

McGorry PD, Hickie IB, Yung AR, Pantelis C, Jackson HJ. Clinical staging of psychiatric disorders: A heuristic framework for choosing earlier, safer and more effective interventions. Aust N Z J Psychiatry. 2006;40(8):616–22. https://doi.org/10.1080/j.1440-1614.2006.01860.x.

McNamara RK, Strawn JR, Chang KD, DelBello MP. Interventions for youth at high risk for bipolar disorder and schizophrenia. Child Adolesc Psychiatr Clin N Am. 2012;21(4):739–51. https://doi.org/10.1016/j.chc.2012.07.009.

Mendlewicz J, Rainer JD. Adoption study supporting genetic transmission in manic–depressive illness. Nature. 1977;268(5618):327–9.

Miklowitz DJ, Schneck CD, Singh MK, Taylor DO, George EL, Cosgrove VE, et al. Early intervention for symptomatic youth at risk for bipolar disorder: A randomized trial of family-focused therapy. J Am Acad Child Adolesc Psychiatry. 2013;52(2):121–31. https://doi.org/10.1016/j.jaac.2012.10.007.

Miller S, Dell'Osso B, Ketter TA. The prevalence and burden of bipolar depression. J Affect Disord. 2014;169:S3–11. https://doi.org/10.1016/S0165-0327(14)70003-5.

Pavuluri MN, Birmaher B, Naylor MW. Pediatric bipolar disorder: a review of the past 10 years. J Am Acad Child Adolesc Psychiatry. 2005;44(9):846–71. https://doi.org/10.1097/01.chi.0000170554.23422.c1.

Perlis RH, Miyahara S, Marangell LB, Wisniewski SR, Ostacher M, DelBello MP, et al. Long-term implications of early onset in bipolar disorder: data from the first 1000 participants in the systematic treatment enhancement program for bipolar disorder (STEP-BD). Biol Psychiatry. 2004;55(9):875–81. https://doi.org/10.1016/j.biopsych.2004.01.022.

Pfennig A, Jabs B, Pfeiffer S, Weikert B, Leopold K, Bauer M. Versorgungserfahrungen bipolarer Patienten in Deutschland: Befragung vor Einführung der S3-Leitlinie zur Diagnostik und Therapie bipolarer Störungen. Nervenheilkunde. 2011;30:333–40.

Pfennig A, Correll CU, Leopold K, Juckel G, Bauer M. Early recognition and intervention for bipolar disorders: State of research and perspectives. Nervenarzt. 2012;83(7):897–902. https://doi.org/10.1007/s00115-012-3589-3.

Pfennig A, Leopold K, Ritter P, Bohme A, Severus E, Bauer M. Longitudinal changes in the antecedent and early manifest course of bipolar disorder - A narrative review of prospective studies. Aust N Z J Psychiatry. 2017;51(5):509–23. https://doi.org/10.1177/0004867417700730.

Post RM, Leverich GS, Kupka RW, Keck PE Jr, McElroy SL, Altshuler LL, et al. Early-onset bipolar disorder and treatment delay are risk factors for poor outcome in adulthood. J Clin Psychiatry. 2010;71(7):864–72. https://doi.org/10.4088/JCP.08m04994yel.

Preisig M, Strippoli MP, Castelao E, Merikangas KR, Gholam-Rezaee M, Marquet P, et al. The specificity of the familial aggregation of early-onset bipolar disorder: A controlled 10-year follow-up study of offspring of parents with mood disorders. J Affect Disord. 2016;190:26–33. https://doi.org/10.1016/j.jad.2015.10.005.

Rios AC, Noto MN, Rizzo LB, Mansur R, Martins FE Jr, Grassi-Oliveira R, et al. Early stages of bipolar disorder: characterization and strategies for early intervention. Braz J Psychiatr. 2015;37(4):343–9. https://doi.org/10.1590/1516-4446-2014-1620.

Schultze-Lutter F, Picker H, Ruhrmann S, Klosterkotter J. The cologne early recognition and intervention center for mental crises (FETZ). Evaluation of Service Use Med Klin (munich). 2008;103(2):81–9. https://doi.org/10.1007/s00063-008-1012-4.

Singh MK. Is there validity to the bipolar prodrome? J Clin Psychiatry. 2015;76(5):e655–6. https://doi.org/10.4088/JCP.14com09502.

Skjelstad DV, Malt UF, Holte A. Symptoms and signs of the initial prodrome of bipolar disorder: A systematic review. J Affect Disord. 2010;126(1–2):1–13. https://doi.org/10.1016/j.jad.2009.10.003.

Smoller JW, Finn CT. Family, twin, and adoption studies of bipolar disorder. Am J Med Genet. 2003;123C(1):48–58. https://doi.org/10.1002/ajmg.c.20013.

Spitzer RL. Psychiatric diagnosis: are clinicians still necessary? Compr Psychiatry. 1983;24(5):399–411. https://doi.org/10.1016/0010-440x(83)90032-9.

Strawn JR, Cotton S, Luberto CM, Patino LR, Stahl LA, Weber WA, et al. Neural function before and after mindfulness-based cognitive therapy in anxious adolescents at risk for developing bipolar disorder. J Child Adolesc Psychopharmacol. 2016;26(4):372–9. https://doi.org/10.1089/cap.2015.0054.

Thiebaut S, Godart N, Radon L, Courtet P, Guillaume S. Crossed prevalence results between subtypes of eating disorder and bipolar disorder: A systematic review of the literature. Encephale. 2019;45(1):60–73. https://doi.org/10.1016/j.encep.2018.06.001

Tohen M, Zarate CA, Hennen J, Khalsa HMK, Strakowski SM, Gebre-Medhin P, et al. The McLean-Harvard First-Episode Mania Study: prediction of recovery and first recurrence. Am J Psychiatry. 2003;160(12):2099–107. https://doi.org/10.1176/appi.ajp.160.12.2099.

van Meter AR, Burke C, Youngstrom EA, Faedda GL, Correll CU. The bipolar prodrome: meta-analysis of symptom prevalence prior to initial or recurrent mood episodes. J Am Acad Child Adolesc Psychiatry. 2016;55(7):543–55. https://doi.org/10.1016/j.jaac.2016.04.017.

Vos T, Flaxman AD, Naghavi M, Lozano R, Michaud C, Ezzati M, et al. Years lived with disability (YLDs) for 1160 sequelae of 289 diseases and injuries 1990–2010: a systematic analysis for the Global Burden of Disease Study 2010. Lancet. 2012;380(9859):2163–96. https://doi.org/10.1016/S0140-6736(12)61729-2.

Wals M, Hillegers MH, Reichart CG, Ormel J, Nolen WA, Verhulst FC. Prevalence of psychopathology in children of a bipolar parent. J Am Acad Child Adolesc Psychiatry. 2001;40(9):1094–102. https://doi.org/10.1097/00004583-200109000-00019.

Wittchen HU, Jacobi F, Rehm J, Gustavsson A, Svensson M, Jönsson B, et al. The size and burden of mental disorders and other disorders of the brain in Europe 2010. Eur Neuropsychopharmacol. 2011;21(9):655–79. https://doi.org/10.1016/j.euroneuro.2011.07.018.

World Medical Association. WMA Declaration of Helsinki - Ethical principles for medical research involving human subjects. 1964. https://www.wma.net/policies-post/wma-declaration-of-helsinki-ethical-principles-for-medical-research-involving-human-subjects/. Accessed 27 Jul 2020.

12

# Improving early recognition and intervention in people at increased risk for the development of bipolar disorder: study protocol of a prospective-longitudinal, naturalistic cohort study (Early-BipoLife)

Andrea Pfennig[1*], Karolina Leopold[2], Julia Martini[1], Anne Boehme[1], Martin Lambert[3], Thomas Stamm[4,5], Felix Bermpohl[4], Andreas Reif[6], Sarah Kittel-Schneider[6], Georg Juckel[7], Andreas J. Fallgatter[8], Tilo Kircher[9], Andreas Jansen[9], Steffi Pfeiffer[1], Christina Berndt[1], Maren Rottmann-Wolf[1], Cathrin Sauer[1], Philipp Ritter[1], Christoph U. Correll[10,11], Andreas Bechdolf[2], Irina Falkenberg[9] and Michael Bauer[1]

**Abstract**

**Background:** Bipolar disorders (BD) belong to the most severe mental disorders, characterized by an early onset and recurrent, severe episodes or a chronic course with poor psychosocial functioning in a proportion of patients. Many patients with BD experience substantial symptomatology months or even years before full BD manifestation. Adequate diagnosis and treatment is often delayed, which is associated with a worse outcome. This study aims to prospectively evaluate and improve early recognition and intervention strategies for persons at-risk for BD.

**Methods:** Early-BipoLife is a prospective-longitudinal cohort study of 1419 participants (aged 15–35 years) with at least five waves of assessment over a period of at least 2 years (baseline, 6, 12, 18 and 24 months). A research consortium of ten university and teaching hospitals across Germany conducts this study. The following risk groups (RGs) were recruited: RG I: help-seeking youth and young adults consulting early recognition centres/facilities presenting ≥ 1 of the proposed risk factors for BD, RG II: in-/outpatients with unipolar depressive syndrome, and RG III: in-/outpatients with attention-deficit/hyperactivity disorder (ADHD). The reference cohort was selected from the German representative IMAGEN cohort. Over the study period, the natural course of risk and resilience factors, early symptoms of BD and changes of symptom severity (including conversion to manifest BD) are observed. Psychometric properties of recently developed, structured instruments on potential risk factors for conversion to BD and subsyndromal symptomatology (Bipolar Prodrome Symptom Scale, Bipolar at-risk criteria, EPI*bipolar*) and biomarkers that potentially improve prediction are investigated. Moreover, actual treatment recommendations are monitored in the participating specialized services and compared to recently postulated clinical categorization and treatment guidance in the field of early BD.

*Correspondence: andrea.pfennig@uniklinikum-dresden.de
[1] Department of Psychiatry and Psychotherapy, Carl Gustav Carus University Hospital, Technische Universität Dresden, Fetscherstraße 74, 01307 Dresden, Germany
Full list of author information is available at the end of the article

**Discussion:** Findings from this study will contribute to an improved knowledge about the natural course of BD, from the onset of first noticeable symptoms (precursors) to fully developed BD, and about mechanisms of conversion from subthreshold to manifest BD. Moreover, these generated data will provide information for the development of evidence-based guidelines for early-targeted detection and preventive intervention for people at risk for BD.

**Keywords:** Bipolar disorder, Early recognition, Early intervention, Risk factor, Prevention, Antecedent, Precursor, Protective, Resilience

## Background

Bipolar disorder (BD) is a severe and disabling mental disorder, characterized by an early onset and recurrent, severe episodes or a chronic course with poor psychosocial functioning in a proportion of patients (Ferrari et al. 2016; Fagiolini et al. 2013). Although efficacious psychopharmacological and psychosocial treatments for manifest BD exist (da Silva Lima et al. 2017; Pfennig et al. 2012a), BD is often diagnosed and treated with a significant delay (up to 10 years on average) (Baldessarini et al. 2003; Pfennig et al. 2011; Dagani et al. 2017). Treatment delay is associated with a worse functional outcome, an elevated risk of suicide (Chen and Dilsaver 1996; Miller et al. 2014; Post et al. 2010) and an inferior response to mood stabilizing drug treatment (Kessing et al. 2014). Improved diagnostic instruments for early recognition and guidelines for early-targeted intervention have the potential to enhance overall disease management or even to prevent conversion to manifest BD (Lish et al. 1994).

Recent evidence from early recognition centers has shown that help-seeking persons at-risk for BD are often already affected by a substantial impairing subsyndromal symptomatology (Leopold et al. 2013a, 2014; Pfennig et al. 2012b). Given the low specificity of individual precursors and early symptoms of BD prior to the first manifest manic episode (Berk et al. 2007), comprehensive criteria defining high-risk profiles need to be assembled. Due to its high heritability (Craddock and Sklar 2009), a positive family history for BD is one of the major risk factors for BD (Duffy et al. 2010, 2014; Smoller and Finn 2003; Mendlewicz and Rainer 1977). Moreover, evidence from prospective clinical and observational studies indicates that depressive and subthreshold (hypo-)manic symptoms may be antecedents or rather first noticeable symptoms of BD (Beesdo et al. 2009; Duffy et al. 2014, 2017; Bechdolf et al. 2012; Mesman et al. 2013; Ryles et al. 2017).

There is a vivid discussion about the association between attention-deficit/hyperactivity disorder (ADHD) and BD. At least a subgroup of patients with ADHD may be at risk to develop BD (Leopold et al. 2012; Faedda et al. 2014; Wang et al. 2016). Additionally, the following factors are discussed as further potential risk factors for BD: (a) a history of critical/stressful life events (Garno et al. 2005; Kessing et al. 2004), (b) childhood anxiety disorders or being anxious/worried/fearful, hyper-alert or sensitive (Lenox et al. 2002; Egeland et al. 2003; Tillman et al. 2003), (c) mood swings and impaired emotional regulation (frequent "ups and downs") (Thompson et al. 2003), (d) changes in sleep and circadian rhythm (Lenox et al. 2002), (e) somatic complaints or medical/physical problems (Egeland et al. 2003), (f) substance (ab-)use or dependence (Rush 2003), and (g) particular personality, temperament and character traits (e.g., extraversion, novelty seeking, creativity, high reward responsiveness and ambitious goal-striving, cyclothymic/hyperthymic temperament) (Duffy et al. 2010; Mesman et al. 2013; Leopold et al. 2012; Pfennig et al. 2017; Egeland et al. 2000; Correll et al. 2014a; Alloy et al. 2012; Kwapil et al. 2000; Blechert and Meyer 2005).

Based on this knowledge, structured instruments have been developed by different research groups to identify persons at risk for BD (Leopold et al. 2012; Bechdolf et al. 2014; Correll et al. 2014b) and to assess initial subsyndromal symptomatology (Bipolar Prodrome Symptom Scale, Correll et al. 2014b), EPI*bipolar*, Leopold et al. 2012), Bipolar at-risk criteria (Bechdolf et al. 2012)/extended BAR criteria (Fusar-Poli et al. 2018). First prospective studies revealed promising results on the psychometric properties of single instruments and the predictive validity regarding the conversion to BD (Bechdolf et al. 2014; Correll et al. 2014b; Fusar-Poli et al. 2018). Bechdolf and colleagues showed a conversion rate to BD of 14.3% within 12 months in people presenting with BAR criteria (Bechdolf et al. 2014), and Birmaher and colleagues found a conversion rate of 25% to BD in children and adolescents with clinically relevant bipolar symptoms that did not fulfil the DSM-IV criteria for bipolar-I or bipolar-II disorder (Birmaher et al. 2006). Conversion rates of patients with unipolar depression range in different studies from 4 to 49% (Geller et al. 2001; Gilman et al. 2012). However, previous samples were small, and the comparison of study results is hampered by heterogeneous risk definition/description and differences in study methodology (e.g., diverse follow-up duration). Standardization of the diagnostic process across specialized early recognition facilities is not formed yet. Moreover, at present protective/resilience factors (Stange et al. 2013) and potential biomarkers (Duffy et al. 2014; Ritter et al. 2016; Kapczinski et al. 2009) are not part of the existing assessment tools (Leopold et al. 2012; Bechdolf et al. 2014; Correll et al. 2014b).

Besides the challenges of early and appropriate diagnostics, prevention as well as early-targeted intervention of BD is crucial, because treatment delay is associated with a worse social adjustment, an increased risk for suicide, increased comorbidity rates, more hospitalizations, and an impaired age-appropriate development (Goldberg and Ernst 2002; Matza et al. 2005). Pharmacological treatment approaches with mood stabilizing agents (lithium and divalproex) in at-risk patients have only been investigated in underpowered studies not showing effectiveness (Findling et al. 2007; Geller et al. 1998). Regarding monotherapy with antidepressants, study data in bipolar at-risk patients are lacking, and there might be a risk for inducing mania. However, in case of depressive, anxiety and/or obsessive symptomatology, antidepressant treatment under close monitoring is in line with guideline recommendations for both, unipolar (DGPPN 2015) and bipolar (DGBS and DGPPN 2019) disorders. A recent review of psychotherapeutic interventions in young at-risk patients (Pfennig et al. 2017) showed promising results. Three studies on the efficacy of early family-focused approaches suggest favorable outcomes such as improved symptoms, a longer duration in remission and a better psychosocial functioning (Miklowitz et al. 2011, 2013; Nadkarni and Fristad 2010). A updated systematic review (Blum 2018) provided evidence for the efficacy of Interpersonal and social rhythm therapy (IPSRT, Goldstein et al. 2018) and Mindfulness-based cognitive therapy (MBCT, Cotton et al. 2016) with improvement in sleep patterns, emotion regulation and a decrease of anxiety, compared to baseline.

Based on the knowledge of risk factors and early clinical features of BD and of the promising research on early targeted interventions, pilot clinical category models and treatment guidance (Berk et al. 2007; Kapczinski et al. 2009; Leopold et al. 2013b; Schneck et al. 2017) have been formulated. Primary treatment recommendations for early (at-risk) stages of BD are psychoeducation, preventive strategies to halt conversion to BD, and strategies on preserving the young person's ability to meet age-appropriate developmental tasks (Berk et al. 2007; Kapczinski et al. 2009; Leopold et al. 2013b). At later stages, the focus changes to symptomatic treatment, and the establishment of adherence and relapse prevention of BD (Berk et al. 2007; Kapczinski et al. 2009; Leopold et al. 2013b). The verification of the suggested models and guidance could enable evidence-based treatment approaches in early stages of BD. A validated model would provide greater utility for testing the efficacy, cost-effectiveness, risk–benefit ratios and feasibility of available interventions (McGorry et al. 2006).

In summary, early recognition of at-risk states for BD is an important clinical field, but the diagnostic process across specialized early recognition facilities has not been standardized yet. First approaches of clinical categorization and treatment guidance have been formulated (Berk et al. 2007; Kapczinski et al. 2009; Leopold et al. 2013b), but no common diagnostic and/or treatment guidelines are available supporting the individual decision-making processes for those in the early stages of BD. This situation impedes the accumulation of superior clinical-epidemiological knowledge regarding the core predictors for conversion to manifest BD and prevention of incident BD.

To address these areas of unmet needs, a prospective, naturalistic cohort study in the age group of 15–35 years was designed to clarify the following research questions, with (a) being the primary question:

- a What is the predictive power of the individual risk factors/constellations in defined risk groups for BD using the existing instruments and recommended at-risk criteria? What is the prevalence of these risk factors and constellations in a representative cohort? How do risk factors interact?
- b What are protective/resilience factors for BD in the proposed age group?
- c What is the association of biomarkers with the clinical outcome?
- d How can the information from (a), (b), and (c) be integrated for further development of existing diagnostic tools for early detection (interviews, risk criteria) and standardization/harmonization of the diagnostic process across centres/facilities?
- e What factors are relevant for treatment decision-making in this naturalistic setting?
- f What information from (a–e) can be used to refine existing category model and treatment guidances?

## Methods

The *Improving early recognition and intervention in people at-risk for development of bipolar disorder* (*Early-BipoLife*) study is a multicentre study conducted by a research consortium of ten university and teaching hospitals across Germany with early recognition centres/facilities and specialised in- and outpatient care. *Early-BipoLife* is funded by the Federal Ministry of Education and Research (BMBF, Grant number: 01EE1404A) and is part of the BipoLife consortium described elsewhere (Ritter et al. 2016; Mühlbauer et al. 2018). The study is conducted according to good clinical practice (GCP) standards and has been approved by the responsible Ethics Committee of the Medical Faculty of the Technische Universität Dresden (No: EK290082014) and all local ethics committees. All participants provided written informed consent after comprehensive information about study aims and procedures.

### Study design and procedures

Early-BipoLife is a naturalistic, prospective-longitudinal observational cohort study of participants aged 15–35 years with at least five waves of assessment over a period of at least 2 years.

From July 2015 until September 2018, help seeking youth and young adults consulting early recognition centres/facilities presenting with at least one of the proposed risk factors for BD as well as in- and outpatients with depressive syndrome or ADHD, respectively, were recruited at the network sites (in Berlin (two sites), Bochum, Dresden, Frankfurt/Main, Hamburg, Marburg, Brandenburg/Neuruppin, Tübingen).

The reference cohort was selected from the German representative IMAGEN cohort (Berlin, Dresden). This cohort is a representative population-based sample of N = 2000 young people from Germany, the United Kingdom, Ireland and France who were recruited at the age 14 years with follow-up assessments at 16 and 18 to 20 years (https://imagen-europe.com). For the Early-BipoLife study assessment, subjects from the IMAGEN cohort were recruited from July 2016 to December 2018. With their informed consent, data from the previous assessments at age 14 and 16 will be used in the present study analyses.

Participants were examined at baseline (BL), and after 6 months (FU1), 12 months (FU2), 18 months (FU3) and 24 months (FU4) with further long-term follow-up (currently up to month 36). At BL, FU2 and FU4, participants are assessed with a comprehensive standardized face-to-face diagnostic procedure by trained academic study personnel (physicians and psychologists). The mean time for completion of the standardized interview and additional questionnaires is approximately 3 to 7 h (mostly conducted over three appointments). FU1 and FU3 are conducted as telephone-interviews with a duration of approximately 30 min. If indicators for change in risk score severity or conversion to BD are registered in the telephone interview, a face-to-face contact with the comprehensive assessment battery is conducted. Interviewers/raters at baseline and follow-up were trained centrally in a 2-day training before starting to recruit at the individual study center, were supervised locally by the principal investigator of the respective study center and were re-trained regularily. Reliability was assessed for the early detection instruments and the SCID. FU-raters were not blinded for risk status. The risk detection instruments use historical information and change to former FU, so to ensure to rate the current risk profile accurately, using historical information was allowed.

The design and procedures of the Early-BipoLife study are displayed at Fig. 1.

Participants further receive the option to participate in the neuroimaging, electroencephalography (EEG), and genomics platform projects within the Early-BipoLife study. Details of the used methods and paradigms are described below and elsewhere (Ritter et al. 2016).

Since individuals not (yet) meeting BD diagnostic criteria may benefit from a structured and supervised diagnostic and decision-making process with tailored symptomatic treatment, all persons in RG I (see below) receive state-of-the-art counselling and treatment according to their individual needs. Although clinical category models and treatment guidance were recently postulated (Berk et al. 2007; Leopold et al. 2013b), it is not clear to what extent those theoretical models are implemented in daily care and how beneficial they are to the individual patient. Due to the naturalistic design of the Early-BipoLife study, the content and the extent of the particular counselling and treatment recommendations are at the discretion of the individual study centre staff and reflect the particular centre's usual care that is based on the clinical experience of the site's clinical experts (Pfennig et al. 2012b). Particular recommendations (e.g., general or specific preventive strategies, psychotherapy, and/or pharmacotherapy) are monitored and analysed during the Early-BipoLife study. A comparison with the recently postulated models and guidance will be conducted (Berk et al. 2007; Kapczinski et al. 2009; Leopold et al. 2013b; Schneck et al. 2017).

### Sampling and initial risk groups

Overall, N = 2279 persons were screened for inclusion and exclusion criteria. For eligibility of participants for the Early-BipoLife study (inclusion and exclusion criteria) see Table 1.

In total, N = 1419 study participants were included in the study. Due to their baseline diagnostic status, risk participants (N = 1229) were assigned to one of the above mentioned risk groups (RG I–III).

### Measures

Core instruments to observe and predict the natural course of disease in terms of change of severity of the risk status are the EPI*bipolar* (Leopold et al. 2012), the BPSS-P (Correll et al. 2014b) and the BAR criteria (Bechdolf et al. 2012)/extended BAR criteria (Fusar-Poli et al. 2018) (see "Core instruments" below). The assessments further include interviewer ratings and self-report scales

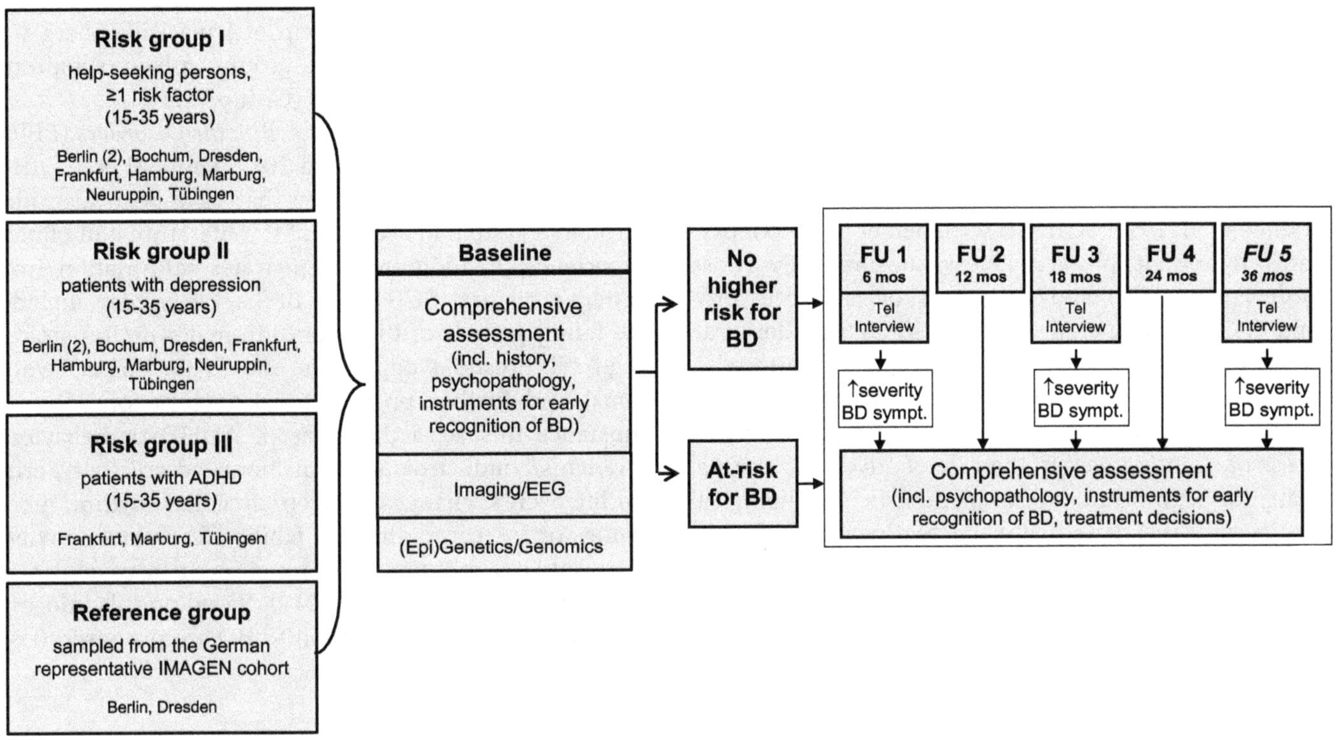


**Fig. 1** Design of the BipoLife-study

**Table 1 Key inclusion and exclusion criteria for study participants of the risk groups I–III**

| | Inclusion criteria | Exclusion criteria |
|---|---|---|
| Risk group I (RG I) | • Age: 15 to 35 years<br>• Consultation of an early recognition centre/facility<br>• Presence of at least one of the proposed risk factors for BD:<br>– Family history of BD<br>– (Sub)threshold affective symptomatology/depressive syndrome<br>– Hypomanic/mood swings<br>– Disturbances of circadian rhythm/sleep other clinical hints | • Diagnosis of: BD, schizoaffective disorder, schizophrenia<br>• Diagnosis of anxiety, obsessive–compulsive or substance dependence disorder that fully explains the whole symptomatology<br>• Limited ability to comprehend the study<br>• Implied expressed negative declaration of intent to participate in the study by a minor and<br>• Acute suicidality |
| Risk group II (RG II) | • Age: 15 to 35 years<br>• In- or outpatients with a depressive syndrome in the context of:<br>– Major depressive disorder<br>– Dysthymic disorder<br>– Cyclothymic disorder<br>– Minor depressive disorder<br>– Recurrent brief depressive disorder<br>– Adjustment disorder with depressed mood<br>– Depressive disorder Not Otherwise Specified (NOS) | |
| Risk group III (RG III) | • Age: 15 to 35 years<br>• In- or outpatients with a clinically confirmed ADHD diagnosis | |

to characterize the development of the risk constellation during the study period and to examine disease progression from subthreshold and threshold symptomatology of BD [EPI*bipolar* (Leopold et al. 2012), BPSS-P (Correll et al. 2014b), BAR (Bechdolf et al. 2012)/extended BAR criteria (Fusar-Poli et al. 2018), SCID-I (Wittchen et al. 1997), IDS-C (Drieling et al. 2007), QIDS–SR16 (Roniger et al. 2015), YMRS (Mühlbacher et al. 2011), ASRM (Bernhard and Meyer 2011)].

The primary outcome of the study is change in illness severity in terms of (a) change of the risk status in the core instruments, (b) initial prescription of a drug with the aim of mood stabilization, (c) conversion to manifest BD, or (d) change in clinical relevant burden of disease or impairment of psychosocial functioning [measured with EPI*bipolar* (Leopold et al. 2012), GAF (Hall 1995), FAST (Riegler et al. 2017; Rosa et al. 2007) and WHOQOL-BREF (Angermeyer et al. 2000)].

Throughout the study, comorbid disorders (SCID-I, Wittchen et al. 1997; SCID-II, Wittchen et al. 1997), psychiatric treatment, physical illness, substance use (Case Report Form, CRF) and symptoms of psychotic prodrome (PQ-16, Ising et al. 2012; SIPS/SOPS, Miller et al. 2003; SPI-A, Schultze-Lutter et al. 2012) are monitored.

There is agreement that resilience is not equal to absence of risk. Resilience has been described as the process of adapting well in the face of adversity, trauma, threats, or significant stress (American Psychological Association 2014). Potential protective/resilience factors assessed include sociodemographic variables (e.g., living with a partner, being employed), resources and self-management skills (measured with FERUS, Jack 2004) as well as help-seeking behaviour (CRF). These are then analysed in relation to perceived stress, stressful life-events and psychosocial functioning.

### Core instruments

Three recently developed structured instruments for potential risk factors/constellations for conversion to BD and initial subsyndromal symptomatology are applied in parallel throughout the study.

The *Bipolar Prodrome Symptom Scale—Prospective* (BPSS-P, © Correll 2013, Correll et al. 2014b) is a semi-structured interview developed based on the DSM-IV criteria for BD and Major Depressive Disorder (MDD) as well as established rating scales for symptoms of the manic, depressive and psychotic spectrum. Moreover, recent literature on risk factors for BD was considered. The BPSS-P assesses the onset and severity of prodromal symptoms in three sections (Mania Symptom Index, Depression Symptom Index, and General Symptom Index). The BPSS-P has good internal consistency, convergent validity and inter-rater reliability (Correll et al. 2014b).

*Bipolar at-risk criteria* (BAR criteria, © Bechdolf 2012, Bechdolf et al. 2012): Bechdolf and colleagues developed a set of ultra-high-risk criteria for BD that comprise subthreshold clinical and behavioral information as well as genetic risk. BAR criteria are met when persons are aged 15–24 years and fulfil the criteria of at least one of the following at-risk groups: sub-threshold mania (Group I), depression plus cyclothymic features (Group II), depression plus genetic risk (Group III). One prospective study revealed promising results regarding the predictive validity of the BAR criteria for conversion to manifest BD (Bechdolf et al. 2012, 2014). The extension of the BAR criteria proposed by the group of Irina Falkenberg was assessed adding the at-risk groups mixed symptoms (Group IV) and mood swings (Group V).

The *Early Phase Inventory for Bipolar Disorders* (EPI*bipolar*, © Pfennig and Leopold 2012, Leopold et al. 2012) captures risk factor categories that have been identified through a systematic review of the literature and clinical experience. It additionally integrates information from patient's history, SCID and BPSS. EPI*bipolar* includes the family history of BD, subsyndromal symptomatology (e.g., subthreshold depressive and (hypo-)manic symptoms) and further proposed risk factors for BD (e.g., substance misuse, a diagnosis of ADHD or behavioral problems/conduct disorder, pronounced creativity, critical life events, changes in sleep/circadian rhythm, mood swings or increased affective lability, fearfulness/anxiety, dissociative symptoms, and impairment in psychosocial functioning, Leopold et al. 2012). Based on this information, risk states for conversion to BD are proposed (risk, high-risk, ultra-high risk).

### Predictors and potential risk and resilience factors for change in severity of BD

Diagnostic and dimensional instruments are listed in Table 2. The following overview operationalizes predictors or potential risk factors for change in the observational outcomes.

#### *Potential risk factors*

- Genetic risk: positive family history (1st or 2nd degree relative with a confirmed diagnosis of BD, major depressive disorder, schizoaffective disorder or schizophrenia) (CRF).
- At least subthreshold affective symptomatology (BPSS-P, Correll et al. 2014b), BAR criteria (Bechdolf et al. 2012), SCID-I (Wittchen et al. 1997).
- Mood swings and affective lability (EPI*bipolar*, Leopold et al. 2012).
- Lifetime and present ADHD or conduct disorder (patient's history; EPI*bipolar*, Leopold et al. 2012).
- Recurrent anxiety (lifetime or present), independent of depressive episodes (EPI*bipolar*, Leopold et al. 2012).
- Specific sleep and circadian rhythm disturbances (EPI*bipolar*, Leopold et al. 2012).
- Substance misuse related to mood swings or affective disturbances (EPI*bipolar*, Leopold et al. 2012).
- Pronounced creativity (BWAS, Welsh and Barron 1949; CAQ, Carson et al. 2005).

**Table 2 Overview of main instruments and assessment waves**

| Constructs and instruments | Self-report (SR)/ interviewer rating (IR) | Baseline | FU1 6 months | FU2 12 months | FU3 18 months | FU4 24 months | FU5 36 months |
|---|---|---|---|---|---|---|---|
| Core instruments for early recognition of bipolar disorders | | | | | | | |
| Early Phase Inventory for bipolar disorders [EPI*bipolar* (Leopold et al. 2012)] | IR | x | (x)[a] | x | (x)[a] | x | (x)[a] |
| Bipolar Prodrome Symptom Scale—Full Prospective [BPSS-FP (Correll et al. 2014b)] | IR | x | (x)[a] | x | (x)[a] | x | (x)[a] |
| Bipolar at-risk Criteria [BAR-Criteria (Bechdolf et al. 2012)] | IR | x | (x)[a] | x | (x)[a] | x | (x)[a] |
| Patient history and mental disorders (DSM, ICD) | | | | | | | |
| Case Report Form (CRF): study tailored questions on family history of BD, age, sex, marital status, family of origin, housing situation, level of education, employment status and nationality | IR | x | | x | | x | |
| Patient history | IR | | x | x | x | x | x |
| Structured Clinical Interview for DSM-IV-TR Disorders [SCID-I (Wittchen et al. 1997)] | IR | x | (x)[a] | x | (x)[a] | x | (x)[a] |
| SCID-II Screening, in case of positive screening Structured Clinical Interview for DSM-IV-TR Axis II Personality Disorders [SCID-II (Wittchen et al. 1997)] | IR | x | | | | | |
| Telephone interview, study tailored questions on symptoms of BD | IR | | x | | x | | x |
| Further instruments for the assessment depressive and manic symptoms | | | | | | | |
| Inventory of Depressive Symptomatology-Clinician [IDS-C (Drieling et al. 2007)] | IR | x | | | | | |
| Quick Inventory of Depressive Symptomatology [QIDS-SR16 (Roniger et al. 2015)] | SR | x | | | | | |
| Young Mania Rating Scale [YMRS (Mühlbacher et al. 2011)] | IR | x | | | | | |
| Altman Self-Rating Mania Scale [ASRM (Bernhard and Meyer 2011; Altman et al. 1997)] | SR | x | | | | | |
| Psychotic features | | | | | | | |
| PQ-16 Screening, in case of ≥ 6 points: Structured Interview for Prodromal Syndroms, German Version [SOPS (Miller et al. 2003)], Schizophrenia Proneness Interview—Adult version [SPI-A (Schultze-Lutter et al. 2012)] | IR | x | | | | | |
| Temperament | | | | | | | |
| Barratt Impulsiveness Scale [BIS (Preuss et al. 2008)] | SR | x | | | | | |
| Temperament Evaluation of Memphis, Pisa, Paris and San Diego—Autoquestionnaire short version [TEMPS-A (Victor et al. 2006)] | SR | x | | | | | |
| Behavioral Inhibition System and Behavioral Activation System [BIS/BAS (Strobel et al. 2001)] | SR | x | | | | | |
| Creativity | | | | | | | |
| Barron Welsh Art Scale [BWAS (Welsh and Barron 1949)] | SR | x | | | | | |
| Creative Achievement Questionnaire [CAQ (Carson et al. 2005)] | SR | x | | | | | |
| Life events and stress | | | | | | | |
| Childhood Trauma Questionnaire [CTQ (Wingenfeld et al. 2010)] and previous life events (study tailored) | SR | x | | | | | |
| Modified Life Events Questionnaire [MLEQ (McLean et al. 2014)] | SR | x | (x)[a] | x | (x)[a] | x | (x)[a] |

**Table 2 (continued)**

| Constructs and instruments | Self-report (SR)/ interviewer rating (IR) | Baseline | FU1 6 months | FU2 12 months | FU3 18 months | FU4 24 months | FU5 36 months |
|---|---|---|---|---|---|---|---|
| Trier Inventory for Chronic Stress [TICS (Schulz et al. 2004)] | SR | x | | | | | |
| Psychosocial functioning and quality of life | | | | | | | |
| Functioning Assessment Short Test [FAST (Riegler et al. 2017; Rosa et al. 2007)] | IR | x | (x)[a] | x | (x)[a] | x | (x)[a] |
| Global Assessment of Functioning Scale [GAF (Hall 1995)] | IR | x | (x)[a] | x | (x)[a] | x | (x)[a] |
| World Health Organization Quality of Life [WHOQOL-BREF (Angermeyer et al. 2000)] | SR | x | (x)[a] | x | (x)[a] | x | (x)[a] |
| Resources and resilience | | | | | | | |
| Questionnaire for resources and self-management skills [FERUS (Jack 2004)] | SR | x | | | | | |

[a] If indicators for change in risk score severity of risk status or conversion to BD are registered in the telephone interview, a face-to-face contact with the comprehensive assessment is conducted

- Stressful life events (CTQ, Wingenfeld et al. 2010); section on post-traumatic stress disorder in the SCID-I, Wittchen et al. 1997).
- Affective temperaments (TEMPS-A, Victor et al. 2006).
- Impulsivity (BIS, Preuss et al. 2008).
- Sensitivity of behavioural inhibition/activation system (BIS/BAS, Strobel et al. 2001).
- Chronic stress (TICS, Schulz et al. 2004).
- Psychosocial functioning (before, during and following a symptomatic episode) (EPI*bipolar*, Leopold et al. 2012) and functional impairment (GAF, Hall 1995; FAST, Riegler et al. 2017; Rosa et al. 2007).

***Further potential influencing factors***

- Sociodemographic factors (including age, sex, marital status, level of education and employment status) (CRF).
- Physical health: somatic diseases, BMI (CRF).
- Resources, resilience and self-management skills (FERUS, Jack 2004).
- Stressor load (MLEQ, McLean et al. 2014)
- Help-seeking behaviour (CRF).
- Quality of life (WHOQOL-BREF, Angermeyer et al. 2000).

**Observational outcomes: change in severity**

Diagnostic and dimensional instruments listed in Table 2 operationalize observational outcomes of this study as follows:

1 Change in severity of risk status: This criterion is met when there is an increase from a lower to a higher risk state (EPI*bipolar*, Leopold et al. 2012), or if the subject scores on more criteria than in the prior assessments (BPSS-P, Correll et al. 2014b; BAR, Bechdolf et al. 2012/extended BAR criteria, Fusar-Poli et al. 2018).

2 Initial prescription of a drug with the aim of mood stabilization: This criterion is fulfilled when one of the recommended mood-stabilizing agents of the German S3 guidelines on diagnostics and therapy of BD (Pfennig et al. 2012a) is initiated with the purpose of mood stabilization (and not solely for the treatment of depression, prevention of recurrent depressive episodes, or to address insomnia).

3 Conversion to manifest BD: A consensus diagnosis of BD (BD-I or BD-II according to DSM-IV criteria, Saß et al. 2012) is based on the information of the SCID-I (Wittchen et al. 1997) and the confirmation by a consensus board of clinically experienced staff members (psychiatrist and psychotherapist) of the respective specialized service centers/facilities. Conversion to BD occurs when diagnostic criteria for BD-I or BD-II are fulfilled for the first time during the follow-up period.

4 Change in burden of disease and psychosocial functioning: This outcome is defined using EPI*bipolar* (Leopold et al. 2012), GAF (Hall 1995) and FAST (Riegler et al. 2017; Rosa et al. 2007) as well as meas-

ures on quality of life (WHOQOL-BREF, Angermeyer et al. 2000). The criterion is met when there is a clinically relevant change in impairment or quality of life compared to the prior assessment.

#### *Biomarkers: neuroimaging, electrophysiology and genetics*

All participants of the Early-BipoLife study are invited to participate in the neuroimaging, EEG and genomics platform projects.

*Neuroimaging: functional magnetic resonance imaging (fMRI)* All participants opting for the neuroimaging part complete an identical test battery including:

- T1-sequence for morphometric analyses.
- Resting-state fMRI sequence.
- Three fMRI activation paradigms:
  - Desire-reason dilemma task using conditioned reward stimuli in different experimental situations, thereby allowing the investigation of subcortical structures of the dopaminergic reward system and their specific functional interactions with prefrontal cortical areas (Diekhof and Gruber 2010).
  - Highly robust emotional face matching paradigm for assessing limbic responsiveness to negative facial expressions (Dannlowski et al. 2012).
  - Cartoon Theory-of-Mind (ToM) task, which robustly activates the ToM network relevant for social cognition, since a dysfunction of the ToM network activated by this task is associated with a genetic risk variant for BD and in relatives of patients with BD (Walter et al. 2011).

For quality assurance, a phantom measurement is performed after each subject to investigate the stability of the magnetic resonance signal.

*Neurophysiology: electroencephalography (EEG)* The EEG battery focusing on neural synchrony in long-range and local oscillatory responses includes cognitive (choice-reaction tasks), perceptive (Kanizsa figures), and emotional (emotional faces) paradigms (Özerdem et al. 2011).

*Genetics and biomaterial* A network-wide phenotyping and biobanking platform was implemented in synergy with the German Association for Psychiatry and Psychotherapy and Psychosomatics (DGPPN) and their DGPPN Cohort (Anderson-Schmidt et al. 2013) infrastructure. Genomic analyses including targeted genotyping of candidate regions, exome sequencing will be performed. Therefore, saliva samples were acquired following consortium-wide SOPs and protocols and all 2D barcoded material is stored at two mirrored sites in Goettingen and Wuerzburg for genomic, transcriptomic, and proteomic analyses.

Details of the used methods and paradigms are described elsewhere (Ritter et al. 2016).

#### Monitoring of treatment

At the end of the baseline assessment as well as the FU2 and FU4, a case conference was held summarizing the findings (regarding established diagnoses and risk status) and the subsequent counselling and treatment procedures within the CRF. As mentioned above, due to the naturalistic design of the Early-BipoLife study, the content and the extent of the particular counselling and treatment recommendations are at the discretion of the individual study centre staff and depict the particular centre's usual care that is based on clinical experiences of the site's clinical experts (Pfennig et al. 2012b). Particular recommendations (e.g., general or specific preventive strategies, psychotherapy, and/or pharmacotherapy) are analysed and compared to the recently proposed models and guidance (Berk et al. 2007; Kapczinski et al. 2009; Leopold et al. 2013b; Schneck et al. 2017).

#### Statistical analysis

To compare each of the risk groups (RG I–III) with the reference group concerning each of the four observational outcomes that depict change in severity, univariate analyses are conducted (e.g., t-tests, Chi squared tests and univariate ANOVA). Univariate analyses are used to determine individual predictors of change in severity, too.

A multivariate logistic regression model is constructed for each measure of change in severity to determine risk factor constellations that are predictive of change in severity with each individual factor also being significant within the model. The analyses use a backward selection approach to ascertain variables that have unique predictive associations with change in severity at an initially liberal threshold of $p < 0.10$. After this, another logistic regression analysis is conducted in which variables found to contribute uniquely to change in severity in the initial series are considered together. Variables that remain significant at $p < 0.05$ in this analysis are then tested for multiplicative (interaction) effects in relation to change in severity. Finally, the identified risk factor(s) are tested regarding their predictive power, calculating sensitivity, specificity, positive predictive value, negative predictive value, and accuracy (e.g., applying ROC analyses).

In addition to the logistic regression model approach, Cox regression analyses are conducted to compare the four study groups concerning time to onset of change in severity, recognizing that individuals will have variable follow-up-times, which will be censored according to a survival analysis approach.

In addition to analysing each risk factor and risk factor constellations, the psychometric properties of the EPI*bipolar*, BPSS-P and BAR criteria are assessed (e.g., Cronbach's alpha, convergent validity). For all three scales the predictive power will be assessed with calculation of sensitivity, specificity, positive predictive value, negative predictive value, and accuracy (e.g., applying ROC analyses).

To analyse the extent to which the treatment recommendations given match published clinical categorization and treatment guidance (Berk et al. 2007; Kapczinski et al. 2009; Leopold et al. 2013b; Schneck et al. 2017) Cohen's kappa statistics are applied.

## Discussion

Early-BipoLife is a naturalistic prospective-longitudinal observational cohort study of 1419 participants who are repeatedly assessed during their most vulnerable and formative years (Leopold et al. 2014; Pfennig et al. 2012b; Lish et al. 1994). This comprehensive design has been developed in order (a) to determine the natural course of potential risk and resilience factors and early symptoms/precursors of BD; (b) to observe the change in severity of early symptomatology of BD as primary outcome (including conversion to manifest BD); (c) to evaluate the predictive power of potential risk factors/precursors of BD and biomarkers as well as psychometric properties of recently introduced instruments for the early identification of persons at-risk for BD; and (d) to investigate currently recommended treatment advices in daily care and compare these with recently proposed clinical categorization and treatment guidance (Berk et al. 2007; Leopold et al. 2012; Kapczinski et al. 2009; Schneck et al. 2017).

To the best of our knowledge, this is the first investigation of a help-seeking cohort of at-risk persons for BD sampled from early recognition centres/facilities as well as in-/outpatient settings. Other research on risk factors for BD mainly focused on the investigation of offspring of persons with manifest BD (Duffy et al. 2007, 2009). For a discussion on differences of studies regarding samples, focus, outcomes and statistical approaches see (Geoffroy and Scott 2017).

Major strengths of the Early-BipoLife study are:

- The sample size (N = 1419) and the high number of assessment points during the particular vulnerable phase of disease development and potential conversion to BD. This design allows for the investigation of the natural course of BD from early signs/precursors and subsyndromal symptomatology to research-facilitated diagnosis of manifest BD.
- The reference sample selected from the German representative IMAGEN cohort provides the opportunity to compare the frequency of the proposed risk protective factors in the risk groups with a non-risk cohort. Additionally, data from the previous IMAGEN prospective assessments at age 14 and 16 can be used to analyse courses with and without development of BD symptomatology.
- The assessment of high-risk criteria for BD, potential predictors and subsyndromal symptomatology (e.g., subthreshold depressive and (hypo-) manic symptoms) using recently published instruments in parallel (Bechdolf et al. 2012; Leopold et al. 2012; Correll et al. 2014b). Those standardized diagnostic assessments are repeatedly conducted face-to-face along with a broad range of dimensional measures (on severity and further relevant factors for the natural course of BD).
- The clinical benefit of the supplementation of clinical diagnostics with information on biomarkers is explored.
- Individual resources, resilience factors and their impact on the development, and manifestation (e.g., age of onset) as well as the course of disease is investigated.
- Results from diagnostic assessments and treatment recommendations are comprehensively discussed in a consensus board of clinical experienced staff members (psychiatrists and psychotherapists).
- Data on treatment recommendations and on the effectiveness of applied treatments to patients at risk for BD are investigated in a non-interventional clinical settings. A recently published clinical categorization and treatment guidance/staging model will ideally be refined according to the results on the real-world effectiveness of the treatments applied as part of usual care within the study.

The study has the following limitations. First, this is a naturalistic follow-up study. As such, we will not be able to test the effectiveness of individual components of the treatments that were recommended and delivered. We consider this a second-generation question for further efficacy studies and wish to focus on more generalizable outcomes to study risk and protective factors for BD without the restrictions of an efficacy design and restricted treatment approaches. Second, adherence to the prescribed treatments is not assessed. The study sample includes patients with depression, ADHD, as well as subjects at increased risk for the development of bipolar disorder. In some of these, psychotropic medication is applied out of which the risk for mania might arise. Individual medication is assessed at baseline and FU and will be attended to in the analysis as effectively as possible. Third, we include mostly university centres and hospitals with specialized BD services. While this approach reduces the generalizability of the findings, it provides a yardstick against which other more usual care settings can be compared. Fourth, the study is conducted in Germany and under German health care conditions, with less generalizability of the pathways to care and treatment approaches as well as related illness trajectories in systems with less access to care. Fifth, not all patients enrolling in the Early-BipoLife study will have a complete neuroimaging, electrophysiology and genetics battery. However, given the large number of expected participants, the generated data will be highly informative. We acquire data on somatic diseases and BMI, but no further information on the subject`s physical health. Sixth, the study sample includes patients with depression, ADHD, as well as subjects at increased risk for the development of bipolar disorder. In some of these, psychotropic medication is applied out of which the risk for mania might arise. Individual medication is assessed at baseline and FU and will be attended to in the analysis as effectively as possible. Seventh, with applying a comprehensive FU assessment, especially hypomanic episodes could be detected that otherwise had been overlooked, or had not been classified as such with coarser questioning. Eighth, the control sample is representative for the young population in Dresden and Berlin, was, however, recruited under different conditions as the risk group subjects, which might affect comparability.

Nevertheless, despite these limitations, the Early-BipoLife study will be one of the largest prospective studies to comprehensively characterize a sample of adolescents and young adults at risk for the development of BD. Results are expected to inform patients, families, clinicians, guideline developers, payers and policy makers alike.

Long-term follow-up beyond the visits predefined in the study is planned to increase confidence in the evaluation of the proposed risk and protective factors and lead to a deeper understanding of early stages of BD. At present, all study centers follow patients up to month 36, an extension study will be applied for at a public sponsor.

## Conclusions

The Early-BipoLife study will provide unprecedented and detailed information about the relationship between recently discussed risk and protective factors and the onset and natural course of BD. Findings expected from the Early-BipoLife study will significantly contribute novel insights into pathomechanisms of disease and beneficial treatment algorithms. This information is crucial to further develop early-targeted primary and secondary prevention and intervention strategies to reduce the risk for conversion to BD and improve outcomes when BD has developed. A validated clinical categorization and treatment guidance/staging model will be able to inform patients, clinicians and researchers additionally about the prognosis and treatment response. It is also of particular interest, which assessment tool(s) or which parts of those will perform best to allow a valid categorization and staging of BD risk.

**Abbreviations**

ADHD: Attention-deficit/hyperactivity disorder; ANOVA: Analysis of variance; ASRM: Altman Self-Rating Mania Scale; BAR: Bipolar at risk; BD: Bipolar disorder; BIS: Barratt Impulsiveness Scale; BIS/BAS: Behavioral Inhibition System and Behavioral Activation System; BL: Baseline visit; BPSS-P: Bipolar Prodrome Symptom Scale-Prospective; BWAS: Barron Welsh Art Scale; CAQ: Creative Achievement Questionnaire; CRF: Case Report Form; CTQ: Childhood Trauma Questionnaire; DGBS: German Association of Bipolar Disorders; DGPPN: German Association for Psychiatry and Psychotherapy and Psychosomatics; EEG: Electroencephalography; EPI*bipolar*: Early Phase Inventory for Bipolar Disorders; FAST: Functioning Assessment Short Test; FERUS: Questionnaire for resources and self-management skills; fMRI: Functional Magnet-resonance-tomography; FU 1: Follow-up 1 visit (6 months); FU 2: Follow-up 2 visit (12 months); FU 3: Follow-up 3 visit (18 months); FU 4: Follow-up 4 visit (24 months); FU 5: Follow-up 5 visit (36 months); GAF: Global Assessment of Functioning Scale; GCP: Good clinical practice; IDS-C: Inventory of Depressive Symptomatology-Clinician; IPSRT: Interpersonal and social rhythm therapy; IR: Interviewer-rating; MBCT: Mindfulness-based cognitive therapy; MLEQ: Modified Life Events Questionnaire; MRI: Magnet-resonance-tomography; PQ-16: Prodromal Questionnaire; QIDS-SR16: Quick Inventory of Depressive Symptomatology-Self Rating; RG: Risk group; ROC: Receiver operating characteristic; SCID-I: Structured Clinical Interview for DSM-IV-TR Disorders; SCID-II: Structured Clinical Interview for DSM-IV-TR Axis II Personality Disorders; SIPS/SOPS: Structured Interview for Prodromal Syndroms, German Version; SPI-A: Schizophrenia Proneness Interview—Adult version; SR: Self-rating; TEMPS-A: Temperament Evaluation of Memphis, Pisa, Paris and San Diego—Autoquestionnaire short version; TICS: Trier Inventory for Chronic Stress; ToM: Theory of Mind; WHOQOL-BREF: World Health Organization Quality of Life—Short Form; YMRS: Young Mania Rating Scale.

**Acknowledgements**

We thank Martin Brüne for supporting the study progress at the study centre Bochum.

**Authors' contributions**

AP, KL and MB designed the study and supervised the multicentre study conduction. AP and KL additionally wrote parts of the manuscript, MB additionally reviewed the manuscript. SP supervised the quality assurance of the study data and reviewed the manuscript. JM analysed the data and wrote parts of the manuscript. CS supervised data analysis. AB recruited study participants, collected data and wrote parts of the manuscript. CB and MRW contributed to the study design, recruited study participants, collected data and reviewed the manuscript. ML, TS, FB, AR, SKS, GJ, AJF, TK, AJ supervised recruitment of study participants and data collection and reviewed the manuscript. AB and CC contributed to the study design and reviewed the manuscript. IF contributed to the study design, supervised recruitment of study participants and data collection and reviewed the manuscript. PR coordinated the project within BipoLife and reviewed the manuscript. All authors read and approved the final manuscript.

**Competing interests**

AP has received speakers honoraria and travel support from Janssen and Lundbeck. KL has been an advisor to and received speakers honoraria and travel support from Janssen, Lundbeck, Otsuka and Recordati. She received grant support from Janssen and Otsuka. ML has held lectures for AstraZeneca, Bristol-Myers Squibb, Lilly Deutschland GmbH, Janssen Cilag GmbH, Lundbeck GmbH, Otsuka Pharma GmbH, Roche Deutschland Holding GmbH, Sanovi Aventis; Grants: AstraZeneca, Bristol-Myers Squibb, Lilly Deutschland GmbH, Janssen Cilag GmbH, Lundbeck, Sanovi Aventis; Consultancy: AstraZeneca, Lilly Deutschland GmbH, Janssen Cilag GmbH, Roche Deutschland Holding GmbH, Trommsdorff GmbH & Co. KG. GJ received speakers honoraria from Janssen. TK received unrestricted educational grants from Bristol-Myers Squibb, Janssen, and Otsuka. CC has been a consultant and/or advisor to or has received honoraria from: Alkermes, Allergan, Angelini, Boehringer-Ingelheim, Gedeon Richter, Gerson Lehrman Group, Indivior, IntraCellular Therapies, Janssen/J&J, LB Pharma, Lundbeck, MedAvante-ProPhase, Medscape, Merck, Neurocrine, Noven, Otsuka, Pfizer, Recordati, Rovi, Servier, Sumitomo Dainippon, Sunovion, Supernus, Takeda, and Teva. He has provided expert testimony for Bristol-Myers Squibb, Janssen, and Otsuka. He served on a Data Safety Monitoring Board for Boehringer-Ingelheim, Lundbeck, Rovi, Supernus, and Teva. He received royalties from UpToDate and grant support from Janssen and Takeda. He is also a shareholder of LB Pharma. ABe acknowledges support for investigator initiated trials from Janssen and Osuka and educational funds and speaker honoraria from Otsuka, Servier, Janssen and Lundbeck.JM, AB, IF, AJF, AJ, SKS, SP, CB, MRW, CS, AR, PR, FB, TS, MB state to have no conflict of interest.

**Author details**

[1] Department of Psychiatry and Psychotherapy, Carl Gustav Carus University Hospital, Technische Universität Dresden, Fetscherstraße 74, 01307 Dresden, Germany. [2] Department of Psychiatry, Psychotherapy and Psychosomatics, Vivantes Klinikum Am Urban, Berlin, Germany. [3] Department of Psychiatry and Psychotherapy, University Medical Center Hamburg-Eppendorf, Hamburg, Germany. [4] Department of Psychiatry and Psychotherapy, Charité Universitätsmedizin Berlin, Berlin, Germany. [5] Department of Psychiatry, Psychotherapy and Psychosomatic, Medical School Brandenburg, Neuruppin, Germany. [6] Department of Psychiatry, Psychosomatics and Psychotherapy, University Hospital Frankfurt, Frankfurt, Germany. [7] Department of Psychiatry and Psychotherapy, LWL-University Hospital Bochum, Ruhr-University Bochum, Bochum, Germany. [8] Department of General Psychiatry and Psychotherapy, University Hospital Tübingen, Tübingen, Germany. [9] Department of Psychiatry and Psychotherapy, University Hospital Marburg, Marburg, Germany. [10] The Donald and Barbara Zucker School of Medicine at Hofstra/Northwell, The Zucker Hillside Hospital, Glen Oaks, NY, USA. [11] Department of Child- and Adolescent Psychiatry, Charité Universitätsmedizin Berlin, Berlin, Germany.

**References**

Alloy LB, Bender RE, Whitehouse WG, Wagner CA, Liu RT, Grant DA, et al. High Behavioral Approach System (BAS) sensitivity, reward responsiveness, and goal-striving predict first onset of bipolar spectrum disorders: a prospective behavioral high-risk design. J Abnorm Psychol. 2012;121(2):339–51.

Altman EG, Hedeker D, Peterson JL, Davis JM. The Altman Self-Rating Mania Scale. Biol. Psychiatry. 1997;42:948–55.

American Psychological Association. The road to resilience. Washington, DC: American Psychological Association; 2014.

Anderson-Schmidt H, Adler L, Aly C, Anghelescu I-G, Bauer M, Baumgärtner J, et al. The "DGPPN-Cohort": a national collaboration initiative by the German Association for Psychiatry and Psychotherapy (DGPPN) for establishing a large-scale cohort of psychiatric patients. Eur Arch Psychiatry Clin Neurosci. 2013;263(8):695–701.

Angermeyer MC, Kilian R, Matschinger H. WHOQOL-100 und WHOQOL-BREF: Handbuch für die deutschsprachige Version der WHO Instrumente zur Erfassung von Lebensqualität. Göttingen: Hogrefe; 2000.

Baldessarini RJ, Tondo L, Hennen J. Treatment-latency and previous episodes: relationships to pretreatment morbidity and response to maintenance treatment in bipolar I and II disorders. Bipolar Disord. 2003;5(3):169–79.

Bechdolf A, Ratheesh A, Wood SJ, Tecic T, Conus P, Nelson B, et al. Rationale and first results of developing at-risk (prodromal) criteria for bipolar disorder. Curr Pharm Des. 2012;18(4):358–75.

Bechdolf A, Ratheesh A, Cotton SM, Nelson B, Chanen AM, Betts J, et al. The predictive validity of bipolar at-risk (prodromal) criteria in help-seeking adolescents and young adults: a prospective study. Bipolar Disord. 2014;16(5):493–504.

Beesdo K, Höfler M, Leibenluft E, Lieb R, Bauer M, Pfennig A. Mood episodes and mood disorders: patterns of incidence and conversion in the first three decades of life. Bipolar Disord. 2009;11(6):637–49.

Berk M, Conus P, Lucas N, Hallam K, Malhi GS, Dodd S, et al. Setting the stage: from prodrome to treatment resistance in bipolar disorder. Bipolar Disord. 2007;9(7):671–8.

Bernhard B, Meyer T. Bipolare Störungen. In: Margraf J, editor. Lehrbuch der Verhaltenstherapie: Band 4: Materialien für die Psychotherapie. Heidelberg: Springer; 2011.

Birmaher B, Axelson D, Strober M, Gill MK, Valeri S, Chiappetta L, et al. Clinical course of children and adolescents with bipolar spectrum disorders. Arch Gen Psychiatry. 2006;63(2):175–83.

Blechert J, Meyer TD. Are measures of hypomanic personality, impulsive nonconformity and rigidity predictors of bipolar symptoms? Br J Clin Psychol. 2005;44(1):15–27.

Blum S. Early psychotherapeutic interventions in children, adolescents and young adults at increased risk for development of bipolar disorder; library of the Technische Universität Dresden. 2018.

Carson SH, Peterson JB, Higgins DM. Reliability, validity, and factor structure of the Creative Achievement Questionnaire. 2005.

Chen YW, Dilsaver SC. Lifetime rates of suicide attempts among subjects with bipolar and unipolar disorders relative to subjects with other Axis I disorders. Biol Psychiatry. 1996;39(10):896–9.

Correll CU, Hauser M, Penzner JB, Auther AM, Kafantaris V, Saito E, et al. Type and duration of subsyndromal symptoms in youth with bipolar I disorder prior to their first manic episode. Bipolar Disord. 2014a;16(5):478–92.

Correll CU, Olvet DM, Auther AM, Hauser M, Kishimoto T, Carrion RE, et al. The Bipolar Prodrome Symptom Interview and Scale-Prospective (BPSS-P): description and validation in a psychiatric sample and healthy controls. Bipolar Disord. 2014b;16(5):505–22.

Cotton S, Luberto CM, Sears RW, Strawn JR, Stahl L, Wasson RS, et al. Mindfulness-based cognitive therapy for youth with anxiety disorders at risk for bipolar disorder: a pilot trial. Early Interv Psychiatry. 2016;10(5):426–34.

Craddock N, Sklar P. Genetics of bipolar disorder: successful start to a long journey. Trends Genet. 2009;25(2):99–105.

da Silva Lima AFB, Cruz L, Cohen M, Zimmermann JJ, de Sousa Miguel SRP. Cost-effectiveness of treatment for bipolar disorders. In: Razzouk D, editor. Mental health economics. Cham: Springer International Publishing; 2017. p. 299–311.

Dagani J, Signorini G, Nielssen O, Bani M, Pastore A, de Girolamo G, et al. Meta-analysis of the interval between the onset and management of bipolar disorder. Can J Psychiatry. 2017;62(4):247–58.

Dannlowski U, Stuhrmann A, Beutelmann V, Zwanzger P, Lenzen T, Grotegerd D, et al. Limbic scars: long-term consequences of childhood maltreatment revealed by functional and structural magnetic resonance imaging. Biol Psychiatry. 2012;71(4):286–93.

DGBS, DGPPN. S3-Leitlinie zur Diagnostik und Therapie Bipolarer Störungen. 2019.

DGPPN. S3-Leitlinie/Nationale Versorgungsleitlinie: Unipolare Depression. 2nd edn. 2015.

Diekhof EK, Gruber O. When desire collides with reason: functional interactions between anteroventral prefrontal cortex and nucleus accumbens underlie the human ability to resist impulsive desires. J Neurosci. 2010;30(4):1488–93.

Drieling T, Schärer LO, Langosch JM. The inventory of depressive symptomatology: German translation and psychometric validation. Int J Methods Psychiatr Res. 2007;16(4):230–6.

Duffy A, Alda M, Crawford L, Milin R, Grof P. The early manifestations of bipolar disorder: a longitudinal prospective study of the offspring of bipolar parents. Bipolar Disord. 2007;9(8):828–38.

Duffy A, Alda M, Hajek T, Grof P. Early course of bipolar disorder in high-risk offspring: prospective study. Br J Psychiatry. 2009;195(5):457–8.

Duffy A, Alda M, Hajek T, Sherry SB, Grof P. Early stages in the development of bipolar disorder. J Affect Disord. 2010;121(1–2):127–35.

Duffy A, Horrocks J, Doucette S, Keown-Stoneman C, McCloskey S, Grof P. The developmental trajectory of bipolar disorder. Br J Psychiatry. 2014;204(2):122–8.

Duffy A, Vandeleur C, Heffer N, Preisig M. The clinical trajectory of emerging bipolar disorder among the high-risk offspring of bipolar parents: current understanding and future considerations. Int J Bipolar Disord. 2017;5(1):37.

Egeland JA, Hostetter AM, Pauls DL, Sussex JN. Prodromal symptoms before onset of manic-depressive disorder suggested by first hospital admission histories. J Am Acad Child Adolesc Psychiatry. 2000;39(10):1245–52.

Egeland JA, Shaw JA, Endicott J, Pauls DL, Allen CR, Hostetter AM, et al. Prospective study of prodromal features for bipolarity in well Amish children. J Am Acad Child Adolesc Psychiatry. 2003;42(7):786–96.

Faedda GL, Serra G, Marangoni C, Salvatore P, Sani G, Vazquez GH, et al. Clinical risk factors for bipolar disorders: a systematic review of prospective studies. J Affect Disord. 2014;168:314–21.

Fagiolini A, Forgione R, Maccari M, Cuomo A, Morana B, Dell'Osso MC, et al. Prevalence, chronicity, burden and borders of bipolar disorder. J Affect Disord. 2013;148(2–3):161–9.

Ferrari AJ, Stockings E, Khoo J-P, Erskine HE, Degenhardt L, Vos T, et al. The prevalence and burden of bipolar disorder: findings from the Global Burden of Disease Study 2013. Bipolar Disord. 2016;18(5):440–50.

Findling RL, Frazier TW, Youngstrom EA, McNamara NK, Stansbrey RJ, Gracious BL, et al. Double-blind, placebo-controlled trial of divalproex monotherapy in the treatment of symptomatic youth at high risk for developing bipolar disorder. J Clin Psychiatry. 2007;68(5):781–8.

Fusar-Poli P, De MA, Rocchetti M, Cappucciati M, Ramella-Cravaro V, Rutigliano G, et al. Semistructured interview for bipolar at risk states (SIBARS). Psychiatry Res. 2018;264:302–9.

Garno JL, Goldberg JF, Ramirez PM, Ritzler BA. Impact of childhood abuse on the clinical course of bipolar disorder. Br J Psychiatry. 2005;186:121–5.

Geller B, Cooper TB, Zimerman B, Frazier J, Williams M, Heath J, et al. Lithium for prepubertal depressed children with family history predictors of future bipolarity: a double-blind, placebo-controlled study. J Affect Disord. 1998;51(2):165–75.

Geller B, Zimerman B, Williams M, Bolhofner K, Craney JL. Bipolar disorder at prospective follow-up of adults who had prepubertal major depressive disorder. Am J Psychiatry. 2001;158(1):125–7.

Geoffroy PA, Scott J. Prodrome or risk syndrome: what's in a name? Int J Bipolar Disord. 2017;5(1):7.

Gilman SE, Dupuy JM, Perlis RH. Risks for the transition from major depressive disorder to bipolar disorder in the National Epidemiologic Survey on Alcohol and Related Conditions. J Clin Psychiatry. 2012;73(6):829–36.

Goldberg JF, Ernst CL. Features associated with the delayed initiation of mood stabilizers at illness onset in bipolar disorder. J Clin Psychiatry. 2002;63(11):985–91.

Goldstein TR, Merranko J, Krantz M, Garcia M, Franzen P, Levenson J, et al. Early intervention for adolescents at-risk for bipolar disorder: a pilot randomized trial of Interpersonal and Social Rhythm Therapy (IPSRT). J Affect Disord. 2018;235:348–56.

Hall RCW. Global assessment of functioning. Psychosomatics. 1995;36(3):267–75.

Ising HK, Veling W, Loewy RL, Rietveld MW, Rietdijk J, Dragt S, et al. The validity of the 16-item version of the Prodromal Questionnaire (PQ-16) to screen for ultra high risk of developing psychosis in the general help-seeking population. Schizophr Bull. 2012;38(6):1288–96.

Jack M. FERUS: Fragebogen zur Erfassung von Ressourcen und Selbstmanagementfähigkeiten. Göttingen: Hogrefe; 2004.

Kapczinski F, Dias VV, Kauer-Sant'Anna M, Frey BN, Grassi-Oliveira R, Colom F, et al. Clinical implications of a staging model for bipolar disorders. Expert Rev Neurother. 2009;9(7):957–66.

Kessing LV, Agerbo E, Mortensen PB. Major stressful life events and other risk factors for first admission with mania. Bipolar Disord. 2004;6(2):122–9.

Kessing LV, Vradi E, Andersen PK. Starting lithium prophylaxis early versus late in bipolar disorder. Br J Psychiatry. 2014;205(3):214–20.

Kwapil TR, Miller MB, Zinser MC, Chapman LJ, Chapman J, Eckblad M. A longitudinal study of high scorers on the hypomanic personality scale. J Abnorm Psychol. 2000;109(2):222–6.

Lenox RH, Gould TD, Manji HK. Endophenotypes in bipolar disorder. Am J Med Genet. 2002;114(4):391–406.

Leopold K, Ritter P, Correll CU, Marx C, Ozgurdal S, Juckel G, et al. Risk constellations prior to the development of bipolar disorders: rationale of a new risk assessment tool. J Affect Disord. 2012;136(3):1000–10.

Leopold K, Pfeiffer S, Correll CU, Bauer M, Pfennig A. Early recognition centers for mental disorders—a complementary supply in the German health system. Psychiatr Prax. 2013a;40(5):264–70.

Leopold K, Pfennig A, Severus E, Bauer M. Prevention of bipolar disorders. Nervenarzt. 2013b;84(11):1310–5.

Leopold K, Ratzer S, Correll CU, Rottmann-Wolf M, Pfeiffer S, Ritter P, et al. Characteristics, symptomatology and naturalistic treatment in individuals at-risk for bipolar disorders: baseline results in the first 180 help-seeking individuals assessed at the Dresden high-risk project. J Affect Disord. 2014;152–154:427–33.

Lish JD, Dimemeenan S, Whybrow PC, Price RA, Hirschfeld RMA. The National Depressive and Manic-Depressive Association (DMDA) Survey of bipolar members. J Affect Disord. 1994;31(4):281–94.

Matza LS, Rajagopalan KS, Thompson CL, de Lissovoy G. Misdiagnosed patients with bipolar disorder: comorbidities, treatment patterns, and direct treatment costs. J Clin Psychiatry. 2005;66(11):1432–40.

McGorry PD, Hickie IB, Yung AR, Pantelis C, Jackson HJ. Clinical staging of psychiatric disorders: a heuristic framework for choosing earlier, safer and more effective interventions. Aust N Z J Psychiatry. 2006;40(8):616–22.

McLean TL, Kotwicki RJ, Harvey PD. A longitudinal analysis of patients' perceptions of life events after discharge from community mental health services. 2014. https://www.skylandtrail.org/Portals/0/PDFs/Skyland-Poster-APA-2014.pdf. Accessed 5 July 2018.

Mendlewicz J, Rainer JD. Adoption study supporting genetic transmission in manic–depressive illness. Nature. 1977;268(5618):327–9.

Mesman E, Nolen WA, Reichart CG, Wals M, Hillegers MH. The Dutch bipolar offspring study: 12-year follow-up. Am J Psychiatry. 2013;170(5):542–9.

Miklowitz DJ, Chang KD, Taylor DO, George EL, Singh MK, Schneck CD, et al. Early psychosocial intervention for youth at risk for bipolar I or II disorder: a one-year treatment development trial. Bipolar Disord. 2011;13(1):67–75.

Miklowitz DJ, Schneck CD, Singh MK, Taylor DO, George EL, Cosgrove VE, et al. Early intervention for symptomatic youth at risk for bipolar disorder: a randomized trial of family-focused therapy. J Am Acad Child Adolesc Psychiatry. 2013;52(2):121–31.

Miller TJ, McGlashan TH, Rosen JL, Cadenhead K, Cannon T, Ventura J, et al. Prodromal assessment with the structured interview for prodromal syndromes and the scale of prodromal symptoms: predictive validity, interrater reliability, and training to reliability. Schizophr Bull. 2003;29(4):703–15.

Miller S, Dell'Osso B, Ketter TA. The prevalence and burden of bipolar depression. J Affect Disord. 2014;169:S3–11.

Mühlbacher M, Egger C, Kaplan P, Simhandl C, Grunze H, Geretsegger C, et al. Relabilität und Übereinstimmungsvalidität der deutschen Version der Young Mania Rating Scale (YMRS-D). Neuropsychiatrie. 2011;25(1):16–25.

Mühlbauer E, Bauer M, Ebner-Priemer U, Ritter P, Hill H, Beier F, et al. Effectiveness of smartphone-based ambulatory assessment (SBAA-BD) including a predicting system for upcoming episodes in the long-term treatment of patients with bipolar disorders: study protocol for a randomized controlled single-blind trial. BMC Psychiatry. 2018;18(1):349.

Nadkarni RB, Fristad MA. Clinical course of children with a depressive spectrum disorder and transient manic symptoms. Bipolar Disord. 2010;12(5):494–503.

Özerdem A, Güntekin B, Atagün I, Turp B, Başar E. Reduced long distance gamma (28–48 Hz) coherence in euthymic patients with bipolar disorder. J Affect Disord. 2011;132(3):325–32.

Pfennig A, Jabs B, Pfeiffer S, Weikert B, Leopold K, Bauer M. Versorgungserfahrungen bipolarer Patienten in Deutschland: befragung vor Einführung der S3-Leitlinie zur Diagnostik und Therapie bipolarer Störungen. Nervenheilkunde. 2011;30:333–40.

Pfennig A, Bschor T, Baghai T, Braunig P, Brieger P, Falkai P, et al. S3 guidelines on diagnostics and therapy of bipolar disorders: development process and essential recommendations. Der Nervenarzt. 2012a;83(5):568–86.

Pfennig A, Correll CU, Leopold K, Juckel G, Bauer M. Early recognition and intervention for bipolar disorders: state of research and perspectives. Der Nervenarzt. 2012b;83(7):897–902.

Pfennig A, Leopold K, Ritter P, Bohme A, Severus E, Bauer M. Longitudinal changes in the antecedent and early manifest course of bipolar disorder—a narrative review of prospective studies. Aust N Z J Psychiatry. 2017;51(5):509–23.

Post RM, Leverich GS, Kupka RW, Keck PE Jr, McElroy SL, Altshuler LL, et al. Early-onset bipolar disorder and treatment delay are risk factors for poor outcome in adulthood. J Clin Psychiatry. 2010;71(7):864–72.
Preuss UW, Rujescu D, Giegling I, Watzke S, Koller G, Zetzsche T, et al. Psychometric evaluation of the German version of the Barratt Impulsiveness Scale. Nervenarzt. 2008;79(3):305–19.
Riegler C, Teismann H, Baune B, Faller H, Störk S, Heuschmann P. Inter-Rater-Reliabilität einer deutschsprachigen Variante des Functioning Assessment Short Test (FAST). In: Gemeinsame Jahrestagung – der Deutschen Gesellschaft für Epidemiologie e.V. (DGEpi), – der Deutschen Gesellschaft für Medizinische Soziologie e.V. (DGMS) und – der Deutschen Gesellschaft für Sozialmedizin und Prävention e.V. (DGSMP). Das Gesundheitswesen. Georg Thieme Verlag KG. 2017.
Ritter PS, Bermpohl F, Gruber O, Hautzinger M, Jansen A, Juckel G, et al. Aims and structure of the German Research Consortium BipoLife for the study of bipolar disorder. Int J Bipolar Disord. 2016;4(1):26.
Roniger A, Späth C, Schweiger U, Klein JP. A psychometric evaluation of the German version of the Quick Inventory of Depressive Symptomatology (QIDS-SR16) in outpatients with depression. Fortschr Neurol Psychiatr. 2015;83(12):e17–22.
Rosa AR, Sánchez-Moreno J, Martínez-Aran A, Salamero M, Torrent C, Reinares M, et al. Validity and reliability of the Functioning Assessment Short Test (FAST) in bipolar disorder. Clin Pract Epidemiol Ment Health. 2007;3:5.
Rush AJ. Toward an understanding of bipolar disorder and its origin. J Clin Psychiatry. 2003;64(Suppl 6):4–8 **(discussion 28)**.
Ryles F, Meyer TD, Adan-Manes J, MacMillan I, Scott J. A systematic review of the frequency and severity of manic symptoms reported in studies that compare phenomenology across children, adolescents and adults with bipolar disorders. Int J Bipolar Disord. 2017;5(1):4.
Saß H, Wittchen HU, Zaudig M, Houben I. Diagnostisches und Statistisches Manual Psychischer Störungen - Textrevision - (DSM-IV-TR). Göttingen: Hogrefe-Verlag. 2012. 1001 Seiten.
Schneck CD, Chang KD, Singh MK, DelBello MP, Miklowitz DJ. A pharmacologic algorithm for youth who are at high risk for bipolar disorder. J Child Adolesc Psychopharmacol. 2017;27(9):796–805.
Schultze-Lutter F, Ruhrmann S, Fusar-Poli P, Bechdolf A, Schimmelmann BG, Klosterkötter J. Basic symptoms and the prediction of first-episode psychosis. Curr Pharm Des. 2012;18(4):351–7.
Schulz P, Schlotz W, Becker P. TICS. Trierer Inventar zum chronischen Stress. Testmappe mit Manual. Göttingen: Hogrefe; 2004.
Smoller JW, Finn CT. Family, twin, and adoption studies of bipolar disorder. Am J Med Genet. 2003;123C(1):48–58.
Stange JP, Boccia AS, Shapero BG, Molz AR, Flynn M, Matt LM, et al. Emotion regulation characteristics and cognitive vulnerabilities interact to predict depressive symptoms in individuals at risk for bipolar disorder: a prospective behavioral high-risk study. Cognit Emot. 2013;27(1):63–84.
Strobel A, Beauducel A, Debener S, Brocke B. Eine deutschsprachige Version des BIS/BAS-Fragebogens von Carver und White. Zeitschrift für Differentielle und Diagnostische Psychologie. 2001;22(3):216–27.
Thompson KN, Conus PO, Ward JL, Phillips LJ, Koutsogiannis J, Leicester S, et al. The initial prodrome to bipolar affective disorder: prospective case studies. J Affect Disord. 2003;77(1):79–85.
Tillman R, Geller B, Bolhofner K, Craney JL, Williams M, Zimerman B. Ages of onset and rates of syndromal and subsyndromal comorbid DSM-IV diagnoses in a prepubertal and early adolescent bipolar disorder phenotype. J Am Acad Child Adolesc Psychiatry. 2003;42(12):1486–93.
Victor D, Sakado K, Mundt C, Kronmüller K-T. Psychometrische Evaluation der deutschen Version des Temperamentsfragebogens TEMPS-A. Psychother Psychosom Med Psychol. 2006;56(2):70–7.
Walter H, Schnell K, Erk S, Arnold C, Kirsch P, Esslinger C, et al. Effects of a genome-wide supported psychosis risk variant on neural activation during a theory-of-mind task. Mol Psychiatry. 2011;16(4):462–70.
Wang L-J, Shyu Y-C, Yuan S-S, Yang C-J, Yang K-C, Lee T-L, et al. Attention-deficit hyperactivity disorder, its pharmacotherapy, and the risk of developing bipolar disorder: a nationwide population-based study in Taiwan. J Psychiatr Res. 2016;72:6–14.
Welsh GS, Barron F. Barron-Welsh art scale. Palo Alto: Consulting Psychologists Press; 1949.
Wingenfeld K, Spitzer C, Mensebach C, Grabe HJ, Hill A, Gast U, et al. Die deutsche Version des Childhood Trauma Questionnaire (CTQ): Erste Befunde zu den psychometrischen Kennwerten. Psychother Psychosom Med Psychol. 2010;60(8):e13.
Wittchen HU, Zaudig M, Fydrich T. SKID. Strukturiertes Klinisches Interview für DSM-IV. Achse I und II. Göttingen: Hogrefe; 1997.

# 13

# Late chronotype predicts more depressive symptoms in bipolar disorder over a 5 year follow-up period

Parisa Vidafar[1], Anastasia K. Yocum[2], Peisong Han[3], Melvin G. McInnis[2] and Helen J. Burgess[1,2*]

**Abstract**

**Background:** There is increasing evidence that bipolar disorder is influenced by circadian timing, including the timing of sleep and waking activities. Previous studies in bipolar disorder have shown that people with later timed daily activities, also known as late chronotypes, are at higher risk for subsequent mood episodes over the following 12–18 months. However, these studies were limited to euthymic patients and smaller sample sizes. The aim of the current study was to further examine baseline chronotype as a potentially important predictor of mood-related outcomes in a larger sample of individuals with bipolar disorder and over the longest follow up period to date, of 5 years. Participants included 318 adults diagnosed with bipolar I and II (19–86 years) who were enrolled in the Prechter Longitudinal Study of Bipolar Disorder.

**Results:** Participants with a late chronotype were found to be more likely to have mild to more severe depressive symptoms (PHQ-9 $\geq$ 5) as captured with PHQ-9 assessments every 2 months over the 5 year follow up period. This higher risk for depressive symptoms remained even after adjusting for age, sex and mood at baseline. Additionally, late chronotypes reported fewer hypomania/mania episodes during the 5 year follow up, as derived from clinical interviews every two years.

**Conclusions:** These results highlight the potential clinical usefulness of a single self-report question, in identifying patients at risk for a more depressive mood course. The results also suggest that circadian phase advancing treatments, that can shift circadian timing earlier, should be explored as a means to reduce depressive symptoms in late chronotypes with bipolar disorder.

**Keywords:** Chronotype, Circadian, Mood

## Background

Bipolar disorder is characterized by pathological mood swings ranging from mania (e.g., high levels of energy, euphoria and minimal sleep need) to depression (e.g., low levels of energy, despair and increased sleep need or disrupted sleep) that are typically periodic but may become chronic (American Psychiatric Association DSM Task Force 2013). Bipolar I and bipolar II affects approximately 2% of the adult population in the United States (Merikangas et al. 2007; Miller et al. 2014), and suicide rates among individuals with bipolar disorder are 15 times higher than the general population (American Psychiatric Association DSM Task Force 2013). The etiology of bipolar disorder is unknown, but likely to be multifaceted (Harrison et al. 2018) and growing evidence suggests that bipolar disorder and the circadian system are intricately linked (Melo et al. 2017).

The gold standard measure of circadian timing in humans is the onset of melatonin secretion, when measured in dim light conditions (dim light melatonin onset,

*Correspondence: bhelen@med.umich.edu
[1] Sleep and Circadian Research Laboratory, Department of Psychiatry, University of Michigan, Rachel Upjohn Building, 4250 Plymouth Rd, Ann Arbor, MI 48109, USA
Full list of author information is available at the end of the article

DLMO) (Klerman et al. 2002; Lewy et al. 1999). The DLMO typically occurs 2–3 h before an individual's habitual sleep onset (Burgess and Fogg 2008), but melatonin must be measured in dim light as otherwise its secretion is suppressed by light (Lewy et al. 1980). The DLMO can be obtained non-invasively from half-hourly or hourly saliva samples, collected in the 6 h or so before habitual sleep onset (Burgess and Fogg 2008). However, the procedures to assess the DLMO requires staff support, considerable participant effort, and the melatonin assay is relatively expensive (Kantermann et al. 2015).

An alternative to measuring the DLMO is to simply ask people about the timing of their behaviors such as sleep and waking activities (their "chronotype") using questionnaires such as the Morningness-Eveningness Questionnaire (MEQ) (Horne and Ostberg 1976) or the Munich ChronoType Questionnaire (MCTQ) (Roenneberg et al. 2003). Previous work has shown that chronotype derived from these questionnaires correlates with the DLMO ($r=0.70$), and thus self-reported chronotype can serve as a proxy measure of circadian timing in humans (Kantermann et al. 2015). As with the DLMO, chronotype usually changes as a function of age. Children demonstrate morningness, or earlier circadian timing, but with the onset of puberty there is more eveningness, or later circadian timing. Eveningness peaks in the early twenties, before a steady return to morningness with increasing age (Fischer et al. 2017). There are also important sex differences in chronotype, with women typically showing earlier circadian timing and more morningness than men, although this difference diminishes after menopause (Fischer et al. 2017; Duffy et al. 2011).

Eveningness, or late chronotype, is well-recognized to be associated with more depressive symptoms in individuals with major depressive disorder and healthy controls (Kitamura et al. 2010; Levandovski et al. 2011; Merikanto et al. 2013; Selvi et al. 2010). People with bipolar disorder have more eveningness than healthy controls (Ahn et al. 2008; Wood et al. 2009; Baek et al. 2016; Mansour et al. 2005; Romo-Nava et al. 2020), even when euthymic (Giglio et al. 2010). Further, more eveningness in people with bipolar disorder was found to be associated with worse depressive symptoms (Wood et al. 2009) and a history of rapid mood swings (Mansour et al. 2005; Romo-Nava et al. 2020). Only two studies have assessed the influence of chronotype on subsequent mood course in bipolar disorder. One study found that in a sample of 104 euthymic individuals with bipolar disorder, those that met criteria for delayed sleep phase disorder (extreme eveningness), were more likely to have a mood episode in the following year (Takaesu et al. 2017). The other study examined baseline chronotype in 80 euthymic individuals with bipolar disorder and measured their subsequent anxiety, behavioral function, and number of mood episodes every month across an 18-month period. Eveningness at baseline significantly predicted poorer behavioral function, increased anxiety levels and a greater number of mood episodes (Melo et al. 2020). These results suggest that assessing chronotype in individuals with bipolar disorder may help identify patients at higher risk for adverse outcomes. As the authors of these previous studies acknowledged, 12–18-months were relatively short periods to assess mood course and the sample sizes were relatively small (Takaesu et al. 2017; Melo et al. 2020). Therefore, the aim of the current study was to further examine baseline chronotype as a potentially important predictor of mood-related outcomes in a larger sample of individuals with bipolar disorder over a longer follow up period. In addition, age and sex were included as important covariates known to impact both chronotype and mood.

## Methods

### Participants

Participants included 318 adults diagnosed with bipolar I and II, aged 19–86 years (see Table 1 for demographics and baseline psychosocial characteristics). All participants were enrolled in the Prechter Longitudinal Study of Bipolar Disorder ("Prechter study"), an observational, open cohort study established in 2005 at the University of Michigan, and had been followed for at least 5 years. The follow up analysis was restricted to 5 years to control

**Table 1** Participant demographics and psychosocial characteristics at baseline

| Baseline characteristics (n = 318) | |
|---|---|
| Age (SD) years | 43.7 (13.3) |
| Sex | |
| Females (number, %) | 223 (70%) |
| Males (number, %) | 95 (30%) |
| Chronotype, n = 318 | |
| Early chronotype (number, %) | 135 (42%) |
| Normal chronotype (number %) | 36 (11%) |
| Late chronotype (number, %) | 147 (46%) |
| PHQ-9 (mean, SD) n = 297 | 8.0 (6.4) |
| PHQ-9 ≥ 5 (number, %) | 190 (64%) |
| GAD-7 (mean, SD) n = 221 | 5.8 (4.4) |
| GAD-7 ≥ 10 (number, %) | 48 (22%) |
| HAM-D (mean, SD) n = 265 | 2.4 (0.7) |
| HAM-D ≥ 10 (number, %) | 100 (38%) |
| YMRS (mean, SD) n = 290 | 3.2 (4.5) |
| YMRS ≥ 12 (number, %) | 15 (5%) |

The mean and SD of each measure at baseline is listed

The sample size and percentage of the sample meeting the defined cut-off score at baseline is also described for the varying duration of the follow up period across participants. The Prechter study gathers phenotypic and biological data with the intention of better understanding the underlying mechanisms of bipolar disorder (McInnis et al. 2018). Participants are continuously recruited into the study by way of online and print advertisements in inpatient and outpatient psychiatric clinics within the University of Michigan Health System, as well as mental health centers and outreach events within the broader community. At enrolment, bipolar I participants were required to have had a history of treatment for a manic episode, and for bipolar II a history of recurrent depression in addition to hypomania. They were assessed via the Diagnostic Interview for Genetic Studies (Nurnberger et al. 1994) and a best estimate process by at least two doctoral level clinicians was used to confirm diagnosis of bipolar I or II using the Diagnostic and Statistical Manual of Mental Disorders (DSM-IV) criteria. All participants were free from neurological disease and active substance dependence at enrollment. Participants provided written informed consent and all study procedures were approved by the University of Michigan Institutional Review Board.

### Measures

#### *Self-report questionnaires*

Chronotype at enrolment was collected using the original version of the Munich Chronotype Questionnaire (Roenneberg et al. 2003). In this questionnaire, one item asks people to rate their chronotype according to a scale (0 = extreme early type, 1 = moderate early type, 2 = slight early type, 3 = normal type, 4 = slight late type, 5 = moderate late type and 6 = extreme late type) which results in seven possible chronotypes. As this item was reported to be in excellent agreement with the total questionnaire score (Roenneberg et al. 2003), which is not easily derived (Kantermann et al. 2015), and the single item could be easily used in clinical practice, the utility of this single item was explored here. The 7 categories were combined into three groups for analysis: (1) early (includes extreme early, moderate early and slight early types, (2) normal, and (3) late (includes slight late, moderate late, and extreme late types).

Depressive symptoms were assessed with the Patient Health Questionnaire (PHQ-9), which is designed to determine the presence and severity of depressive symptoms over the previous two-week period (Kroenke et al. 2001). The PHQ-9 was initially collected at enrollment ("baseline") and thereafter administered every two months. A score $\geq 5$ was used to determine the presence of mild or more severe depressive symptoms.

The Generalized Anxiety Disorder Scale (GAD-7) was administered at enrollment and then every two months to assess for the severity of anxiety symptoms over the past two weeks (Spitzer et al. 2006). A score $\geq 10$ was used to determine the presence of moderate or higher levels of anxiety.

#### *Clinician administered interviews*

The Hamilton Depression Rating Scale (HAM-D) was used to assess depressive symptoms at enrollment and thereafter every two years. The HAM-D is typically considered the gold standard assessment for measuring the presence and severity of depressive symptoms over the past week (Hamilton 1960; Rohan et al. 2016). A score $\geq 10$ was used to determine the presence of depressive symptoms (Hamilton 1960).

The Young Mania Rating Scale (YMRS) was administered at enrollment and thereafter annually to assess manic symptoms. During the YMRS interview, individuals were asked about how they have been feeling over the past week. A score $\geq 12$ was used to determine the presence of some manic symptoms (Young et al. 1978).

Every two years after enrollment, participants were interviewed with the Longitudinal Interval Follow-up Evaluation (LIFE), which measures the course of psychiatric disorders (Keller et al. 1987). From the LIFE interview several additional measures were derived: the number of hypomania/mania episodes, the number of depressive episodes, the number of hospitalizations and the number of suicide attempts, that had occurred since the last LIFE assessment.

#### *Data analysis*

To characterize mood-related outcomes following the baseline assessment, the number of assessments above a set score were divided by the total number of assessments of that same measure, for each participant. This generated a proportion metric for each measure and for each participant, whereby a higher proportion indicated a worse mood-related outcome. This approach helped account for the different frequencies with which the measures were assessed (from every two months to two years). So for example, for depressive symptoms, the number of assessments where PHQ-9 was $\geq 5$ was divided by the total number of PHQ-9 assessments for each participant. Similarly, the number of assessments with a HAM-D score $\geq 10$ was divided by the total number of HAM-D assessments. For anxiety symptoms, the number of assessments with GAD-7 $\geq 10$ were divided by the total number of GAD-7 assessments. For manic symptoms, the number of assessments where YMRS $\geq 12$ was divided by the total number of YMRS assessments. The LIFE interview outcomes were coded as the number of hypomania/mania episodes and depressive episodes during the follow up period, and whether at least one psychiatric hospitalization or suicide attempt had occurred during the follow up (to account for the low rate of psychiatric hospitalizations and suicide attempts during the follow up).

The influence of chronotype on subsequent mood-related outcomes estimated with a proportion were analyzed with a multivariate Poisson regression using "normal chronotype" as a reference group. The Poisson regression model explicitly takes the total number of assessments for each measure into account. The model included adjustment for age and sex (females used as a reference group) which are important influences on chronotype and mood. The model also adjusted for the baseline score, to determine if the assessment of chronotype provided any additional predictive utility for mood-related outcomes, above and beyond the baseline score of that specific measurement tool. For the LIFE interview measures of number of mood episodes, and whether a psychiatric hospitalization or suicide attempt had occurred at all during the follow up period, the data was analyzed using logistic regression. Baseline YMRS score was included in the models assessing hypomania/mania, suicide attempts and psychiatric hospitalizations, and baseline PHQ-9 score was included in the models assessing depressive episodes, suicide attempts and psychiatric hospitalizations. All of the data was analyzed using the R software (https://cran.r-project.org/).

## Results

The sample of bipolar I and II participants were mostly female, and on average middle aged (Table 1). Only about 1 in 10 participants identified as having a normal chronotype, with most reporting either a late or early chronotype. The distribution of chronotype according to age and sex in the sample indicated that at least compared to early chronotypes, the late chronotypes were younger, with almost half of males and females being a late chronotype (Fig. 1).

At baseline, almost two-thirds of the sample reported at least some mild depressive symptoms on the PHQ-9. Fewer participants were identified with depressive symptoms using the HAM-D, which may have reflected the higher cut-off score of 10 or more. About a quarter of the sample reported moderate anxiety symptoms on the GAD-7. Only a small minority of participants had manic symptoms at baseline, as reflected on the YMRS. Some participants did not complete all scheduled assessments, and the final sample size for each measure is shown in Table 1. Missing data ranged from 6.6% for the PHQ-9 to 30.5% for the GAD-7, mostly due to the GAD-7 not being included in the Prechter study until March 2012. The average number of follow up assessments per participant were 22.6 for the PHQ-9, 9.9 for the GAD-7, 2.4 for the HAM-D and 3.6 for the YMRS. On average each participant completed 2.4 LIFE interviews.

The regression results indicated that younger adults with bipolar disorder I and II were more likely to have depressive and anxiety symptoms on the PHQ-9 and GAD-7 during the follow up period, although the magnitude of this effect was very small and likely not clinically meaningful (Table 2). Similarly, those participants with higher scores on the GAD-7, HAM-D and YMRS at baseline were slightly more likely to have a higher proportion of assessments with GAD-7 $\geq$ 10, HAM-D $\geq$ 10 and YMRS $\geq$ 12 during the follow up period. Late chronotype predicted a higher proportion of assessments of PHQ-9 $\geq$ 5 during the follow up period, even after adjusting for age, sex and baseline score. On average in all chronotypes, there was a decrease from the baseline PHQ-9 to the average PHQ-9 during follow up, reflecting a reduction in depressive symptoms while participating in the Prechter study (Fig. 2). Notably, as compared to the early and normal chronotypes, the late chronotypes started with the highest average PHQ-9 at baseline and decreased on average by less than 0.5 during the follow up period to reach close to the average baseline PHQ-9 score of the early chronotypes.

In terms of the LIFE interview variables, hypomania/mania episodes were less frequent in late chronotypes, and hypomania/mania episodes were more frequent in males and in those with a higher baseline YMRS score (Table 3). Depressive episodes were slightly more likely to occur in those with a higher baseline PHQ-9 score. No effects of age, sex, baseline scores or early or late chronotype were observed on the occurrence of a suicide attempt. However, males and those with a lower PHQ-9 score at baseline were less likely to have a psychiatric hospitalization during the follow up period (Table 4).

## Discussion

The results of this study indicate that people with bipolar I and II who self-identify as late chronotypes, have a higher frequency of depressive symptoms over a 5 year follow up. Thus bipolar patients with late chronotype are at increased risk for a more depressive mood course over time, even after adjusting for the effects of age, sex and mood at baseline. This result was observed with the bimonthly administration of the PHQ-9, but not with the HAM-D or LIFE interviews. The HAM-D assessed depressive symptoms over the past week, but was only assessed every 2 years and therefore could have more easily missed detecting depressive symptoms. The LIFE interview would have captured depressive episodes, but does rely on participant recall of the previous 2 years, and detects depressive episodes, which are likely more severe than the mild depressive symptoms detected with a

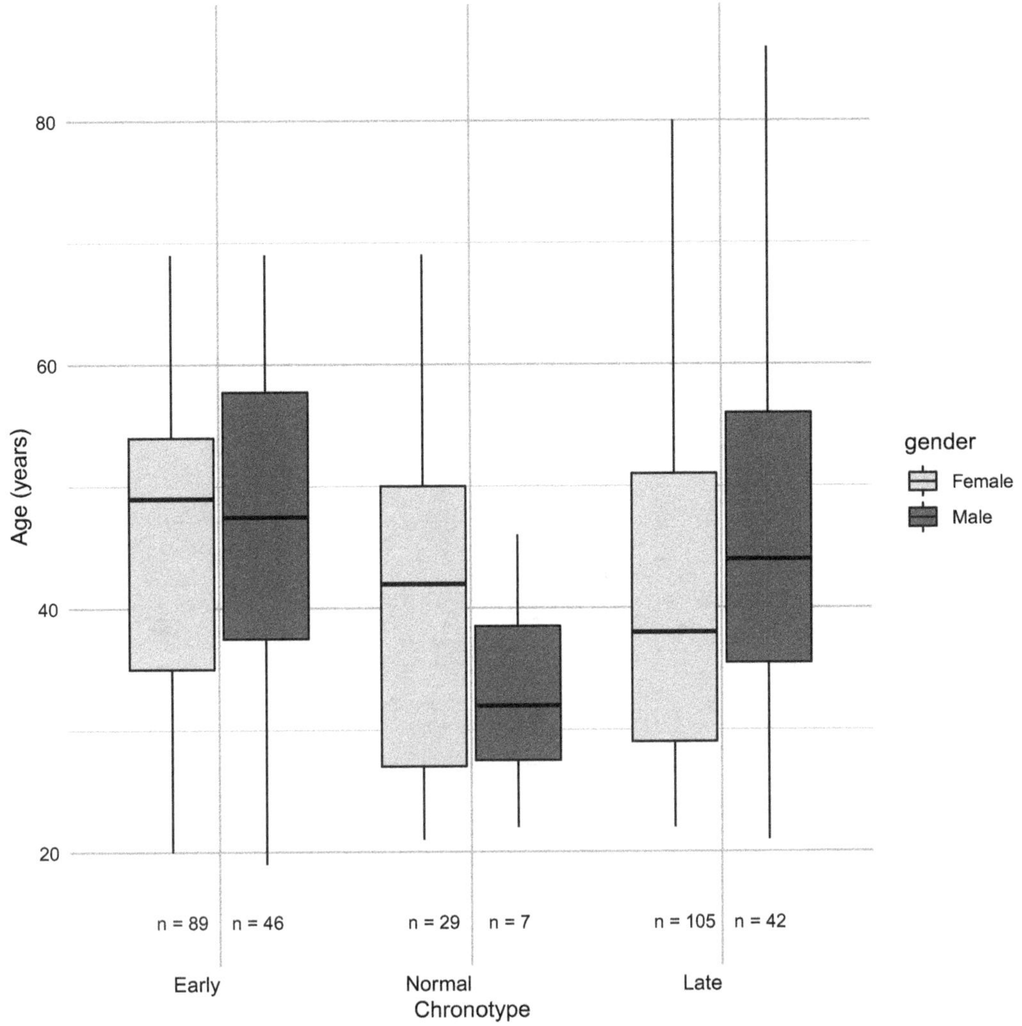


**Fig. 1** Boxplots of age is shown for each sex within each of the three chronotypes. The maximum and minimum age is shown by the top and bottom of the vertical lines, the interquartile range is represented by the box, and median by the horizontal line. Compared to early chronotypes, late chronotypes were more likely to be younger and male

**Table 2** Results of a model using age, sex, baseline score and chronotype to predict the rate of mood assessments above a predefined score during the follow up period

| | Rate ratio [95% CI] | | | | |
|---|---|---|---|---|---|
| | **Age (years)** | **Sex (male)** | **Baseline score** | **Early chronotype** | **Late chronotype** |
| PHQ-9 ≥ 5 | **0.995 [0.992–0.997]** | 1.069 [0.980- 1.166] | 0.996 [0.990–1.00] | 1.115 [0.977—1.272] | **1.290 [1.135–1.466]** |
| GAD-7 ≥ 10 | **0.995 [0.992–0.998]** | 0.945 [0.854–1.045] | **1.034 [1.024–1.043]** | 1.003 [0.871–1.155] | 1.034 [0.903–1.185] |
| HAM-D ≥ 10 | 1.002 [0.993–1.012] | 1.162 [0.905–1.492] | **1.084 [1.071–1.098]** | 0.826 [0.564–1.210] | 0.794 [0.547–1.151] |
| YMRS ≥ 12 | 1.001 [0.985–1.018] | 0.822 [0.525–1.286] | **1.164 [1.133–1.195]** | 0.973 [0.485–1.951] | 0.968 [0.486–1.929] |

Females and normal chronotype were used as reference groups

Bold RRs are significant at $p < 0.01$

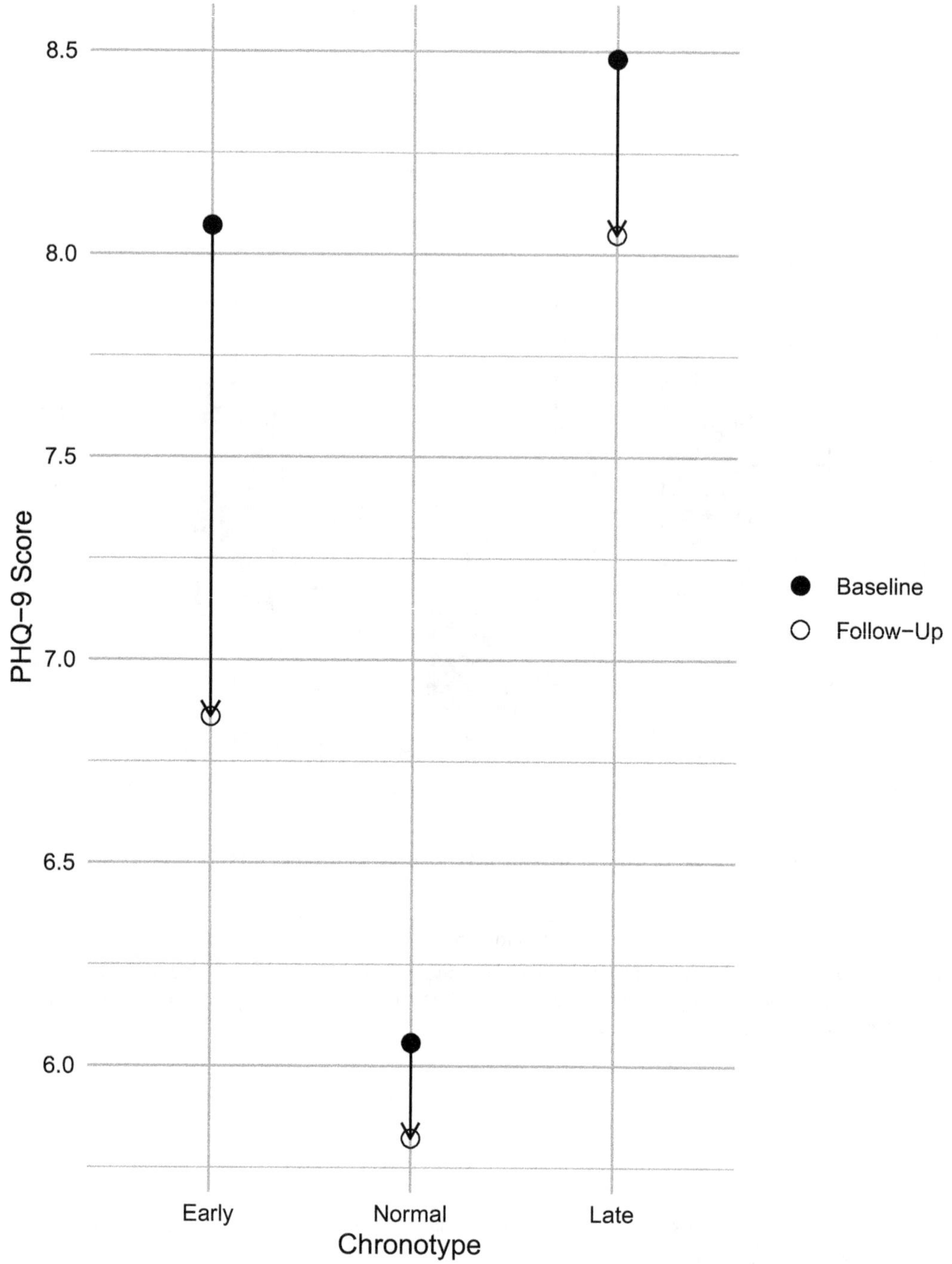


**Fig. 2** The mean baseline PHQ-9 score and mean follow up PHQ-9 score of early, normal, and late chronotypes

PHQ-9 threshold of 5. Notably the average PHQ-9 score at baseline and follow up in the late chronotype group remained under 10 (Fig. 2), further highlighting that the depressive symptoms were on average, mild. Interestingly, late chronotype was also associated with a reduced likelihood of hypomania/mania episodes on the LIFE interview, an effect that was also seen with the YMRS, although this was not statistically significant. This result raises the interesting possibility that late chronotype could be protective against manic relapse and symptoms, which should be explored in further research (Table 5).

This study of the impact of chronotype on subsequent mood course in people with bipolar disorder is the largest study to date, in a sample three times that of previous studies and with a follow up period more than three times as long (Takaesu et al. 2017; Melo et al. 2020). In both previous studies, late chronotype predicted more mood episodes in the following 12–18 months, but hypomania/mania episodes or symptoms were not distinguished from depressive episodes or symptoms due to limited statistical power. Our results suggest that late chronotype predominantly increases the risk for a depressive mood course rather than a hypomania/mania mood course. One previous study also reported that late chronotypes had more anxiety symptoms during follow up (Melo et al. 2020), but this effect was not detected in the current study possibly due to the smaller number of GAD-7 assessments. Both previous studies only included individuals who were euthymic at baseline, whereas in the current study all participants were included and baseline mood was adjusted for in the analyses. Thus the current results are relevant to any patient with bipolar disorder regardless of current mood state, and not only to euthymic patients.

The association between late chronotype (reflecting later or delayed circadian timing) and a greater likelihood of depressive symptoms is not unique to bipolar disorder, having been observed in individuals with major depressive disorder and even in healthy controls (Kitamura et al. 2010; Levandovski et al. 2011; Merikanto et al. 2013; Selvi et al. 2010). Indeed, there is preliminary evidence from a double-blinded randomized study in healthy controls, that even small circadian phase delays of only 30 min, can reduce people's overall sense of well-being (Yang et al. 2001). Others have reported that people with bipolar disorder have more eveningness, or are more likely to be a late chronotype, than healthy controls (Ahn et al. 2008; Wood et al. 2009; Baek et al. 2016; Mansour et al. 2005), even when they are euthymic (Giglio et al. 2010). Furthermore, when chronotype was assessed in people with bipolar disorder at two to three time points over two to four years, evening or late chronotype

**Table 3** Results of a model using age, sex, baseline YMRS score and chronotype to predict the number of hypomania/mania episodes during the follow up period as derived from the LIFE interview

| | Rate ratio [95% CI] | | | | |
|---|---|---|---|---|---|
| | **Age (years)** | **Sex (male)** | **YMRS** | **Early chronotype** | **Late chronotype** |
| Hypomania/mania | 0.999 [0.995–1.002] | **1.142 [1.034–1.260]** | **1.050 [1.041–1.060]** | 0.921 [0.797–1.065] | **0.747 [0.646–0.863]** |

Females and normal chronotype were used as reference groups

Bold RRs are significant at $p < 0.01$

**Table 4** Results of a model using age, sex, baseline PHQ-9 score and chronotype to predict the number of depressive episodes during the follow up period as derived from the LIFE interview

| | Rate ratio [95% CI] | | | | |
|---|---|---|---|---|---|
| | **Age (years)** | **Sex (male)** | **PHQ-9** | **Early chronotype** | **Late chronotype** |
| Depression | 0.997 [0.992–1.001] | 0.961 [0.848–1.090] | **1.051 [1.043–1.059]** | 0.984 [0.825–1.173] | 0.946 [0.796–1.124] |

Females and normal chronotype were used as reference groups

Bold RRs are significant at $p < 0.01$

**Table 5** Results of a model using age, sex, chronotype, baseline PHQ-9 and YMRS scores to predict occurrence of a suicide attempt or psychiatric hospitalization during the follow up period as derived from the LIFE interview

| | Odds ratio [95% ci] | | | | | |
|---|---|---|---|---|---|---|
| | **Age (years)** | **Sex (male)** | **PHQ-9** | **YMRS** | **Early chronotype** | **Late chronotype** |
| Suicide attempts | 1.012 [0.976–1.048] | 0.513 [0.145–1.820] | 1.057 [0.997–1.120] | 0.954 [0.836–1.089] | 0.610 [0.181–2.054] | 0.539 [0.165–1.767] |
| Psychiatric hospitalizations | 0.988 [0.972–1.004] | **0.321 [0.166–0.619]** | **1.067 [1.040–1.095]** | 1.020 [0.971–1.066] | 1.052 [0.568–1.948] | 0.877 [0.482–1.594] |

Females and normal chronotype were used as reference groups

Bold ORs are significant at $p < 0.01$

was found to be a stable characteristic, irrespective of mood state (Wood et al. 2009; Seleem et al. 2015). Together, these findings suggest the possibility that eveningness or late chronotype may be a trait marker of bipolar disorder (Seleem et al. 2015).

The finding that people with bipolar disorder who self-identified as being a late chronotype, had a more depressive mood course over the following 5 years, even after adjusting for sex, age and baseline score, raises the possibility that treatments that phase advance or shift circadian timing earlier, may help reduce depressive symptoms in people with bipolar disorder. Indeed, others have suggested circadian timing as a target for improving the mood course in bipolar disorder (Takaesu et al. 2017). Morning light treatment is well-recognized to phase advance circadian rhythms, and has antidepressant properties (Al-Karawi and Jubair 2016). Morning bright light treatment has been found to be antidepressant in people with bipolar disorder, but concerns over inducing mania have led to recommendations to administer light treatment in the middle of the day rather than the morning (Sit et al. 2018), the timing of which does not typically lead to large phase advances (Khalsa et al. 2003). Interestingly, low doses of melatonin (e.g. 0.5 mg) in the few hours before habitual bedtime are well-recognized to phase advance the circadian clock without the sleepiness side effect often associated with melatonin (Burgess et al. 2010). While higher doses of melatonin taken at bedtime have been tested in people with bipolar disorder as a sleep aid (Baandrup et al. 2011) and to improve cardiometabolic health (Mostafavi et al. 2017), it remains to be determined if melatonin, when used to phase advance circadian timing, can improve mood course in people with bipolar disorder. While the five years of follow up in this study is meaningfully longer than the previous studies (Takaesu et al. 2017; Melo et al. 2020), the granularity and frequency of the data collection nonetheless remains modest. The gathering of self-reported mood symptoms every two months and an in-person clinical assessment every two years may still have not accurately captured the nuanced daily to weekly variability in mood in people with bipolar disorder. Additionally, the restriction of the data analysis to those participants with at least 5 years of follow up means that more recently enrolled participants in the Prechter study were not included in this study. Further, chronotype was self-reported and subject to bias at the individual level, with no objective markers of sleep or circadian timing to verify the self-report. For analytical reasons the chronotype categories were collapsed from seven to three groups, which may have obscured any differences due to the intensity of chronotype, such as between the extreme, moderate and slight late chronotypes. Lastly, we note only 11% of the participants identified as a 'normal chronotype', with the remainder of the sample reporting being some degree of an early type (42%) or late type (46%). This is not dissimilar to results from the largest cross-sectional study to date of chronotype in bipolar disorder (n=773), where only 16% identified as being neither a morning or evening type, with the rest reporting as a morning type (35%) or evening type (49%) (Romo-Nava et al. 2020).

## Conclusions

This study replicates the findings that people with bipolar disorder who identify as late chronotypes have a worse mood course over the following years. Specifically, this study found that late chronotypes had a higher rate of mild or more severe depressive symptoms as assessed bimonthly with the PHQ-9 over 5 years. Conversely, late chronotypes were less likely to experience a hypomania/mania episode over 5 years. These results highlight the importance of frequent assessments with sensitive instruments over prolonged periods to better capture mood course in bipolar disorder over time. Future research could examine if the influence of late chronotype on disease course also extends to other significant life outcomes including productivity and employment.

**Acknowledgements**

With gratitude, we acknowledge The University of Michigan Prechter Bipolar Longitudinal Research participants and thank the research team of the Prechter Bipolar Research Program for their contributions in the collection and stewardship of the data used in this publication.

**Authors' contributions**

PV, AY, PH and HB assisted with data analysis. All authors assisted with manuscript preparation. All authors read and approved the final manuscript.

**Author details**

[1]Sleep and Circadian Research Laboratory, Department of Psychiatry, University of Michigan, Rachel Upjohn Building, 4250 Plymouth Rd, Ann Arbor, MI 48109, USA. [2]Depression Center, Department of Psychiatry, University of Michigan, Ann Arbor, MI 48109, USA. [3]Department of Biostatistics, School of Public Health, University of Michigan, Ann Arbor, MI 48109, USA.

**References**

Ahn YM, Chang J, Joo YH, Kim SC, Lee KY, Kim YS. Chronotype distribution in bipolar I disorder and schizophrenia in a Korean sample. Bipolar Disord. 2008;10(2):271–5.

Al-Karawi D, Jubair L. Bright light therapy for nonseasonal depression: meta-analysis of clinical trials. J Affect Disord. 2016;198:64–71.

American Psychiatric Association DSM Task Force. Diagnostic and statistical manual of mental disorders : DSM-5. 5th ed. Arlington, VA: American Psychiatric Association; 2013.

Baandrup L, Fagerlund B, Jennum P, Lublin H, Hansen JL, Winkel P, et al. Prolonged-release melatonin versus placebo for benzodiazepine discontinuation in patients with schizophrenia: a randomized clinical trial—the SMART trial protocol. BMC Psychiatry. 2011;11:160.

Baek JH, Kim JS, Kim MJ, Ryu S, Lee K, Ha K, et al. Lifetime characteristics of evening-preference and irregular bed-rise time are associated with lifetime seasonal variation of mood and behavior: comparison between individuals with bipolar disorder and healthy controls. Behav Sleep Med. 2016;14(2):155–68.

Burgess HJ, Fogg LF. Individual differences in the amount and timing of salivary melatonin secretion. PLoS ONE. 2008;3(8):e3055-e.

Burgess HJ, Revell VL, Molina TA, Eastman CI. Human phase response curves to three days of daily melatonin: 0.5 mg versus 3.0 mg. J Clin Endocrinol Metab. 2010;95(7):3325–31.

Duffy JF, Cain SW, Chang AM, Phillips AJ, Munch MY, Gronfier C, et al. Sex difference in the near-24-hour intrinsic period of the human circadian timing system. Proc Natl Acad Sci U S A. 2011;108(Suppl 3):15602–8.

Fischer D, Lombardi DA, Marucci-Wellman H, Roenneberg T. Chronotypes in the US—Influence of age and sex. PLoS ONE. 2017;12(6):e0178782.

Giglio LM, Magalhaes PV, Andersen ML, Walz JC, Jakobson L, Kapczinski F. Circadian preference in bipolar disorder. Sleep Breath. 2010;14(2):153–5.

Hamilton M. A rating scale for depression. J Neurol Neurosurg Psychiatry. 1960;23(1):56–62.

Harrison PJ, Geddes JR, Tunbridge EM. The emerging neurobiology of bipolar disorder. Trends Neurosci. 2018;41(1):18–30.

Horne JA, Ostberg O. A self-assessment questionnaire to determine morningness-eveningness in human circadian rhythms. Int J Chronobiol. 1976;4(2):97–110.

Kantermann T, Sung H, Burgess HJ. Comparing the morningness-eveningness questionnaire and munich chronotype questionnaire to the dim light melatonin onset. J Biol Rhythms. 2015;30(5):449–53.

Keller MB, Lavori PW, Friedman B, Nielsen E, Endicott J, McDonald-Scott P, et al. The longitudinal interval follow-up evaluation. A comprehensive method for assessing outcome in prospective longitudinal studies. Arch Gen Psychiatry. 1987;44(6):540–8.

Khalsa SBS, Jewett ME, Cajochen C, Czeisler CA. A phase response curve to single bright light pulses in human subjects. J Physiol. 2003;549(3):945–52.

Kitamura S, Hida A, Watanabe M, Enomoto M, Aritake-Okada S, Moriguchi Y, et al. Evening preference is related to the incidence of depressive states independent of sleep-wake conditions. Chronobiol Int. 2010;27(9–10):1797–812.

Klerman EB, Gershengorn HB, Duffy JF, Kronauer RE. Comparisons of the variability of three markers of the human circadian pacemaker. J Biol Rhythm. 2002;17(2):181–93.

Kroenke K, Spitzer RL, Williams JB. The PHQ-9: validity of a brief depression severity measure. J Gen Intern Med. 2001;16(9):606–13.

Levandovski R, Dantas G, Fernandes LC, Caumo W, Torres I, Roenneberg T, et al. Depression scores associate with chronotype and social jetlag in a rural population. Chronobiol Int. 2011;28(9):771–8.

Lewy AJ, Wehr T, Goodwin F, Newsome D, Markey S. Light suppresses melatonin secretion in humans. Science. 1980;210(4475):1267–9.

Lewy AJ, Cutler NL, Sack RL. The endogenous melatonin profile as a marker for circadian phase position. J Biol Rhythm. 1999;14(3):227–36.

Mansour HA, Wood J, Chowdari KV, Dayal M, Thase ME, Kupfer DJ, et al. Circadian phase variation in bipolar I disorder. Chronobiol Int. 2005;22(3):571–84.

McInnis MG, Assari S, Kamali M, Ryan K, Langenecker SA, Saunders EFH, et al. Cohort profile: the Heinz C. Prechter longitudinal study of bipolar disorder. Int J Epidemiol. 2018;47(1):28–28n.

Melo MCA, Abreu RLC, Linhares Neto VB, de Bruin PFC, de Bruin VMS. Chronotype and circadian rhythm in bipolar disorder: a systematic review. Sleep Med Rev. 2017;34:46–58.

Melo MC, Garcia RF, Araújo CF, Luz JH, Bruin PF, Bruin VM. Chronotype in bipolar disorder: an 18-month prospective study. Braz J Psychiatry. 2020;42(1):68–71.

Merikangas KR, Akiskal HS, Angst J, Greenberg PE, Hirschfeld RMA, Petukhova M, et al. Lifetime and 12-month prevalence of bipolar spectrum disorder in the National Comorbidity Survey replication. Arch Gen Psychiatry. 2007;64(5):543–52.

Merikanto I, Lahti T, Kronholm E, Peltonen M, Laatikainen T, Vartiainen E, et al. Evening types are prone to depression. Chronobiol Int. 2013;30(5):719–25.

Miller S, Dell'Osso B, Ketter TA. The prevalence and burden of bipolar depression. J Affect Disord. 2014;169(1):S3–11.

Mostafavi SA, Solhi M, Mohammadi MR, Akhondzadeh S. Melatonin for reducing weight gain following administration of atypical antipsychotic olanzapine for adolescents with bipolar disorder: a randomized, double-blind, placebo-controlled trial. J Child Adolesc Psychopharmacol. 2017;27(5):440–4.

Nurnberger JI, Jr., Blehar MC, Kaufmann CA, York-Cooler C, Simpson SG, Harkavy-Friedman J, et al. Diagnostic interview for genetic studies. Rationale, unique features, and training. NIMH Genetics Initiative. Arch Gen Psychiatry. 1994;51(11):849–59; discussion 63–4.

Roenneberg T, Wirz-Justice A, Merrow M. Life between clocks: daily temporal patterns of human chronotypes. J Biol Rhythms. 2003;18(1):80–90.

Rohan KJ, Rough JN, Evans M, Ho SY, Meyerhoff J, Roberts LM, et al. A protocol for the Hamilton Rating Scale for Depression: item scoring rules, rater training, and outcome accuracy with data on its application in a clinical trial. J Affect Disord. 2016;200:111–8.

Romo-Nava F, Blom TJ, Cuellar-Barboza AB, Winham SJ, Colby CL, Nunez NA, et al. Evening chronotype as a discrete clinical subphenotype in bipolar disorder. J Affect Disord. 2020;266:556–62.

Seleem MA, Merranko JA, Goldstein TR, Goldstein BI, Axelson DA, Brent DA, et al. The longitudinal course of sleep timing and circadian preferences in adults with bipolar disorder. Bipolar Disord. 2015;17(4):392–402.

Selvi Y, Aydin A, Boysan M, Atli A, Agargun MY, Besiroglu L. Associations between chronotype, sleep quality, suicidality, and depressive symptoms in patients with major depression and healthy controls. Chronobiol Int. 2010;27(9–10):1813–28.

Sit DK, McGowan J, Wiltrout C, Diler RS, Dills JJ, Luther J, et al. Adjunctive bright light therapy for bipolar depression: a randomized double-blind placebo-controlled Trial. Am J Psychiatry. 2018;175(2):131–9.

Spitzer RL, Kroenke K, Williams JB, Löwe B. A brief measure for assessing generalized anxiety disorder: the GAD-7. Arch Intern Med. 2006;166(10):1092–7.

Takaesu Y, Inoue Y, Ono K, Murakoshi A, Futenma K, Komada Y, et al. Circadian rhythm sleep-wake disorders as predictors for bipolar disorder in patients with remitted mood disorders. J Affect Disord. 2017;220:57–61.

Wood J, Birmaher B, Axelson D, Ehmann M, Kalas C, Monk K, et al. Replicable differences in preferred circadian phase between bipolar disorder patients and control individuals. Psychiatry Res. 2009;166(2–3):201–9.

Yang CM, Spielman AJ, D'Ambrosio P, Serizawa S, Nunes J, Birnbaum J. A single dose of melatonin prevents the phase delay associated with a delayed weekend sleep pattern. Sleep. 2001;24:272–81.

Young RC, Biggs JT, Ziegler VE, Meyer DA. A rating scale for mania: reliability, validity and sensitivity. Br J Psychiatry. 1978;133:429–35.

# 14

# A pilot investigation of emotional regulation difficulties and mindfulness-based strategies in manic and remitted bipolar I disorder and major depressive disorder

Christie W. Musket[1], Natasha S. Hansen[2], Keith M. Welker[3], Kirsten E. Gilbert[4] and June Gruber[2*]

**Abstract**

**Background:** Both bipolar disorder and major depressive disorder are characterized by difficulties in emotion regulation. Little is known about which specific emotion regulatory patterns may be transdiagnostic versus disorder specific, and how such patterns change as a function of current mood states.

**Methods:** This preliminary investigation examined specific patterns of self-reported trait emotion regulation difficulties and mindfulness-based regulations strategies across four groups: remitted adults with bipolar I disorder (BD-remitted; $n = 32$), currently manic adults with bipolar I disorder (BD-manic; $n = 19$), remitted adults with major depressive disorder (MDD-remitted; $n = 32$), and healthy controls (CTL; $n = 30$).

**Results:** All three clinical groups reported significantly greater difficulties with emotion regulation and decreased overall mindfulness-based strategies.

**Conclusions:** These results suggest that increased emotion regulation difficulties, decreased mindfulness, and increased emotion-driven impulsivity may be transdiagnostic across mood disorders and states, and that impulsivity may be particularly impaired during periods of mania.

**Keywords:** Emotion regulation, Emotional awareness, Impulsivity, Mindfulness, Bipolar disorder, Major depressive disorder

## Background

Emotion regulation is defined as the set of actions that individuals take (either consciously or unconsciously) to affect their emotional experience (Gross and Jazaieri 2014). Emotion regulation can be either adaptive or maladaptive (i.e., can either improve or worsen individuals' functioning or internal experience). An expanding literature highlights the prevalence and severity of emotion regulation difficulties across many different psychopathologies, including major depression and bipolar disorder (Gross and Jazaieri 2014; Aldao et al. 2010). In spite of the prevalence of such difficulties, there is a lack of research examining the similarities and differences in specific aspects of emotion dysregulation within and across mood disorders.

Bipolar disorder (BD) and major depressive disorder (MDD) are severe and chronic mood disorders. Disruptions in emotion regulation have been proposed as critical predictors of the etiology and maintenance of both BD and MDD (e.g., Alloy et al. 2009; Gruber 2011). However, less is known about whether emotion regulation patterns are stable across time or vary as a function of current mood state. For bipolar disorder in particular,

*Correspondence: june.gruber@colorado.edu
[2] Department of Psychology and Neuroscience, University of Colorado, Boulder, 345 UCB, Muenzinger D321C, Boulder, CO 80309-0345, USA
Full list of author information is available at the end of the article

there is a dearth of research exploring the pattern emotion dysregulation in manic states. Furthermore, it is not known if such regulatory patterns are transdiagnostic across mood disorders. The goal of this pilot study was to begin to examine self-reported emotion regulation patterns across bipolar and unipolar mood disorders.

**Emotion regulation and mood disorders**

BD is centrally characterized not only by extreme emotion fluctuation but also by impaired emotion regulation (Gruber 2011). Individuals with remitted BD tend to use more maladaptive emotion regulation strategies known to amplify emotional distress, including suppression and rumination (Gruber et al. 2013; Wolkenstein et al. 2014). Remitted BD individuals also tend to engage in maladaptive emotion-related impulsivity, which is associated with increased manic symptom severity and poorer global functioning (e.g., (Muhtadie et al. 2014). These findings suggest that problematic emotion regulation is a central feature of BD. However, little research has been conducted to determine whether or not such findings are state-specific (i.e., persist across mood phases in BD). Emotion regulation deficits are also a central feature of MDD (Rottenberg et al. 2005). Individuals with remitted MDD use more maladaptive emotion regulation strategies compared to individuals without any psychiatric diagnoses (Garnefski and Kraaij 2006; Joormann 2010), and have a tendency to up-regulate negative emotion intensity and fail to maintain positive emotion intensity (Gruber et al.. 2014). It still remains unclear whether or not such features are disorder-specific to unipolar depression or transdiagnostic across mood disorders.

One concept central to emotion regulation is mindfulness. Mindfulness is a mental state defined by bringing awareness to the present moment and accepting thoughts and feelings as they arise without immediate reaction or judgment (e.g., Kabat-Zinn 1990). Mindfulness has been shown to facilitate adaptive emotion regulation, and to promote physical and psychological well being (e.g., Kang et al. 2013). Recent work suggests that mindfulness-based emotion regulation strategies may help reduce mood symptom severity in both BD and MDD (Deckersbach et al. 2012; Teasdale et al. 2000; Hanssen et al. 2019). Individuals with BD even appear to benefit emotionally and physiologically from engaging in mindfulness-based instructions in laboratory studies (Gilbert et al. 2013). One key aspect of mindfulness as it relates to the process of regulating emotions is emotional awareness, or the extent to which an individual is conscious of his/her present emotional state. The ability to notice and accurately distinguish between different emotions has been proposed as a first step in regulating emotions adaptively (Vine and Aldao 2014). Despite its probable role in adaptive emotion regulation, emotional awareness remains largely unexplored in BD and MDD. Moreover, although some preliminary work has found that those with BD and MDD may not differ from controls in their self-reported awareness of emotional states (Rheenen et al. 2015), other research has suggested that deficits in identifying and differentiating between emotions are a transdiagnostic feature of mood disorders (Vine and Aldao 2014).

The present study examined self-reported patterns of trait difficulties with emotion regulation, and mindfulness-based emotion regulation strategies across four groups: currently hypomanic/manic BD I (BD-manic), remitted BD I (BD-remitted), remitted MDD (MDD-remitted), and healthy non-psychiatric control (CTL) adults. Aim 1 examined group differences in trait emotion regulation difficulties. Based on prior research indicating that both BD and MDD are characterized by difficulties with emotion regulation (Gruber 2011; Rottenberg et al. 2005; Rheenen et al. 2015; Giovanelli et al. 2013), we predicted that all three clinical groups would exhibit greater trait emotion regulation difficulties compared to the CTL group. Aim 2 examined group differences in trait mindfulness-based regulation strategies. For Aim 2, we examined two competing perspectives: The first is that there should be decreased mindfulness-based strategies across remitted and symptomatic phases of BD and MDD as compared to healthy controls, based on work suggesting that mood disorders are characterized by difficulties in emotion differentiation (e.g., Vine and Aldao 2014), and that increasing mindfulness reduces both manic and depressive mood symptoms (Deckersbach et al. 2012; Teasdale et al. 2000). The second perspective posits intact emotion awareness (one aspect of mindfulness) across remitted and symptomatic phases in both BD and MDD based on research that suggests no significant deficit in self-reported emotional awareness in BD and MDD (Das et al. 2014; Ehring et al. 2008).

## Method

### Participants

Participants between the ages of 18–60 were recruited via posted flyers or online advertisements (e.g., www.craigslist.org) from the greater New Haven, CT area. Participants responded to one of three separate study advertisements: a study on "emotion and mood" for healthy controls, on "bipolar disorder and emotion" for the BD group, and on "history of depression and emotion" for the MDD group. Interested participants completed a brief phone screen with a trained researcher and were invited to the laboratory for a diagnostic evaluation to determine final study eligibility (see below).

**Table 1 Demographic and clinical characteristics**

| | BD-remitted (*n* = 32) | BD-manic (n = 19) | MDD-remitted (*n* = 32) | CTL (*n* = 30) |
|---|---|---|---|---|
| Demographic characteristics | | | | |
| Age (yrs) | 29.30 (8.80) | 35.93 (13.00) | 31.23 (11.38) | 31.93 (9.36) |
| Female | 65.60% | 57.90% | 64.50% | 63.3% |
| Caucasian | 90.60% | 100% | 90.60% | 90.00% |
| Education (Yrs) | 14.95 (2.39) | 14.67 (2.38) | 15.13 (2.26) | 15.95 (2.37) |
| Employment status | | | | |
| Full-time | 12.50% | 21.10% | 18.80% | 36.70% |
| Part-time | 34.40% | 15.80% | 31.30% | 30.00% |
| Unemployed (not student) | 15.60% | 47.40% | 21.90% | 16.70% |
| Unemployed (student) | 37.50% | 5.30% | 28.10% | 13.30% |
| Marital status | | | | |
| Single (no relationship) | 56.30% | 15.80% | 37.50% | 40.00% |
| Single (in relationship) | 9.40% | 42.10% | 28.10% | 33.30% |
| Live-in partner | 3.10% | 0% | 3.10% | 6.70% |
| Married | 28.10% | 15.80% | 12.50% | 16.70% |
| Divorced or widowed | 3.10% | 26.30% | 18.80% | 3.30% |
| Annual income | | | | |
| < $10 K | 18.80% | 47.40% | 15.60% | 13.30% |
| $10 K–$25 K | 18.80% | 15.80% | 18.80% | 10.00% |
| $26 K–$50 K | 31.30% | 21.10% | 40.60% | 26.70% |
| $51 K–$75 K | 3.10% | 10.50% | 12.50% | 20.00% |
| $76 K–$100 K | 15.60% | 5.30% | 3.10% | 16.70% |
| > $100 K | 12.50% | 0% | 9.40% | 13.30% |
| Clinical characteristics | | | | |
| YMRS | 1.88 (1.90) | 15.00 (5.48) | 1.72 (1.87) | 1.17 (1.05) |
| IDS-C | 4.22 (3.27) | 17.68 (8.45) | 5.03 (2.79) | 2.00 (1.98) |
| GAF | 75.78 (5.91) | 61.42 (8.64) | 79.03 (6.82) | 88.03 (3.03) |
| # Comorbid disorders | 0.50 (0.84) | 1.63 (1.54) | 0.78 (0.94) | – |
| # Medications | 2.03 (1.52) | 1.65 (1.11) | 0.53 (0.84) | – |
| Age at depression onset (Yrs) | 16.57 (7.08) | 13.32 (4.62) | 16.09 (7.26) | – |
| Depression duration (Yrs) | 14.29 (10.07) | 22.92 (15.39) | 15.34 (10.36) | – |
| # Depressive episodes | 14.87 (23.28) | 9.50 (17.19) | 5.47 (7.35) | – |
| Age at Mania Onset (Yrs) | 19.72 (6.74) | 17.13 (9.28) | – | – |
| Mania duration (Yrs) | 11.13 (9.86) | 19.97 (15.96) | – | – |
| # Manic episodes | 12.33 (25.55) | 46.45 (40.73) | – | – |

*BD-remitted* Bipolar I disorder remitted group, *BD-manic* Bipolar I disorder manic group, *MDD* Major depressive disorder remitted group, *CTL* Healthy control group, *YMRS* Young Mania Rating Scale, *IDS-C* Inventory to Diagnose Depression, *GAF* Global Assessment of Functioning, *Age at Onset* Age of first depressive or manic episode, *#Comorbid Disorders* the number of current DSM-IV-TR Axis I comorbidities, Mean values are displayed with standard deviations in parentheses where applicable

The study sample consisted of four groups of individuals who met the following DSM-IV criteria: currently remitted BD type I (BD-remitted; $n = 32$), currently manic BD type I (BD-manic, $n = 19$), currently remitted MDD (MDD; $n = 32$), and healthy controls with no current or past Axis I disorders (CTL; $n = 30$). Exclusion criteria included a lifetime history of neurological disease, severe head trauma, stroke, autoimmune disorder, severe medical illness, and alcohol or substance abuse in the past six months. Given that both BD and MDD are highly comorbid with other disorders, participants in the three clinical groups were not excluded based on comorbidities other than substance abuse or dependence within the past 6 months. Demographic and clinical data are presented in Table 1.

## Measures of clinical functioning

### Diagnostic evaluation

Diagnoses were established using the Structured Clinical Interview for DSM-IV (SCID-IV; First et al. 2007), administered by a licensed clinical psychologist, trained clinical psychology doctoral student, or trained post-baccalaureate fellow. Illness duration, age of onset, and lifetime number of depressive and manic mood episodes were also obtained. Following common practices in inter-rater reliability in our lab (e.g., Gruber and Weinstock 2018; Ong et al. 2017), a large subset ($n=91$; 81%) of videotaped interviews was reviewed by a second rater to evaluate the reliability of diagnostic ratings. These ratings were discussed at a group consensus meeting and scoring adjustments were made as necessary. Final ratings between the interviewer and consensus rater matched 100% ($\kappa=1.00$) of primary diagnoses.

### Mood symptoms

Current symptoms of depression were measured using the Inventory of Depressive Symptomatology (IDS-C; Trivedi et al. 2004), a 30-item clinician-rated assessment with scores ranging from 0 to 84, with higher scores indicating more depressive symptomatology. Current symptoms of mania were measured using the Young Mania Rating Scale (YMRS; (Young et al. 1978), an 11-item clinician-rated scale with scores ranging from 0 to 60, with higher scores indicating more manic symptomatology. Remitted status for the BD-remitted, MDD-remitted, and CTL groups was confirmed using the SCID-IV current mood disorder module criteria and scores below standardized cutoffs on the IDS-C ($\leq 11$) and YMRS ($\leq 7$). Current manic status for the BD-manic group was confirmed using SCID-IV criteria for a current manic episode ($n=16$) or hypomanic episode ($n=3$)[1] in the past month, as well scores above the YMRS cutoff ($>7$) in the past week. Intra-class correlations (ICCs) for the same subset of participants were strong for the YMRS (ICC=0.98) and IDS-C (ICC=0.97).

### Global functioning

Participants' occupational, social, and psychological functioning within the past week was assessed using the Global Assessment of Functioning scale (GAF; *DSM-IV Axis V*), which ranges from 1 (lowest level of functioning) to 100 (highest level of functioning). GAF ICCs for a large subset of study participants ($n=91$) was high (=0.86).

[1] Unless otherwise specified, parallel results emerged when running analyses with and without the smaller hypomanic subgroup excluded in the BD group.

### Difficulties in emotion regulation scale

The Difficulties in Emotion Regulation Scale (DERS; Gratz and Roemer 2004) is a 36-item questionnaire that provides an assessment of self-reported emotion regulation difficulties. Items (e.g., "When I'm upset, I have difficulty getting work done," "I have difficulty making sense out of my feelings") were rated using a 5-point Likert scale (1=almost never, 5=almost always). The DERS is made up of six subscales: Non-acceptance (i.e., a tendency to pass negative judgment on one's own distress); Goals (i.e., trouble accomplishing goals while upset); Strategies (i.e., limited access to emotion regulation strategies); Impulse (i.e., the tendency to lose control of behaviors when emotionally upset); Awareness (i.e., attentiveness to one's emotions); and Clarity (i.e., confusion about what one is feeling). Higher scores are associated with increased difficulties in emotion regulation.

### Five-facet mindfulness questionnaire

The Five-Facet Mindfulness Questionnaire (FFMQ; Baer et al. 2006) is a 39-item self-report measure of mindfulness strategies in daily life, with higher scores indicating greater use of mindfulness. Items (e.g., "I perceive my thoughts and emotions without having to react to them," "Even when I'm feeling terribly upset, I can find a way to put it into words") were rated on a 5-point Likert scale (1=never or rarely true, 5=very often or always true). The FFMQ comprises five subscales (Cronbach's $\alpha s \geq 0.76$) including (1) Acting with Awareness (i.e., remaining present in the moment), (2) Non-reacting (i.e., avoiding reflexive reactions to emotions), (3) Non-judging (i.e., non-judgmental attitude towards one's emotions), (4) Observing (i.e., the tendency to pay attention to current emotional states), and (5) Describing (i.e., the ability to describe emotions in words).

## Procedure

Participants provided informed consent and were administered a structured clinical interview by a trained interviewer. Next, participants completed a series of experimental tasks not relevant to the present investigation followed by self-report questionnaires, which included the measures of emotion awareness and regulation strategies reported in the present study. Participants were then debriefed and compensated in cash ($10 per hour) for participation.

## Results

Demographic information and clinical characteristics are provided in Table 1. Groups did not differ on age, gender, ethnicity, or education. For the main hypotheses, we completed analyses both with and without current symptom covariates (IDSC and YMRS), noting where analyses

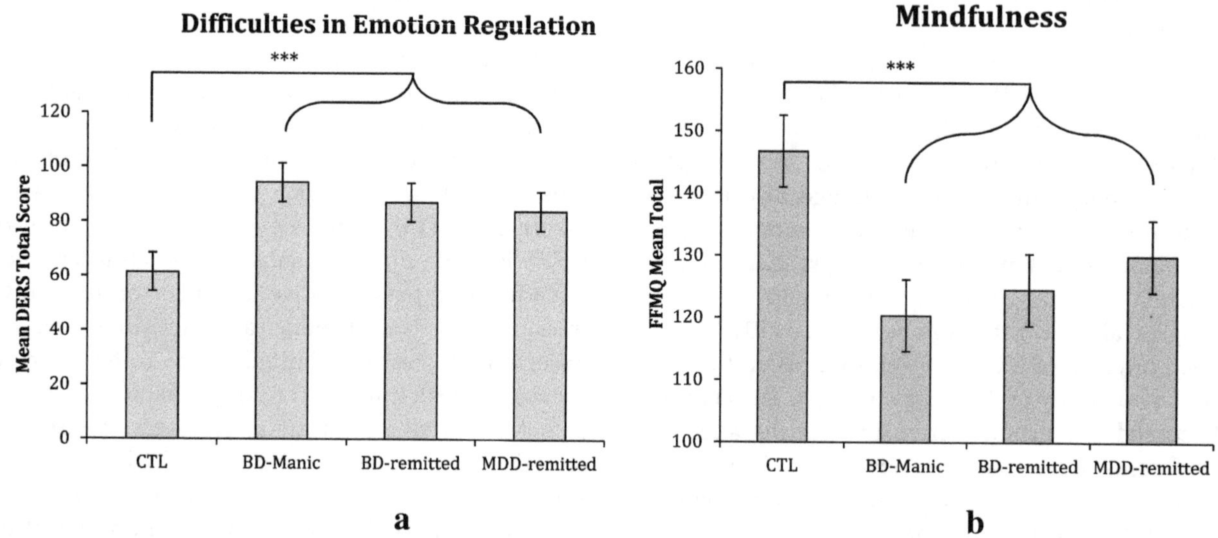


**Fig. 1** Group differences in total scores for difficulties in emotion regulation (**a**) and mindfulness-based regulation strategies (**b**). Error bars represent standard errors of the mean. *$p<.05$, **$p<.01$, ***$p<.001$

differed with the inclusion of covariates.[2] Effect sizes of mean differences are presented in the metric of Cohen's *d*.

Our first aim examined group differences in emotion regulation difficulties (based on the DERS total score). Consistent with our predictions, all three clinical groups reported greater difficulties in emotion regulation compared with the CTL group. As seen in Fig. 1a, for difficulties in emotion regulation, there was a main effect of Group ($F(3, 108)=14.18$, $p<0.001$). Post-hoc analyses confirmed that, relative to the CTL group ($M=61.33$, $SD=15.61$), the BD-remitted ($M=86.97$, $SD=21.92$, $d=1.35$), MDD-remitted ($M=83.75$, $SD=18.72$, $d=1.30$), and BD-manic ($M=94.28$, $SD=21.79$, $d=1.74$) groups had significantly greater difficulties in emotion regulation ($p$'s$<0.001$). No other group differences were significant ($p$'s$\geq 0.21$). As seen in in Table 2, post-hoc analyses indicated that the three clinical groups differed from the CTL group (i.e., reported significantly greater emotion regulation difficulties) on the non-acceptance, goals, impulse, and strategies subscales of the DERS; as above, the clinical groups did not differ from one another. Furthermore, the BD-remitted and MDD-remitted groups also reported greater difficulties on the clarity subscale than the CTL group. No group differences emerged on the awareness subscale.

Our second aim examined group differences in mindfulness-based regulation strategies based on the FFMQ total score. Consistent with our predictions, all three clinical groups reported decreased use of mindfulness compared to the CTL group. As seen in Fig. 1b, there was a main effect of Group ($F(3, 107)=10.47$, $p<0.001$) for trait mindfulness, which was characterized by significantly decreased mindfulness in the BD-manic ($M=120.37$, $SD=20.98$, $d=1.46$), BD-Remitted ($M=124.53$, $SD=19.36$, $d=1.30$), and MDD-Remitted ($M=129.93$, $SD=19.97$, $d=0.96$) groups relative to the CTL group ($M=146.73$, $SD=14.56$, $p$'s$<0.001$); however, the clinical groups did not differ from one another. As seen in in Table 2, post-hoc analyses of the FFMQ subscales indicated that the three clinical groups differed from the CTL group (i.e., scored significantly lower on) on the non-reactivity, acting with awareness, describing, and non-judging subscales of the FFMQ; as above, the clinical groups did not differ from one another. No group differences emerged on the observing subscale.

## Discussion

The present study investigated group differences in trait emotion regulation and mindfulness-based regulation strategies in a sample of adults with currently manic BD, remitted BD, remitted MDD, and a healthy non-psychiatric control group. Our results suggest that all three clinical groups reported greater difficulty regulating their emotions and used fewer mindfulness-based regulation

[2] We suggest that any results based on the inclusion of symptom scores as covariates be interpreted with caution given that controlling for current symptoms to minimize between-group variability violates important statistical assumptions (e.g., (Baer et al. 2006)). In addition it is theoretically questionable given a primary aim was to examine group differences as a function of symptom severity (i.e., comparing our manic BD group to remitted BD and MDD groups). Nonetheless we present these results for full transparency. Thus we did not control for current symptoms in the present analyses.

**Table 2 Descriptive statistics for FFMQ and DERS by diagnostic group**

| | BD-remitted ($n=32$) | BD-manic ($n=19$) | MDD-remitted ($n=32$) | CTL ($n=30$) | Main effect of group |
|---|---|---|---|---|---|
| FFMQ | | | | | |
| Non-reactivity | 20.72 (4.33)$^{a}$ | 19.63 (4.68)$^{b}$ | 21.28 (5.13)$^{c}$ | 24.23 (3.99)$^{a,b,c}$ | $F(3, 109)=4.99, p=.003$ |
| Observing | 25.53 (7.00) | 26.89 (9.00) | 26.75 (7.53) | 26.80 (13.72) | $F(3, 109)=.35, p=.788$ |
| Acting with awareness | 22.13 (5.89)$^{a}$ | 20.12 (5.77)$^{b,f}$ | 23.19 (5.58)$^{c,f}$ | 30.00 (3.92)$^{a,b,c}$ | $F(3, 109)=17.63, p<.001$ |
| Describing | 28.31 (6.78)$^{a}$ | 27.95 (7.86)$^{b}$ | 29.19 (5.57)$^{c}$ | 33.53 (4.70)$^{a,b,c}$ | $F(3, 109)=4.96, p=.003$ |
| Non-Judging | 27.84 (8.77)$^{a}$ | 25.79 (8.16)$^{b}$ | 28.90 (5.99)$^{c}$ | 33.83 (5.49)$^{a,b,c}$ | $F(3, 107)=5.98, p=.001$ |
| DERS | | | | | |
| Non-acceptance | 13.25 (5.25)$^{a}$ | 14.67 (7.34)$^{b}$ | 13.09 (4.90)$^{c}$ | 9.90 (4.86)$^{a,b,c}$ | $F(3, 108)=3.54, p=.017$ |
| Goals | 15.34 (4.29)$^{a}$ | 16.67 (5.59)$^{b}$ | 15.53 (4.47)$^{c}$ | 10.80 (4.21)$^{a,b,c}$ | $F(3, 108)=8.87, p<.001$ |
| Impulse | 12.69 (4.80)$^{a,d}$ | 16.94 (7.22)$^{b,d,f}$ | 12.03 (4.30)$^{f}$ | 8.03 (2.51)$^{a,b,c}$ | $F(3, 108)=14.15, p<.001$ |
| Awareness | 15.03 (5.00) | 14.94 (4.72) | 13.66 (4.04) | 12.80 (4.43) | $F(3, 108)=1.58, p=.199$ |
| Strategies | 18.66 (7.98)$^{a}$ | 20.55 (7.09)$^{b}$ | 18.56 (6.94)$^{c}$ | 10.87 (3.38)$^{a,b,c}$ | $F(3, 107)=10.94, p<.001$ |
| Clarity | 12.00 (5.09)$^{a}$ | 10.28 (3.78) | 11.09 (2.99)$^{c}$ | 8.87 (3.78)$^{a,c}$ | $F(3, 108)=3.75, p=.013$ |

*BD-remitted* Bipolar I disorder remitted group, *BD-manic* Bipolar I disorder manic group, *MDD* major depressive disorder remitted group, *CTL* healthy control group, *FFMQ* Five Facet Mindfulness Questionnaire (higher scores = increased mindfulness), *DERS* Difficulties in Emotion Regulation Scale (higher scores = more difficulties in emotion regulation). Mean scores are displayed with standard deviations in parentheses. In each row, means sharing a superscript letter (*a, b, c, d, or e*) were significantly different in pairwise group comparisons ($p<.05$): $^{a}$BD-remitted significantly different from CTL; $^{b}$BD-manic significantly different from CTL; $^{c}$MDD-remitted significantly different from CTL; $^{d}$BD-remitted significantly different from BD-manic; $^{e}$BD-remitted significantly different from MDD; $^{f}$BD-manic significantly different from MDD-remitted

strategies in their everyday lives compared with individuals without a psychiatric history. However, the three mood-disordered groups did not differ significantly from one another in either overall emotion regulation or mindfulness-based regulation strategies. Post-hoc examination of individual subscales generally suggested these patterns were consistent across distinct facets of emotion regulation difficulties and mindfulness. Together, these results indicate that BD and MDD are both characterized by increased levels of emotion regulation difficulties, as well as decreased mindfulness, compared to the healthy control group. Interestingly, this pattern seems to be transdiagnostic and consistent regardless of current mood state.

## Conclusions

This preliminary investigation sheds light on emerging evidence regarding patterns of emotion regulation strategies across mood disorders. First, this work is consistent with a growing body of work documenting increased emotion regulation difficulties (including emotion-relevant impulsivity), and decreased utilization of adaptive mindfulness-based strategies, in mood disorders (e.g., Gruber 2011; Gruber et al. 2013; Wolkenstein et al. 2014; Muhtadie et al. 2014; Rottenberg et al. 2005; Garnefski and Kraaij 2006; Joormann 2010; Gruber et al. 2014; Hanssen et al. 2019; Gilbert et al. 2013; Vine and Aldao 2014; Rheenen et al. 2015; Giovanelli et al. 2013; Park et al. 2014; Weinstock et al. 2018), and importantly extends this work by examining bipolar and unipolar mood-disordered groups within a single study and with the additional inclusion of currently hypomanic/manic bipolar individuals. Interestingly, post-hoc analyses exploring individual facets of emotion regulation and mindfulness-based strategies suggested that the emotion awareness subscales on both the DERS and FFMQ were not significantly different between groups. This suggests that mood-disordered individuals may not exhibit differences from non-psychiatric controls in their tendency to notice and pay attention to what they are feeling. This is surprising considering that, in the present investigation, such individuals self-reported difficulties with putting their feelings into words and endorsed an increased tendency to judge and react negatively to their own feelings. Further work is warranted to examine the extent to which intact awareness, as well as prior exposure to mindfulness-based strategies and interventions, may contribute to the etiology and course of mood symptomatology. Additional work in larger sample sizes using multivariate analytic approaches might also reveal unique versus common underlying factors across distinct types of emotion regulation strategies.

Some limitations of the present research design should be mentioned. First, we note that although the sample sizes were larger than those from previous studies on this topic and relatively large considering the severe nature of the psychiatric groups recruited, the present sample sizes were still somewhat small. Power analyses (using standard estimates of adequate power of 0.80) suggest that our sample size was adequately powered to detect a medium to large effect size (i.e., $\eta_p^2 \geq 0.11$), but it is possible that we may have failed to detect more subtle effects. Future studies with larger sample sizes are an important next step to examine the generalizability of these findings. Second, although the current research identifies group differences in mindfulness and emotional regulation, without a longitudinal design or the inclusion of interventions aimed at modulating emotional awareness and regulation strategies, the current research is not designed to elucidate the etiological role of emotional awareness and regulation in the trajectory of BD and MDD. Third, while our study has provided first-step pilot data suggesting that emotion regulation difficulties and deceased mindfulness may be a more trait-like rather than state-dependent feature of mood disturbance, further work is necessary to examine underlying mechanisms that give rise to these observed patterns. Given our outpatient manic BD participants endorsed mild to moderate symptom severity, future work replicating these findings in acutely manic as well as currently depressed BD individuals would be informative. Fourth, the study relied on self-report measures and additional research obtaining converging results using behavioral and neurophysiological indices of emotion regulation is warranted (e.g., Miller and Chapman 2001). In addition, while this study provided valuable insights regarding self-reported measures of emotion regulation and mindfulness, it will be critical to examine how such findings translate to everyday life. An examination of state-specific regulatory patterns that target the regulation of specific positive and negative emotion states within BD and MDD would be a useful expansion of the current research. Finally, forthcoming research could explore the effectiveness of mindfulness training in reducing impulsivity and increasing emotional awareness in individuals with BD and MDD. Such work may help uncover the possible causal role that emotion regulation and mindfulness may play in the etiology and severity of affective disorders.

#### Acknowledgements
We thank Amanda Purcell, Amelia Aldao, Yoona Kang, Elizabeth Reeves, Franziska Goer, Winfield Call, and Colin Bosma for their assistance with data collection.

#### Authors' contributions
JG and KEG designed the study and oversaw data collection. CWM, NSH, KMW, KEG and JG conceptualized the ideas behind this manuscript. CWM, NSH, and KMW led analyses. NSH, KMW, and JG drafted the initial manuscript and CWM led substantive revisions to the manuscript. All authors read and approved the final manuscript.

#### Author details
[1] Department of Psychology, University of Pittsburgh, Pittsburgh, USA.
[2] Department of Psychology and Neuroscience, University of Colorado, Boulder, 345 UCB, Muenzinger D321C, Boulder, CO 80309-0345, USA. [3] Department of Psychology, University of Massachusetts, Boston, USA. [4] Department of Psychiatry, Washington University in St. Louis, St. Louis, USA.

#### References
Aldao A, Nolen-Hoeksema S, Schweizer S. Emotion regulation strategies across psychopathology: a meta-analytic review. Clin Psychol Rev. 2010;30:217–37.

Alloy LB, Abramson LY, Walshaw PD, Gerstein RK, Keyser JD, Whitehouse WG, et al. Behavioral approach system (BAS)–relevant cognitive styles and bipolar spectrum disorders: concurrent and prospective associations. J Abnorm Psychol. 2009;118(3):459.

Baer RA, Smith GT, Hopkins J, Krietemeyer J, Toney L. Using self report assessment methods to explore facets of mindfulness. Assessment. 2006;13(1):27–45.

Das P, Calhoun V, Malhi GS. Bipolar and borderline patients display differential patterns of functional connectivity among resting state networks. Neuroimage. 2014;2014(98):73–81.

Deckersbach T, Hölzel BK, Eisner LR, Stange JP, Peckham AD, Dougherty DD, et al. Mindfulness-Based Cognitive Therapy for nonremitted patients with bipolar disorder. CNS Neurosci Ther. 2012;18(2):133–41.

Ehring T, Fischer S, Schnülle J, Bösterling A, Tuschen-Caffier B. Characteristics of emotion regulation in recovered depressed versus never depressed individuals. Pers Individ Dif. 2008;44(7):1574–84.

First MB, Spitzer RL, Gibbon M, Williams J. Structured Clinical Interview for DSM-IV-TR Axis I Disorders, Research Version, Patient Edition (SCID-IV). New York, NY: Biometrics Research, New York State Psychiatric Institute; 2007.

Garnefski N, Kraaij V. Relationships between cognitive emotion regulation strategies and depressive symptoms: a comparative study of five specific samples. Pers Individ Dif. 2006;40(8):1659–69.

Gilbert KE, Nolen-Hoeksema S, Gruber J. Positive emotion dysregulation across mood disorders: How amplifying versus dampening predicts emotional reactivity and illness course. Behav Res Ther. 2013;51(11):736–41.

Giovanelli A, Hoerger M, Johnson SL, Gruber J. Impulsive responses to positive mood and reward are related to mania risk. Cogn Emot. 2013;27(6):1091–104.

Gratz KL, Roemer L. Multidimensional assessment of emotion regulation and dysregulation: development, factor structure, and initial validation of the difficulties in emotion regulation scale. J Psychopathol Behav Assess. 2004;26(1):41–54.

Gross JJ, Jazaieri H. Emotion, emotion regulation, and psychopathology: an affective science perspective. Clin Psychol Sci. 2014;2:387–401.

Gruber J. When feeling good can be bad: positive emotion persistence (PEP) in bipolar disorder. Curr Dir Psychol Sci. 2011;20(4):217–21.

Gruber J, Weinstock LM. Interrater reliability in bipolar disorder research: current practices and suggestions for enhancing best practices. Int J Bipolar Disorders. 2018;6(1):1–3.

Gruber J, Kogan A, Mennin D, Murray G. Real-world emotion? An experience-sampling approach to emotion experience and regulation in bipolar I disorder. J Abnorm Psychol. 2013;122(4):971–83.

Hanssen I, van Dord MI, Compen FR, Geurts DEM, Schellekens MPJ, Speckens AEM. Exploring the clinical outcome of mindfulness-based cognitive therapy for bipolar and unipolar depressive patients in routine clinical practice: A pilot study. International Journal of Bipolar Disorders. 2019;7(1):18.

Joormann J. Cognitive inhibition and emotion regulation in depression. Curr Dir Psychol Sci. 2010;19(3):161–6.

Kabat-Zinn J. Full catastrophe living: The program of the stress reduction clinic at the University of Massachusetts Medical Center. New York: Delta; 1990.

Kang Y, Gruber J, Gray JR. Mindfulness and de-automatization. Emot Rev. 2013;5(2):192–201.

Gruber J, Dutra SJ, Hay AC, Devlin HC. Positive emotion disturbance across disorders. In: Shiota MN, Tugade M, Kirby L, eds. Handbook of Positive Psychology. New York; Guilford Press, 2014.

Miller GA, Chapman JP. Misunderstanding analysis of covariance. J Abnorm Psychol. 2001;110(1):40–8.

Muhtadie L, Johnson SL, Carver CS, Gotlib IH, Ketter TA. A profile approach to impulsivity in bipolar disorder: the key role of strong emotions. Acta Psychiat Scand. 2014;129(2):100–8.

Ong DC, Zaki J, Gruber J. Increased cooperative behavior across remitted bipolar I disorder and major depression: Insights utilizing a behavioral economic trust game. J Abnorm Psychol. 2017;126(1):1.

Park J, Ayduk O, O'Donnell L, Chun J, Gruber J, Kamali M, et al. Regulating the high: cognitive and neural processes underlying positive emotion regulation in Bipolar I Disorder. Clin Psychol Sci. 2014;1:1–14.

Rottenberg J, Gross JJ, Gotlib IH. Emotion context insensitivity in major depressive disorder. J Abnorm Psychol. 2005;114(4):627–39.

Teasdale JD, Segal ZV, Williams JMG, Ridgeway VA, Soulsby JM, Lau MA. Prevention of relapse/recurrence in major depression by mindfulness-based cognitive therapy. J Consult Clin Psychol. 2000;68(4):615–23.

Trivedi MH, Rush AJ, Ibrahim HM, Carmody TJ, Biggs MM, Suppes T, et al. The inventory of depressive symptomatology, clinician rating (IDS-C) and SELF-REPORT (IDS-SR), and the quick inventory of depressive symptomatology, clinician rating (QIDS-C) and self-report (QIDS-SR) in public sector patients with mood disorders: A psychometric evaluation. Psychol Med. 2004;34(01):73–82.

Van Rheenen TE, Murray G, Rossell SL. Emotion regulation in bipolar disorder: Profile and utility in predicting trait mania and depression propensity. Psychiatry Res. 2015;225(3):425–32.

Vine V, Aldao A. Impaired emotional clarity and psychopathology: A transdiagnostic deficit with symptom-specific pathways through emotion regulation. J Soc Clin Psychol. 2014;33(4):319–42.

Weinstock LM, Chou T, Celis-deHoyos C, Miller IW, Gruber J. Reward and punishment sensitivity and emotion regulation processes differentiate bipolar and unipolar depression. Cogn Ther Res. 2018;42(6):794–802.

Wolkenstein L, Zwick JC, Hautzinger M, Joormann J. Cognitive emotion regulation in euthymic bipolar disorder. J Affect Disord. 2014;160:92–7.

Young RC, Biggs JT, Ziegler VE, Meyer DA. A rating scale for mania: reliability, validity and sensitivity. Br J Psychiatry. 1978;133(5):429–35.

# 15

# A comprehensive assessment of personality traits and psychosocial functioning in parents with bipolar disorder and their intimate partners

Lisa Serravalle[1], Vanessa Iacono[1], Sheilagh Hodgins[2,3] and Mark A. Ellenbogen[1*]

**Abstract**

**Background:** Individuals with bipolar disorder (BD) often possess maladaptive traits and present with various difficulties in psychosocial functioning. However, little is known about the intimate partners of adults with bipolar disorder (BD) and how mental illnesses other than BD within couples may further complicate the picture. Such knowledge is needed to inform both couple and family interventions.

**Methods:** Participants were parents whose children were enrolled in a prospective study: 55 with BD and their partners, and 47 healthy control couples. All completed diagnostic interviews, and questionnaires describing personality traits, negative life events, coping skills, social support, marital adjustment and inter-partner verbal aggression. Parents with BD and healthy control parents were compared, as were the intimate partners. A series of exploratory analyses focused on the average measures within couples, with and without BD, and took account of comorbid personality disorders among those with BD and major depressive disorder among their partners.

**Results:** Intimate partners of adults with BD, relative to healthy control partners, presented with more mental disorders, higher neuroticism, lower extraversion, more emotion-focused coping, smaller social networks, less satisfaction with their social networks, and little, satisfying social contact. Additionally, they reported less consensus and satisfaction in their marital relationships, and engaged in more verbal aggression towards their partners. Participants with BD showed similar, more extreme, characteristics. Marital distress and verbal aggression were greatest among couples with an adult having BD and a comorbid personality disorder or a partner with major depressive disorder.

**Conclusion:** This study contributes to the literature by demonstrating that *both* parents with BD and their intimate partners exhibit high levels of mental illness, maladaptive personality traits and psychosocial difficulties, thus limiting their partners' ability to provide support and stability in the these high risk families. Moreover, mental illnesses other than BD may contribute to marital problems within couples. Some statistical analyses, particularly those involving comorbid conditions, were under-powered in this study. As clinical implications, the current study suggests that *both* individuals with BD and their partners could benefit from interventions aimed at lowering emotionality and verbal aggression, and increasing social support and effective coping skills.

**Keywords:** Bipolar disorder, Intimate partners, Personality, Psychosocial functioning, Marital adjustment

*Correspondence: mark.ellenbogen@concordia.ca
[1] Centre for Research in Human Development, Concordia University, Montréal, Canada
Full list of author information is available at the end of the article

## Background

Bipolar disorder (BD), a chronic and debilitating condition, is ranked among the top ten leading causes of disability worldwide (World Health Organization 2001). In addition to the incapacitating effects of acute symptoms, persons with BD display maladaptive personality traits and impaired psychosocial functioning between episodes (Hodgins et al. 2002). Adults with BD also experience high levels of dependent negative life events (Bender et al. 2010; Ellenbogen and Hodgins 2004), and engage in ineffective coping strategies to address stressful situations (Fletcher et al. 2013; Moon et al. 2014). Additionally, there is evidence to suggest individuals with BD have difficulty establishing and maintaining social support networks that could aid in buffering stress (Beyer et al. 2003; Eidelman et al. 2012). Further complicating the picture, individuals with BD present with high rates of personality disorders (PDs; Brieger et al. 2003; Fan and Hassell 2008; George et al. 2003). Among adults with BD, those with comorbid disorders, relative to those without, show greater impairment in interpersonal functioning (Carpenter et al. 1995; Loftus and Jaeger 2006). Taken together, individuals with BD present with stable maladaptive traits and experience recurring stress which they are unable to effectively cope with and further compounded by low levels of social support. Targeting these factors with effective treatments could potentially improve the course of BD and ameliorate the child-rearing environment. To inform such interventions, more information is needed about these factors within the family context.

Many adults with BD form intimate relationships that they report to be unsatisfactory (Whisman 2007) and characterized by verbal aggression from their partner (Lam et al. 2005). Moreover, divorce rates are two to three times higher in adults with BD relative to the general population (Kogan et al. 2004; Suppes et al. 2001). One factor contributing to marital instability in these couples may be the presence of a major affective disorder in the partner, which is approximately three-to-four times greater in partners of adults with, than without, BD (Butterworth and Rodgers 2008; Mathews and Reus 2001; Nordsletten et al. 2016). Little else is known about the characteristics of the intimate partners selected by adults with BD. There is some evidence to suggest that partners of individuals having BD may also display dysfunctional psychosocial patterns, such as adopting ineffective coping styles (Borowiecka-Karpiuk et al. 2014). Therefore, the intimate partner's personality traits, dependent negative life events, coping skills and social support could potentially lessen or exacerbate maladaptive behaviours of their spouse, and be associated with marital adjustment and family functioning.

The intimate partners of adults with BD play key roles within the family context, particularly in rearing children. Relative to the children of families with parents having no mental disorders, the offspring in families with a parent having BD are at increased risk of developing internalizing and externalizing problems in childhood, interpersonal difficulties, risky sexual behaviors, low occupational competence, and mental disorders (Bella et al. 2011; Duffy et al. 2014; Nijjar et al. 2014; Ostiguy et al. 2009,2012; Shaw et al. 2005). In addition to genetic effects (Kieseppä et al. 2004; Song et al. 2015), parents with BD and their partners may contribute to poor functioning and increased risk for mental disorders among their offspring by adopting suboptimal parenting practices and maladaptive behaviors, often associated with high neuroticism, that contribute to a chaotic home environment (Ellenbogen and Hodgins 2004; Iacono et al. 2018). However, intimate partners of parents with BD might mitigate some of these negative effects in the home. For example, intimate partners could help individuals with BD identify signs of developing episodes, provide support for taking medication, and encourage participation in programs aimed at reducing maladaptive behaviors, and increasing effective coping skills and social support. Indeed psychosocial interventions, including those which include family members in the treatment of BD, have been shown to improve outcomes (Miklowitz 2006; Rea et al. 2003). Therefore, intimate partners may also be key participants in family-based interventions aimed at promoting healthy development of the offspring of parents with BD (OBD). To date, there are few empirical studies of intimate partners of individuals with BD. Thus, gaining knowledge of the psychosocial functioning and maladaptive traits of the intimate partners of parents with BD is needed.

The present study examined the mental health, personality traits, negative life events, coping skills, social support, marital adjustment and verbal aggression of adults with and without BD and their intimate partners. Participants were the parents and their spouses or intimate partners who participated in a prospective longitudinal study of families in the province of Quebec (Canada) having a parent with BD or parents with no mental disorder. The study included a comprehensive assessment of families (Ellenbogen and Hodgins 2004; Rende et al. 2005), their relatives (via a structured family history interview) and their offspring who were between 4 and 14 years of age, followed by a second assessment of the offspring approximately 11 years later (Nijjar et al. 2014; Ostiguy et al. 2012). The present study utilizes data collected in parents during the initial assessment and is different from a previous publication that focused on the effects of parents' levels of neuroticism on measure of the family environment and their offspring (Ellenbogen and Hodgins 2004). As the first goal, to confirm and extend past findings, parents with BD were compared to healthy control parents. To meaningfully characterize the intimate partners of adults with BD, they were compared to partners of healthy control adults. In a second set of analyses, we focused on couples, to assess family-wide risk, comparing those with one partner with BD and those with two healthy control partners. Since comorbid PDs are common among adults with BD (Brieger et al. 2003; Fan and Hassell 2008; George et al. 2003), we conducted exploratory analyses to determine if couples that included a partner with BD and a PD differed from those without the comorbid disorder. Finally, given the elevated rate of major depressive disorder (MDD) among partners of adults with BD (Butterworth and Rodgers 2008; Mathews and Reus 2001; Nordsletten et al. 2016), we compared couples in which one partner presented BD with and without a partner with MDD to healthy couples.

## Methods

### Participants

Fifty-eight parents with BD and their 62 intimate partners from were recruited from psychiatric outpatient clinics and support groups in the province of Québec (Canada). Using community advertisements, healthy control parents (52 index parents and 48 spouses/intimate partners), who were free of any *current* Axis-I disorder or a history of affective disorder, were recruited from the same geographic regions as parents with BD. Six parents from families having a parent with BD and 10 parents from the control group were excluded from the study or dropped out prior to completing the baseline assessment. Thus, the final study sample included 102 index parents (55 BD and 47 control) and 102 intimate partners (59 BD and 43 control) from 204 parents participating in a prospective study comparing the development of children of parents with BD and children of healthy control parents (Ellenbogen and Hodgins 2004; Ostiguy et al. 2012). The majority of intimate partners were biological parents of the OBD with the exception of eight stepparents (4 males) in the families with a parent having BD. Eleven families consisted of single-parent families (7 BD, 2 males). Among the control families, one parent was randomly designated as an index parent. At the time of the assessments, index parents with BD, their intimate partners, index control parents, and their intimate partners had a mean age of 39.25 ($SD=5.35$), 39.41 ($SD=5.06$), 38.15 ($SD=5.24$) and 38.28 ($SD=4.18$) years respectively. Parent education level (number of years), used as a proxy of socioeconomic status, was 13.87 ($SD=2.96$), 13.86 ($SD=3.39$), 15.98 ($SD=2.88$) and 15.35 ($SD=2.65$) for index parents with BD, their intimate partners, index control parents, and their intimate partners respectively.

Diagnoses were confirmed using a semi-structured diagnostic assessment (see below) and psychiatric records. Some healthy control parents did meet criteria for *past* mental illness and personality disorders: 6 (13%) drug abuse/dependence, 2 (4%) anxiety disorders, 1 (2%) avoidant PD, 1 (2%) obsessive–compulsive PD and 1 (2%) PD NOS. For inclusion, all parents were required to have at least one biological child between 4 to 14 years of age, be fluent in English or French, and have been raised and educated in Canada. Parents who presented with a chronic medical condition, physical handicap, or below-average intelligence quotient ($IQ<70$) were excluded. Parents were mostly Caucasian, middle-class, and French Canadian.

## Measures

### Diagnostic interviews

#### *The structured clinical interview for DSM-III-R (SCID-I; Spitzer et al. 1992)*

The SCID-I, a valid and reliable diagnostic instrument, was used to assess parents' mental health (e.g., Zanarini and Frankenburg 2001). Independent inter-rater agreements were obtained on 15% of the interviews. Agreement between clinicians was excellent as indicated by the kappa coefficients for diagnoses of bipolar disorder, 1.0, and other mood disorders 1.0, (lifetime and current).

#### *The structured clinical interview for DSM-IV axis II personality disorders (SCID-II; Gibbon et al. 1997)*

The SCID-II was also administered to parents to assess the presence of personality disorders.

### Questionnaires

#### *NEO personality inventory-revised (NEO PI-R; Costa and McCrae 1992)*

The NEO PI-R is a self-report personality inventory. It includes 240 items measuring levels of trait neuroticism, extraversion, agreeableness, openness to experience, and conscientiousness using a Likert scale ranging from 1 (*strongly disagree*) to 5 (*strongly agree*). Studies have demonstrated high internal consistency (Chronbach's $\alpha=.89$ to .95), convergent and discriminant validity, as well as temporal stability of the NEO PI-R (Costa et al. 2000; Costa and McCrae 1992). Similar psychometric proprieties have been reported for its French translation (Rolland et al. 1998).

#### *Dyadic Adjustment Scale (DAS; Spanier 1976)*

The DAS is a 32-item, self-report questionnaire which evaluates overall relationship quality over the previous year within couples. The four subscales include consensus (agreement on matters important to the relationship), affectional expression (expression of affection and sexual desire), satisfaction (satisfaction with the relationship and commitment to its continuance), and cohesion (common interests and activities). Participants respond to each item using a Likert scale, with higher values indicating greater relationship quality. The DAS has adequate internal consistency (Chronbach's $\alpha = .70$ to .95). The DAS has been validated for its use in both English and French (Bouchard et al. 1991; Spanier and Thompson 1982). The DAS was only administered to parents with a current intimate partner.

#### *Revised conflict tactics scales (CTS2; Straus et al. 1996)*

The CTS2 measures self-reported levels of verbal and physical aggression within couples. Parents were asked to identify how often each of the 78 items occurred during the previous year. Adequate internal consistency, construct validity, and test–retest reliability have been demonstrated for the CTS2 (Straus and Mickey 2012; Vega and O'Leary 2007). Given the low base rate of physical violence, only levels of verbal aggression were utilized. The CTS2 was administered only to parents with a current intimate partner.

#### *Arizona social support interview schedule (ASSIS; Barrera 1980; Barrera et al. 1981)*

The ASSIS is a semi-structured interview containing 30 questions pertaining to the structural components of a participant's social network (size and frequency of contact) and the adequacy of social support (satisfaction). Internal consistency (Chronbach's $\alpha = 0.74 - 0.78$) for the ASSIS are adequate (Barrera 1980; Barrera et al. 1981).

#### *Psychiatric epidemiological research interview—Life Events Scale (PERI Life Events Scale; Dohrenwend et al. 1978)*

The PERI Life Events Scale measures participants' self-reported experiences of positive and negative life events which are coded as being dependent (e.g. divorce) or independent (e.g. a death in the family) of the participant's own behaviour. Only negative dependent and independent life events were utilized due to their associations with mental illness (Kendler et al. 2010; Risch et al. 2009).

#### *Coping inventory for stressful situation—adult (CISS; Endler and Parker 1994)*

Parents rated the extent to which they engaged in 48 different coping activities following stressful situations using a five-point scale ranging from 1 (*Not at all*) to 5 (*Very Much*). Standardized $T$ scores for three primary styles of coping (task-oriented, emotion-focused, and avoidance-oriented) were obtained. High internal consistency (Chronbach's $\alpha = .78 - .88$) and temporal stability have been reported for the CISS (Brands et al. 2014).

### Procedure

Data for the current study was collected from October 1994 to May 1997. Following a telephone screening, parents with BD were administered the SCID and SCID-II interviews in the laboratory or at their homes, as well as the NEO PI-R, CISS, ASSIS, DAS, and CTS2. Parents with BD were euthymic during testing. The intimate partners of parents with BD also completed the same interviews and questionnaires independently. The same procedure was undergone for healthy controls. Subsamples of parents and their intimate partners were contacted at a later date to complete the PERI-Life Event Scale. Informed written consent was obtained from all parents and procedures were approved by the Ethics Committee of the Université de Montréal (Montréal, Canada).

### Data analysis

Data were screened and corrected for outliers (the values of outliers was reduced or increased to three standard deviations from the mean) and distributional anomalies that violated statistical assumptions. A series of Multivariate Analysis of Covariance (MANCOVA) tests were conducted to examine differences in personality traits, negative life events, coping skills, social support, marital adjustment and verbal aggression between BD and healthy control index parents, and the partners of parents with BD and healthy control partners. MANCOVAs were also conducted to explore differences between couples with a parent having BD and a comorbid PD, couples having a parent with BD and no comorbid PD and healthy control couples. Similar analyses were conducted to examine the effects of having an intimate partner with a history of MDD in couples with a parent having BD. Due to the issue of non-independence and to obtain a global estimate of couple functioning, the latter analyses used mean scores across all available parents when there was more than one parent in a family. For the measure of verbal aggression at the couple level, we averaged the mean levels of verbal aggression towards and from partners (i.e., inter-partner verbal aggression). Education, a proxy for socio-economic status, was used as a covariate for all analyses. For all analyses, we focus on contrast analyses comparing groups across dependent variables of interest rather than multivariate omnibus tests, as the latter was not of interest in the present study (Kline 2008). From the effect size (Cohen's d = 0.51) observed in a previous study of this population (Iacono et al. 2018), we estimated that the effect size was in the medium range ($f^2 = .15$, $R^2$ increment of .06 to .07). Therefore, a sample size of 92 was estimated to be sufficient to detect group differences in the aforementioned MANOVA analyses with power 0.80 and an alpha level of 0.05.

## Results

### Personality traits, negative life events, coping skills, social support, marital adjustment and inter-partner verbal aggression

#### *Index parents with BD and healthy control partners*

Of the index parents with BD, 15 (27%) also presented with PDs. As presented in Table 1, index parents with BD differed from index healthy controls on the majority of measures. Parents with BD, relative to index healthy controls, obtained higher scores for neuroticism, as well as lower scores for agreeableness and for conscientiousness. The effect size for neuroticism was particularly large, as group membership accounted for 25% of the residual variance. Relative to healthy index controls, parents with BD

**Table 1 Comparisons of personality traits, psychosocial functioning, and marital adjustment of index parents with bipolar disorder (BD) and index healthy control parents and of intimate partners of parents with BD and intimate partners of healthy control parents**

| | Index parents | | | | Intimate partners | | | |
|---|---|---|---|---|---|---|---|---|
| | BD | Healthy control | | | Of adults with BD | Of healthy controls | | |
| | *M* (SD) | *M* (SD) | *F* | $\eta^2$ | *M* (SD) | *M* (SD) | *F* | $\eta^2$ |
| **Personality (NEO-PI-R)[a]** | *n*=55 | *n*=47 | | | *n*=59 | *n*=43 | | |
| Neuroticism | 60.40 (12.70) | 45.11 (8.80) | 33.41** | .25 | 50.49 (10.20) | 44.58 (8.70) | 7.41** | .07 |
| Extraversion | 48.47 (9.11) | 51.45 (7.35) | 1.62 | .02 | 47.10 (7.87) | 52.67 (7.22) | 11.08** | .10 |
| Openness | 50.95 (10.50) | 52.85 (8.65) | .01 | .00 | 48.20 (8.35) | 50.98 (7.04) | .99 | .01 |
| Agreeableness | 49.56 (9.74) | 54.04 (6.74) | 4.08* | .04 | 51.19 (8.41) | 49.67 (8.77) | 1.14 | .01 |
| Conscientiousness | 44.44 (11.10) | 50.43 (6.07) | 6.25* | .06 | 50.18 (9.84) | 51.42 (7.74) | .19 | .00 |
| **Negative life events (LES)[b]** | *n*=48 | *n*=32 | | | *n*=28 | *n*=33 | | |
| Dependent | 2.83 (1.98) | 1.09 (1.28) | 13.41** | .15 | 1.93 (1.33) | 1.58 (1.56) | .90 | .02 |
| Independent | .44 (.62) | .31 (.59) | .89 | .01 | .32 (.55) | .39 (.55) | .25 | .00 |
| **Coping skills (CISS)[c]** | *n*=55 | *n*=47 | | | *n*=58 | *n*=43 | | |
| Task-oriented | 44.80 (10.80) | 51.60 (9.75) | 5.82* | .06 | 49.40 (8.85) | 51.88 (8.11) | .98 | .01 |
| Emotion-focused | 55.27 (10.40) | 46.70 (8.68) | 11.39** | .10 | 49.90 (8.79) | 45.63 (7.51) | 5.69* | .06 |
| Avoidance-oriented | 53.04 (11.90) | 44.62 (9.24) | 15.10** | .13 | 48.34 (9.63) | 46.37 (10.6) | 1.07 | .01 |
| **Social support (ASSI)[d]** | *n*=55 | *n*=47 | | | *n*=59 | *n*=43 | | |
| Size of social network | 10.04 (6.66) | 17.85 (13.80) | 7.65** | .07 | 10.25 (7.74) | 16.60 (12.40) | 8.66** | .08 |
| Satisfaction with social network | 25.53 (3.56) | 28.30 (2.01) | 17.78** | .15 | 25.98 (3.46) | 28.23 (2.45) | 11.80** | .11 |
| Amount of social contact | 6.27 (6.98) | 12.47 (11.8) | 7.08** | .07 | 7.61 (7.91) | 12.65 (11.8) | 5.47* | .05 |
| Satisfaction with social contact | 4.25 (.95) | 4.74 (.61) | 6.40* | .06 | 4.14 (.97) | 4.63 (.691) | 7.09** | .07 |
| **Marital adjustment (DAS)[e]** | *n*=38 | *n*=45 | | | *n*=43 | *n*=40 | | |
| Consensus | 50.87 (7.80) | 53.62 (5.66) | 2.46 | .03 | 49.77 (8.12) | 52.88 (6.54) | 4.89* | .06 |
| Affectional expression | 8.24 (2.50) | 9.31 (1.81) | 7.05** | .08 | 8.00 (2.66) | 9.10 (2.41) | 3.47 | .04 |
| Satisfaction | 35.71 (7.70) | 39.56 (4.46) | 5.54* | .07 | 32.63 (8.90) | 39.53 (4.83) | 17.49** | .18 |
| Cohesion | 13.79 (5.48) | 16.18 (3.51) | 4.94* | .06 | 13.81 (5.49) | 15.68 (4.04) | 3.60 | .04 |
| **Verbal aggression (CTS)[f]** | *n*=38 | *n*=45 | | | *n*=44 | *n*=41 | | |
| From partner | 18.39 (21.60) | 8.62 (11.60) | 3.97* | .05 | 14.98 (21.00) | 10.61 (10.8) | .41 | .01 |
| Towards partner | 16.71 (21.90) | 8.73 (9.78) | 3.76 | .05 | 23.73 (26.80) | 8.95 (9.31) | 8.11** | .09 |

T-scores were used for the Personality and Coping Skills subcategories, *$p<.05$, **$p<.01$

BD: bipolar disorder

[a] From the NEO Personality Inventory-Revised

[b] From the Life Events Scale

[c] From the Coping Inventory of Stressful Situations

[d] From the Arizona Social Support Interview

[e] From the Dyadic Adjustment Scale

[f] From the Conflict Tactic Scale

reported more dependent negative life events ($\eta^2=.15$). Parents with BD also reported less effective coping strategies compared to index healthy controls. In particular, 10 and 13% of the residual variance in emotion-focused and avoidance-oriented coping, respectively, was explained by group membership. Index parents with BD reported low social support, including smaller networks, less satisfaction, and fewer contacts, relative to index healthy controls. Group differences were largest (15% of the residual variance) for satisfaction with social network. Index parents with BD displayed less affection to their partner, were less satisfied with their relationship and perceived it as less cohesive, than index healthy control parents. Group membership explained between 6–8% of the residual variance in each of these areas of marital adjustment. Finally, parents with BD reported elevated levels of verbal aggression from their partner relative to healthy controls. `

#### *Partners of index parents with BD and healthy control partners*

The intimate partners of parents with BD and healthy control partners also differed. Among the intimate partners of parents with BD, 18 (31%) presented past or current major depression, 9 (15%) past or current alcohol abuse/dependence, 6 (10%) past or current drug abuse/dependence, 6 (10%) past or current anxiety disorders, 5 (8%) past or present eating disorders, 1 (2%) borderline PD, 1 (2%) avoidant PD, 1 (2%) narcissistic PD, 1 (2%) schizotypal PD, and 2 (3%) passive aggressive PD. As presented in Table 1, partners of index parents with BD, relative to healthy control partners, obtained higher scores for neuroticism and lower scores for extraversion, accounting for 10 and 7% of the residual variance respectively. Partners of parents with BD engaged in more emotion-focused coping relative to partners of healthy control index parents, with group membership explaining 5% of the residual variance.

Intimate partners of parents with BD also reported smaller social networks, less satisfaction with their social networks, and less satisfying social contact than the partners of healthy control parents. Similar to parents with BD, group differences were largest (11% of the residual variance) for satisfaction with social network. Additionally, they reported less consensus (6% of the residual variance) and satisfaction (18% of the residual variance) in their marital relationships, and engaged in more verbal aggression towards their partners (9% of the residual variance). Low couple satisfaction reported by the intimate partners of parents with BD, given the large effect size, was particularly robust.

In sum, index parents with BD differed from healthy control index parents as to high levels of maladaptive personality traits, dependent negative life events, ineffective coping skills, low levels of social support, unsatisfying marriages, and verbal abuse from their spouse. Their intimate partners differed from the healthy control partners to a lesser extent, but significantly as to the same personality traits, the use of emotion-focused coping skills, low levels of social support, as well as unsatisfactory marital relationships and verbally abusing their spouse.

#### *Exploratory analyses comparing personality traits, negative life events, coping skills, social support, and marital adjustment and inter-partner abuse of couples with and without a partner with BD*

The next series of analyses compared mean scores of couples with and without a partner with BD. As presented in Table 2, couples with one partner with BD, as compared to healthy control couples, obtained higher scores for neuroticism, lower scores for extraversion and conscientiousness. The couples with a partner with BD reported more dependent negative life events and more ineffective coping skills, less social support, poorer marital adjustment and more verbal aggression than healthy control couples .

#### *Couples in which one partner presents BD and a PD*

As presented in Table 3, couples that included a partner with BD and a PD as compared to those with BD and no PD, obtained lower scores for avoidant coping (22% of the variance), and reported less consensus (12% of the variance) and satisfaction (20% of the variance) with their marital relationship. Notably, the proportion of residual variance explained by group membership was 1.3 to 2 times greater than in the analyses which compared *all* couples with a parent having BD vs. controls (see Table 2). Increased inter-partner violence was found in couples with a parent having BD and a PD relative to healthy control couples; this difference was not found between couples with a BD parent and no PD and control couples. Approximately 5% of the residual variance in inter-partner violence was explained by group membership. On most measures, however, both types of couples with a partner with BD differed from healthy couples.

#### *Couples in which one partner presents BD and one MDD*

As presented in Table 4, among the couples with one partner with BD, those that included a partner with MDD differed on only two measures from the couples without MDD: lower scores for agreeableness (6% of the variance) and less affection in the marital relationship (16% of the variance). These two findings are noteworthy. In the previous analyses comparing all couples with BD vs. controls (Table 2), group membership accounted for none or only 7% of the residual variance in agreeableness and marital affection, respectively. Generally, relative to healthy control couples, the couples with one partner with BD, with and without a partner with MDD, were similar.

**Table 2 Comparisons of personality traits, psychosocial functioning and marital adjustment of couples with and without a partner with bipolar disorder**

| | Couples | | | |
|---|---|---|---|---|
| | One partner with BD | Two healthy control partners | | |
| | *M* (SD) | *M* (SD) | *F* | $\eta^2$ |
| **Personality (NEO-PI-R)[a]** | ***n*=58** | ***n*=47** | | |
| Neuroticism | 55.37 (7.43) | 44.94 (7.35) | 35.86** | .26 |
| Extraversion | 47.88 (6.45) | 52.10 (5.56) | 7.80** | .07 |
| Openness | 49.68 (7.70) | 52.10 (6.46) | .13 | .00 |
| Agreeableness | 50.11 (6.81) | 52.16 (5.71) | .51 | .01 |
| Conscientiousness | 47.12 (7.73) | 51.06 (5.45) | 6.21* | .06 |
| **Negative life events (LES)[b]** | ***n*=48** | ***n*=33** | | |
| Dependent | 2.55 (1.47) | 1.32 (1.17) | 13.17** | .14 |
| Independent | .40 (.48) | .35 (.40) | .61 | .01 |
| **Coping skills (CISS)[c]** | ***n*=57** | ***n*=47** | | |
| Task-oriented | 46.93 (7.43) | 51.60 (7.20) | 5.51* | .05 |
| Emotion-focused | 52.56 (7.13) | 46.19 (6.08) | 13.41** | .12 |
| Avoidance-oriented | 51.33 (8.15) | 45.38 (7.60) | 14.20** | .12 |
| **Social support (ASSI)[d]** | ***n*=58** | ***n*=47** | | |
| Size of social network | 10.16 (5.72) | 17.20 (9.22) | 12.52** | .11 |
| Satisfaction with social network | 25.75 (2.89) | 28.27 (1.85) | 21.07** | .17 |
| Amount of social contact | 7.00 (6.02) | 12.45 (8.10) | 8.73** | .08 |
| Satisfaction with social contact | 4.19 (.76) | 4.70 (.50) | 10.33** | .09 |
| **Marital adjustment (DAS)[e]** | ***n*=45** | ***n*=46** | | |
| Consensus | 50.39 (6.72) | 53.52 (5.44) | 6.51* | .07 |
| Affectional expression | 8.08 (2.41) | 9.23 (1.95) | 6.65* | .07 |
| Satisfaction | 34.07 (7.80) | 39.72 (4.22) | 15.83** | .15 |
| Cohesion | 14.04 (4.89) | 16.15 (3.32) | 5.25* | .06 |
| **Verbal aggression (CTS)[f]** | ***n*=45** | ***n*=45** | | |
| Inter-partner | 18.45 (19.47) | 9.44 (9.34) | 3.46 | .04 |

Due to non-independence of data and to obtain a global estimate of couple functioning, mean scores across all available parents. when there was more than one parent in a family were used (number of single-parent families = 11 (7 BD))

T-scores were used for the Personality and Coping Skills subcategories, *p<.05, **p<.01

BD: bipolar disorder

[a] From the NEO Personality Inventory-Revised

[b] From the Life Events Scale

[c] From the Coping Inventory of Stressful Situations

[d] From the Arizona Social Support Interview

[e] From the Dyadic Adjustment Scale

[f] From the Conflict Tactic Scale

## Discussion

The present study compared parents having BD and their intimate partners with healthy control parents and their partners on a comprehensive battery of psychosocial measures important for adaptive family functioning, including mental disorders, personality traits, negative life events, coping skills, social support, marital adjustment, and verbal aggression. To assess family-wide risk, we conducted exploratory analyses examining the same variables within couples rather than individuals, comparing couples having a parent with BD with those having no mental disorders. Notably, comorbid personality

**Table 3 Comparisons of personality traits, psychosocial functioning and marital adjustment of couples with a partner with bipolar disorder, with and without a comorbid personality disorder, and healthy control couples**

| | Couples | | | | | Couples with a partner with BD and PD vs healthy control couples | Couples with a partner with BD no PD vs healthy control couples | Couples with a partner with BD and PD vs couples with a partner with BD no PD |
|---|---|---|---|---|---|---|---|---|
| | One partner with BD | | Two healthy control partners | | | | | |
| | PD | No PD | | | | | | |
| | $M$ (SD) | $M$ (SD) | $M$ (SD) | $F$ | $\eta^2$ | | | |
| **Personality (NEO-PI-R)[a]** | $n=21$ | $n=37$ | $n=47$ | | | | | |
| Neuroticism | 58.52 (7.40) | 53.59 (6.93) | 44.94 (7.35) | 20.37** | .29 | ✓ | ✓ | |
| Extraversion | 45.59 (6.18) | 49.17 (6.31) | 52.10 (5.56) | 5.79** | .10 | ✓ | | |
| Openness | 48.79 (9.44) | 50.18 (6.60) | 52.10 (6.46) | .07 | .00 | | | |
| Agreeableness | 49.29 (6.58) | 50.58 (6.98) | 52.16 (5.71) | .27 | .01 | | | |
| Conscientiousness | 47.90 (7.55) | 46.68 (7.90) | 51.06 (5.45) | 3.45* | .06 | | ✓ | |
| **Negative life events (LES)[b]** | $n=18$ | $n=30$ | $n=33$ | | | | | |
| Dependent | 2.22 (1.34) | 2.75 (1.53) | 1.32 (1.17) | 7.81** | .17 | | ✓ | |
| Independent | .50 (.49) | .33 (.48) | .35 (.41) | 1.60 | .04 | | | |
| **Coping skills (CISS)[c]** | $n=21$ | $n=36$ | $n=47$ | | | | | |
| Task-oriented | 45.83 (6.31) | 47.57 (8.03) | 51.60 (7.20) | 2.81 | .05 | ✓ | ✓ | |
| Emotion-focused | 53.72 (6.54) | 51.88 (7.47) | 46.19 (6.08) | 6.71** | .12 | ✓ | ✓ | |
| Avoidance-oriented | 46.72 (4.99) | 54.01 (8.48) | 45.38 (7.60) | 13.93** | .22 | | ✓ | ✓ |
| **Social support (ASSI)[d]** | $n=21$ | $n=37$ | $n=47$ | | | | | |
| Size of social network | 9.17 (5.47) | 10.73 (5.86) | 17.20 (9.22) | 6.20** | .11 | ✓ | ✓ | |
| Satisfaction with social network | 26.04 (2.90) | 25.59 (2.92) | 28.27 (1.85) | 10.84** | .18 | ✓ | ✓ | |
| Amount of social contact | 5.87 (6.44) | 7.64 (5.77) | 12.44 (8.10) | 4.41** | .08 | ✓ | ✓ | |
| Satisfaction with social contact | 4.10 (.80) | 4.24 (.74) | 4.70 (.47) | 5.25** | .09 | ✓ | ✓ | |
| **Marital adjustment (DAS)[e]** | $n=19$ | $n=26$ | $n=46$ | | | | | |
| Consensus | 48.35 (7.07) | 51.88 (6.16) | 53.52 (5.44) | 5.89** | .12 | ✓ | | ✓ |
| Affectional expression | 7.78 (1.84) | 8.31 (2.78) | 9.23 (1.95) | 3.84* | .08 | ✓ | | |
| Satisfaction | 31.68 (8.08) | 35.81 (7.25) | 39.72 (4.22) | 10.88** | .20 | ✓ | ✓ | ✓ |
| Cohesion | 13.14 (4.72) | 14.69 (5.00) | 16.15 (3.32) | 3.50* | .07 | ✓ | | |
| **Verbal aggression (CTS)[f]** | $n=19$ | $n=26$ | $n=45$ | | | | | |
| Inter-partner | 22.85 (19.60) | 15.24 (19.12) | 9.44 (9.34) | 2.31 | .05 | ✓ | | |

Due to non-independence of data and to obtain a global estimate of couple functioning, mean scores across all available parents were used for these analyses when there was more than one parent in a family [number of single-parent families = 11 (7 BD)]

T-scores were used for the Personality and Coping Skills subcategories, $^{*}p < .05$, $^{**}p < .01$

BD: bipolar disorder; PD: personality disorder; ✓: significant group difference

[a] From the NEO Personality Inventory-Revised

[b] From the Life Events Scale

[c] From the Coping Inventory of Stressful Situations

[d] From the Arizona Social Support Interview

[e] From the Dyadic Adjustment Scale

[f] From the Conflict Tactic Scale

**Table 4 Comparisons of personality traits and psychosocial functioning of couples in which one partner presents BD and the other major depression, couples in which one partner presents BD and the other no major depression, and healthy control couples**

| | Couples | | | | | Couples with a partner with BD and MDD vs healthy control couples | Couples with a partner with BD no MDD vs healthy control couples | Couples with a partner with BD and MDD vs couples with a partner with BD no MDD |
|---|---|---|---|---|---|---|---|---|
| | One partner with BD | | Two healthy control partners | | | | | |
| | MDD | No MDD | | | | | | |
| | *M* (SD) | *M* (SD) | *M* (SD) | *F* | $\eta^2$ | | | |
| **Personality (NEO-PI-R)[a]** | *n*=18 | *n*=40 | *n*=47 | | | | | |
| Neuroticism | 57.07 (7.13) | 54.61 (7.53) | 44.94 (7.35) | 18.82** | .27 | ✓ | ✓ | |
| Extraversion | 48.02 (6.64) | 47.81 (6.44) | 52.10 (5.56) | 3.87* | .07 | | ✓ | |
| Openness | 49.49 (7.06) | 49.76 (8.06) | 52.10 (6.46) | .08 | .00 | | | |
| Agreeableness | 47.34 (8.41) | 51.35 (5.64) | 52.16 (5.71) | 3.09* | .06 | ✓ | | ✓ |
| Conscientiousness | 48.00 (6.05) | 46.7 (8.42) | 51.06 (5.45) | 3.30* | .06 | | ✓ | |
| **Negative life events (LES)[b]** | *n*=16 | *n*=32 | *n*=33 | | | | | |
| Dependent | 2.25 (1.30) | 2.70 (1.54) | 1.32 (1.17) | 7.19** | .16 | ✓ | ✓ | |
| Independent | .38 (.50) | .41 (.48) | .35 (.41) | .33 | .01 | | | |
| **Coping skills (CISS)[c]** | *n*=18 | *n*=39 | *n*=47 | | | | | |
| Task-oriented | 46.28 (6.21) | 47.23 (7.99) | 51.60 (7.20) | 2.85 | .05 | ✓ | | |
| Emotion-focused | 51.98 (6.02) | 52.83 (7.65) | 46.19 (6.08) | 6.74** | .12 | ✓ | ✓ | |
| Avoidance-oriented | 51.26 (7.21) | 51.36 (8.64) | 45.38 (7.60) | 7.03** | .12 | ✓ | ✓ | |
| **Social support (ASSI)[d]** | *n*=18 | *n*=40 | *n*=47 | | | | | |
| Size of social network | 9.42 (5.42) | 10.50 (5.89) | 17.20 (9.22) | 6.39** | .11 | ✓ | ✓ | |
| Satisfaction with social network | 26.22 (2.73) | 25.54 (2.97) | 28.27 (1.85) | 10.98** | .18 | ✓ | ✓ | |
| Amount of social contact | 6.23 (4.92) | 7.34 (6.49) | 12.45 (8.10) | 4.52** | .08 | ✓ | ✓ | |
| Satisfaction with social contact | 4.19 (.686) | 4.19 (.80) | 4.70 (.496) | 5.12** | .09 | ✓ | ✓ | |
| **Marital adjustment (DAS)[e]** | *n*=15 | *n*=30 | *n*=47 | | | | | |
| Consensus | 49.97 (5.33) | 50.60 (7.39) | 53.52 (5.44) | 3.27* | .07 | ✓ | ✓ | |
| Affectional expression | 6.72 (2.94) | 8.77 (1.79) | 9.23 (1.95) | 8.34** | .16 | ✓ | | ✓ |
| Satisfaction | 32.83 (6.65) | 34.68 (8.35) | 39.72 (4.22) | 8.34** | .16 | ✓ | ✓ | |
| Cohesion | 13.21 (5.10) | 14.45 (4.82) | 16.15 (3.32) | 3.06 | .07 | ✓ | | |
| **Verbal aggression (CTS)[f]** | *n*=15 | *n*=30 | *n*=45 | | | | | |
| Inter-partner | 20.95 (16.63) | 17.28 (20.93) | 9.44 (9.34) | 2.02 | .05 | | | |

Due to non-independence of data and to obtain a global estimate of couple functioning, mean scores across all available parents were used for these analyses when there was more than one parent in a family [number of single-parent families = 11 (7 BD)]

T-scores were used for the Personality and Coping Skills subcategories, *p < .05, **p < .01

BD: bipolar disorder; MDD: major depression disorder; ✓: significant group difference

[a] From the NEO Personality Inventory-Revised

[b] From the Life Events Scale

[c] From the Coping Inventory of Stressful Situations

[d] From the Arizona Social Support Interview

[e] From the Dyadic Adjustment Scale

[f] From the Conflict Tactic Scale

disorders among the participants with BD and the presence of MDD in their partners were examined, in order to determine how these two factors, in conjunction with increased heritability (Merikangas et al. 1988), might impact the family environment.

In line with previous research (Bender et al. 2010; Fletcher et al. 2013; MacQueen et al. 2001), parents with BD displayed more maladaptive personality traits, more dependent stressful life events, ineffective coping strategies, smaller social networks and fewer social contacts that provided lower levels of satisfaction than healthy control parents. In addition, they reported that their marital relationships were unsatisfactory and that they were verbally abused by their partners. Thus, even between acute episodes of BD, these parents seem to elicit high levels of stress. Moreover, they demonstrate ineffective coping strategies and receive little social support from those around them, including their intimate partners.

As a unique focus of the present study, the intimate partners of the parents with BD differed in multiple ways from the partners of healthy control parents. Consistent with the literature on assortative mating (Butterworth and Rodgers 2008; Mathews and Reus 2001; Nordsletten et al. 2016), 56% of the partners of parents with BD presented current or past axis I disorders, and 10% presented axis II disorders. Additionally, they presented high levels of neuroticism, low levels of extraversion, and frequent use of emotion-focused coping, relative to healthy control partners. The intimate partners of the parents with BD also had few contacts outside the couple, and thereby little social support, while acknowledging that their marital relationship was unsatisfactory and characterized by high levels of verbal abuse. Marital problems, high levels of emotion-focused coping and failure to establish social support networks by the partners of adults with BD may result from a heightened perception of the burden imposed by their partners (Borowiecka-Karpiuk et al. 2014; Perlick et al. 2007, 2016; Reinares et al. 2006). Alternatively, or additionally, the maladaptive behaviors of the partners, like those of adults with BD, may be associated with high levels of neuroticism. For example, individuals high in neurotic traits tend to respond to stress with negative affect (Jacobs et al. 2011) that in turn is linked to emotion-focused coping strategies. Similarly, neuroticism is associated with depression symptoms that are in turn linked to low levels of social support (Stice et al. 2004).

The portrait of the intimate partners of parents with BD indicates that they confer risk for mental disorders, neuroticism, and low psychosocial functioning in the OBD, rather than providing a buffering effect. The presence of heritable mental disorders and neuroticism among the intimate partners of parents with BD suggest that they also may transmit genes to the OBD that increase their liability for similar disorders and the trait of neuroticism (Kieseppä et al. 2004; Song et al. 2015). Importantly, the presence of high neuroticism in both parents has been associated with negative outcomes in their offspring (Ellenbogen et al. 2010). Indeed, parents' neuroticism is associated prospectively with poor interpersonal functioning and higher rates of risky sexual behaviours in late adolescence and early adulthood among their offspring (Ostiguy et al. 2012; Nijjar et al. 2016). Further, OBD show greater sensitivity to their parents' emotionality than offspring of healthy control parents (Ostiguy et al. 2012). Moreover, the intimate partners of parents with BD, but not the parents with BD, reported decreased extraversion compared to healthy controls. This finding is important as low extraversion is associated with negative health outcomes, anxiety disorders, and depressive symptoms, all of which might exacerbate an already stressful home environment (Bienvenu et al. 2007; Hakulinen et al. 2015).

Taken together, the present findings indicate that both parents model maladaptive behaviors such as emotion-focused coping skills, and experience low social support and marital difficulties. Therefore, these findings suggest that parents with BD *and* their intimate partners may benefit from individual treatments aimed at developing effective coping skills, social support networks, and a satisfying marital relationship. These findings are consistent with and further support the use of efficacious adjunct interventions for BD targeting families, such as Family-Focused Therapy for BD, rather than pharmacotherapy alone (Miklowitz et al. 2003, 2017). Interventions targeting neuroticism in both parents, although more difficult, might be particularly pertinent given its robust associations with environmental outcomes (Tang et al. 2009).

Contrasting individual parent reports of marital adjustment in the dyad revealed interesting differences in perspective. Similar to previous research (Lam et al. 2005; Whisman 2007), both parents with BD and their intimate partners reported low marital satisfaction relative to healthy controls. However, differences in partner reports surfaced with regards to other aspects of marital functioning. Parents with BD, but not their intimate partners, qualified their relationships as having infrequent expressions of affection and sexual desire and few common activities and interests within the couple, relative to healthy controls. This result concurs with previous studies reporting heightened difficulties adjusting to the shifts in sexual arousal/desire during manic and depressive episodes of the affected partner, as reported by their intimate partners (Lam et al. 2005). Consistent with previous literature (Perlick et al. 2016), intimate partners of parents with BD often experience depressive symptoms themselves, which includes decreased interest for activities and sex. Therefore, this may be another way by which the partner with BD may be unsatisfied in these areas of their relationship. From the perspective of the intimate partner of adults with BD, difficulties in marital adjustment are driven by disagreements on what is important in their relationship. This may be a result of the burden of caregiving often experienced by intimate partners of patients with BD, including increased responsibilities in maintaining finances, household routines, and childcare (Perlick et al. 2007).

Surprisingly, the presence of comorbid PDs in adults with BD, or MDD in their partner, altered few of the differences between couples with BD and healthy control couples. Specifically, inter-partner verbal abuse was greatest among couples with BD and PDs, which is consistent with studies showing high rates of personality disorder among domestic violence perpetrators (Gibbons et al. 2011). Marital difficulties in couples with BD and comorbid PD or a partner with MDD were greater than couples with BD only. These findings suggest that the marital adjustment and verbal abuse associated with BD may be driven, in part, by mental disorders other than BD within these couples. With respect to PD, this is not surprising as symptoms of PDs in an intimate partner within community samples have been associated with marital dysfunction and low satisfaction (South et al. 2008; Whisman and Schonbrun 2009).

Although this is, to the best of our knowledge, the first comprehensive study of parents having BD and their intimate partners, there are a number of study limitations. The results of the study can only be generalized to middle-class and Caucasian parents with BD and their partners who care for children. These individuals may differ from other adults with BD who have no children, or families living in poverty or from minority communities. For example, the participants with BD in the current study showed lower rates of anxiety disorders than previously reported among adults with BD (McElroy et al. 2001). Another limitation is the relatively small sample size that may have prevented the detection of effects when taking account of mental disorders other than BD in couples. Therefore, readers should mainly focus on effect sizes when interpreting these results and interpret small effects sizes with caution. Finally, except for the assessment of mental health and personality disorders, the study relies solely of self-report measures. Observational methods or ratings from other sources would strengthen the reported findings.

## Conclusion

In conclusion, adults with BD appear to select intimate partners with similar maladaptive personality traits, ineffective coping skills and who demonstrate high levels of verbal aggression. Moreover, both adults with BD and their intimate partners report a paucity of social support. These findings indicate that the intimate partners, as well as the partners with BD, could *both* benefit from individual treatments aimed at lowering emotionality and verbal aggression, increasing social support, and improving effective coping skills. Not surprisingly, both partners in these couples report difficulties and low levels of satisfaction in their relationships, which was further exacerbated (along with verbal aggression) by comorbid PDs and or a having a partner with MDD. Thus, the present findings indicate that couple and family therapy are also warranted. Many of the suggested intervention might improve family functioning and by extension the health of their children. Indeed, strong social support systems in parents with BD during middle childhood were found to act as a protective factor against the future development of substance use symptoms in OBD in early adulthood (Trespalacios et al. manuscript in preparation).

**Acknowledgements**
We thank Dr. Micheline Lapalme and Catherine Laroche for their invaluable assistance on this project, and all the families for so graciously taking the time to participate in our research.

**Authors' contributions**
LS ran the statistical analyses. LS and VI produced the first draft of the manuscript. Professors ME and SH designed the study and edited the manuscript. All authors read and approved the final manuscript.

**Author details**
[1] Centre for Research in Human Development, Concordia University, Montréal, Canada. [2] Département de Psychiatrie, Université de Montréal, Montréal, Canada. [3] Department of Clinical Neuroscience, Karolinska Institute, Stockholm, Sweden.

**References**

Barrera M. A method for the assessment of social support networks in community survey research. Connections. 1980;3:8–13.

Barrera M, Sandler IN, Ramsay TB. Preliminary development of a scale of social support: studies on college students. Am J Community Psychol. 1981;9:435–47. https://doi.org/10.1007/BF00918174.

Bella T, Goldstein T, Axelson D, Obreja M, Monk K, Hickey MB, Goldstein B, Brent D, Diler RS, Kupfer D, Sakolsky D. Psychosocial functioning in offspring of parents with bipolar disorder. J Affect Disord. 2011;133:204–11. https://doi.org/10.1016/j.jad.2011.03.022.

Bender RE, Alloy LB, Sylvia LG, Uroševic S, Abramson LY. Generation of life events in bipolar spectrum disorders: a re-examination and extension of the stress generation theory. J Clin Psychol. 2010;66:907–26. https://doi.org/10.1002/jclp.20705.

Beyer JL, Kuchibhatla M, Looney C, Engstrom E, Cassidy F, Krishnan KRR. Social support in elderly patients with bipolar disorder. Bipolar Disord. 2003;5:22–7. https://doi.org/10.1034/j.1399-5618.2003.00016.x.

Bienvenu OJ, Hettema JM, Neale MC, Prescott CA, Kendler KS. Low extraversion and high neuroticism as indices of genetic and environmental risk for social phobia, agoraphobia, and animal phobia. Am J Psychiatry. 2007;164:1714–21. https://doi.org/10.1176/appi.ajp.2007.06101667.

Borowiecka-Karpiuk J, Dudek D, Siwek M, Jaeschke R. Spousal burden in partners of patients with major depressive disorder and bipolar disorder. Psychiatr Pol. 2014;48:773–87.

Bouchard G, Sabourin S, Lussier Y, Wright J, Boucher C. La structure factorielle de la version français de l'Échelle d'adjustemente dyadique. Can J Counselling Psychother/Revue canadienne de counseling et de psychothér. 1991;25:4–11.

Brands IM, Köhler S, Stapert SZ, Wade DT, van Heugten CM. Psychometric properties of the Coping Inventory for Stressful Situations (CISS) in patients with acquired brain injury. Psychol Assess. 2014;26:848. https://doi.org/10.1037/a0036275.

Brieger P, Ehrt U, Marneros A. Frequency of comorbid personality disorders in bipolar and unipolar affective disorders. Compr Psychiatry. 2003;44:28–34. https://doi.org/10.1053/comp.2003.50009.

Butterworth P, Rodgers B. Mental health problems and marital disruption: is it the combination of husbands and wives' mental health problems that predicts later divorce? Soc Psychiatry Psychiatr Epidemiol. 2008;43:758–63. https://doi.org/10.1007/s00127-008-0366-5.

Carpenter D, Clarkin JF, Glick ID, Wilner PJ. Personality pathology among married adults with bipolar disorder. J Affect Disord. 1995;34:269–74. https://doi.org/10.1016/0165-0327(95)00024-H.

Costa PT, McCrae RR. Normal personality assessment in clinical practice: The NEO Personality Inventory. Psychol Assess. 1992;4:5. https://doi.org/10.1037/1040-3590.4.1.5.

Costa PT Jr, Herbst JH, McCrae RR, Siegler IC. Personality at midlife: stability, intrinsic maturation, and response to life events. Assessment. 2000;7:365–78. https://doi.org/10.1177/107319110000700405.

Dohrenwend BS, Askenasy AR, Krasnoff L, Dohrenwend BP. Exemplification of a method for scaling life events: the PERI Life Events Scale. J Health Soc Behav. 1978. https://doi.org/10.2307/2136536.

Duffy A, Alda M, Crawford L, Milin R, Grof P. The early manifestations of bipolar disorder: a longitudinal prospective study of the offspring of bipolar parents. Bipolar Disord. 2007;9:828–38. https://doi.org/10.1111/j.1399-5618.2007.00421.x.

Duffy A, Horrocks J, Doucette S, Keown-Stoneman C, McCloskey S, Grof P. The developmental trajectory of bipolar disorder. Br J Psychiatry. 2014;204:122–8. https://doi.org/10.1192/bjp.bp.113.126706.

Eidelman P, Gershon A, Kaplan K, McGlinchey E, Harvey AG. Social support and social strain in inter-episode bipolar disorder. Bipolar Disord. 2012;14:628–40. https://doi.org/10.1111/j.1399-5618.2012.01049.x.

Eley TC, Plomin R. Genetic analyses of emotionality. Curr Opin Neurobiol. 1997;7:279–84. https://doi.org/10.1016/S0959-4388(97)80017-7.

Ellenbogen MA, Hodgins S. The impact of high neuroticism in parents on children's psychosocial functioning in a population at high risk for major affective disorder: A family environmental pathway of intergenerational risk. Dev Psychopathol. 2004;16:113–36. https://doi.org/10.1017/S0954579404044438.

Ellenbogen MA, Ostiguy CS, Hodgins S. Intergenerational effects of high neuroticism in parents and their public health significance. Am Psychol. 2010. https://doi.org/10.1037/a0018512.

Endler NS, Parker JD. Assessment of multidimensional coping: Task, emotion, and avoidance strategies. Psychol Assess. 1994;6:50. https://doi.org/10.1037/1040-3590.6.1.50.

Fan AH, Hassell J. Bipolar disorder and comorbid personality psychopathology: a review of the literature. J Clin Psychiatry. 2008;69:1794–803. https://doi.org/10.4088/JCP.v69n1115.

Fletcher K, Parker GB, Manicavasagar V. Coping profiles in bipolar disorder. Compr Psychiatry. 2013;54:1177–84. https://doi.org/10.1016/j.comppsych.2013.05.011.

George EL, Miklowitz DJ, Richards JA, Simoneau TL, Taylor DO. The comorbidity of bipolar disorder and axis II personality disorders: prevalence and clinical correlates. Bipolar Disord. 2003;5:115–22. https://doi.org/10.1034/j.1399-5618.2003.00028.x.

Gibbon M, Spitzer RL, Williams JB, Benjamin LS, First MB. Structured clinical interview for DSM-IV axis II personality disorders (SCID-II). Am Psych Pub. 1997. https://doi.org/10.1521/pedi.1997.11.3.279.

Gibbons P, Collins M, Reid C. How useful are indices of personality pathology when assessing domestic violence perpetrators? Psychol Assess. 2011;23:164. https://doi.org/10.1037/a0021289

Hakulinen C, Elovainio M, Pulkki-Råback L, Virtanen M, Kivimäki M, Jokela M. Personality and depressive symptoms: individual participant meta-analysis of 10 cohort studies. Depress Anxiety. 2015;32:461–70. https://doi.org/10.1002/da.22376.

Hodgins S, Faucher B, Zarac A, Ellenbogen MA. Children of parents with bipolar disorder: a population at high risk for major affective disorders. Child Adolesc Psychiatr Clin N Am. 2002;11:533–53. https://doi.org/10.1016/S1056-4993(02)00002-0.

Iacono V, Beaulieu L, Hodgins S, Ellenbogen MA. Parenting practices in middle childhood mediate the relation between growing up with a parent having bipolar disorder and offspring psychopathology from childhood into early adulthood. Dev Psychopathol. 2018;30:635–49. https://doi.org/10.1017/S095457941700116X.

Jacobs N, Van Os J, Derom C, Thiery E, Delespaul P, Wichers M. Neuroticism explained? From a non-informative vulnerability marker to informative person–context interactions in the realm of daily life. Br J Clin Psychol. 2011;50:19–32. https://doi.org/10.1348/014466510X491397.

Kendler KS, Kessler RC, Walters EE, MacLean C, Neale MC, Heath AC, Eaves LJ. Stressful life events, genetic liability, and onset of an episode of major depression in women. Focus. 2010;8:459–70. https://doi.org/10.1176/foc.8.3.foc459.

Kieseppä T, Partonen T, Haukka J, Kaprio J, Lönnqvist J. High concordance of bipolar I disorder in a nationwide sample of twins. Am J Psychiatry. 2004;161:1814–21. https://doi.org/10.1176/ajp.161.10.1814.

Kline RB. Becoming a behavioral science researcher: a guide to producing research that matters. New York: Guilford Press; 2008.

Kogan JN, Otto MW, Bauer MS, Dennehy EB, Miklowitz DJ, Zhang HW, Ketter T, Rudorfer MV, Wisniewski SR, Thase ME, Calabrese J. Demographic and diagnostic characteristics of the first 1000 patients enrolled in the Systematic Treatment Enhancement Program for Bipolar Disorder (STEP-BD). Bipolar Disord. 2004;6:460–9. https://doi.org/10.1111/j.1399-5618.2004.00158.x.

Lam D, Donaldson C, Brown Y, Malliaris Y. Burden and marital and sexual satisfaction in the partners of bipolar patients. Bipolar Disord. 2005;7:431–40. https://doi.org/10.1111/j.1399-5618.2005.00240.x.

Loftus ST, Jaeger J. Psychosocial outcome in bipolar I patients with a personality disorder. J Nerv Ment Dis. 2006;194:967–70. https://doi.org/10.1097/01.nmd.0000243814.35854.10.

MacQueen GM, Young LT, Joffe RT. A review of psychosocial outcome in patients with bipolar disorder. Acta Psychiatr Scand. 2001;103:163–70. https://doi.org/10.1034/j.1600-0447.2001.00059.x.

Mathews CA, Reus VI. Assortative mating in the affective disorders: a systematic review and meta-analysis. Compr Psychiatry. 2001;42:257–62. https://doi.org/10.1053/comp.2001.24575.

McElroy SL, Altshuler LL, Suppes T, Keck PE Jr, Frye MA, Denicoff KD, Nolen WA, Kupka RW, Leverich GS, Rochussen JR, Rush AJ. Axis I psychiatric comorbidity and its relationship to historical illness variables in 288 patients with bipolar disorder. Am J Psychiatry. 2001;158:420–6. https://doi.org/10.1176/appi.ajp.158.3.420.

Merikangas KR, Weissman MM, Prusoff BA, John K. Assortative mating and affective disorders: psychopathology in offspring. Psychiatry. 1988;51(1):48–57. https://doi.org/10.1080/00332747.1988.11024379.

Miklowitz DJ. A review of evidence-based psychosocial interventions for bipolar disorder. J Clin Psychiatry. 2006;67:28–33.

Miklowitz DJ, George EL, Richards JA, Simoneau TL, Suddath RL. A randomized study of family-focused psychoeducation and pharmacotherapy in the outpatient management of bipolar disorder. Arch Gen Psychiatry. 2003;60:904–12. https://doi.org/10.1001/archpsyc.60.9.904.

Miklowitz DJ, Schneck CD, Walshaw PD, Garrett AS, Singh MK, Sugar CA, Chang KD. Early intervention for youth at high risk for bipolar disorder: a multisite randomized trial of family-focused treatment. Early Intervent Psychiatry. 2017. https://doi.org/10.1111/eip.12463.

Moon E, Chang JS, Choi S, Ha TH, Cha B, Cho HS, Park JM, Lee BD, Lee YM, Choi Y, Ha K. Characteristics of stress-coping behaviors in patients with bipolar disorders. Psychiatry Res. 2014;218:69–74. https://doi.org/10.1016/j.psychres.2014.03.047.

Nijjar R, Ellenbogen MA, Hodgins S. Personality, coping, risky behavior, and mental disorders in the offspring of parents with bipolar disorder: a comprehensive psychosocial assessment. J Affect Disord. 2014;166:315–23. https://doi.org/10.1016/j.jad.2014.04.047.

Nijjar R, Ellenbogen MA, Hodgins S. Sexual risk behaviors in the adolescent offspring of parents with bipolar disorder: prospective associations with parents' personality and externalizing behavior in childhood. J Abnorm Child Psychol. 2016;44:1347–59. https://doi.org/10.1007/s10802-015-0112-x.

Nordsletten AE, Larsson H, Crowley JJ, Almqvist C, Lichtenstein P, Mataix-Cols D. Patterns of nonrandom mating within and across 11 major psychiatric disorders. JAMA Psychiatry. 2016;73:354–61. https://doi.org/10.1001/jamapsychiatry.2015.3192.

Ostiguy CS, Ellenbogen MA, Linnen AM, Walker EF, Hammen C, Hodgins S. Chronic stress and stressful life events in the offspring of parents with bipolar disorder. J Affect Disord. 2009;114:74–84. https://doi.org/10.1016/j.jad.2008.08.006.

Ostiguy CS, Ellenbogen MA, Walker CD, Walker EF, Hodgins S. Sensitivity to stress among the offspring of parents with bipolar disorder: a study of daytime cortisol levels. Psychol Med. 2011;41:2447–57. https://doi.org/10.1017/S0033291711000523.

Ostiguy CS, Ellenbogen MA, Hodgins S. Personality of parents with bipolar disorder and interpersonal functioning among their offspring: A prospective 10-year study. Dev Psychopathol. 2012;24:573–87. https://doi.org/10.1017/S095457941200017X.

Perlick DA, Rosenheck RA, Miklowitz DJ, Chessick C, Wolff N, Kaczynski R, Ostacher M, Patel J, Desai R. Prevalence and correlates of burden among caregivers of patients with bipolar disorder enrolled in the Systematic Treatment Enhancement Program for Bipolar Disorder. Bipolar Disord. 2007;9:262–73. https://doi.org/10.1111/j.1399-5618.2007.00365.x.

Perlick DA, Berk L, Kaczynski R, Gonzalez J, Link B, Dixon L, Grier S, Miklowitz DJ. Caregiver burden as a predictor of depression among family and friends who provide care for persons with bipolar disorder. Bipolar Disord. 2016;18:183–91. https://doi.org/10.1111/bdi.12379.

Rea MM, Tompson MC, Miklowitz DJ, Goldstein MJ, Hwang S, Mintz J. Family-focused treatment versus individual treatment for bipolar disorder: results of a randomized clinical trial. J Consult Clin Psychol. 2003;71:482. https://doi.org/10.1037/0022-006X.71.3.482.

Reinares M, Vieta E, Colom F, Martinez-Aran A, Torrent C, Comes M, Goikolea JM, Benabarre A, Daban C, Sánchez-Moreno J. What really matters to bipolar patients' caregivers: sources of family burden. J Affect Disord. 2006;94:157–63. https://doi.org/10.1016/j.jad.2006.04.022.

Rende R, Hodgins S, Palmour R, Faucher B, Allaire JF. Familial overlap between bipolar disorder and psychotic symptoms in a Canadian cohort. Can J Psychiatry. 2005;50:189–94. https://doi.org/10.1177/070674370505000401.

Risch N, Herrell R, Lehner T, Liang KY, Eaves L, Hoh J, Griem A, Kovacs M, Ott J, Merikangas KR. Interaction between the seonin transporter gene (5-HTTLPR), stressful life events, and risk of depression: a meta-analysis. JAMA. 2009;301:2462–71. https://doi.org/10.1001/jama.2009.878.

Rolland JP, Parker WD, Stumpf H. A psychometric examination of the French translations of NEO-PI-R and NEO-FFI. J Pers Assess. 1998;71:269–91. https://doi.org/10.1207/s15327752jpa7102_13.

Shaw JA, Egeland JA, Endicott J, Allen CR, Hostetter AM. A 10-year prospective study of prodromal patterns for bipolar disorder among Amish youth. J Am Acad Child Adolesc Psychiatry. 2005;44:1104–11. https://doi.org/10.1097/01.chi.0000177052.26476.e5.

Song J, Bergen SE, Kuja-Halkola R, Larsson H, Landén M, Lichtenstein P. Bipolar disorder and its relation to major psychiatric disorders: a family-based study in the Swedish population. Bipolar Disord. 2015;17:184–93. https://doi.org/10.1111/bdi.12242.

South SC, Turkheimer E, Oltmanns TF. Personality disorder symptoms and marital functioning. J Consult Clin Psychol. 2008;76:769. https://doi.org/10.1037/a0013346.

Spanier GB. Measuring dyadic adjustment: new scales for assessing the quality of marriage and similar dyads. J Marital Fam. 1976. https://doi.org/10.2307/350547.

Spanier GB, Thompson L. A confirmatory analysis of the dyadic adjustment scale. J Marital Fam. 1982. https://doi.org/10.2307/351593.

Spitzer RL, Williams JB, Gibbon M, First MB. The structured clinical interview for DSM-III-R (SCID): I: history, rationale, and description. Arch Gen Psychiatry. 1992;49:624–9. https://doi.org/10.1001/archpsyc.1992.01820080032005.

Stice E, Ragan J, Randall P. Prospective relations between social support and depression: differential direction of effects for parent and peer support? J Abnorm Psychol. 2004;113:155. https://doi.org/10.1037/0021-843X.113.1.155.

Straus MA, Mickey EL. Reliability, validity, and prevalence of partner violence measured by the conflict tactics scales in male-dominant nations. Aggress Violent Behav. 2012;17:463–74. https://doi.org/10.1016/j.avb.2012.06.004.

Straus MA, Hamby SL, Boney-McCoy S, Sugarman DB. The revised conflict tactics scales (CTS2) development and preliminary psychometric data. J Fam Issues. 1996;17:283–316. https://doi.org/10.117/019251396017003001.

Suppes T, Leverich GS, Keck PE Jr, Nolen WA, Denicoff KD, Altshuler LL, McElroy SL, Rush AJ, Kupka R, Frye MA, Bickel M. The Stanley Foundation Bipolar Treatment Outcome Network: II. demographics and illness characteristics of the first 261 patients. J Affect Disord. 2001;67:45–59. https://doi.org/10.1176/appi.ajp.158.3.420.

Tang TZ, DeRubeis RJ, Hollon SD, Amsterdam J, Shelton R, Schalet B. Personality change during depression treatment: a placebo-controlled trial. Arch Gen Psychiatry. 2009;66:1322–30. https://doi.org/10.1001/archgenpsychiatry.2009.166.

Trespalacios F, Yong Ping E, Serravalle L, and Ellenbogen MA. Social support moderates the development of psychopathology in the offspring of parents with bipolar disorder: a 10-year longitudinal study (in preparation).

Vega EM, O'Leary KD. Test–retest reliability of the revised Conflict Tactics Scales (CTS2). J Fam Violence. 2007;22:703–8. https://doi.org/10.1007/s10896-007-9118-7.

Whisman MA. Marital distress and DSM-IV psychiatric disorders in a population-based national survey. J Abnorm Psychol. 2007;116:638. https://doi.org/10.1037/0021-843X.116.3.638.

Whisman MA, Schonbrun YC. Social consequences of borderline personality disorder symptoms in a population-based survey: marital distress, marital violence, and marital disruption. J Pers Disord. 2009;23:410–5. https://doi.org/10.1521/pedi.2009.23.4.410.

World Health Organization. The World Health Report 2001—Mental health: new understandings, new hope. Geneva: Author; 2001.

Zanarini MC, Frankenburg FR. Olanzapine treatment of female borderline personality disorder patients: a double-blind, placebo-controlled pilot study. J Clin Psychiatry. 2001;62:849–54. https://doi.org/10.4088/JCP.v62n1103.

# 16

# Executive functioning but not IQ or illness severity predicts occupational status in bipolar disorder

Julia Drakopoulos[1], Timea Sparding[1*], Caitlin Clements[2,3,4], Erik Pålsson[1] and Mikael Landén[1,3]

**Abstract**

**Background:** Bipolar disorder is associated with significant functional deficits including occupational functioning. Despite the high rates of unemployment and sick leave in the patient population, only a limited number of studies have examined factors associated with occupational functioning in bipolar disorder. The aim of the study was to investigate the relative importance of demographic, clinical, and neuropsychological factors on occupational dysfunction in bipolar disorder.

**Methods:** A sample of 120 partially or fully remitted bipolar disorder I and II patients were included in the study. Patients were stratified into an active and an inactive group based on the number of hours per week working or studying. Active (n = 86) and inactive (n = 34) patients were compared with respect to demographic factors, clinical characteristics, medication, measures of psychosocial functioning, and cognitive functioning (i.e., IQ and executive functions). No other cognitive domains were examined.

**Results:** Univariate analyses revealed better overall cognitive function in active patients in terms of IQ and executive functioning. However, only executive functioning accounted for a significant amount of the variance in occupational status when other significant predictors were taken into account.

**Conclusions:** Executive functioning was a more powerful predictor of occupational status in bipolar disorder patients than IQ and other clinical factors, including illness severity.

**Keywords:** Employment, Observational study, Neuropsychological tests, Bipolar disorder, Cognitive dysfunction, Executive function

## Background

Bipolar disorder is one of the leading causes of disability worldwide, which incurs higher costs on the health care system and society than most other illnesses (Murray and Lopez 1997). The bulk of societal costs of bipolar disorders are due to indirect costs such as sick-leave, unemployment, and early retirement (Ekman et al. 2013). This is because as many as 30 to 60% of patients with bipolar disorder do not regain full occupational or social functioning after illness onset (MacQueen et al. 2001). Functional recovery also lags behind recovery from clinical symptoms and may be incomplete despite the absence of mood symptoms (Goldberg et al. 1995).

Employment is an important area of functioning. Factors previously associated with poor occupational or functional outcome in bipolar disorder include the number of affective episodes (MacQueen et al. 2000; Zimmerman et al. 2010), lingering subsyndromal depression (Dickerson et al. 2004; Bonnín et al. 2010; Burdick et al. 2010), history of psychiatric hospitalizations (Dickerson et al. 2004; Burdick et al. 2010; Gutiérrez-Rojas et al. 2011), total symptom severity (Goetza et al. 2007), age

*Correspondence: timea.sparding@vgregion.se
[1] Department of Psychiatry and Neurochemistry, Institute of Neuroscience and Physiology, The Sahlgrenska Academy, University of Gothenburg, Sahlgrenska University Hospital, Blå Stråket 15, 413 45 Gothenburg, Sweden
Full list of author information is available at the end of the article

(Depp et al. 2012), educational attainment (Reed et al. 2010), age at onset (Perlis et al. 2009), history of psychotic symptoms (Tohen et al. 1990, 2000), and comorbid psychiatric conditions such as panic disorder and substance abuse (Hajek et al. 2005; Zimmerman et al. 2010).

Cognitive performance is another domain that has been linked to poor occupational functioning (Mur et al. 2009; Gilbert and Marwaha 2013; Ryan et al. 2013; Bonnín et al. 2014). Executive functions seem to be particularly important for psychosocial functioning and practical tasks of daily life (Lezak 2012). Bipolar disorder patients feature cognitive impairments (mainly deficits in attention, verbal memory, and executive functioning) on group level that persist during euthymia (Robinson et al. 2006; Mur et al. 2007; Palsson et al. 2013; Sparding et al. 2015a, b; Salarvan et al. 2019).

It is important to establish factors influencing occupational functioning in order to tailor and optimize care management in bipolar disorder. Previous research has linked clinical, demographic, and cognitive factors to occupational functioning, but their relative influence remains unclear. The aim of the current study was to investigate the relative importance of demographic, clinical and neuropsychological factors on occupational dysfunction in bipolar disorder.

## Methods

### Subjects

The present study is part of the St. Göran Bipolar Project, which is an interdisciplinary, prospective, longitudinal study of bipolar disorder conducted in Sweden. Patients were recruited and examined at the Northern Stockholm Mental Health Service and followed over time. The methods of this study have been outlined in detail previously (Rydén et al. 2009a; b; Ekman et al. 2010). Briefly, patients were examined at a time when the patient was considered stable with respect to mood symptoms by the treating physician. This means that patients were not in an acute depressive or hypomanic episode, but not always completely asymptomatic. Patients were diagnosed using the Affective Disorder Evaluation (ADE) and the Mini International Neuropsychiatric Interview (M.I.N.I.) (Sheehan et al. 1998). The ADE is a semi-structured interview that was employed in the Systematic Treatment Enhancement Program of Bipolar Disorder (STEP-BD) project (Sachs et al. 2003). It includes an adapted version of the affective module of the Structural Clinical Interview for DSM-IV (SCID). The M.I.N.I. was used to screen for other psychiatric disorders. A final best estimate diagnosis was determined by a consensus panel of experienced psychiatrists. Bipolar disorder severity was rated by an experienced clinician using the Clinical Global Impression (CGI) rating scale (Guy 1976). To screen for alcohol and substance abuse, patients completed two self-report questionnaires: the Alcohol Use Disorders Identification Test (AUDIT) (Saunders et al. 1993) and the Drug Use Disorders Identification Test (DUDIT) (Berman et al. 2005). Data on medication were collected from either the baseline diagnostic assessment or the somatic examination, depending on which appointment occurred closest in time to the neuropsychological testing.

The retirement age for the guaranteed pension scheme in Sweden is 65 years. The current study therefore included participants aged 18 to 64 years who met DSM-IV criteria for bipolar I or II disorder ($n = 120$). Only data for individuals with $\leq 14$ on the Montgomery-Åsberg Depression Rating Scale (MADRS) (Asberg and Schalling 1979) and the Young Ziegler Mania Rating Scale (YMRS) (Young et al. 1978) were included in the present study. The reason for choosing 14 as the cut off on MADRS and YMRS was to strike a balance between excluding patients with manifest mood symptoms while keeping patients with subsyndromal lingering symptoms, which is prevalent in bipolar disorder (Judd et al. 2002).

There were no cases of intellectual disability, nor any somatic disorders of clinical significance that might affect cognitive performance (such as stroke or other neurological disorders) in this cohort. Patients with current alcohol or substance dependency were excluded, but patients with a history of alcohol or substance abuse were retained in order to study the natural course of the disorder and to obtain a representative clinical sample.

The project was approved by Stockholm Regional Ethical Review Board, and all participants provided written and oral informed consent.

#### Neuropsychological assessments

In the overarching St. Göran bipolar study, the participants completed a broad neuropsychological test battery (Sparding et al. 2015a, b) to assess cognitive functioning. For the purpose of this study, we preselected the *Wechsler Adult Intelligence Scale III* as a measure of general cognitive ability (Wechsler 1997), and the *Delis–Kaplan Executive Function System* (Delis et al. 2001) as measures of executive functions. No other cognitive domains were examined.

The Wechsler Adult Intelligence Scale (WAIS-III) is the most widely used intelligence quotient (IQ) test and is composed of 10 verbal and non-verbal performance tests: Information, Similarities, Vocabulary, Arithmetic, Digit Span, Block Design, Matrix Reasoning, Picture Completion, Digit Symbol-Coding, and Symbol Search. The subtests generate a measure of general intelligence (mean value = 100; standard deviation = 15). The Vocabulary subtest is frequently used as proxy for premorbid IQ (Martinez-Aran et al. 2007; Ryan et al. 2013; Bonnín et al. 2014).

The Delis–Kaplan Executive Function System (D-KEFS) is a normed and standardized set of nine subtests used to evaluate key components of executive function, including mental flexibility, concept formation, problem solving, and inhibition. Most subtests include one baseline task (condition 1) followed by more difficult tasks/conditions. The latter tasks are considered to be the primary measures of executive functioning. We used five individual tests from the D-KEFS:

i. The *Color-Word Interference Test,* which corresponds to the Stroop Color Word Test and measures the ability to inhibit automatic verbal responses, in this case by reading names of colors (e.g., red, blue, green) printed in incongruent font colors. The test conditions are: (1): Color Naming, (2): Word Reading, (3): Inhibition, and (4): Inhibition/Switching.
ii. The *Verbal Fluency Test* measures the ability to produce as many words as possible from a given category in 60 s. The categories are either phonemic (i.e., words beginning with a specified letter) or semantic (i.e., objects such as animals or fruit). Test results provide information about language skills and verbal processing ability, as well as problem solving and inhibition. The test conditions are: (1): Letter Fluency, (2): Category Fluency, and (3): Category Switching.
iii. The *Design Fluency Test* evaluates the subjects' ability to draw as many different designs as possible in 60 s by connecting a set of printed dots. The executive functions required for the test include the capacity of initiating problem-solving behavior, cognitive flexibility, and inhibition of automatic responses. The test conditions are: (1): Filled Dots, (2): Empty Dots Only, (3): Switching.
iv. The *Trail Making Test* (TMT) contains measures of cognitive flexibility, visual attention, and motor speed. The test requires the subject to connect a sequence of 25 consecutive numbers and/or letters as fast as possible. In TMT 2, the subject connects a number sequence only. In TMT 4, which is similar to TMT B, the subject alternates between numbers and letters (e.g., 1-A, 2-B, etc.). The test conditions are: (1): Visual scanning, (2): Number Sequencing, (3): Letter Sequencing, (4): Number-Letter Switching, and (5): Motor Speed.
v. The Tower Test assesses planning and spatial problem-solving abilities such as the ability to inhibit perseverative and impulsive responses. Visual attention and visual-spatial ability are fundamental skills required for this task.

### Assessment of occupational status

We had access to categorized information on occupational functioning. The alternatives were (i) working or studying more than 50% time in a competitive employment (or educational) setting; (ii) working or studying in a competitive employment (or educational) setting 50% time or less (which in Sweden usually means receiving early retirement benefit, or temporary or permanent sick-leave benefits at $\geq$ 50%), (iii) unemployed, (iv) supported employment, (v) idle. The sample was divided into two groups according to their current occupational status: active versus inactive. Active patients ($n = 86$) included the highest functioning group including subjects who held a competitively-obtained occupation, or were university students, at > 50% (i.e., working/studying more than 20 h per week). Inactive patients ($n = 34$) included all the other options, i.e., subjects who were unemployed, received early retirement benefit, or were on temporary or permanent sick-leave at $\geq$ 50% (i.e., working/studying 20 h or less per week). This group also included subjects who held supported employments (i.e., outside the open labor market), or were enrolled in vocational rehabilitation programs.

### Assessment of psychosocial functioning

We used scores from both the symptom and function domains of the Global Assessment of Functioning (GAF) Scale (Luborsky 1975) to assess overall functioning. The Sheehan Disability Scale (Sheehan 1983) was administered to obtain information about patients' subjective assessment of psychosocial dysfunction following their illness. This scale is a composite of three self-rated items designed to assess the extent to which three major areas in life are compromised by psychiatric symptomatology. The patient rates the extent to which his or her (1) work or school, (2) social life or leisure activities, and (3) home life or family responsibilities are impaired by his or her symptoms on a 10-point visual analogue scale (0 = not at all, 1–3 = mildly, 4–6 = moderately, 7–9 = markedly, 10 = extremely).

### Statistical procedures

Data analyses were carried out with the statistical package IBM SPSS 23.0 for Windows (IBM Corp. Armonk, NY). We first examined which variables were different between the groups of active and inactive patients. Between-group differences in demographic and clinical characteristics were evaluated with univariate analyses of variance (ANOVAs) by examining a single factor of the group (active vs. inactive). Pearson's Chi-square tests were run for dichotomous and categorical variables.

For cognitive measures, Analyses of Covariance (ANCOVAs) were performed for each test to investigate differences between the active and inactive group. Effect sizes were calculated with the formula for partial eta squared ($\eta^2$). Current medication with benzodiazepines was used as a covariate because a significantly higher proportion of patients in the inactive group were prescribed such drugs. Scaled scores were used as outcome measures because they account for group differences in age. Two-tailed tests were performed for all analyses, and statistical significance was defined as $p < 0.05$.

A composite measure of executive function was created using principal component analysis (PCA) using the SIMCA software (SIMCA-P 13.0 software, Umetrics AB, Umeå, Sweden). A PCA reduces data dimensions and summarizes systematic variation in a model by aggregating variables in 'components' or 'latent variables' that describe the correlations structure (Eriksson et al. 2013). By creating a PCA-model, it is possible to (i) examine measures that are highly correlated, (ii) look at all the executive tests together without losing any test specific information, (iii) avoid problems with mass significance. A total of 11 subtest scores were selected from five D-KEFS tests: the *Tower Test*, the *Verbal Fluency Test*, the *Color Word Test*, the *Design Fluency Test*, and the *Trail Making Test*. All test conditions were included, except the baseline tasks and non-executive measures (i.e., TMT Motor Speed, which did not differ between the groups [$p = 0.112$]). 18 subjects (12 active, 6 inactive) were automatically excluded from the analysis as they had completed less than 50% of the tests. Two parameters are important to consider when evaluating a principal component: goodness of fit (R2), which expresses the explained variation, and goodness of prediction (Q2), which expresses the power to anticipate data, either internally or externally (Eriksson et al. 2013).

The first principal component (PC1) was thereafter used as an executive functioning score as a predictor in the binary logistic regression models to predict occupational status. Each test's loading (P1) reveals how much each test contributes to the latent variable, executive functioning. We conducted three successive logistic regressions to estimate the relative influence of executive functions, IQ, and clinical variables to predict occupational status (active vs. inactive). In the first model, only executive functioning (PC1) was used as predictor variable. In the second model, IQ was added. The active and the inactive group differed in age, but we did not add age and sex into the logistic regression model because the cognitive variables (IQ and the PC of executive functioning) were in scaled scores already adjusted for age and sex. In the third model, we added clinical variables that differed significantly between groups in the univariate analyses: history of psychotic symptoms, history of involuntary psychiatric care (i.e., being sectioned under the Mental Health Act), and current benzodiazepine use. All clinical variables were categorical and coded 1 or 0 ("yes" = 1, "no" = 0). Variance of inflation tests performed to control for multicollinearity did not reveal conflicting relations between the covariates.

## Results

The characteristics of the 86 active and 34 inactive patients are displayed in Table 1. Subjects in the inactive group were slightly older than the active group. A significantly larger proportion of the inactive patients had a history of psychotic symptoms, and had at least one involuntary hospitalization (i.e., had been sectioned under the Mental Health Act). The use of benzodiazepines was more prevalent in the inactive group than the active group (44% vs. 20%, $p < 0.05$). No other group differences were observed with respect to comorbid conditions, bipolar subtype, age at illness onset, subsyndromal symptomatology (as measured with YMRS and MADRS), number of previous depressive or manic episodes, or bipolar disorder severity as rated with CGI. The inactive patients showed worse functioning as measured by the GAF symptom and function scales, as well as all three dimensions of the Sheehan Disability Scale.

The ANCOVAs showed differences between the active and inactive group in the majority of cognitive tests, where active patients performed better overall. Active patients also showed a significantly higher IQ than inactive patients (109 vs. 101, $p = 0.014$).

The PCA model created with 11 D-KEFS executive functioning subtests was significant ($R2X = 0.611$; $Q2X = 0.415$). The executive functioning subtests loaded robustly on the first principal component ($R2 = 0.464$; $Q2 = 0.329$; Table 2).

Three logistic regressions were run to evaluate the relative influence of executive functioning in predicting occupational status (active vs. inactive). In the first regression model (Table 3), we only used our composite measure of executive functioning as predictor. It demonstrated that the odds of a person to be in the inactive group decreased by 36% as the principal component score increased by 1.

The second logistic regression (Table 4) was used to evaluate the additional impact of IQ. IQ did not make a unique statistically significant contribution to the model ($p = 0.183$) despite a considerably higher rate of correctly classified inactive patients in this model compared to the previous one (42.3% vs. 25.0%).

**Table 1 Demographic, clinical, functional, and pharmacological variables**

| | Active (n=86) | Inactive (n=34) | Statistics F | *p*-value |
|---|---|---|---|---|
| Demographics, mean (SD) | | | | |
| Age, years | 35.3 (10.8) | 40.0 (13.5) | 4.01 | 0.048 |
| Clinical features, mean (SD) | | | | |
| Age at onset, years | 16.2 (3.8) | 16.4 (4.6) | 0.07 | 0.793 |
| Age at first therapy, years | 26.7 (8.0) | 24.6 (10.7) | 1.14 | 0.288 |
| Total number of manic episodes | 2.0 (3.6) | 2.4 (3.1) | 0.35 | 0.556 |
| Total number of depressive episodes | 9.2 (14.0) | 13.3 (15.1) | 2.03 | 0.157 |
| MADRS score | 3.4 (3.2) | 4.0 (3.8) | 0.54 | 0.463 |
| YMRS score | 1.7 (2.4) | 2.1 (3.0) | 0.50 | 0.483 |
| GAF symptom score | 69.7 (9.7) | 63.1 (9.0) | 11.54 | 0.001 |
| GAF function score | 69.7 (9.7) | 63.9 (9.5) | 8.63 | 0.004 |
| CGI (total) | 4.5 (0.9) | 4.6 (1.2) | 0.41 | 0.524 |
| Sheehan disability scale[a], mean (SD) | | | | |
| Work/school | 4.2 (3.4) | 7.1 (3.4) | 14.41 | < 0.001 |
| Social life | 3.6 (3.2) | 5.6 (2.7) | 7.71 | 0.007 |
| Family life/home responsibilities | 2.6 (2.9) | 5.2 (2.3) | 17.80 | < 0.001 |
| | **Active (n=86)** | **Inactive (n=34)** | $\chi^2$ | ***p*-value** |
| Sex, no. (%) | | | 0.57 | 0.451 |
| Female | 52 (60.5) | 18 (52.9) | | |
| Male | 34 (39.5) | 16 (47.1) | | |
| Diagnosis, no. (%) | | | 1.09 | 0.297 |
| Bipolar I disorder | 54 (63.5) | 25 (73.5) | | |
| Bipolar II disorder | 31 (36.5) | 9 (26.5) | | |
| University studies | 52 (61.2) | 15 (44.1) | 2.87 | 0.090 |
| Comorbidity, no. (%) | | | | |
| ADHD | 11 (15.7) | 6 (22.2) | 0.57 | 0.450 |
| Anxiety disorder[b] | 15 (17.4) | 10 (29.4) | 2.12 | 0.146 |
| Clinical features, no. (%) | | | | |
| Lifetime history of psychotic symptoms | 43 (50.6) | 24 (70.6) | 3.95 | 0.047 |
| History of involuntary psychiatric care | 38 (44.7) | 22 (64.7) | 3.87 | 0.049 |
| History of alcohol abuse | 16 (19.5) | 9 (26.5) | 0.69 | 0.407 |
| History of substance abuse | 9 (10.8) | 6 (18.2) | 1.13 | 1.129 |
| Type of current medication, no. (%) | | | | |
| Lithium | 53 (61.6) | 20 (58.8) | 0.08 | 0.777 |
| Antidepressants | 32 (37.2) | 15 (44.1) | 0.49 | 0.485 |
| Anticonvulsants | 24 (27.9) | 15 (44.1) | 2.92 | 0.088 |
| Antipsychotics | 23 (26.7) | 9 (26.5) | 0.00 | 0.976 |
| Central stimulants | 2 (2.3) | 3 (8.8) | 2.58 | 0.108 |
| Benzodiazepines | 17 (19.8) | 15 (44.1) | 7.39 | 0.007 |

*MADRS* Montgomery-Åsberg Depression Rating Scale, *YMRS* Young Ziegler Mania Rating Scale, *GAF* Global Assessment of Functioning Scale, *CGI* Clinical Global Impression Rating Scale

[a] Sheehan Disability Scale is a self-report scale in which patients rate to what extent their functioning in three different life areas is impaired by psychiatric symptomatology (0 = not at all, 1–3 = mildly, 4–6 = moderately, 7–9 = markedly, 10 = extremely)

[b] Anxiety disorders include the following DSM-IV diagnoses: generalized anxiety disorder, panic disorder, agoraphobia, social anxiety disorder, obsessive–compulsive disorder, and post-traumatic stress disorder

**Table 2 Neurocognitive assessment for all participants**

| | | Active | Inactive | Statistics F | d.f. | *p*-value | $\eta^2$ |
|---|---|---|---|---|---|---|---|
| WAIS-III | | | | | | | |
| Full scale IQ | | 109.0 (1.6) | 101.3 (2.6) | 6.311 | 1 | 0.014 | 0.06 |
| Premorbid IQ (vocabulary) | | 11.8 (0.3) | 10.9 (0.4) | 3.086 | 1 | 0.082 | – |
| D-KEFS | | | | | | | |
| Principal component (PC) | | | | | | | |
| Test included in PC1 | Loading on PC1 (P1) | | | | | | |
| Color word 3 | 0.325713 | 10.3 (0.3) | 7.6 (0.6) | 16.225 | 1 | < 0.001 | 0.14 |
| Color word 4 | 0.326118 | 10.0 (0.3) | 8.4 (0.6) | 6.057 | 1 | 0.016 | 0.06 |
| Verbal fluency 2 | 0.340796 | 13.0 (0.5) | 10.9 (0.8) | 5.010 | 1 | 0.027 | 0.05 |
| Verbal fluency 3—correct responses | 0.334285 | 11.8 (0.4) | 10.1 (0.6) | 4.944 | 1 | 0.028 | 0.05 |
| Verbal fluency 3—switching accuracy | 0.30624 | 12.1 (0.4) | 9.6 (0.6) | 12.161 | 1 | 0.001 | 0.10 |
| Design fluency 2 | 0.22314 | 11.4 (0.4) | 10.2 (0.6) | 2.542 | 1 | 0.114 | – |
| Design fluency 3 | 0.26376 | 11.3 (0.3) | 9.9 (0.5) | 5.028 | 1 | 0.027 | 0.05 |
| TMT 2 | 0.303005 | 9.7 (0.4) | 7.6 (0.6) | 7.415 | 1 | 0.008 | 0.07 |
| TMT 3 | 0.309674 | 10.0 (0.3) | 8.0 (0.6) | 8.206 | 1 | 0.005 | 0.08 |
| TMT 4 | 0.330988 | 9.7 (0.3) | 7.9 (0.6) | 7.438 | 1 | 0.008 | 0.07 |
| Tower test | 0.221951 | 11.2 (0.4) | 9.4 (0.7) | 4.360 | 1 | 0.040 | 0.05 |

Results from WAIS-III and D-KEFS subtests are scaled scores, for which the average range is 9-11 (low average scores = 7–8; high average scores = 12–13). The average range for WAIS-III Full Scale IQ is 85–115

*WAIS-III* Wechsler Adult Intelligence Scale, *D-KEFS* Delis–Kaplan Executive Function System

**Table 3 Logistic regression predicting likelihood of an inactive occupational status (executive functioning as only predictor)**

| | *p*-value | OR | 95% CI |
|---|---|---|---|
| Executive functions | < 0.001 | 0.64 | 0.51–0.80 |
| Constant | < 0.001 | 0.31 | |

Occupational status as a dichotomized dependent variable (inactive = 1; active = 0). Executive functions (composite measure) as the only covariate. Cox and Snell's $R^2 = 0.17$. Nagelkerke's $R^2 = 0.25$. The model correctly classified 73.5% of the cases, with 91.9% of the active patients and 25.0% of the inactive patients correctly classified, n = 102

**Table 4 Logistic regression predicting likelihood of an inactive occupational status (executive functioning and IQ as predictors)**

| | *p*-value | OR | 95% CI |
|---|---|---|---|
| Executive functions | < 0.001 | 0.53 | 0.38–0.76 |
| WAIS-III–IQ | 0.183 | 1.04 | 0.98–1.10 |
| Constant | 0.090 | 0.01 | |

Occupational status as a dichotomized dependent variable (inactive = 1; active = 0). Executive functions (composite measure) and Full Scale IQ (measured with WAIS-III) as covariates. A test of the full model with the two predictors against the constant-only model was significant (omnibus Chi-square = 21.05, df = 2, $p < 0.001$.), Cox and Snells $R^2 = 0.20$. Nagelkerke's $R^2 = 0.29$. The model correctly classified 81.1% of patients (95.7% of the active patients and 42.3% of the inactive patients were correctly classified, n = 95

**Table 5 Logistic regression predicting likelihood of an inactive occupational status (cognitive and clinical factors as predictors)**

| | *p*-value | OR | 95% CI |
|---|---|---|---|
| Executive functions | 0.001 | 0.55 | 0.38–0.78 |
| WAIS-III–IQ | 0.196 | 1.04 | 0.98–1.10 |
| History of psychosis | 0.240 | 0.41 | 0.09–1.81 |
| Involuntary care | 0.245 | 2.46 | 0.54–11.2 |
| Benzodiazepines | 0.224 | 0.47 | 0.14–1.58 |
| Constant | 0.135 | 0.01 | |

Occupational status as a dichotomized dependent variable (inactive = 1; active = 0) and five covariates, including Executive functions (composite measure) and Full Scale IQ (measured with WAIS-III). Categorical covariates are prior history of psychotic symptoms (yes = 1; no = 0), history of involuntary care (i.e. if ever sectioned under the Mental Health Act; yes = 1; no = 0), and benzodiazepines (yes = 1; no = 0). The full model significantly predicted an inactive occupational status (omnibus Chi-square = 24.11, df = 5, $p < 0.001$). Cox and Snell's $R^2 = 0.23$ Nagelkerke's $R^2 = 0.33$. The model correctly classified 78.7% of the patients (92.6% of the active patients and 42.3% of the inactive patients were correctly classified), n = 94

The third logistic regression was used to evaluate the additional impact of both IQ and clinical factors. No clinical variables made a statistically significant contribution to the model ($p$ values > 0.05). Only executive function significantly predicted occupational status ($p = 0.001$). The odds of a person to be in the inactive group decreased by 45% as each principal component score increased by 1. None of the other variables made a unique, significant contribution to the model (Table 5).

## Discussion

The high rate of occupational dysfunction is a major issue in bipolar disorder. Here we studied the relative influence of clinical, demographic, and cognitive factors on occupational status by comparing bipolar disorder patients that worked or studied (active group) with those who did not (inactive group). We found that executive functioning was a stronger determinant of occupational functioning than general cognitive functioning (IQ) and other important clinical factors, including illness severity. In fact, executive functioning was the only factor that accounted for a significant amount of the variance in occupational status when clinical factors and IQ was taken into account. Taken together, our results suggest that poor executive functioning is the main factor associated with occupational dysfunction in bipolar disorder patients.

When individual predictors were considered separately, our findings align with previous cross-sectional and longitudinal studies that assessed the relationship with occupational status in bipolar disorder. First, psychotic symptoms during affective episodes and hospitalizations have been linked to a worse occupational and functional outcome in previous studies (Dickerson et al. 2004; Burdick et al. 2010; Gutiérrez-Rojas et al. 2011). We find similar differences regarding both lifetime history of psychotic symptoms and previous hospitalizations between the active and the inactive group. Second, general cognitive ability has been strongly associated with occupational status in both clinical and control samples (Schmidt and Hunter 2004). In line with this, we found in univariate analyses that the active group had significantly higher IQ than inactive patients. The groups did not, however, differ regarding premorbid IQ. Third, previous studies have found an association between executive functioning test scores and occupational status in bipolar disorder (Mur et al. 2008; Baune and Malhi 2015) similar to our findings. Finally, we found a higher prescription of benzodiazepines in the inactive patients.

Importantly, however, we demonstrate that none of the above variables significantly predict occupational status above and beyond the influence of executive functions. In terms of cognitive functioning, it was particularly notable that IQ was not a significant predictor of occupational status when compared to the model with executive function alone, further demonstrating the strong relationship between executive functioning and occupational status in bipolar disorder.

Instead, cognitive flexibility and inhibitory control as measured by condition 3 of the Color Word Test, the Verbal Fluency Test, and the Trail Making Test captured the largest differences between active and inactive patients ($\eta^2 = 0.08–0.14$). Cognitive flexibility is needed to adjust thinking and behavior in response to changing demands, and inhibitory control function facilitates inhibition of a dominant response in favor of one that is consistent with a long-term goal (Delis et al. 2001). Tests measuring these executive processes also stood out in previous studies predicting the occupational status of bipolar disorder patients (Ryan et al. 2013; Bonnín et al. 2014; O'Donnell et al. 2017).

The construct of executive functioning generally describes the integrated cognitive processes responsible for planning, initiating, sequencing, and monitoring complex goal-directed behavior (Royall et al. 2002). Different measures of executive function generally correlate strongly with each other but less with IQ (Friedman et al. 2006). Executive impairments are considered to be more disabling than other cognitive deficits as they affect many aspects of behavior (Lezak 2012). Despite this, the ecological validity of executive functioning performance tests has been questioned by ADHD researchers, who have found that self-report ratings were better predictors of occupational impairment (Barkley and Murphy 2010). The fact that our study clearly captured executive deficits in the inactive group suggests that executive function test scores do reflect real-life executive impairments and can be useful in clinical assessment.

The finding that occupationally inactive bipolar disorder patients manifest executive cognitive deficits has clinical implications. Early identification these impairments could give valuable information about the individuals' ability to return to his/her work, and guide which possible adaptions could be made in the workplace. Some cognitive remediation programs have been developed and shown promising results on occupational and social outcomes (Sanchez-Moreno et al. 2017).

### Strengths and limitations

Strengths of this study include that we defined occupational functioning by means of actual time working (or studying), which provides a hard outcome of functioning. Our study also involved a meticulous clinical characterization, including well-established neuropsychological tests. The participants were representative of bipolar disorder patients receiving psychiatric care, as nearly all patients with this diagnosis in the catchment area were referred to the Bipolar Affective Disorder unit for treatment by the time of enrollment. Finally, our study complements the literature with data from a

Scandinavian cohort in a field where most studies have been conducted by research groups in the US and Spain.

We also acknowledge a number of limitations. First, it should be noted that 72% of the subjects were occupationally active, which is a rather high number compared with previous reports (MacQueen et al. 2001). A possible explanation is that the catchment area of the recruiting clinic includes districts in Stockholm where the unemployment rates are lower than in the rest of the country, and the mean incomes above the Swedish average. Second, our analyses did not investigate the relative prediction of executive functioning compared to other cognitive functions previously found to predict occupational status in bipolar disorder patients, such as verbal memory (Dickerson et al. 2004), visual memory (Mur et al. 2009), and processing speed (Burdick et al. 2010). Future studies should further explore the relative contributions of these factors. Third, a potential source of bias is that 12 active and 6 inactive participants were excluded from the PCA because they had completed less than 50% of the tests. However, the proportion of excluded participants did not differ between the groups (Fisher exact test statistic value $=0.3585$, $p>0.05$). Fourth, the difference between measures of premorbid IQ and Full Scale IQ may indicate that the inactive group has declined in cognitive functioning. Our study did not investigate whether such decline predicted occupational status. The last and most important limitation is the cross-sectional design. We cannot determine if executive dysfunction causes occupational disability or if unemployment worsens executive functioning.

## Conclusions

Bipolar disorder patients with worse executive functioning are more likely to be occupationally inactive. These deficits can be identified with neuropsychological tests and should be targeted in treatment and rehabilitation.

#### Acknowledgements

We wish to thank all participants of this study. We also thank the staff at St. Göran Affective Bipolar Disorder unit, including data manager Mathias Kardell.

#### Authors' contributions

JD, TS and ML conceived and designed the study. JD analyzed the data and wrote the first draft of the manuscript. JD, TS, CC, EP, and ML interpreted the data and contributed to the writing of the final manuscript. All authors agreed with the results and conclusions of this article. All authors read and approved the final manuscript.

#### Author details

[1] Department of Psychiatry and Neurochemistry, Institute of Neuroscience and Physiology, The Sahlgrenska Academy, University of Gothenburg, Sahlgrenska University Hospital, Blå Stråket 15, 413 45 Gothenburg, Sweden. [2] Department of Psychology, University of Pennsylvania, 3720 Walnut Street, Philadelphia, PA 19104, USA. [3] Department of Medical Epidemiology and Biostatistics, Karolinska Institutet, Stockholm, Sweden. [4] Center for Autism Research, The Children's Hospital of Philadelphia, 2716 South St, Philadelphia, PA 19104, USA.

#### References

Asberg M, Schalling D. Construction of a new psychiatric rating instrument, the Comprehensive Psychopathological Rating Scale (CPRS). Prog Neuropsychopharmacol. 1979;3:405–12.

Barkley RA, Murphy KR. Impairment in occupational functioning and adult ADHD: the predictive utility of executive function (EF) ratings versus EF tests. Arch Clin Neuropsychol. 2010;25:157–73.

Baune BT, Malhi GS. A review on the impact of cognitive dysfunction on social, occupational, and general functional outcomes in bipolar disorder. Bipolar Disord. 2015;17(Suppl 2):41–55.

Berman AH, Bergman H, Palmstierna T, Schlyter F. Evaluation of the drug use disorders identification test (DUDIT) in criminal justice and detoxification settings and in a Swedish population sample. Eur Addict Res. 2005;11:22–31.

Bonnín CM, Martínez-Arán A, Torrent C, Pacchiarotti I, Rosa AR, Franco C, et al. Clinical and neurocognitive predictors of functional outcome in bipolar euthymic patients: a long-term, follow-up study. J Affect Disord. 2010;121:156–60.

Bonnín CM, Torrent C, Goikolea JM, Reinares M, Solé B, Valentí M, et al. The impact of repeated manic episodes and executive dysfunction on work adjustment in bipolar disorder. Eur Arch Psychiatry Clin Neurosci. 2014;264:247–54.

Burdick KE, Goldberg JF, Harrow M. Neurocognitive dysfunction and psychosocial outcome in patients with bipolar I disorder at 15-year follow-up. Acta Psychiatr Scand. 2010;122:499–506.

Delis DC, Kaplan E, Kramer JH. Delis–Kaplan executive function system (D-KEFS) examiner's manual. San Antonio: The Psychological Corporation; 2001.

Depp CA, Mausbach BT, Bowie C, Wolyniec P, Thornquist MH, Luke JR, et al. Determinants of occupational and residential functioning in bipolar disorder. J Affect Disord. 2012;136:812–8.

Dickerson FB, Boronow JJ, Stallings CR, Origoni AE, Cole S, Yolken RH. Association between cognitive functioning and employment status of persons with bipolar disorder. Psychiatr Serv. 2004;55:54–8.

Ekman CJ, Lind J, Rydén E, Ingvar M, Landén M. Manic episodes are associated with grey matter volume reduction a voxel-based morphometry brain analysis. Acta Psychiatr Scand. 2010;122:507–15.

Ekman M, Granstrom O, Omerov S, Jacob J, Landen M. The societal cost of bipolar disorder in Sweden. Soc Psychiatry Psychiatr Epidemiol. 2013;48:1601–10.

Eriksson L, Byrne T, Johansson E, Trygg J, Wikström C. Multi- and megavariate data analysis: basic principles and applications. Malmö: MKS Umetrics; 2013.

Friedman NP, Miyake A, Corley RP, Young SE, Defries JC, Hewitt JK. Not all executive functions are related to intelligence. Psychol Sci. 2006;17:172–9.

Gilbert E, Marwaha S. Predictors of employment in bipolar disorder: a systematic review. J Affect Disord. 2013;145:156–64.

Goetza I, Tohen M, Reed C, Lorenzo M, Vieta E. Functional impairment in patients with mania: baseline results of the EMBLEM study. Bipolar Disord. 2007;9:45–52.

Goldberg JF, Harrow M, Grossman LS. Course and outcome in bipolar affective disorder: a longitudinal follow-up study. Am J Psychiatry. 1995;152:379–84.

Gutiérrez-Rojas L, Jurado D, Gurpegui M. Factors associated with work, social life and family life disability in bipolar disorder patients. Psychiatry Res. 2011;186:254–60.

Guy W. ECDEU Assessment Manual for Psychopharmacology. Rockville, MD, US Department of Health, Education, and Welfare Public Health Service Alcohol, Drug Abuse, and Mental Health Administration. 1976.

Hajek T, Slaney C, Garnham J, Ruzickova M, Passmore M, Alda M. Clinical correlates of current level of functioning in primary care-treated bipolar patients. Bipolar Disord. 2005;7:286–91.

Judd LL, Akiskal HS, Schettler PJ, Endicott J, Maser J, Solomon DA, et al. The long-term natural history of the weekly symptomatic status of bipolar I disorder. Arch Gen Psychiatry. 2002;59:530–7.

Lezak MD. Neuropsychological assessment. New York: Oxford University Press; 2012.

Luborsky L. Clinicians' judgments of mental health: specimen case descriptions and forms for the health-sickness rating scale. Bull Menninger Clin. 1975;39:448–80.

MacQueen GM, Young LT, Robb JC, Marriott M, Cooke RG, Joffe RT. Effect of number of episodes on wellbeing and functioning of patients with bipolar disorder. Acta Psychiatr Scand. 2000;101:374–81.

MacQueen GM, Young LT, Joffe RT. A review of psychosocial outcome in patients with bipolar disorder. Acta Psychiatr Scand. 2001;103:163–70.

Martinez-Aran A, Vieta E, Torrent C, Sanchez-Moreno J, Goikolea JM, Salamero M, et al. Functional outcome in bipolar disorder: the role of clinical and cognitive factors. Bipolar Disord. 2007;9:103–13.

Mur M, Portella MJ, Mártinez-Arán A, Pifarré J, Vieta E. Persistent neuropsychological deficit in euthymic bipolar patients: executive function as a core deficit. J Clin Psychiatry. 2007;68:1078–86.

Mur M, Portella MJ, Martínez-Arán A, Pifarré J, Vieta E. Long-term stability of cognitive impairment in bipolar disorder: a 2-year follow-up study of lithium-treated euthymic bipolar patients. J Clin Psychiatry. 2008;69:712–9.

Mur M, Portella MJ, Martinez-Aran A, Pifarre J, Vieta E. Influence of clinical and neuropsychological variables on the psychosocial and occupational outcome of remitted bipolar patients. Psychopathology. 2009;42:148–56.

Murray CJ, Lopez AD. Alternative projections of mortality and disability by cause 1990–2020: global Burden of Disease Study. Lancet. 1997;349:1498–504.

O'Donnell LA, Deldin PJ, Grogan-Kaylor A, McInnis MG, Weintraub J, Ryan KA, et al. Depression and executive functioning deficits predict poor occupational functioning in a large longitudinal sample with bipolar disorder. J Affect Disord. 2017;215:135–42.

Palsson E, Figueras C, Johansson AG, Ekman CJ, Hultman B, Ostlind J, et al. Neurocognitive function in bipolar disorder: a comparison between bipolar I and II disorder and matched controls. BMC Psychiatry. 2013;13:165.

Perlis RH, Dennehy EB, Miklowitz DJ, Delbello MP, Ostacher M, Calabrese JR, et al. Retrospective age at onset of bipolar disorder and outcome during two-year follow-up: results from the STEP-BD study. Bipolar Disord. 2009;11:391–400.

Reed C, Goetz I, Vieta E, Bassi M, Haro JM. Work impairment in bipolar disorder patients—results from a two-year observational study (EMBLEM). Eur Psychiatry. 2010;25:338–44.

Robinson LJ, Thompson JM, Gallagher P, Goswami U, Young AH, Ferrier IN, et al. A meta-analysis of cognitive deficits in euthymic patients with bipolar disorder. J Affect Disord. 2006;93:105–15.

Royall DR, Lauterbach EC, Cummings JL, Reeve A, Rummans TA, Kaufer DI, et al. Executive control function: a review of its promise and challenges for clinical research: a report from the committee on research of the American Neuropsychiatric Association. J Neuropsychiatry Clin Neurosci. 2002;14:377–405.

Ryan KA, Vederman AC, Kamali M, Marshall D, Weldon AL, McInnis MG, et al. Emotion perception and executive functioning predict work status in euthymic bipolar disorder. Psychiatry Res. 2013;210:472–8.

Rydén E, Johansson C, Blennow K, Landén M. Lower CSF HVA and 5-HIAA in bipolar disorder type 1 with a history of childhood ADHD. J Neural Transm. 2009a;116:1667–74.

Rydén E, Thase ME, Stråht D, Åberg-Wistedt A, Bejerot S, Landén M. A history of childhood attention-deficit hyperactivity disorder (ADHD) impacts clinical outcome in adult bipolar patients regardless of current ADHD. Acta Psychiatr Scand. 2009b;120:239–46.

Sachs GS, Thase ME, Otto MW, Bauer M, Miklowitz D, Wisniewski SR, et al. Rationale, design, and methods of the Systematic Treatment Enhancement Program for bipolar disorder. Biol Psychiatry. 2003;53:1028–42.

Salarvan S, Sparding T, Clements C, Ryden E, Landen M. Neuropsychological profiles of adult bipolar disorder patients with and without comorbid attention-deficit hyperactivity disorder. Int J Bipolar Disord. 2019;7:14.

Sanchez-Moreno J, Martinez-Aran A, Vieta E. Treatment of functional impairment in patients with bipolar disorder. Curr Psychiatry Rep. 2017;19:3.

Saunders JB, Aasland OG, Babor TF, de la Fuente JR, Grant M. Development of the alcohol use disorders identification test (AUDIT): WHO Collaborative Project on early detection of persons with harmful alcohol consumption-II. Addiction. 1993;88:791–804.

Schmidt FL, Hunter J. General mental ability in the world of work: occupational attainment and job performance. J Pers Soc Psychol. 2004;86:162–73.

Sheehan DV. The anxiety disease. New York: Charles Scribner and Sons; 1983.

Sheehan DV, Lecrubier Y, Sheehan KH, Amorim P, Janavs J, Weiller E, et al. The Mini-International Neuropsychiatric Interview (M.I.N.I.): the development and validation of a structured diagnostic psychiatric interview for DSM-IV and ICD-10. J Clin Psychiatry. 1998;59:22–33.

Sparding T, Silander K, Pålsson E, Östlind J, Sellgren C, Ekman CJ, et al. Cognitive functioning in clinically stable patients with bipolar disorder I and II. PLoS ONE. 2015a;10:13.

Sparding T, Silander K, Pålsson E, Östlind J, Sellgren C, Ekman CJ, et al. Cognitive functioning in clinically stable patients with bipolar disorder I and II. PLoS ONE. 2015b;10:e0115562.

Tohen M, Waternaux CM, Tsuang MT. Outcome in Mania. A 4-year prospective follow-up of 75 patients utilizing survival analysis. Arch Gen Psychiatry. 1990;47:1106–11.

Tohen M, Hennen J, Zarate CM Jr, Baldessarini RJ, Strakowski SM, Stoll AL, et al. Two-year syndromal and functional recovery in 219 cases of first-episode major affective disorder with psychotic features. Am J Psychiatry. 2000;157:220–8.

Wechsler D. WAIS-III administration and scoring manual. San Antonio: The Psychological Corporation; 1997.

Young RC, Biggs JT, Ziegler VE, Meyer DA. A rating scale for mania: reliability, validity and sensitivity. Br J Psychiatry. 1978;133:429–35.

Zimmerman M, Galione JN, Chelminski I, Young D, Dalrymple K, Ruggero CJ. Sustained unemployment in psychiatric outpatients with bipolar disorder: frequency and association with demographic variables and comorbid disorders. Bipolar Disord. 2010;12:720–6.

# 17

# Impact of modification to DSM-5 criterion A for hypomania/mania in newly diagnosed bipolar patients: findings from the prospective BIO study

Mette U. Fredskild[1], Sharleny Stanislaus[1], Klara Coello[1], Sigurd A. Melbye[1], Hanne Lie Kjærstad[1], Kimie Stefanie Ormstrup Sletved[1], Trisha Suppes[2], Maj Vinberg[1,3,4] and Lars Vedel Kessing[1,3*]

**Abstract**

**Background:** DSM-IV states that criterion A for diagnosing hypomania/mania is mood change. The revised DSM-5 now states that increased energy or activity must be present alongside mood changes to diagnose hypomania/mania, thus raising energy/activity to criterion A. We set out to investigate how the change in criterion A affects the diagnosis of hypomanic/manic visits in patients with a newly diagnosed bipolar disorder.

**Results:** In this prospective cohort study, 373 patients were included (median age = 32; IQR, 27–40). Women constituted 66% (n = 245) of the cohort and 68% of the cohort (n = 253) met criteria for bipolar type II, the remaining patients were diagnosed bipolar type I. Median number of contributed visits was 2 per subject (IQR, 1–3) and median follow-up time was 3 years (IQR, 2–4). During follow-up, 127 patients had at least one visit with fulfilled DSM-IV criterion A. Applying DSM-5 criterion A reduced the number of patients experiencing a hypomanic/manic visit by 62% at baseline and by 50% during longitudinal follow-up, compared with DSM-IV criterion A. Fulfilling DSM-5 criterion A during follow-up was associated with higher modified young mania rating scale score (OR = 1.51, CL [1.34, 1.71], $p < 0.0001$) and increased number of visits contributed (OR = 1.86, CL [1.52, 2.29], $p < 0.0001$).

**Conclusion:** Applying the stricter DSM-5 criterion A in a cohort of newly diagnosed bipolar patients reduced the number of patients experiencing a hypomanic/manic visit substantially, and was associated with higher overall young mania rating scale scores, compared with DSM-IV criterion A. Consequently, fewer hypomanic/manic visits may be detected in newly diagnosed bipolar patients with applied DSM-5 criterion A, and the upcoming ICD-11, which may possibly result in longer diagnostic delay of BD as compared with the DSM-IV.

**Keywords:** Bipolar disorder, Diagnostic and Statistical Manual of Mental Disorders Version IV (DSM-IV), Diagnostic and Statistical Manual of Mental Disorders 5th edition (DSM-5), Mood, Irritability, Energy, Activity, The International Classification of Diseases 10 (ICD-10), The International Classification of Diseases 11 (ICD-11)

*Correspondence: lars.vedel.kessing@regionh.dk
[1] Copenhagen Affective Disorders Research Centre (CADIC), Psychiatric Centre Copenhagen, Department O, 6233, Rigshospitalet, Blegdamsvej 9, 2100 Copenhagen, Denmark
Full list of author information is available at the end of the article

## Background

The introduction of the Diagnostic and Statistical Manual of Mental Disorders 5th edition (DSM-5) (Association AP 2013) has in many ways changed the diagnostic criteria for bipolar disorder (BD). Several iterations of the DSM, including DSM-IV, emphasized mood abnormalities (*elevated, expansive or irritable mood*) as the cardinal symptom (criterion A) for a hypomanic/manic episode, and listed psychomotor disturbances (activity) as one of the seven criterion B symptoms (Association AP 1994). However, the revised DSM-5, which was published in 2013, now states that increased energy or activity must be present alongside mood disturbances to diagnose a hypomanic/manic episode, thus raising psychomotor disturbances to criterion A (Association AP 2013) (see Table 1). The argument behind the modification of criterion A was that it might improve specificity when making the diagnosis of hypomania/mania, and consequently, BD.

The International Classification of Diseases (ICD) is following in the footsteps of the DSM definitions. The ICD-10 definition of hypomania (F30.0)/mania (F30.1) highlighted mood abnormalities as criterion A (like DSM-IV) in the diagnostic criteria for research version (WHO 1992a) while the clinical descriptions and diagnostic guidelines version does not operate with A and B criteria (WHO 1992b). However, the newly online released ICD-11, like DSM-5, includes increased energy or activity as criterion A alongside mood abnormalities (WHO 2020).

Few studies have investigated the impact of the modification to DSM-5 criterion A for the diagnosis of hypomanic/manic episodes but only in cohorts of more chronic patients with more progressed and longer duration recurrent bipolar disorder. The STEP-BD study (Machado-Vieira et al. 2017), from the US, found that applying DSM-5 criterion A reduced the identified number of hypomanic/manic episodes by 48% when looking at baseline visits only (point prevalence), compared with DSM-IV criterion A. A study by our group of 907 chronic bipolar patients, from the US and Europe, found a 34% reduction in the number of patients experiencing a hypomanic/manic visit during follow up when DSM-5 criterion A was applied (Fredskild et al. 2019). On the other hand, the BDRN study (Gordon-Smith et al. 2017), from the UK, found that up to 94% of patients with a *lifetime* diagnosis of DSM-IV BD also met lifetime DSM-5 criteria for BD. All three mentioned studies have in common that they investigated populations of more chronic bipolar patients with more progressed and longer duration recurrent bipolar disorder. Results from the three mentioned studies suggest that the reduction in the diagnostic prevalence of hypomania/mania, and consequently BD, is highest earlier in the course of bipolar illness (a 34–48% reduction) but may diminish during lifetime (to a 6% reduction).

Thus, a knowledge gap remains, regarding how the introduction of DSM-5 criteria for BD affects the diagnostic prevalence of hypomanic/manic visits in newly diagnosed bipolar patients and potentially prolong the diagnostic gap from first symptoms to diagnosis.

Therefore, in a cohort of newly diagnosed patients with BD, we aimed to quantitatively determine the point prevalence of patients fulfilling criterion A of a hypomanic/manic visit according to DSM-IV and DSM-5 at baseline and during longitudinal follow up. Furthermore, we aimed to investigate if any of the covariates available could predict DSM-5 diagnosis. Lastly, we explored the individual association between manic symptoms available from the Young Mania Rating Scale (YMRS) to understand the relationship between present manic symptoms and the transition from DSM-IV to DSM-5 diagnosis of hypomania/mania.

We hypothesized that applying DSM-5 criterion A would lower the number of hypomanic/manic visits significantly, both at baseline and during follow-up and that no association between sex, age and DSM-5 diagnosis would be found. Lastly, we hypothesized that mood abnormalities (mood elevation and irritability) and energy/activity would show a strong association.

This study is of high importance as the consequences of modification to DSM-5 criterion A are still unknown and have never been looked at in a population of newly diagnosed bipolar patients. This study will help us understand the impact of the current modification to DSM-5

**Table 1** DSM and study definitions

| | DSM definition of criterion A for a hypomanic/manic episode | Study defined criterion A for a hypomanic/manic visit based on YMRS[a] |
|---|---|---|
| DSM-IV | *"A distinct period of abnormally and persistently elevated, expansive or irritable mood"* | Item 1[b] $\geq 2$ and/or Item 5[d] $\geq 4$ |
| DSM-5 | *"A distinct period of abnormally and persistently elevated, expansive or irritable mood AND persistently increased activity or energy"* | Item 1 $\geq 2$ and/or Item 5 $\geq 4$ ***AND*** Item 2[c] $\geq 2$ |

[a] Young Mania Rating Scale (11-item)

[b] Item 1: Mood elevation

[c] Item 2: Energy/activity

[d] Item 5: Irritability

criterion A for newly diagnosed bipolar patients, and hopefully help us understand the patient's disease-trajectory in the light of DSM-5.

## Methods

### Study design and aim

The present study is a prospective cohort study investigating follow-up data on newly diagnosed patients with BD. The overall aim of the present study is to elucidate the clinical consequences of the modification to the current DSM-5 criterion A when focusing on newly diagnosed bipolar patients.

### Setting of the study

The present study investigated data from the ongoing longitudinal Bipolar Illness Onset study (BIO), which aims to identify biomarkers for BD (Kessing et al. 2017). Details on methods and procedures in the BIO-study are fully described elsewhere (Kessing et al. 2017). The BIO-study protocol was approved by the Committee on Health Research Ethics of the Capital region of Denmark (Protocol No. H-7-2014-007) and the Danish Data Protection Agency, Capital Region of Copenhagen (RHP-2015-023). All participants provided written informed consent. The BIO-study complied with the Declaration of Helsinki principles (Seoul, October 2008).

### Participants

We included 373 patients with newly diagnosed BD. Recruitment of participants took place at the outpatient Copenhagen Affective Disorder Clinic from June 2015 to November 2019. The Clinic provides treatment for patients with newly diagnosed BD and receives patients from the Capital region of Denmark, an area covering 1.6 million and all the psychiatric centers in the Region (Kessing et al. 2013). All patients referred to the clinic as newly diagnosed bipolar patients were routinely asked for inclusion in the BIO-study.

At baseline, the initial diagnostic assessment of participants was conducted by an experienced specialist in psychiatry using the Structures Clinical Interview for DSM-IV-TR Axis I Disorders (First et al. 1996), categorizing patients into bipolar disorder I (BD I) or bipolar disorder II (BD II). The diagnosis of a single manic episode or BD was confirmed in a semi-structured research-based interview by M.Ds or M.Scs in Psychology Ph.D. students using the Schedules for Clinical Assessment in Neuropsychiatry (SCAN) providing an ICD-10 diagnosis (WHO 1992b). Inclusion criteria were an ICD-10 diagnosis of BD or a single manic episode and age 15–70 years.

No attempts to balance the prevalence of bipolar subtypes were taken. Patients with BD not otherwise specified and patients with cyclothymia were not offered treatment in the Clinic and thus not included in the BIO-study. Exclusion criteria were organic BD secondary to brain injury.

Patients with BD received treatment as usual in the clinic without interference from study investigators.

Besides the clinical assessment at inclusion (baseline), patients were assessed during remitted depressive, manic or mixed phases and and once yearly for up to 5 years of follow up.

### Procedures

At each assessment the severity of manic and/or depressive symptoms were evaluated using the 11-item clinician administered Young Mania Rating Scale (YMRS) (Young et al. 1978) and the 17-item Hamilton Depression Rating Scale (HAMD-17) (Hamilton 1960), respectively, covering the precceding 3 days. Both rating scales have been extensively validated for assessing manic and depressive symptoms, respectively (Young et al. 1978; Bech 2012). Patients were required to have a completed YMRS score at their first visit (baseline) to be included in the present study, as this was the basis of inclusion criteria.

### Definitions

We used the same methodology and definitions as in our prior publication on patients with more chronic BD (). The individual ratings on item 1 (Mood), item 2 (Energy/Activity) and item 5 (Irritability) on the 11-item YMRS allowed an evaluation of the presence of fulfilled criterion A of hypomania/mania according to DSM definition (see Table 1).

A score equal or above 2 on item 1 (Mood) was considered reflective of increased/elevated mood. A score equal or above 2 on item 2 (Energy/Activity) was considered reflective of increased motor activity or energy. A score equal or above 4 on item 5 (Irritability) was considered reflective of increased irritability (see Table 1).

Thus, study definition of fulfilling DSM-IV criterion A for a hypomanic/manic visit was defined as item 1 (Mood) $\geq 2$ and/or item 5 (Irritability) $\geq 4$, presumably adequate to meet the DSM-IV definition of criterion A. Study definition of fulfilled DSM-5 criterion A for a hypomanic/manic visit was defined as item 1 (Mood) $\geq 2$ and/or item 5 (Irritability) $\geq 4$ AND item 2 $\geq 2$ (Energy/Activity), presumably adequate to meet the DSM-5 definition of criterion A (see Table 1).

Depressive symptoms were defined as an HAMD-17 total score $\geq 15$.

### Statistical analyses

A total of 849 visits by 373 participants were analyzed. Data analyses were performed based on participants (373 patients) using logistic regression models and based on visits (849 visits) using linear mixed-effects models.

Descriptive data were presented as median and interquartile range (IQR) or count and percentage (%). A power of 80% and a significance level of alfa = 0.05 were chosen for all statistical analyses. Results from analyses were presented as odds ratios with 95% confidence limits.

All statistical analyses were performed using software programs (SAS Enterprise Guide version 7.15, SAS institute, Cary, North Carolina).

#### Missing data

One subject had missing data on the variables "age of onset" and "age at first hypomanic/manic episode" and additional one subject had missing data on "delay in diagnosis". These missing data were handled by single imputation with the median value of the cohort. Twelve subjects had missing data on family history of BD, 4 had missing data on no. of previous hospitalizations/admissions, and 4 had missing data on education years. These missing data were likewise handled by imputation before inclusion in the logistic regression model. A maximum of 7 missing values on the individual YMRS items were present throughout all visits (849) and were handled in the mixed model analysis.

#### Logistic regression

A modified YMRS score for each visit was calculated based on the total YMRS score, minus item 1, 2, and 5, as these items were used to define the outcome, i.e., DSM-IV and DSM-5 criterion A. The mean modified YMRS score was found for each participant as a mean of the modified YMRS scores across their visits.

Logistic regression models were performed in order to investigate if any of independent variables could predict DSM-5 Criterion A fulfillment during follow-up. The outcome was defined as fulfilling DSM-5 criterion A at least once during follow-up in study (yes/no). Univariate and multivariable analyses were performed, and data were represented unadjusted and fully adjusted for bipolar subtype, sex, no. of visits contributed, age first hypomanic/manic episode (years), no. of visits with depressed symptoms, mean modified YMRS total score, family history of BD, delay in diagnosis, education years. BD subtype, family history of BD, and sex were treated as binary variables, whereas the remaining variables were treated as continuous variables in the univariate and multivariable analysis. Variables included in the multivariable analysis were included based on clinical relevance and/or significance in univariate analysis ($p < 0.2$). Bonferroni correction was conducted to correct for multiple testing.

#### Mixed models

Based on visits, we examined the association between individual items on the YMRS. Visits data (849 visits) represent repeated measures data and were analyzed accordingly, using generalized linear mixed-effects models, specifying each participant as random effect. The data represented zero-inflated data. Thus, the outcome was dichotomized, and the mixed models were specified as binomial.

The first analysis investigated the individual YMRS items (predictors) and their association with experiencing increased mood (outcome variable). The outcome variable mood (item 1) was defined as elevated (> 0) and not elevated (= 0). Univariate as well as multivariable linear mixed-effects models were conducted, and results presented unadjusted and fully adjusted for the other YMRS items. The analysis was repeated with irritability (item 5) as the outcome.

The analyses were specified with mood and irritability, respectively, as outcome variable, the individual YMRS items as predictors, and a random intercept for each participant to account for multiple observations made on the same subject.

## Results

#### Demographic and clinical characteristics

We included 373 patients (median age = 32; IQR 27–40; 66% were female (n = 245) and 32% (n = 120) met criteria for BD I. A total of 849 visits by the 373 patients were included.

The median age at onset of BD was 18 (IQR, 15–22). Median number of visits contributed by each subject in the study was 2 (IQR, 1–3), corresponding to a median follow-up time in months by each subject of 41 months (IQR, 26–50) (see Table 2).

#### DSM-IV and DSM-5 criterion A

***Baseline/first visit***

At baseline (the participant's first visit), 86 patients fulfilled criterion A of a hypomanic/manic visit according to DSM-IV criterion A (mood and/or irritability). Of the 86 patients, 33 patients fulfilled DSM-5 criterion A (mood and/or irritability AND energy/activity) of a hypomanic/manic visit, a reduction of 62% at baseline (see Table 2).

The median of the modified YMRS total score at baseline was 5 (IQR, 2–8) in the group of 86 patients who fulfilled DSM-IV criterion A and 8 (IQR, 4–10) in the group of 33 patients who fulfilled DSM-5 criterion A (see Table 2).

**Table 2** Sociodemographic and clinical characteristics

| Patients, n | 373 |
|---|---|
| Total visits | 849 |
| Sex | |
| Male, n (%) | 128 (34%) |
| Female, n (%) | 245 (66%) |
| Bipolar subtype | |
| BD I, n (%) | 120 (32%) |
| BD II, n (%) | 253 (68%) |
| Years of education, median (IQR) | 15 (13–17) |
| No. of previous hospitalizations/admissions, median (IQR) | 0 (0–1) |
| Family history of BD[a], n (%) | 56 (16%) |
| Age (years), median (IQR) | 32 (27–40) |
| Age at onset (years)[b], median (IQR) | 18 (15–22) |
| Age at first hypomanic/manic episode (years)[c], median (IQR) | 21 (17–27) |
| Illness duration (years)[d], median (IQR) | 10 (6–16) |
| Delay in diagnosis (years)[e], median (IQR) | 5 (2–11) |
| Follow up time in study (months), median (IQR) | 41 (26–50) |
| Follow up time in study (years), median (IQR) | 3 (2–4) |
| No. of visits contributed per patient, median (IQR) | 2 (1–3) |
| YMRS total score, median (IQR) | 3 (0–6) |
| Modified YMRS total score[f], median (IQR) | 1 (0–4) |
| No. of patients fulfilling a depressed visit through follow up (Hamilton $\geq$ 15), n (%) | 135 (36%) |
| No. of patients fulfilling a visit with DSM-IV criterion A for hypomania/mania through follow up, n (%) | 127 (34%) |
| No. of patients fulfilling a visit with DSM-5 criterion A for hypomania/mania through follow up, n (%) | 63 (17%) |
| **Baseline visits (first visit by each subject), n** | 373 |
| YMRS total score at first visit, median (IQR) | 3 (0–6) |
| Modified YMRS total score at first visit, median (IQR) | 1 (0–4) |
| No. of patients fulfilling DSM-IV criterion A for hypomania/mania at baseline, n (%) | 86 (23%) |
| No. of patients fulfilling DSM-5 criterion A for hypomania/mania at baseline, n (%) | 33 (9%) |
| YMRS total score for participants fulfilling DSM-IV criterion A at first visits, median (IQR) | 10 (7–14) |
| Modified YMRS total score for participants fulfilling DSM-IV criterion A at first visits, median (IQR) | 5 (2–8) |
| YMRS total score for participants fulfilling DSM-5 criterion A at first visits, median (IQR) | 14 (10–16) |
| Modified YMRS total score for participants fulfilling DSM-5 criterion A at first visits, median (IQR) | 8 (4–10) |
| No. of patients with a depressive episode at first visit (Hamilton $\geq$ 15) at baseline, n (%) | 101 (27%) |

[a] Family history of BD: Mother, father or sibling with bipolar disorder

[b] Age at onset: From birthdate to first episode of depression, mania, hypomania or mixed episode

[c] Age at first hypomanic/manic episode: From birthdate to first mania, hypomania or mixed episode

[d] Illness duration: From first episode (depression, mania, hypomania or mixed episode) to date of inclusion

[e] Delay in diagnosis: From the time where the first mania, hypomania or mixed episode occurred to date of the diagnosis of a single manic or mixed episode or a diagnosis of BD

[f] Modified YMRS total score = total score minus item 1, item 2 and item 5

#### *Follow up*

During follow-up, 127 subjects had at least one visit fulfilling DSM-IV criterion A of a hypomanic/manic visit. Applying DSM-5 criterion A, 63 subjects had at least one visit fulfilling DSM-5 criterion A of hypomania/mania corresponding to a reduction of 50% in the number of subjects who experienced a hypomanic/manic visit according to criterion A during follow-up in the study when applying DSM-5 criterion A (see Table 2).

#### Multivariable logistic regression

We investigated if any of the demographic and clinical variables could predict DSM-5 diagnosis of hypomania/mania according to DSM-5 criterion A during follow-up. The multivariable logistic regression model revealed that

**Table 3** Logistic regression—prediction of DSM-5 criterion A fulfillment in 373 subjects

| Variable | OR | 95% CL | p-value |
|---|---|---|---|
| Age (years) | | | |
| Univariate analysis | 0.99 | 0.97, 1.02 | 0.65 |
| Sex (Male vs female) | | | |
| Univariate analysis | 0.95 | 0.53, 1.68 | 0.86 |
| Multivariate analysis[f] | 0.79 | 0.37, 1.67 | 0.53 |
| No. of visits contributed | | | |
| Univariate analysis | 1.51 | 1.31, 1.75 | <0.0001 |
| Multivariate analysis[f] | 1.86 | 1.52, 2.29 | <0.0001** |
| Bipolar subtype (BD I vs BD II) | | | |
| Univariate analysis | 1.50 | 0.85, 2.61 | 0.16 |
| Multivariate analysis[f] | 1.64 | 0.82, 3.27 | 0.16 |
| Age at onset (years)[a] | | | |
| Univariate analysis | 0.97 | 0.92, 1.01 | 0.11 |
| Age first hypomanic/manic episode (years)[b] | | | |
| Univariate analysis | 0.96 | 0.92, 0.99 | 0.03 |
| Multivariate analysis[f] | 0.99 | 0.94, 1.04 | 0.57 |
| Delay in diagnosis (years)[c] | | | |
| Univariate analysis | 1.02 | 0.99, 1.06 | 0.15 |
| Multivariate analysis[f] | 1.03 | 0.98, 1.07 | 0.25 |
| No. of visits with depressed symptoms | | | |
| Univariate analysis | 1.34 | 0.99, 1.81 | 0.06 |
| Multivariate analysis[f] | 0.78 | 0.51, 1.19 | 0.24 |
| Mean modified YMRS total score[d] | | | |
| Univariate analysis | 1.38 | 1.24, 1.52 | <0.0001 |
| Multivariate analysis[f] | 1.51 | 1.34, 1.71 | <0.0001** |
| Number of previous hospitalizations/ admissions | | | |
| Univariate analysis | 0.92 | 0.74, 1.14 | 0.44 |
| Education years | | | |
| Univariate analysis | 0.92 | 0.83, 1,02 | 0.12 |
| Multivariate analysis[f] | 0.90 | 0.78, 1.03 | 0.13 |
| Family history of BD[e] (no vs yes) | | | |
| Univariate analysis | 0.79 | 0.35, 1.77 | 0.57 |
| Multivariate analysis[f] | 0.71 | 0.26, 1.97 | 0.52 |

[a] Age at onset: From birthdate to first episode of depression, mania, hypomania or mixed episode

[b] Age at first hypomanic/manic episode: From birthdate to first mania, hypomania or mixed episode

[c] Delay in diagnosis: From first mania, hypomania or mixed episode to date of BD diagnosed

[d] Mean of the modified YMRS total score (YMRS total score minus item 1, item 2 and item 5) across patient visits

[e] Family history of BD: Mother, father or sibling with bipolar disorder

[f] Adjusted for bipolar subtype, sex, no. of visits contributed, age first hypomanic/manic episode (years), no. of visits with depressed symptoms, mean modified YMRS total score, family history of BD, delay in diagnosis, education years

** Remained statistically significant after Bonferroni correction for multiple testing in the multivariate analysis ($p<0.006$)

the number of visits contributed and the mean modified YMRS total were associated with DSM-5 diagnosis according to criterion A during follow-up (see Table 3). For every 1 visit contributed, the odds of DSM-5 diagnosis according to criterion A, increased by 86% after adjustment (adjusted OR [95% CL] 1.86 [1.52, 2.29], $p>0.0001$). For every 1 increasement in mean modified YMRS total score, the odds of DSM-5 diagnosis increased by 51% after adjustment (adjusted OR [95% CL] 1.51 [1.34, 1.71], $p>0.0001$).

Age at first hypomanic/manic episode was associated with fulfilling DSM-5 diagnosis according to criterion A in univariate analysis (OR = 0.96, 95% CL [0.92, 0.99], $p=0.03$), but after adjustment in the multivariable analysis, this association was no longer statistically significant (OR = 0.99, 95% CL [0.94, 1.04], $p=0.57$).

Delay in diagnosis, no. of visits with depressed symptoms, and education years all showed a borderline statiscal significant association with DSM-5 diagnosis according to criterion A in univariate analysis but these associations were no longer statistically significant after adjustment in the multivariable analysis (see Table 3).

We did not find any statistically significant associations between sex, age, bipolar subtype, no. of previous hospitalizations/admissions, family history of BD and DSM-5 diagnosis according to criterion A.

Sensitivity analyses were performed, stratifying based on bipolar subtype and sex, respectively, however, this did not change the results.

### Association between individual YMRS items

#### *Mood*

We investigated the individual hypomanic/manic symptoms (individual YMRS items) and their relationship with mood elevation (see Table 4). In the univariate analysis all items except item 11 (Insight) showed association with mood elevation before adjustment. After adjustment and Bonferroni correction, only item 2 (Energy/Activity), item 3 (Sexual Interest), item 4 (Sleep), and item 6 (Speech), remained statistically significantly associated with item 1 (Mood) with a $p\text{-value}<0.005$. For every 1-value increasement in Energy/Activity on item 2, the odds of experiencing elevated mood increased by 2.5 times in the adjusted model (adjusted OR [95% CL] 2.5 [1.8, 3.4]) (see Table 4).

#### *Irritability*

We investigated the individual hypomanic/manic symptoms (individual YMRS items) and their relationship with irritability (see Table 5). In the univariate analysis all items except item 11 (Insight) showed an association with irritability before adjustment. After adjustment and Bonferroni correction, only item 7 (Language-Thought

**Table 4** Odds ratios of experiencing elevated mood depending on the different manic symptoms (YMRS items) during 849 visits

| | | OR | 95% confidence limts | Range of scale in data set[a] |
|---|---|---|---|---|
| Item 1 (Mood) | x | x | X | 0–4 |
| Item 2 (Energy/activity) | Unadjusted | 4.9 | (3.8, 6.2) | 0–4 |
| | Adjusted[b] | 2.5* | (1.8, 3.4)* | |
| Item 3 (Sexual interest) | Unadjusted | 4.3 | (3.3, 5.6) | 0–3 |
| | Adjusted | 2.2* | (1.6, 3.2)* | |
| Item 4 (Sleep) | Unadjusted | 2.7 | (2.2, 3.4) | 0–4 |
| | Adjusted | 1.6* | (1.2, 2.1)* | |
| Item 5 (Irritability) | Unadjusted | 1.4 | (1.2, 1.5) | 0–6 |
| | Adjusted | 0.9 | (0.7, 1.1) | |
| Item 6 (Speech) | Unadjusted | 2.9 | (2.4, 3.4) | 0–6 |
| | Adjusted | 2.0* | (1.6, 2.4)* | |
| Item 7 (Language-Thought Disorder) | Unadjusted | 2.2 | (1.9, 2.7) | 0–4 |
| | Adjusted | 1.3 | (1.0, 1.7) | |
| Item 8 (Content) | Unadjusted | 2.2 | (1.8, 2.7) | 0–8 |
| | Adjusted | 1.2 | (0.9, 1.6) | |
| Item 9 (Aggression) | Unadjusted | 1.7 | (1.1, 2.4) | 0–5 |
| | Adjusted | 0.8 | (0.5, 1.6) | |
| Item 10 (Appearance) | Unadjusted | 2.4 | (1.4, 4.2) | 0–4 |
| | Adjusted | 0.5 | (0.2, 1.3) | |
| Item 11 (Insight) | Unadjusted | 1.5 | (0.9, 2.4) | 0–6 |
| | Adjusted | 0.7 | (0.3, 1.5) | |

Outcome Mood > 0 vs mood = 0

[a] Range of scale: observed minimum and maximum values of the individual YMRS items in data set

[b] Adjusted model is adjusted for all the remaining YMRS items: Item 2, item 3, item 4, item 5, item 6, item 7, item 8, item 9, item 10, item 11

* Remained statistically significant after adjustment and Bonferroni correction for multiple testing ($p < 0.005$)

Disorder) remained statistically significantly associated with irritability with a p-value < 0.005. For every 1-value increasement in Language-Thought Disorder on Item 7, the odds of experiencing increased irritability was increased 1.5-fold after adjustment (adjusted OR [95% CL] 1.5 [1.3, 1.9]) (see Table 5).

Overall, Tables 4, 5 illustrate and substantiate that elevated mood is associated with activity, which is not the case for irritability.

## Discussion

DSM-5 criterion A for hypomania/mania now includes the requirement of increased energy or activity in addition to mood change. The clinical consequences of the modification to the current DSM-5 criterion A for hypomania/mania has never been investigated in newly diagnosed bipolar patients. Elucidating the consequences of applied DSM-5 criterion A for newly diagnosed bipolar patients can help us understand the disease-trajectory of newly diagnosed bipolar patients in the light of DSM-5, and soon ICD-11 criteria.

In the present study of 373 newly diagnosed BD patients we revealed 3 overall findings. First, we found that applying DSM-5 criterion A reduced the number of patients experiencing a hypomanic/manic visit by 62% at baseline and by 50% during longitudinal follow-up, compared with DSM-IV criterion A. Second, fulfilling DSM-5 criterion A for a hypomanic/manic visit during follow-up was associated with higher scores on the YMRS and associated with increased number of contributed visits. Third, the individual association between manic symptoms available from the Young Mania Rating Scale showed a significant association between elevated mood (item 1) and energy/activity (item 2), sexual interest (item 3), decreased need for sleep (item 4), and speech (item 6). Irritability (item 5) showed a significant association with language-thought disorder (item 7).

The decrease in diagnostic prevalence (62% at baseline and by 50% during follow-up) with applied DSM-5 criterion A is clinically significant in a cohort of newly diagnosed bipolar patients. Previous studies of more chronic bipolar patients also point toward a decrease in both baseline prevalence and longitudinal diagnostic prevalence with applied DSM-5 criterion A for hypomania/mania, however the decrease in the prevalence of BD using DSM-5 compared with DSM-IV was smaller (34%

**Table 5** Odds ratios of experiencing irritability depending on the different manic symptoms (YMRS items) during 849 visits

| | | OR | 95% confidence limits | Range of scale[a] |
|---|---|---|---|---|
| Item 1 (Mood) | Unadjusted | 1.6 | (1.4, 2.0) | 0–4 |
| | Adjusted[b] | 1.1 | (0.8, 1.4) | |
| Item 2 (Energy/activity) | Unadjusted | 1.6 | (1.4, 2.0) | 0–4 |
| | Adjusted | 1.1 | (0.8, 1.4) | |
| Item 3 (Sexual interest) | Unadjusted | 1.6 | (1.3, 2.1) | 0–3 |
| | Adjusted | 1.2 | (0.9, 1.6) | |
| Item 4 (Sleep) | Unadjusted | 1.6 | (1.3, 2.0) | 0–4 |
| | Adjusted | 1.3 | (1.0, 1.6) | |
| Item 5 (Irritability) | X | x | x | 0–6 |
| Item 6 (Speech) | Unadjusted | 1.4 | (1.2, 1.5) | 0–6 |
| | Adjusted | 1.1 | (0.9, 1.2) | |
| Item 7 (Language-Thought Disorder) | Unadjusted | 1.8 | (1.6, 2.2) | 0–4 |
| | Adjusted | 1.5* | (1.3, 1.9)* | |
| Item 8 (Content) | Unadjusted | 1.5 | (1.3, 1.8) | 0–8 |
| | Adjusted | 1.0 | (0.8, 1.3) | |
| Item 9 (Aggression) | Unadjusted | 2.5 | (1.4, 4.5) | 0–5 |
| | Adjusted | 2.2 | (1.1, 4.2) | |
| Item 10 (Appearance) | Unadjusted | 2.4 | (1.3, 4.6) | 0–4 |
| | Adjusted | 1.2 | (0.6, 2.6) | |
| Item 11 (Insight) | Unadjusted | 1.2 | (0.8, 1.9) | 0–6 |
| | Adjusted | 0.7 | (0.4, 1.3) | |

Outcome irritability > 0 vs irritability = 0

[a] Range of scale: observed minimum and maximum values of the individual YMRS items in data set

[b] Adjusted model is adjusted for all the remaining YMRS items: Item 1, Item 2, item 3, item 4, item 6, item 7, item 8, item 9, item 10, item 11

[*] Remained statistically significant after adjustment and Bonferroni correction for multiple testing ($p < 0.005$)

(Fredskild et al. 2019) and 48% (Machado-Vieira et al. 2017)) than in our study of newly diagnosed patients with BD (62% at baseline).

More severe manic symptoms (i.e., higher YMRS score) were associated with DSM-5 diagnosis during follow-up. These results may indicate that the stricter DSM-5 criterion A captures the more severe and evident hypomanic/manic visits but cuts off 50% of previously detected visits by DSM-IV criterion A.

Number of contributed visits per patient was associated with fulfillment of DSM-5 criterion A, suggesting that patients over time, were more likely to have a hypomanic/manic visit detected according to DSM-5 criterion A.

These results are in line with findings from our previous study on more chronic bipolar patients also showing that both higher YMRS scores and number of contributed visits were associated with DSM-5 diagnosis according to criterion A (Fredskild et al. 2019). Consequently, with the DSM-5 criterion A less severe BD may be overlooked, especially early during the course of illness. This may possibly result in a longer diagnostic delay (Dagani et al. 2017; Baldessarini et al. 2007), as patients may not fulfill criteria for BD until later stages of the illness. Consequently, treatment interventions will be delayed likely with poorer outcomes (Kessing et al. 2013, 2014; Kessing 2019). Nevertheless, it should be noted that in the present study we did not prove a direct association between delay in diagnosis and fulfilling DSM-5 criterion A.

The individual association between manic symptoms available from the YMRS showed a strong association between mood and energy/activity after adjustment, however, irritability and energy/activity did not prove any significant association after adjustment. This could potentially be part of the explanation of why some of the DSM-IV diagnosed hypomanic/manic visits (elevated, expansive, or irritable mood) no longer fulfill DSM-5 criterion A (elevated, expansive, or irritable mood AND energy or activity), as irritability and energy/activity did not prove an association in our data after adjustment.

### Strengths and limitations

Our study is based on updated data from the ongoing longitudinal BIO-study, including a large cohort of well-characterized patients with newly diagnosed BD. Our cohort seems representative of newly diagnosed bipolar patients with a median age of illness onset of 18 years and a median delay in diagnosis of 5 years (Dagani et al. 2017; Baldessarini et al. 2007).

The decrease in prevalence of hypomanic and manic visits from DSM-IV to DSM-5 criterion A was larger than in previous studies, this could be explained by the present study had predominance of BD II patients (68%), and the comparable studies had a majority of BD I patients (Machado-Vieira et al. 2017; Fredskild et al. 2019). The large proportion of patients with bipolar disorder, type II in the present sample reflect that a substantial proportion of patients were reffered to the Copenhagen Affective Disorder Clinic from primary care including private psychiatrists and general practice.

Standardized, validated rating scales were used to evaluate both manic and depressive symptoms, YMRS and Hamilton 17-items, respectively, as undertaken by trained M.Ds or M.Scs in Psychology Ph.D. students. The assessment of fulfilled DSM-IV and DSM-5 criterion A were based solely on the YMRS scores on individual items, thus individual YMRS scores served as a proxy for evaluating the presence/absence of a hypomanic/manic visit, although the YMRS rating scale is not designed as a diagnostic tool but rather a rating scale measuring the overall symptom severity of individual manic symptoms. We used YMRS because this scale includes specific items on both mood, activity and irritability that are all criterion A symptoms. In this regard, it should be noted that the majority of patients included in the study did not present with a mood episode at baseline (see Table 2) and the findings were based on limited observations of patients (median visits = 2; IQR, 1–3) and a period of observation with the use of scales during approximately yearly visits of a 3 days look-back. We do not have detailed data from the Structures Clinical Interview for DSM-IV-TR Axis I Disorders (First et al. 1996) so we were not able to directly compare DSM-IV-TR and DSM-5 diagnoses.

It is evident from these and our prior data (Fredskild et al. 2019) that inclusion during a mood episode and more frequent visits and a longer follow-up period would have resulted in a higher concordance between DSM-5 and DSM-IV diagnoses of hypomania/mania and BD.

Furthermore, the present study only evaluated hypomania/mania according to criterion A and did not incorporate the time frame or the criterion B symptoms in the assessment of hypomania/mania. However, criterion A is the gate criterion to evaluate the presence/absence of a manic/hypomanic state according to DSM and thus must be fulfilled in order to continue to criterion B.

Lastly, the present study incorporated an explorative analysis of associations between DSM-5 criterion A fulfillment and clinical characteristics/demographics. Our logistic regression models included multiple testing and thus an increased risk of a random significant finding (type I error). However, this was minimized by applying Bonferroni correction for multiple testing.

On the other hand, several of our predictors showed borderline significance in the logistic regression model, which can either be a random finding, or the result of a too small sample size to detect an actual difference (type II error). Nevertheless, our findings are consistent with results from a cohort of more chronic bipolar patients published by our study group (Fredskild et al. 2019).

## Conclusions

In this prospective cohort study, applying DSM-5 criterion A for hypomania/mania reduced the diagnostic prevalence of hypomanic/manic visits by 62% at baseline and by 50% during longitudinal follow-up, compared with DSM-IV criterion A. Fulfilling DSM-5 criterion A was associated with more severe manic symptoms and increased during follow-up. Overall, fewer hypomanic/manic visits may be detected in newly diagnosed bipolar patients with applied DSM-5 criterion A, and the hypomanic/manic visits detected may be of more severe character, possibly overlooking less evident hypomanic/manic episodes. Consequently, the DSM-5 and the upcoming ICD-11, may possibly result in longer diagnostic delay of BD as compared with the DSM-IV.

### Abbreviations

BD: Bipolar disorder; BD I: Bipolar disorder I; BD II: Bipolar disorder II; BIO: Bipolar Illness Onset study; CADIC: Copenhagen Affective Disorder Clinic; DSM-IV: Diagnostic and Statistical Manual of Mental Disorders version IV; DSM-5: Diagnostic and Statistical Manual of Mental Disorders 5th edition; ICD-10: The International Classification of Diseases 10; ICD-11: The International Classification of Diseases 11.

### Acknowledgements

Not applicable.

### Authors' contributions

MUF has together with SS and LVK designed the study, carried out the primary statistical analyses, and drafted the first version and subsequent versions of the work including interpretation of data. KC, SAM, HLK and KSO have recruited the study participants and have together with TS and MV substantively revised the work and contributed to the interpretation of data. All authors read and approved the final manuscript.

### Competing interests

Lars Vedel Kessing has in the past 3 years been a consultant for Lundbeck. Maj Vinberg has in the past 3 years been a consultant for Lundbeck, Janssen Cilag and Sunovion.Trisha Suppes has in the past 3 years reported: Grants from Merck, National Institute on Drug Abuse, National Institute of Health, VA Cooperative Studies Program, and VA OR&D PRIME Care, Palo Alto Health Sciences, Stanley Medical Research Institute, Pathways Genomics. Consulting fees from Allergan, Inc., Intracellular Therapies, Sunovion Pharmaceuticals, Inc., and Impel NeuroPharma Inc. Honoraria from CME Institute (Physicians Postgraduate Press, Inc.) and CMEology. Royalties from American Psychiatric Association

Publishing, Hogrefe Publishing, Jones and Bartlett, and Wolters Kluwer Health (UpToDate). Travel reimbursement from Sunovion Pharmaceuticals, Inc.The remaining authors declare no conflicts of interest.

**Author details**
[1] Copenhagen Affective Disorders Research Centre (CADIC), Psychiatric Centre Copenhagen, Department O, 6233, Rigshospitalet, Blegdamsvej 9, 2100 Copenhagen, Denmark. [2] Department of Psychiatry & Behavioral Sciences, Stanford University School of Medicine, Palo Alto, CA, USA. [3] Department of Clinical Medicine, Faculty of Health and Medical Sciences, University of Copenhagen, Copenhagen, Denmark. [4] Psychiatric Research Unit, Psychiatric Centre North Zealand, Hillerød, Denmark.

**References**

Association. AP. Diagnostic and Statistical manual of mental disorders: DSM-IV. 4th ed. Washington: American Psychiatric Association; 1994.

Association. AP. Diagnostic and statistical manual of mental disorders. 5th ed. Arlington: American Psychiatric Publishing; 2013.

Baldessarini RJ, Tondo L, Baethge CJ, Lepri B, Bratti IM. Effects of treatment latency on response to maintenance treatment in manic-depressive disorders. Bipolar Disord. 2007;9(4):386–93.

Bech P. Clinical psychometrics. Chicester: Wiley-Blackwell; 2012. p. 1–202.

Dagani J, Signorini G, Nielssen O, Bani M, Pastore A, Girolamo G, et al. Meta-analysis of the interval between the onset and management of bipolar disorder. Can J Psychiatry Revue canadienne de psychiatrie. 2017;62(4):247–58.

First MBGM, Spitzer RL, Williams JBW. Structured clinical interview for DSM-IV Axis I Disorders—Research Version (SCID-I). New York: Biometrics Research Department, New York State Psychiatric Institute; 1996.

Fredskild MU, Mintz J, Frye MA, McElroy SL, Nolen WA, Kupka R, et al. Adding increased energy or activity to criterion (A) of the DSM-5 definition of hypomania and mania: effect on the diagnoses of 907 patients from the bipolar collaborative network. J Clin Psychiatry. 2019;80(6).

Gordon-Smith K, Jones LA, Forty L, Craddock N, Jones I. Changes to the diagnostic criteria for bipolar disorder in DSM-5 make little difference to lifetime diagnosis: findings from the U.K. Bipolar Disorder Research Network (BDRN) Study. Am J Psychiatry. 2017;174(8):803.

Hamilton M. A rating scale for depression. J Neurol Neurosurg Psychiatry. 1960;23(1):56–62.

Kessing LV. What is early intervention in bipolar disorder? Recommendation of a pragmatic way focusing on early intervention in patients with newly diagnosed bipolar disorder. Bipolar Disord. 2019;21(2):168–9.

Kessing LV, Hansen HV, Hvenegaard A, Christensen EM, Dam H, Gluud C, et al. Treatment in a specialised out-patient mood disorder clinic v. standard out-patient treatment in the early course of bipolar disorder: randomised clinical trial. Br J Psychiatry. 2013;202(3):212–9.

Kessing LV, Vradi E, Andersen PK. Starting lithium prophylaxis early v late in bipolar disorder. Br J Psychiatry. 2014;205(3):214–20.

Kessing LV, Munkholm K, Faurholt-Jepsen M, Miskowiak KW, Nielsen LB, Frikke-Schmidt R, et al. The Bipolar Illness Onset study: research protocol for the BIO cohort study. BMJ Open. 2017;7(6):e015462.

Machado-Vieira R, Luckenbaugh DA, Ballard ED, Henter ID, Tohen M, Suppes T, et al. Increased activity or energy as a primary criterion for the diagnosis of bipolar mania in DSM-5: findings from the STEP-BD study. Am J Psychiatry. 2017;174(1):70–6.

WHO. The ICD-10 classification of mental and behavioural disorders: diagnostic criteria for research. Geneva: World Health Organisation; 1992a.

WHO. The ICD-10 classification of mental and behavioural disorders: clinical descriptions and diagnostic guidelines. Genova: World Health Organization; 1992b.

WHO. International classification of diseases for mortality and morbidity statistics (11th Revision). Version 09/2020. https://icd.who.int/browse11/l-m/en.

Young RCBJ, Ziegler VE, Meyer DA. A rating scale for mania: reliability, validity and sensitivity. Br J Psychiatry. 1978;133:429–35.

# 18

# Chronic kidney disease in lithium-treated patients, incidence and rate of decline

Arjan M. Van Alphen[1], Tessa M. Bosch[2], Ralph W. Kupka[3] and Rocco Hoekstra[4*]

**Abstract**

**Background:** Lithium-induced nephropathy is a known long-term complication, sometimes limiting the use of lithium as mood stabilizer. The aim of this study is to establish the incidence of chronic kidney disease and the rate of decline of renal function in patients using lithium and to identify risk factors.

**Methods:** We selected 1012 patients treated with lithium from the laboratory database of the Antes Centre for Mental Health Care spanning a period from 2000 to 2015. Serum lithium and creatinine concentrations were retrieved and eGFR was calculated using the 4-variable CKD-EPI formula. We calculated the incidence of renal insufficiency and the rate of decline. We compared patients with and without chronic kidney disease (CKD) stage 3 regarding duration of lithium exposure.

**Results:** Incidence of chronic kidney disease was 0.012 cases per exposed patient-year. Average decline of eGFR was 1.8 ml/min/year in patients who developed chronic kidney disease stage 3. Incidence of chronic kidney disease stage 4 was only 0.0004 per patient year. No cases of end stage renal disease were found in this cohort. Odds of reaching chronic kidney disease stage 3 were increased with longer duration of lithium exposure.

**Conclusions:** The use of lithium seems to be related to a higher incidence of chronic kidney disease. Longer duration of lithium exposure significantly increased the risk of renal failure.

**Keywords:** Lithium, Kidney, Renal failure, Nephropathy, Chronic kidney disease

## Background

After decades of use, lithium is still considered to be the gold standard therapy for bipolar disorders. Not only is lithium effective for managing acute manic or depressive episodes in bipolar disorder, it also acts as a prophylactic agent in prevention of such episodes, and has an independent anti-suicidal effect (Severus et al. 2018; Smith and Cipriani 2017). Patients using lithium salts may experience several side effects: hypothyroidism, hyperparathyroidism, nephrogenic diabetes insipidus, and decline in renal function (Gitlin 2016). The occurrence of renal failure is especially problematic in the long term. Not only is renal failure a risk factor for occurrence of cardiovascular disease, it can also make it necessary to weigh the balance between pros and cons of continuing lithium therapy.

Some uncertainty remains about the incidence of renal failure in patients treated with lithium salts. Although several reports suggest little effect of lithium on renal function, other studies estimate prevalence of chronic kidney disease (CKD) amongst lithium users between 10 and 35% (Presne et al. 2003; Lepkifker et al. 2004; Bassilios et al. 2008; Bendz et al. 2010; Aprahamian et al. 2014; Aiff et al. 2015; Tondo et al. 2017). Data about the occurrence of lithium-induced end-stage renal disease (ESRD) are sparse (Presne et al. 2003; Bendz et al. 2010; Aiff et al. 2015; Tondo et al. 2017). Nielsen et al. (2018) reviewed several large observational studies and suggested that surveillance bias might play a role. Poorer renal outcome was found in older studies while in more recent studies no end-stage renal failure was found, probably due to improved monitoring. Risk factors for renal failure seem

*Correspondence: r.hoekstra@anteszorg.nl
[4] Outpatient Clinic for Bipolar Disorders, Antes Centre for Mental Health Care, Rotterdam, The Netherlands
Full list of author information is available at the end of the article

to be higher lithium levels, duration of lithium therapy, lower initial eGFR, older age and medical comorbidity (Tondo et al. 2017; Davis et al. 2018).

It is important to more accurately define exact incidence of lithium nephropathy and contributing risk factors to better inform patients of their risk. The aim of the present study is to establish the incidence of chronic kidney disease and the course of renal function in patients treated with lithium salts.

## Methods

### Study population

The laboratory database of the Antes Centre for Mental Health Care in Rotterdam, the Netherlands, was screened for patients who used lithium. Data could be retrieved between 2000 and 2015. A total of 1751 patients were identified in whom serum lithium was measured. Patients were deemed to be on chronic lithium therapy when a minimum of 5 serum lithium measurements were available, leaving 1151 patients. Another 139 patients were excluded because eGFR was 60 ml/min or less at the initiation of lithium therapy or the start of our database in January 2000. Ultimately 1012 patients were included for analysis. Data on eGFR were available from the onset of therapy in 531 patients who started lithium after January 2000. The remaining 481 patients had initiated treatment prior to January 2000 and no data on eGFR were available between the onset of lithium therapy and the year 2000.

eGFR was calculated for each serum creatinine value, using the 4-variable CKD EPI formula. The date at which lithium was initiated or discontinued was retrieved from psychiatric records. Because we had several creatinine measurements we could calculate the average decline of the eGFR per year in the first 10 years after onset of lithium therapy. Chronic kidney disease was defined as CKD stage 3, meaning an eGFR less than 60 ml/min/1.73 $m^2$. Threshold had to be met on at least two consecutive measurements spanning a 30 day period, for an individual to be considered having chronic kidney disease. The occurrence of CKD stage 3B (eGFR between 30 and 45 ml/min/1.73 $m^2$) and CKD stage 4 (eGFR between 15 and 30 ml/min/1.73 $m^2$) were also reported.

We calculated the incidence of CKD in the whole group. In the subgroup of patients who started lithium treatment after the year 2000, we used a paired T-test to compare the eGFR at the start of the therapy between the patients who developed CKD and those who did not. The cumulative incidence of CKD was described using a Kaplan–Meier curve. A binary logistic regression model was used with chronic kidney disease as the dependent variable. The model included gender, age at initiation of lithium therapy and duration of lithium exposure. SPSS® Statistics 18 was used for statistical analysis. p-values $< 0.05$ were considered statistically significant.

## Results

1012 patients treated with lithium were identified for analysis from the database. Of the study population 55% was female. Mean age at onset of lithium therapy was 44.4 years ($\pm$13.4). The average duration of lithium therapy was 9.2 years ($\pm$8.4). In 118 patients eGFR declined below 60 ml/min/1.73 $m^2$ after the year 2000, this comprised 12% of the study population. In this subgroup 60% was female, the mean age at the start of lithium therapy was 48 years ($\pm$12) and the average duration of lithium therapy was 12.4 years ($\pm$8.4). The incidence of an eGFR decline below 60 ml/min was 0.012 per exposed patient year. Incidence for the occurrence of chronic kidney disease stage 4 (eGFR < 30 ml/min) was only 0.0004 per patient year. No cases of end stage renal disease (eGFR < 15 ml/min) were documented in this cohort.

On average eGFR declined 1.8 ml/min/year in the 118 patients who met our target for chronic kidney disease. In the remaining 894 patients eGFR declined only 0.5 ml/min/year. A Kaplan–Meier analysis estimated median time to reaching CKD stage 3 at 40.9 years as shown in Fig. 1. Approximately 10% of patients met our criterion for chronic kidney disease within 5 years after initiation of lithium therapy. A total of 224 patients (13.2%) used lithium more than 20 years without developing CKD. Figure 2 presents the distribution of patients at different CKD stages by the years of lithium exposure.

In the subgroup of patients who started with lithium therapy after 2000, patients who developed CKD had a mean eGFR of 69.8 ml/min at the start of treatment. Patients who did not show a decline of eGFR below 60 ml/min ($\pm$12.2) had a mean eGFR of 80.0 ml/min ($\pm$15.7) at the start of treatment. This difference was statistically significant with a p-value of 0.004.

Age at the start of lithium therapy (odds ratio 1.03 (C.I. 1.007–1.06, $p=0.014$)), and duration of lithium exposure (odds ratio 1.03, C.I. 1.01–1.05, $p=0.003$) were associated with a decline in renal function. Mean lithium levels were about the same in patients who developed CKD in different stages (e.g. stage 3: $n=118$; mean lithium level 0.71 mmol/l, SD 0.12) and those who did not ($n=894$; mean lithium level 0.70 mmol/l, SD 0.11).

## Discussion

We performed a naturalistic retrospective observational cohort study of the incidence of chronic kidney disease in lithium-treated patients, to address a major concern of patients and clinicians about long-term lithium treatment. Our results suggest that the incidence of chronic kidney disease, defined as an eGFR below 60 ml/min, in

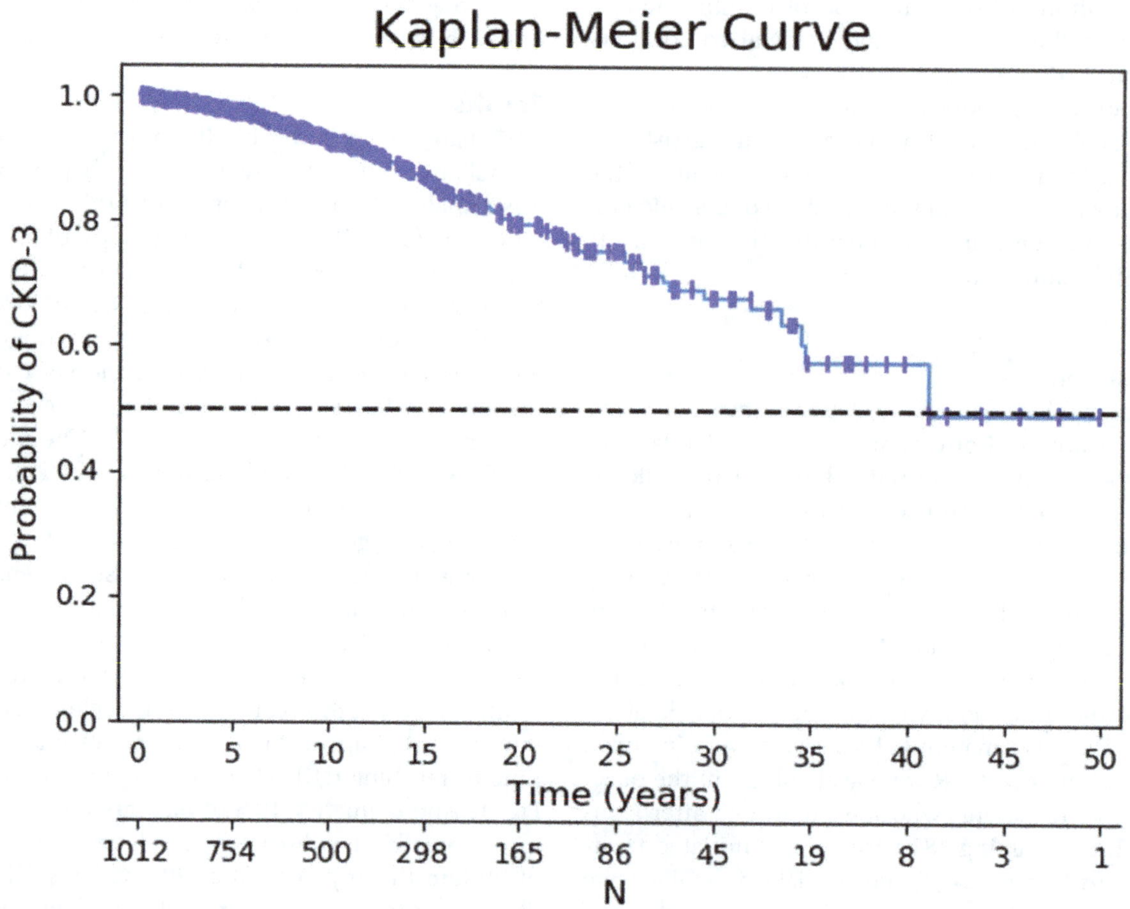


**Fig. 1** Kaplan Meier curve of CKD-free survival in lithium treated patients

patients treated with lithium is 0.012 per patient-year. The incidence in our population is therefore 1.3 times higher than that of the general population in the Netherlands, where an incidence of CKD stage 3 or more of 0.0093 per person-year was found in a group with a comparable age as our patients (van Blijderveen et al. 2014). This difference is probably explained by ours being a highly selected population of psychiatric patients. In our study population lithium use is an obvious risk factor for CKD but from the current data we cannot conclude it is the sole explanation for an increased incidence rate.

In total 12% of patients reached CKD stage 3 which is comparable to previous studies (Aiff et al. 2015; Tondo et al. 2017). Patients with CKD stage 3 had a mean decline of renal function of 1.8 ml/min/year which is slightly lower than most previous reports (Presne et al. 2003; Tondo et al. 2017). Decline in renal function appears to be most pronounced in the initial years after the start of lithium therapy.

The occurrence of chronic kidney disease stage 4 is rare and end-stage renal disease did not occur at all in our cohort. One possible explanation might be discontinuation of lithium therapy as eGFR approaches 40 ml/min lithium, following recommendations of current clinical guidelines. When lithium is discontinued, follow up of renal function is sometimes transferred to the nephrologist, most probably in the hospital in the same region using the same laboratory, but in an individual case outside our region, making creatinine values unavailable to our database.

Duration of lithium exposure and age at onset of lithium therapy, were found to increase odds of developing CKD stage 3. The same risk factors were found in some other studies (Bocchetta et al. 2013; Davis et al. 2018). From our data longer duration of lithium exposure seem to predispose to decline in renal function. Our analysis suggests, however, that its contribution is relatively low with an increased odds of only 1.03 per exposed patient year.

In clinical practice the treating psychiatrist monitors lithium levels frequently and if necessary adjust the dose to keep those levels in the therapeutic range. Therefore, although mean lithium levels were the same in all groups, we think we cannot conclude that fluctuations in lithium levels don't contribute to an increased risk for developing CKD.

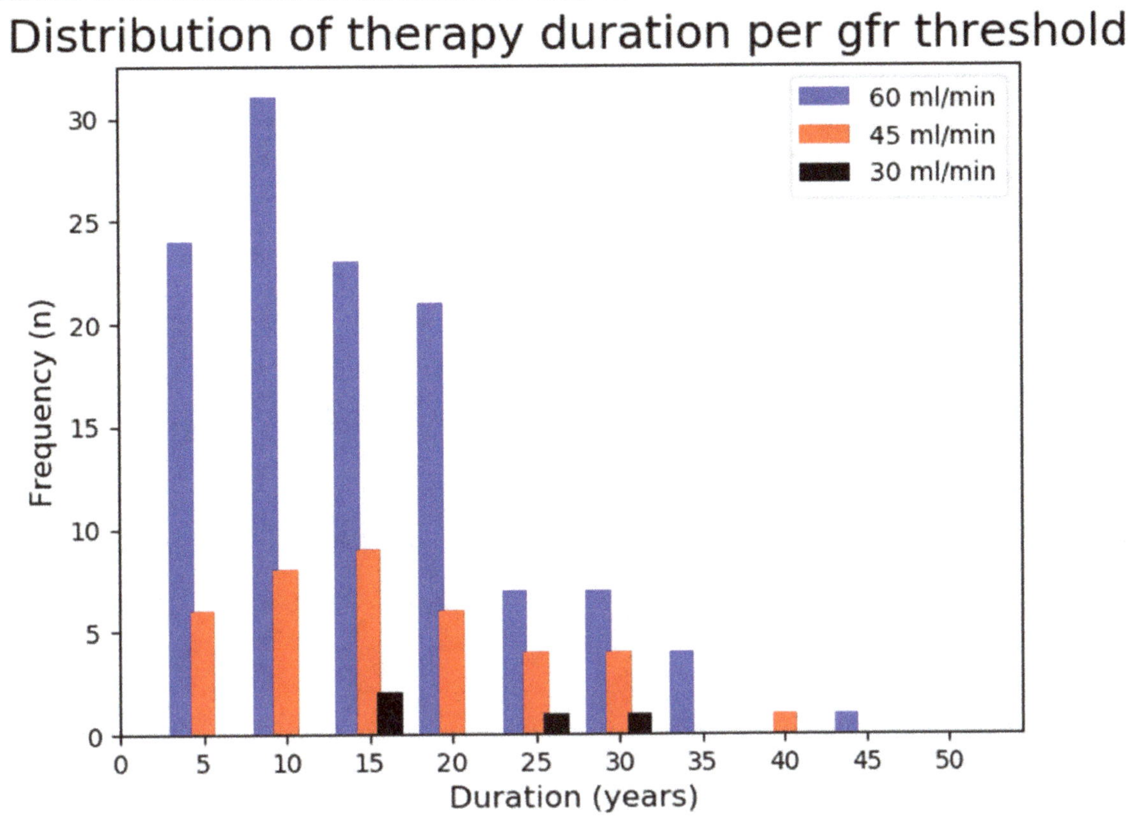


**Fig. 2** Distribution of therapy duration per GFR threshold

As suggested by Nielsen et al. (2018) we think closely monitoring lithium levels and renal functioning can largely prevent the occurrence of chronic kidney disease stage 4 and end stage renal failure. If done so, our analysis suggests that long term use of lithium may be considered only an additional risk factor for the occurrence of chronic kidney disease. Rather than focussing on lithium as the main cause of renal failure, monitoring and management of hypertension and diabetes mellitus, as well as other risk factors associated with cardiovascular morbidity, should receive more attention in clinical practice. This may improve renal survival in this category of patients and hence allow them to continue their lithium treatment for a longer period of time, maintaining stability of bipolar disorder and associated better quality of life.

## Conclusions

When carefully monitored the use of lithium seem to cause chronic kidney disease only in a minority of patients. Severe and end-stage renal failure probably occurs seldom.

### Abbreviations

CKD: Chronic kidney disease; CKD-EPI: Chronic kidney disease epidemiology collaboration; eGFR: Estimated glomerular filtration rate; ESRD: End-stage renal disease.

### Acknowledgements

We thank Martijn Kuijper for his assistance with the statistical analyses.

### Authors' contributions

AA, TB and RH contributed to the design of the study, acquisition, analysis and interpretation of the data and the draft of the manuscript. RK reviewed the manuscript. All authors read and approved the final manuscript.

### Author details

[1] Department of Nephrology, Maasstad Hospital, Rotterdam, The Netherlands. [2] Department of Hospital Pharmacy, Maasstad Hospital, Rotterdam, The Netherlands. [3] Dept. of Psychiatry & Amsterdam Public Health Research Institute, Amsterdam UMC, Vrije Universiteit, Amsterdam, The Netherlands. [4] Outpatient Clinic for Bipolar Disorders, Antes Centre for Mental Health Care, Rotterdam, The Netherlands.

### References

Aiff H, Attman PO, Aurell M, Bendz H, Ramsauer B, Schon S, Svetlund J. Effects of 10 to 30 years of lithium treatment on kidney function. J Psychopharmacol. 2015;29(5):608–14.

Aprahamian I, Santos FS, dos Santos B, Talib L, Diniz BS, Radanovic M, et al. Long-term, low-dose lithium treatment does not impair renal function in the elderly: a 2-year randomized, placebo-controlled trial followed by single-blind extension. J Clin Pcychiatry. 2014;75(7):e672–8.

Bassilios N, Martel P, Godard V, Froissart M, Grünfeld JP, Stengel B, Réseau Néphropar. Monitoring of glomerular filtration rate in lithium-treated outpatients—an ambulatory laboratory database surveillance. Nephrol Dial Transplant. 2008;23(2):562–5.
Bendz H, Schon S, Attman PO, Aurell M. Renal failure occurs in chronic lithium treatment but is uncommon. Kidney Int. 2010;77(3):219–24.
Bocchetta A, Ardau R, Carta P, Ligas F, Sardu C, Pani A, et al. Duration of lithium treatment is a risk factor for reduced glomerular function: a cross-sectional study. BMC Med. 2013;11:33.
Davis J, Desmond M, Berk M. Lithium and nephrotoxicity: a literature review of approaches to clinical management and risk stratification. BMC Nephrol. 2018;19(1):305.
Gitlin M. Lithium side effect and toxicity: prevalence and management strategies. Int J Bipolar Disord. 2016;4(1):27.
Lepkifker E, Sverdlik A, Iancu I, Ziv R, Segev S, Kotler M. Renal insufficiency in long-term lithium treatment. J Clin Psychiatry. 2004;65(6):850–6.
Nielsen RE, Kessing LV, Nolen WA, Licht RW. Lithium and renal impairment: a review on a still hot topic. Pharmacopsychiatry. 2018;51(5):200–5.
Presne C, Fakhouri F, Noël LH, Stengel B, Even C, Kreis H, Mignon F, Grünfeld JP. Lithium-induced nephropathy: rate of progression and prognostic factors. Kidney Int. 2003;64(2):585–92.
Severus E, Bauer M, Geddes J. Efficacy and effectiveness of lithium in the long term treatment of bipolar disorders: an update 2018. Pharmacopsychiatry. 2018;51(5):173–6.
Smith KA, Cipriani A. Lithium and suicide in mood disorders. Bipolar Disord. 2017;19(7):575–86.
Tondo L, Abramowicz M, Alda M, Bauer M, Bocchetta A, Bolzani L, Calkin CV, Chillotti C, Hidalgo-Mazzei D, Manchia M, Müller-Oerlinghausen B, Murru A, Perugi G, Pinna M, Quaranta G, Reginaldi D, Reif A, Ritter P Jr, Rybakowski JK, Saiger D, Sani G, Selle V, Stamm T, Vázquez GH, Veeh J, Vieta E, Baldessarini RJ. Long-term lithium treatment in bipolar disorder: effects on glomerular filtration rate and other metabolic parameters. Int J Bipolar Disord. 2017;5(1):27.
van Blijderveen JC, Straus SM, Zietse R, Stricker BH, Sturkenboom MC, Verhamme KM. A population-based study on the prevalence and incidence of chronic kidney disease in the Netherlands. Int Urol Nephrol. 2014;46:583–92.

# 19

# Is the 4-factor model of symptomology equivalent across bipolar disorder subtypes?

Norm O'Rourke[1*], Andrew Sixsmith[2], Tal Michael[3] and Yaacov G. Bachner[1]

**Abstract**

**Background:** Research with the $BDS_x$ (Bipolar Disorder Symptom Scale) suggests a 4-factor structure of responses: two depression (cognitive, somatic) and two hypo/mania factors (elation/loss of insight, affrontive symptoms). The two depression and two hypo/mania factors are correlated; and affrontive symptoms of hypo/mania (e.g., furious, disgusted, argumentative) are positively correlated with both depression factors suggesting pathways for mixed symptom presentation. This grouping of affrontive symptoms of hypo/mania organically emerged in exploratory research and has subsequently been supported in confirmatory analyses between samples and over time. The $BDS_x$ has been clinically validated with BD outpatients.

**Results:** Over 19 days, we recruited an international sample of 784 adults with BD using micro-targeted, social media advertising (M = 44.48 years, range 18–82). All participants indicated that they had BD (subtype, if known) and had been diagnosed with BD (month, year). This sample size was sufficient to confirm the 4-factor model across subtypes and compare the three (BD I, BD II, BD NOS). Responses to 19 of 20 $BDS_x$ items were psychometrically consistent across BD subtypes. Only responses to the 'hopeless' item were significantly higher for those with BD II.

**Conclusions:** When comparing models, it appears that affrontive symptoms are significantly and uniformly associated with hypo/mania and both depression factors across subtypes. In contrast to BD diagnostic criteria, this suggests that affrontive symptoms are central to the clinical presentation of hypo/mania and mixed symptomology across BD subtypes.

**Keywords:** Affrontive symptoms, $BDS_x$, Bipolar disorder, BD subtypes, Invariance analyses, Scale validation

## Background

Despite the efficacy of pharmacotherapy (Osher et al. 2010), the long-term course of bipolar disorder (BD) is characterized by frequent relapse, often with residual or subthreshold symptoms (Samalin et al. 2016; Treuer and Tohen 2010). BD is a leading cause of global disability (Catala-Lopez et al. 2013). Population growth and aging are further contributing to BD burden (Ferrari et al. 2016).

*Correspondence: ORourke@bgu.ac.il
[1] Department of Public Health and Multidisciplinary Center for Research On Aging, Ben-Gurion University of the Negev, P.O. Box 653, 8410501 Be'er Sheva, Israel
Full list of author information is available at the end of the article

### Bipolar disorder subtypes

Those with BD I (previously, manic-depressive disorder; Phillips and Kupfer 2013) experience both episodes of major depression and mania with psychosis or loss of contact with reality (e.g., perceived special abilities). The negative effects of mania can endure long after (e.g., severed relationships, debts, exhausted savings).

Those with BD II also experience major depression, but more limited hypomania as opposed to full mania (Serretti and Olgiati 2005). Similar to BD I, those with BD II are euthymic most of the time (Saunders and Goodwin 2010) yet they may experience more episodes of depression, of longer duration and greater severity compared to BD I (Tondo et al. 2017).

The symptoms of those with BD not otherwise specified (BD NOS) do not fit cleanly within the criteria or other subtypes (Towbin et al. 2013). BD NOS is a catch-all category more than a defined subtype. The term, unspecified bipolar disorder is today preferred (APA; American Psychiatric Association 2013).

Those with cyclothymia do not meet criteria for either BD I or II (Van Meter et al. 2012); however, subclinical symptoms can extend over years. Cyclothymia may be the most prevalent BD subtype though the least frequently diagnosed (Van Meter et al. 2017); some, however, question whether if cyclothymia is in fact a distinct disorder (Parens and Johnston 2010).

#### 4-factor model of BD symptomology

For the BADAS (Bipolar Affective Disorder and older Adults) Study, a sample of 1010 adults with BD were asked to indicate the extent to which 114 mood and symptom adjectives corresponded to how felt at that moment (O'Rourke et al. 2018). This pool of items was compiled by an expert team of clinicians and BD researchers. A 4-factor solution emerged from separate exploratory analyses (independent samples), confirmed over time (O'Rourke et al. 2016) and across age groups (O'Rourke et al. 2018). Each of these 4 factors are directly and indirectly related to quality of life with BD (O'Rourke et al. 2021).

This 4-factor model is composed of two correlated depression factors (cognitive, somatic symptoms) and two correlated hypo/mania factors (affrontive symptoms, elation/loss of insight). Affrontive symptoms of hypo/mania are also correlated with both depression factors suggestive of a mixed-symptom clinical presentation (American Psychiatric Association 2013). These symptoms reflect a confrontational, interpersonal expression of BD symptomology. See Fig. 1.

#### Affrontive symptoms of hypo/mania

Recent research with BD participants indicates that affrontive symptoms of hypo/mania are correlated with negative partner mood (O'Rourke and King 2019), more so than other $BDS_x$ factors. However, this effect is not statistically significant when couples are physically apart, only when together (i.e., same GPS coordinates), supporting the construct validity of this hostile, interpersonal cluster of symptoms. By contract, the traditional elation/loss of insight factor, more consistent with euphoric mania, appears to have little impact on partner mood (O'Rourke and King 2019).

Another possibility is that affrontive symptoms are not hypo/mania at all, but instead agitated depression. Irritability and anger outbursts occur under both definitions, but there is an interpersonal aspect to affrontive symptoms absent from current understanding of agitated depression. And as noted by Serra et al. (2019), agitation co-occurs with depression not hypo/mania, in particular, decreased libido, poor concentration, and suicidal ideation. With agitated depression, patients sometimes describe an underlying sense of anxiety or unease; with affrontive symptoms, the driving emotion is anger, often rage.

#### Impact of BD on others

It is well documented that BD negatively affects others (Maskill et al. 2010; Maji et al. 2012; Perlick et al. 2008; Srivastava et al. 2010). Symptoms of depression appear to have greater impact that hypo/mania (Perlick et al. 1999; O'Rourke and King 2019) and suicidal ideation appears to impact friends and family most adversely (Chessick et al. 2009).

Despite the apparent significance of these interpersonal symptoms, discussion is limited in the research literature and largely absent from diagnostic criteria (i.e., near exclusive focus on individual, not interpersonal behavior). Affrontive symptoms may qualify as atypical features as DSM 5 lists interpersonal reaction sensitivity as one example (previously interpersonal rejection sensitivity; Peng et al. 2016). Yet affrontive symptoms are proactive not reactive (e.g., suspicious, hostile, argumentative).

For this study, we set out to independently replicate the 4-factor model across BD subtypes (BD I, BD II, BD NOS), assuming that affrontive symptoms would emerge with each. Moreover, we assumed that this affrontive factor would be correlated with elation/loss of insight and both depression factors (cognitive and somatic symptoms), suggesting that these affrontive symptoms are consistent across BD subtypes, and core to the clinical presentation of hypo/mania.

### Methods

#### Participant recruitment

We recruited a global sample of 784 English-speaking adults: 218 with BD I, 277 with BD II and 289 with BD NOS. Responses from 37 respondents with cyclothymia were set aside as too few for latent variable analyses (less than 5%). This study was undertaken with the approval of the Research Ethics Board at Simon Fraser University, Burnaby (BC), Canada.

Data were collected over 19 days using social media advertising micro-targeted to Facebook users with BD. Participants were drawn from a global population of 6.2 million English-speaking, adult Facebook users with 'bipolar disorder interests' (e.g., members of online BD support networks). To expedite data collection, one randomly selected participant (in Ireland) received a $500 lottery prize.

As described elsewhere more thoroughly (King et al. 2014), machine-generated algorithms calculated by social

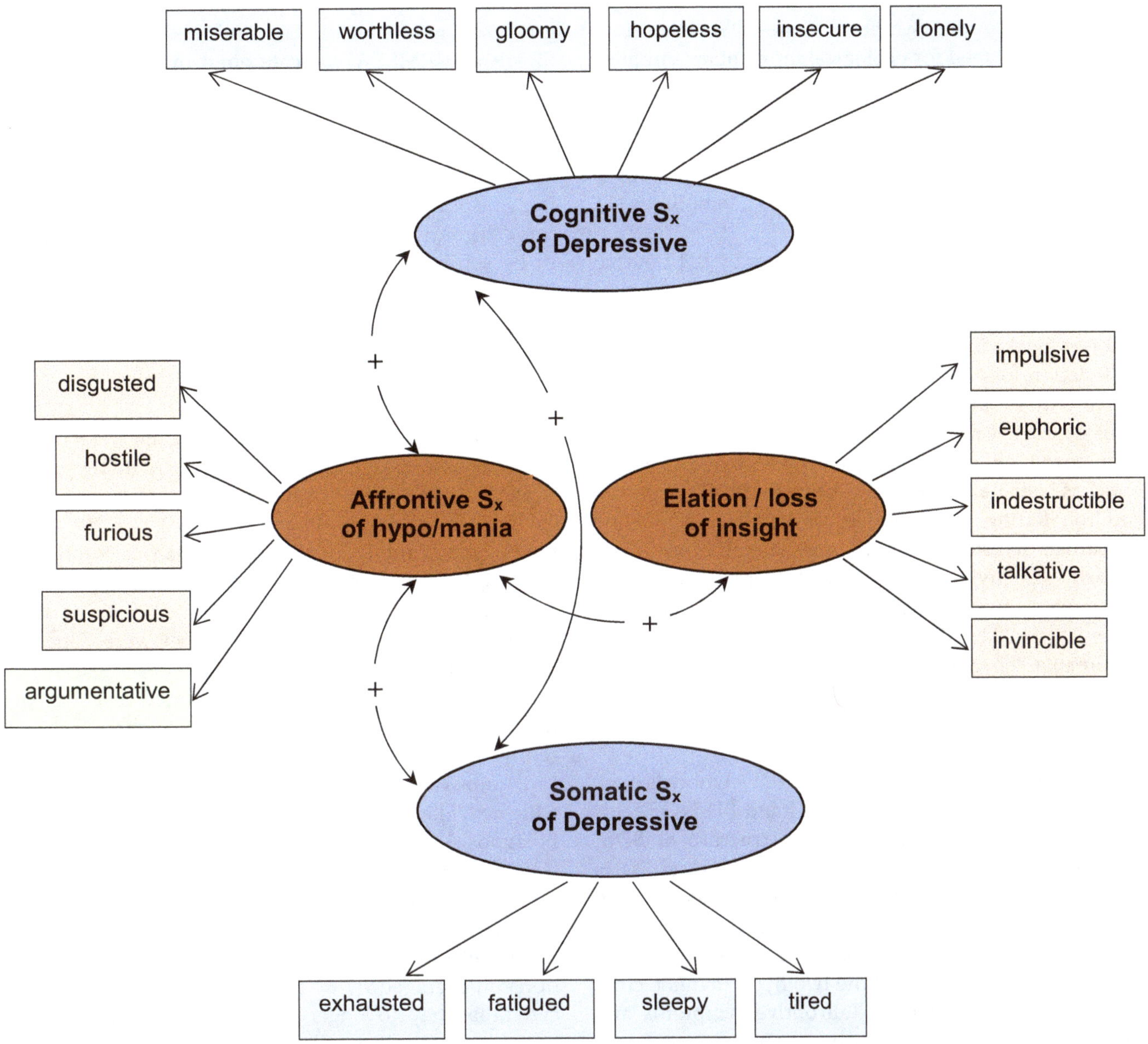


**Fig. 1** 4-factor model of BD symptomology

media platforms are unique not so much for their sensitivity but specificity (i.e., exclusion of those who do not have BD). Persons recruited via Facebook are unlikely representative of the population but we can be confident these are persons with BD because only persons with BD received advertisements.

### Validity check

To corroborate that participants were in fact persons with BD, they were asked to list all prescribed BD medications. Most specified 1+ mood stabilizer (58.9%) and 1+ antidepressant (64.4%) whereas smaller numbers listed 1+ anxiolytic (38.9%) and 1+antipsychotic (38.3%). By category, lithium ($n = 78$), bupropion ($n = 43$), clonazepam ($n = 55$), and quetiapine ($n = 68$) were the medications most commonly listed by participants (i.e., mood stabilizer, antidepressant, anxiolytic and antipsychotic, respectively).

Participants were also asked to categorize each of these medications (mood stabilizers, antidepressants, anxiolytics, antipsychotics, other/specify): 96% correctly specified and categorized both mood stabilizers and anxiolytics, 97% for antidepressants, and 86% for antipsychotics. This high level of accuracy fosters confidence that participants, in fact, are persons with BD.

### $BDS_x$

The Bipolar Disorder Symptom Scale (O'Rourke et al. 2016) was developed for ecological momentary sampling of BD symptoms in the moment. Based on the format of the PANAS (Positive and Negative Affect Scale; Watson et al. 1988); respondents indicate the extent to which to each of 20-items describes how they feel right now, at this moment, ranging from not at all (0), sometimes (1), to a lot (2).

Internal consistency of $BDS_x$ responses by BD I outpatients was recorded as $\alpha = 0.90$ for the depression subscale (cognitive + somatic symptoms; Osher et al. 2020) but lower for the hypo/mania subscale at $\alpha = 0.76$ (affrontive + elation/loss of insight; Kraun et al. 2020). This difference may be due to lower frequency of hypo/manic versus depressive symptoms (Judd et al. 2002).

Concurrent validity of $BDS_x$ responses by BD I outpatients has been demonstrated relative to the self-reported Hamilton Rating Scale for Depression (HAMD-6) and the Altman Self-Rating Mania Scale (Kraun et al. 2020). Similarly, sensitivity (and specificity) are high for the $BDS_x$ depression subscale at 88% (and 76%), respectively (Osher et al. 2020). Sensitivity is lower at 57% for the $BDS_x$ mania subscale (90% specificity) but higher sensitivity than the Altman scale (vs. 43%; Osher et al. 2020).

### Analytical procedures

Separate confirmatory factor analytic (CFA) models were computed for those with BD I, BD II and BD NOS. This allowed us to replicate the 4-factor structure of $BDS_x$ responses as previously reported (O'Rourke et al. 2016; O'Rourke et al. 2018). Each of the 20 items was assumed to load on its respective depression or hypo/mania factor. We assumed that the two depression factors (cognitive and affective symptoms) and the two hypo/mania factors were significantly correlated (affrontive symptoms and elation/loss of insight). Affrontive symptoms of hypo/mania factor were also assumed to correlate with both depression factors, consistent with mixed features specifier as defined by DSM 5 (American Psychiatric Association 2013). Models were computed using the maximum likelihood method of parameter estimation.

We report three goodness-of-fit-indices: an incremental, an absolute, and a parsimonious fit index. The comparative fit index (CFI) is an incremental index representing the extent to which a hypothesized model is a better fit to data than the null model. The standardized root mean square residual (SRMR) is an absolute index which represents the standardized difference between observed and predicted correlations within a hypothesized model. Finally, the root mean square error of approximation (RMSEA) is a parsimony index which represents the extent to which a hypothesized model fits data relative to the general population. Coefficient values greater than 0.94 for the CFI, and less than 0.055 for the SRMR and RMSEA, indicate good model fit (O'Rourke and Hatcher 2013).

### Comparing BD subtypes

We then conducted invariance analyses to compare $BDS_x$ item responses and compared covariance between factors. Affrontive symptoms of hypo/mania were assumed to be similarly correlated with other BD factors across subtypes. Descriptive statistics were computed with SPSS v24; CFA and invariance analyses were computed with AMOS v22.

## Results

The sample was composed of 215 men and 564 women; 5 indicated another gender (e.g., transsexual). They ranged in age from 18 to 82 years ($M$ = 44.48, $SD$ = 13.50), with 11.75 years of education on average (SD = 5.76). Participants lived in the U.S. (41.6%), Canada (30.7%), the U.K. (15.6%), Ireland (5%), Australia/New Zealand (3.7%), and South Africa (4%) with the remaining 3% living in ten other countries; 90% reported that they were Caucasian. See Table 1

Thirty percent of participants indicated that they were married; almost as many indicated that there were currently single (28%). A further 20% were partnered (e.g., civil union) and 18% separated or divorced. Only 2% were widowed. Slightly more men than women indicated a BD I diagnosis, $\chi^2$ [df = 4] = 9.75, $p$ = 0.05.

Participants were diagnosed with BD 10.91 years ago on average ($SD$ = 9.55, range 1 month–61.17 years), they had 1.17 comorbid conditions ($SD$ = 1.41, range 0–6), and were currently prescribed 0.88 psychotropic medications on average ($SD$ = 1.54, range 0–15). Several indicated that they no longer take psychotropic medications; instead, they self-medicate with marijuana and avoid clinical contact.

### BD subtypes

We recruited 218 participants with BD I, 277 with BD II, and 289 with BD NOS. Subtypes did not differ in participant age [$F$ (2772) = 1.74, $p$ = 0.18] or number of comorbid psychiatric conditions, $F$ (2781) = 1.74, $p$ = 0.18. However, those with BD II were diagnosed somewhat more recently (M = 9.72 years) than other subtypes [$F$ (2716) = 3.34, $p$ = 0.03] and were somewhat more educated that those with BD NOS, $F$ (2777) = 3.95, $p$ = 0.02. Those with BD II were also prescribed more psychotropic medications than other participants, $F$ (2781) = 8.76, $p$ < 0.01.

Of note, responses to depression factors did not differ across BD subtypes. And elation/loss of insight was

**Table 1** Descriptive statistics and $BDS_x$ response levels by BD subtype (n = 784)

| | BD I (M, SD, α) n = 218 | | BD II (M, SD, α) n = 277 | | BD NOS (M, SD, α) n = 289 | |
|---|---|---|---|---|---|---|
| Descriptive features | | | | | | |
| Years of age | 43.68 (13.9) | | 43.87 (13.1) | | 45.66 (13.6) | |
| Duration of $D_x$ | 11.85 (11.0)* | | 9.72 (8.85)** | | 11.39 (8.89)* | |
| Years of education | 11.89 (5.92) | | 12.32 (5.96)* | | 11.03 (5.37)* | |
| Comorbid $D_x$ | 1.05 (1.37) | | 1.25 (1.47) | | 1.18 (1.38) | |
| Psychotropic $R_x$ | 0.86 (1.72)* | | 1.16 (1.70)** | | 0.62 (1.16)* | |
| $BDS_x$ response levels | | | | | | |
| Cognitive $S_x$ depression | 11.94 (3.57) | .90 | 12.15 (3.75) | .91 | 12.68 (3.40) | .90 |
| Somatic $S_x$ depression | 8.84 (2.59) | .88 | 9.27 (2.48) | .87 | 9.11 (2.43) | .85 |
| Elation/loss of insight | 7.21 (2.51)* | .79 | 6.63 (2.12)** | .73 | 7.32 (2.39)* | .74 |
| Affrontive $S_x$ of mania | 8.20 (2.85)* | .82 | 8.00 (2.89)* | .85 | 8.81 (2.94)** | .83 |

*Duration of $D_x$* years since BD diagnosis; *Comorbid $D_x$* number of comorbid psychiatric conditions; *Psychotropic $R_x$* number of prescribed psychotropic medications

* Significantly differs from one other group

** Significantly differs from both other groups

significantly higher for those with BD I than BD II [not BD NOS; $F\ (2781) = 6.91, p = 0.01$] as we would expect as this factor measures traditional features of mania (e.g., euphoric, talkative, invincible). By contrast, affrontive symptoms of hypo/mania were significantly higher for those with BD NOS than BD I and II, F (2781) = 5.94, $p < 0.01$ consistent with mixed symptom presentation. See Table 1.

### 4-factor model, each BD subtype

Confirmatory factor analytic (CFA) models were computed separately to replicate the 4-factor model across BD subtypes. Each $BDS_x$ item was assumed to load significantly on its respective depression or hypo/mania factor (i.e., critical ratio values > |1.96|) and the two depression and two hypo/mania factors were assumed to be positively correlated. In accord with existing research, affrontive symptoms were also assumed also to correlate positively with both depression factors. See Fig. 1.

These findings emerged first for those with BD I, $\chi^2$ ($df = 158$) = 261.74, $p < 0.01$. Goodness of fit was calculated after correcting for correlated error between 9 of 210 possible pairs. The Comparative Fit Index (CFI ≥ 0.95; CFI = 0.95) and root mean square error of approximation were both within ideal parameters for this model (RMSEA ≤ 0.055; RMSEA = 0.055, 0.043 < RMSEA $CL_{90}$ < 0.067) whereas the standardized root mean square residual (SRMR ≤ 0.010; SRMR = 0.095) was adequate. Statistic power for this model was estimated at 0.99 ($n = 218$, $df = 158$). See Table 2.

Similar results emerged for those with BD II, $\chi^2$ ($df = 157$) = 281.45, $p < 0.01$. Again the CFI (0.96) and RMSEA (0.054; 0.043 < RMSEA $CL_{90}$ < 0.064) are within ideal parameters. The SRMR (0.063) is adequate yet statistical power is again high ($d = 0.99$; $n = 277$, $df = 157$).

Lastly, we replicated the 4-factor model with those diagnosed as BD NOS, $\chi^2$ ($df = 158$) = 278.16, $p < 0.01$. And as with other subtypes, the CFI (0.96) and RMSEA (0.051; 0.041 < RMSEA $CL_{90}$ < 0.061) were in ideal limits and the SRMR (0.069) was adequate; power was high; $d = 0.99$; n = 289, df = 158.

### Factor structure comparisons

With baseline models computed independently for those with BD I, BD II and BD NOS, we were then able to compare the 4-factor latent structure. Specifically, we compared the strength of association between factors to determine if the latent structure is consistent across BD subtypes. This was what we found. That is, both depression and both hypo/mania factors are similarly associated; moreover, covariance between affrontive symptoms of hypo/mania, cognitive and somatic symptoms of depression are is statistically indistinguishable across subtypes. In other words, affrontive symptoms appear universal to the clinical presentation of hypo/mania. Associations are similar with elation/loss of insight and depression factors (cognitive, somatic symptoms). The 4-factor model including affrontive symptoms are consistent across BD subtypes. See Table 3.

### $BDS_x$ item consistency

Lastly we compared items responses across BD subtypes to examine the psychometric properties of $BDS_x$ scale

**Table 2** 4-factor model of $BDS_x$ responses—BD I, BD II, BD NOS

| $BDS_x$ factors and items | BD I ($n$ = 218) | BD II ($n$ = 277) | BD NOS ($n$ = 289) |
|---|---|---|---|
| Cognitive $S_x$ of depression | | | |
| 1. Miserable | 0.85 (10.5) | 0.87 (11.7) | 0.83 (13.0) |
| 9. Worthless | 0.87 (10.8) | 0.86 (11.6) | 0.79 (12.3) |
| 13. Gloomy | 0.78 (9.93) | 0.80 (11.0) | 0.79 (12.4) |
| 19. Hopeless | 0.24 (3.44) | 0.38 (5.90)[a] | 0.18 (3.07)[a] |
| 11. Insecure | 0.83 (10.2) | 0.76 (10.7) | 0.75 (11.7) |
| 17. Lonely | 0.65 (10.5) | 0.63 (11.7) | 0.70 (13.0) |
| Somatic $S_x$ of depression | | | |
| 12. Fatigued | 0.87 (12.6) | 0.87 (15.4) | 0.86 (15.0) |
| 9. Sleepy | 0.65 (11.6) | 0.61 (11.7) | 0.58 (9.72) |
| 15. Exhausted | 0.89 (12.8) | 0.86 (15.3) | 0.86 (15.0) |
| 3. Tired | 0.74 (12.6) | 0.79 (15.4) | 0.77 (15.0) |
| Affrontive $S_x$ of mania | | | |
| 4. Hostile | 0.80 (10.5) | 0.80 (14.4) | 0.78 (11.6) |
| 8. Furious | 0.76 (10.3) | 0.81 (11.3) | 0.76 (11.3) |
| 5. Disgusted | 0.62 (8.58) | 0.67 (11.5) | 0.66 (9.17) |
| 18. Suspicious | 0.70 (9.20) | 0.61 (10.3) | 0.70 (10.5) |
| 20. Argumentative | 0.70 (10.5) | 0.80 (14.4) | 0.69 (11.6) |
| Elation/loss of insight | | | |
| 6. Impulsive | 0.72 (10.0) | 0.83 (11.4) | 0.73 (8.71) |
| 16. Euphoric | 0.80 (11.3) | 0.81 (11.3) | 0.78 (8.93) |
| 10. Indestructible | 0.76 (10.6) | 0.69 (12.7) | 0.57(9.53) |
| 2. Talkative | 0.48 (6.91) | 0.42 (6.40) | 0.45 (6.33) |
| 14. Invincible | 0.74 (10.0) | 0.69 (11.4) | 0.60 (8.71) |
| Goodness of fit | | | |
| RMSEA ($CL_{90}$) | 0.055 (0.043–0.067) | 0.054 (0.043–0.064) | 0.051 (0.041–0.061) |
| SRMR | 0.095 | 0.063 | 0.069 |
| CFI | 0.95 | 0.96 | 0.96 |

[a] Significantly differs from one other group

[**] Significantly differs from both other groups

responses. Responses were equivalent for 19 of 20 items across BD subtypes; only responses to the 'hopeless' item significantly differed. More precisely, those with BD II reported significantly higher hopelessness than those with BD NOS ($\beta = 0.38$ vs. $\beta = 0.18$). See Table 2. This finding is noteworthy as hopelessness is associated with suicide risk, suggesting that participants with BD II may be at greater risk of self-harm (Neufeld and O'Rourke 2009). See Table 4.

## Discussion

The results of this study provide further support for the 4-factor model of BD symptomology. This model was replicated independently with BD I, BD II and BD NOS participants in which affrontive symptoms of hypo/mania are correlated with elation/loss of insight and both depression factors. This presentation of depressive symptomology as correlated cognitive and somatic factors is consistent with unipolar depression research (Ward 2006).

Less consistent with existing research is our result suggesting that affrontive symptoms are central to the clinical presentation of hypo/mania across BD subtypes. Unlike elation/loss of insight, this facet of hypo/mania is correlated with both cognitive and somatic factors, which indicates ways in which mixed symptomology can present. As we noted, affrontive symptoms were significantly greater for those with BD NOS compared to participants with BD I and BD II.

Our findings also provide psychometric support for the $BDS_x$ across BD subtypes. As we noted, responses to 19 of 20 items were equivalent across subtypes; only responses to the 'hopeless' item were significantly greater by those with BD II. For a separate study (O'Rourke et al. 2018), participants 50+ years of age were later asked if they had made one or more suicide attempts ($n$ = 103): 43% and

**Table 3** 4-Factor model of $BDS_x$ responses, between BD subtype comparisons

| | $\chi^2$ | df | $\Delta\chi^2$ | Δdf | SRMR | CFI | RMSEA ($CL_{90}$) |
|---|---|---|---|---|---|---|---|
| Baseline | 837.02 | 474 | – | – | 0.098 | 0.95 | 0.031 (0.028–0.035) |
| Cognitive-somatic | | | | | | | |
| BDI–BD II | 837.04 | 475 | 0.02 | 1 | 0.098 | 0.95 | 0.031 (0.028–0.035) |
| BDI–BD NOS | 837.55 | 475 | 0.53 | 1 | 0.099 | 0.95 | 0.031 (0.028–0.035) |
| BDII–BD NOS | 837.42 | 475 | 0.4 | 1 | 0.098 | 0.95 | 0.031 (0.028–0.035) |
| BD I, BD II, NOS | 837.68 | 476 | 0.66 | 2 | 0.098 | 0.95 | 0.031 (0.028–0.035) |
| Elation-affrontive | | | | | | | |
| BDI–BD II | 839.94 | 477 | 2.26 | 1 | 0.098 | 0.95 | 0.031 (0.028–0.035) |
| BDI–BD NOS | 838.86 | 477 | 1.18 | 1 | 0.099 | 0.95 | 0.031 (0.028–0.035) |
| BDII–BD NOS | 837.88 | 477 | 0.2 | 1 | 0.098 | 0.95 | 0.031 (0.028–0.035) |
| BD I, BD II, NOS | 840.05 | 478 | 2.37 | 2 | 0.098 | 0.95 | 0.031 (0.028–0.035) |
| Cognitive-affrontive | | | | | | | |
| BDI–BD II | 840.06 | 479 | 0.01 | 1 | 0.098 | 0.95 | 0.031 (0.028–0.035) |
| BDI–BD NOS | 840.09 | 479 | 0.04 | 1 | 0.098 | 0.95 | 0.031 (0.028–0.035) |
| BDII–BD NOS | 840.17 | 479 | 0.12 | 1 | 0.098 | 0.95 | 0.031 (0.028–0.035) |
| BD I, BD II, NOS | 840.18 | 480 | 0.13 | 2 | 0.098 | 0.96 | 0.031 (0.027–0.034) |
| Somatic-affrontive | | | | | | | |
| BDI–BD II | 840.22 | 481 | 0.04 | 1 | 0.097 | 0.96 | 0.031 (0.027–0.034) |
| BDI–BD NOS | 840.26 | 481 | 0.08 | 1 | 0.098 | 0.96 | 0.031 (0.027–0.034) |
| BDII–BD NOS | 840.43 | 481 | 0.25 | 1 | 0.098 | 0.96 | 0.031 (0.027–0.034) |
| BD I, BD II, NOS | 840.45 | 482 | 0.27 | 2 | 0.098 | 0.96 | 0.031 (0.027–0.034) |

45% of BD NOS and BD I reported a prior attempt (15 of 35, and 10 of 22, respectively); by contrast, the majority of participants with BD II reported one or more attempt (28 of 46, or 61%). While these percentages apply only to older participants who agreed to follow up contact, they are consistent with our finding that those with BD II reported feeling more hopeless than other participants. This finding appears to differ from other research showing no difference in suicide risk by BD subtype (Tondo et al. 2016; Undurraga et al. 2011). Further study is warranted.

### Limitations and future research

The results of this study suggest that the 4-factor model of symptomology applies to those with BD I, BD II and BD NOS. This includes affrontive symptoms of hypo/mania. These results need to be replicated with those with cyclothymia and participants diagnosed in accord with DSM 5 or ICD 10 criteria.

We recruited a large sample allowing us to compare BD subtypes. This was achieved by recruiting an international sample of adults with BD. Social media recruitment remains a somewhat novel methodology but is especially well-suited to low prevalence populations like BD (King et al. 2014). Notably, this also enabled us to recruit participants who avoid clinical contact in contrast to most BD research.

International data collection also allowed us to (somewhat) address a fundamental measurement challenge with BD research. Specifically, most with BD are euthymic most of the time, depressed sometimes and hypo/manic sporadically (Saunders and Goodwin 2010). As reported by Osher et al. (2020), just 16% of BD outpatients presented as depressed and 14% with hypo/mania at routine biannual clinical visits over 6-months. In other words, without large samples, it is unlikely to have sufficient numbers to identify and measure hypo/mania. It is therefore easy to underreport the psychometric efficacy of hypo/mania in small, mostly asymptomatic BD samples. Differences in internal consistency for the depression versus hypo/mania subscale may be due to lower overall frequency of hypo/mania in this and most BD outpatient samples.

These findings contribute to a growing body of research pointing to the existence of an interpersonal, aggressive cluster of hypo/mania symptoms unacknowledged in current diagnostic criteria. Our results suggest that these symptoms are consistent across subtypes and correlated with all other BD factors. Further research is needed with inpatient samples and participants recruited using more traditional means (vs. mood disorders clinic patients).

**Table 4** BDS$_x$ item comparisons—BD I, BD II, BD NOS

| | $\chi^2$ | df | $\Delta\chi^2$ | Δdf | SRMR | CFI | RMSEA ($CL_{90}$) |
|---|---|---|---|---|---|---|---|
| Cognitive S$_x$ of depression | | | | | | | |
| 1. Miserable | 842.46 | 484 | 2.01 | 2 | 0.098 | 0.96 | 0.031 (0.028–0.035) |
| 9. Worthless | 846.45 | 486 | 3.99 | 2 | 0.098 | 0.95 | 0.031 (0.028–0.035) |
| 13. Gloomy | 846.48 | 488 | 0.03 | 2 | 0.098 | 0.96 | 0.031 (0.027–0.034) |
| 19. Hopeless | | | | | | | |
| BDI–BD II | 850.03 | 489 | 3.55 | 1 | 0.098 | 0.95 | 0.031 (0.028–0.035) |
| BDI–BD NOS | 846.57 | 489 | 0.09 | 1 | 0.098 | 0.95 | 0.031 (0.028–0.035) |
| BDII–BD NOS | 851.85 | 489 | 5.37* | 1 | 0.098 | 0.95 | 0.031 (0.028–0.035) |
| BD I, BD II, NOS | 852.69 | 490 | 6.21* | 2 | 0.098 | 0.95 | 0.031 (0.028–0.035) |
| 11. Insecure | 853.65 | 492 | 0.96 | 2 | 0.098 | 0.95 | 0.031 (0.027–0.034) |
| 17. Lonely | 853.65 | 492 | 1.64 | 2 | 0.098 | 0.95 | 0.031 (0.027–0.034) |
| Somatic S$_x$ of depression | | | | | | | |
| 12. Fatigued | 853.83 | 494 | 0.18 | 2 | 0.098 | 0.96 | 0.031 (0.028–0.035) |
| 9. Sleepy | 854.16 | 496 | 0.33 | 2 | 0.097 | 0.96 | 0.030 (0.027–0.034) |
| 15. Exhausted | 856.24 | 498 | 2.08 | 2 | 0.097 | 0.96 | 0.030 (0.027–0.034) |
| 3. Tired | 856.24 | 498 | 0.37 | 2 | 0.097 | 0.96 | 0.030 (0.027–0.034) |
| Affrontive S$_x$ of mania | | | | | | | |
| 4. Hostile | 860.07 | 500 | 3.83 | 2 | 0.097 | 0.96 | 0.030 (0.027–0.034) |
| 8. Furious | 860.75 | 502 | 0.68 | 2 | 0.097 | 0.96 | 0.030 (0.027–0.034) |
| 5. Disgusted | 861.1 | 504 | 0.35 | 2 | 0.097 | 0.96 | 0.030 (0.027–0.034) |
| 18. Suspicious | 866.67 | 506 | 5.57 | 2 | 0.097 | 0.95 | 0.030 (0.027–0.034) |
| 20. Argumentative | 866.67 | 506 | 2.84 | 2 | 0.097 | 0.95 | 0.030 (0.027–0.034) |
| Elation/loss of Insight | | | | | | | |
| 6. Impulsive | 867.55 | 508 | 0.88 | 2 | 0.097 | 0.96 | 0.030 (0.027–0.033) |
| 16. Euphoric | 869.23 | 510 | 1.68 | 2 | 0.098 | 0.96 | 0.030 (0.027–0.033) |
| 10. Indestructible | 871.83 | 512 | 2.6 | 2 | 0.098 | 0.96 | 0.030 (0.027–0.033) |
| 2. Talkative | 873.02 | 514 | 0.27 | 2 | 0.098 | 0.96 | 0.030 (0.027–0.033) |
| 14. Invincible | 840.45 | 514 | 1.19 | 2 | 0.098 | 0.96 | 0.030 (0.027–0.033) |

**Acknowledgements**

We thank the many BADAS Study participants from 30 countries across the globe, who graciously responded to study questionnaires.

**Authors' contributions**

The BADAS Study was conceived by Drs. NO'R and AS. The first draft was written and all analyses completed by Drs. NO'R and DBK. All authors contributed to the editing and revision process. All authors read and approved the final manuscript.

**Author details**

[1]Department of Public Health and Multidisciplinary Center for Research On Aging, Ben-Gurion University of the Negev, P.O. Box 653, 8410501 Be'er Sheva, Israel. [2]STAR Institute, Simon Fraser University, Vancouver, BC, Canada. [3]School of Public Health, Faculty of Health Sciences, Ben-Gurion University of the Negev, Be'er Sheva, Israel.

**References**

American Psychiatric Association. Diagnostic and statistical manual of mental disorders (DSM-5). Washington: American Psychiatric Pub; 2013.

Catala-Lopez F, Genova-Maleras R, Vieta E, Tabares-Seisdedos R. The increasing burden of mental and neurological disorders. Eur Neuropsychopharma. 2013;23(11):1337–9.

Chessick CA, Perlick DA, Miklowitz DJ, Dickinson LM, Allen MH, Morris CD, Gonzalez JM, Marangell LB, Cosgrove V, Ostacher M, STED-BD Family Experience Collaborative Study Group. Suicidal ideation and depressive symptoms among bipolar patients as predictors of the health and well-being of caregivers. Bipolar Disord. 2009;11(8):876–84.

Ferrari AJ, Stockings E, Khoo JP, Erskine HE, Degenhardt L, Vos T, Whiteford HA. The prevalence and burden of bipolar disorder: findings from the Global Burden of Disease Study 2013. Bipolar Disord. 2016;18(5):440–50.

Judd LL, Akiskal HS, Schettler PJ, Endicott J, Maser J, Solomon DA, Leon AC, Rice JA, Keller MB. The long-term natural history of the weekly symptomatic status of bipolar I disorder. Arch Gen Psychiatr. 2002;59(6):530–7.

King DB, O'Rourke N, DeLongis A. Social media recruitment and online data collection: a beginner's guide and best practices for accessing low-prevalence and hard-to-reach populations. Can Psychol. 2014;55(4):240–9. https://doi.org/10.1037/a0038087.

Kraun L, O'Rourke N, Osher Y, Bersudsky Y, Belotherkovsky D, Bachner YG. Is the 6-item, self-report HAM-D an effective depression screening measure with bipolar disorder? Perspect Psychiatr Care. 2020. https://doi.org/10.1111/ppc.12509.

Maji KR, Sood M, Sagar R, Khandelwal SK. A follow-up study of family burden in patients with bipolar affective disorder. Int J Soc Psychiatr. 2012;58(2):217–23.

Maskill V, Crowe M, Luty S, Joyce P. Two sides of the same coin: caring for a person with bipolar disorder. J Psychiatr Ment Health Nurs. 2010;17(6):535–42.

Neufeld E, O'Rourke N. Impulsivity and hopelessness as predictors of suicide-related ideation among older adults. Can J Psychiatr. 2009;54(10):684–92. https://doi.org/10.1177/070674370905401005.

O'Rourke N, Hatcher L. A step-by-step approach to using SAS for factor analysis and structural equation modeling. Cary: SAS Institute; 2013.

O'Rourke N, King DB. Within-couple analyses of bipolar disorder symptoms and partner mood over time. Eur Congr Psychol. 2019;21:1114.

O'Rourke N, Sixsmith A, King DB, Yaghoubi-Shahir H, Canham SL, BADAS Study Team. Development and validation of the $BDS_x$: a brief measure of mood and symptom variability for use with adults with bipolar disorder. Int J Bipolar Disord. 2016;4(1):8. https://doi.org/10.1186/s40345-016-0048-2.

O'Rourke N, Bachner YG, Canham SL, Sixsmith A, BADAS Study Team. Measurement equivalence of the $BDS_x$ scale with young and older adults with bipolar disorder. Psychiatr Res. 2018;263:245–9. https://doi.org/10.1016/j.psychres.2017.10.024.

O'Rourke N, Sixsmith A, Kirshner G, Osher Y. Perceived cognitive failures and quality of life for older adults with bipolar disorder. J Affect Disord. 2021;287:433–40.

O'Rourke N, Heisel MJ, Canham SL, Sixsmith A, Yaghoubi-Shahir H, King DB. Psychometric validation of the Geriatric Suicide Ideation Scale (GSIS) among older adults with bipolar disorder. Aging Ment Health. 2018;22(6):794–801. https://doi.org/10.1080/13607863.2017.1317333.

Osher Y, Bersudsky Y, Belmaker RH. The new lithium clinic. Neuropsychobiology. 2010;62(1):17–26.

Osher Y, Bersudsky Y, O'Rourke N, Belotherkovsky D, Bachner YG. Clinical validation of the $BDS_x$ scale with bipolar disorder outpatients. Arch Psychiatr Nurs. 2020;34(1):49–52. https://doi.org/10.1016/j.apnu.2019.11.002.

Parens E, Johnston J. Controversies concerning the diagnosis and treatment of bipolar disorder in children. Child Adol Psychiatr Ment Health. 2010;4(1):9. https://doi.org/10.1186/1753-2000-4-9.

Peng D, Huang Y, Jiang K. Atypical features and bipolar disorder. Shanghai Arch Psychiatr. 2016;28(3):166–8. https://doi.org/10.11919/j.issn.1002-0829.216002.

Perlick D, Rosenheck RR, Clarkin JF, Sirey JA, Raue P, Greenfield S, Struening E. Burden experienced by care-givers of persons with bipolar affective disorder. Brit J Psychiatr. 1999;175(1):56–62.

Perlick DA, Rosenheck RA, Miklowitz DJ, Kaczynski R, Link B, Ketter T, Wisniewski W, Wolff N, Sachs G, STEP-BD Family Experience Collaborative Study Group. Caregiver burden and health in bipolar disorder: a cluster analytic approach. J Nerv Ment Disease. 2008;196(6):484–91.

Phillips ML, Kupfer DJ. Bipolar disorder diagnosis: challenges and future directions. Lancet. 2013;381(9878):1663–71. https://doi.org/10.1016/S0140-6736(13)60989-7.

Samalin L, de Chazeron I, Vieta E, Bellivier F, Llorca PM. Residual symptoms and specific functional impairments in euthymic patients with bipolar disorder. Bipolar Disord. 2016;18(2):164–73. https://doi.org/10.1111/bdi.12376.

Saunders KE, Goodwin GM. The course of bipolar disorder. Adv Psychiatr Treat. 2010;16(5):318–28.

Serra F, Gordon-Smith K, Perry A, Fraser C, Di Florio A, Craddock N, Jones I, Jones L. Agitated depression in bipolar disorder. Bipolar Disord. 2019;21(6):547–55.

Serretti A, Olgiati P. Profiles of "manic" symptoms in bipolar I, bipolar II and major depressive disorders. J Affect Disord. 2005;84(2–3):159–66.

Srivastava S, Bhatia MS, Sharma V, Rajender G, Kumar P. Health-related quality of life in bipolar disorder patients and their caregivers. Int J Ment Health. 2010;39(4):3–15.

Tondo L, Pompili M, Forte A, Baldessarini RJ. Suicide attempts in bipolar disorders: comprehensive review of 101 reports. Acta Psychiatr Scand. 2016;133(3):174–86. https://doi.org/10.1111/acps.12517.

Tondo L, Vazquez GH, Baldessarini RJ. Depression and mania in bipolar disorder. Curr Neuropharmacol. 2017;15(3):353–8.

Towbin K, Axelson D, Leibenluft E, Birmaher B. Differentiating bipolar disorder–not otherwise specified and severe mood dysregulation. J Am Acad Child Adol Psychiatr. 2013;52(5):466–81.

Treuer T, Tohen M. Predicting the course and outcome of bipolar disorder: a review. Euro Psychiatr. 2010;25(6):328–33.

Undurraga J, Baldessarini RJ, Valenti M, Pacchiarotti I, Vieta E. Suicidal risk factors in bipolar I and II disorder patients. J Clin Psychiatr. 2011;73(6):778–82. https://doi.org/10.4088/JCP.11m07041.

Van Meter AR, Youngstrom EA, Findling RL. Cyclothymic disorder: a critical review. Clin Psychol Rev. 2012;32(4):229–43.

Van Meter AR, Youngstrom EA, Birmaher B, Fristad MA, Horwitz SM, Frazier TW, Arnold LE, Findling RL. Longitudinal course and characteristics of cyclothymic disorder in youth. J Affect Disord. 2017;215:314–22.

Ward LC. Comparison of factor structure models for the Beck Depression Inventory–II. Psychol Assess. 2006;18(1):81–8. https://doi.org/10.1037/1040-3590.18.1.81.

Watson D, Clark LA, Tellegen A. Development and validation of brief measures of positive and negative affect: the PANAS scales. J Person Soc Psychol. 1988;54(6):1063–70. https://doi.org/10.1037/0022-3514.54.6.1063.

# Permissions

All chapters in this book were first published by Springer; hereby published with permission under the Creative Commons Attribution License or equivalent. Every chapter published in this book has been scrutinized by our experts. Their significance has been extensively debated. The topics covered herein carry significant findings which will fuel the growth of the discipline. They may even be implemented as practical applications or may be referred to as a beginning point for another development.

The contributors of this book come from diverse backgrounds, making this book a truly international effort. This book will bring forth new frontiers with its revolutionizing research information and detailed analysis of the nascent developments around the world.

We would like to thank all the contributing authors for lending their expertise to make the book truly unique. They have played a crucial role in the development of this book. Without their invaluable contributions this book wouldn't have been possible. They have made vital efforts to compile up to date information on the varied aspects of this subject to make this book a valuable addition to the collection of many professionals and students.

This book was conceptualized with the vision of imparting up-to-date information and advanced data in this field. To ensure the same, a matchless editorial board was set up. Every individual on the board went through rigorous rounds of assessment to prove their worth. After which they invested a large part of their time researching and compiling the most relevant data for our readers.

The editorial board has been involved in producing this book since its inception. They have spent rigorous hours researching and exploring the diverse topics which have resulted in the successful publishing of this book. They have passed on their knowledge of decades through this book. To expedite this challenging task, the publisher supported the team at every step. A small team of assistant editors was also appointed to further simplify the editing procedure and attain best results for the readers.

Apart from the editorial board, the designing team has also invested a significant amount of their time in understanding the subject and creating the most relevant covers. They scrutinized every image to scout for the most suitable representation of the subject and create an appropriate cover for the book.

The publishing team has been an ardent support to the editorial, designing and production team. Their endless efforts to recruit the best for this project, has resulted in the accomplishment of this book. They are a veteran in the field of academics and their pool of knowledge is as vast as their experience in printing. Their expertise and guidance has proved useful at every step. Their uncompromising quality standards have made this book an exceptional effort. Their encouragement from time to time has been an inspiration for everyone.

The publisher and the editorial board hope that this book will prove to be a valuable piece of knowledge for researchers, students, practitioners and scholars across the globe.

# List of Contributors

**Ross J. Baldessarini**
Department of Psychiatry, Harvard Medical School, Boston, MA, USA
International Consortium for Bipolar & Psychotic Disorders Research, McLean Hospital, Belmont, MA, USA

**Gustavo H. Vázquez**
International Consortium for Bipolar & Psychotic Disorders Research, McLean Hospital, Belmont, MA, USA
Department of Psychiatry, Queen's University School of Medicine, Kingston, ON, Canada

**Leonardo Tondo**
Department of Psychiatry, Harvard Medical School, Boston, MA, USA
International Consortium for Bipolar & Psychotic Disorders Research, McLean Hospital, Belmont, MA, USA
Lucio Bini Mood Disorder Center, Cagliari, Sardinia, Italy

**Francis Bennett and Andrew Close**
Institute of Neuroscience, Newcastle University, Newcastle upon Tyne, UK

**Sophie Hodgetts**
School of Psychology, University of Sunderland, Sunderland, UK

**Mark Frye**
Department of Psychiatry & Psychology, Mayo Clinic, Rochester, MN, USA

**Heinz Grunze**
PMU Nuremberg & Psychiatrie Schwäbisch Hall, Schwäbisch Hall, Germany

**Paul Keck**
Linder Center of Hope, Mason, OH, USA
Biological Psychiatry Program, University of Cincinnati Medical College, Cincinnati, OH, USA

**Ralph Kupka and Susan McElroy**
Department of Psychiatry, VU University Medical Center, Amsterdam, The Netherlands

**Willem Nolen**
University of Groningen, University Medical Center Groningen, Groningen, The Netherlands

**Robert Post**
Bipolar Collaborative Network, Bethesda, MD, USA

**Lars Schärer**
Department of Psychiatry, and Psychotherapy Medical Center, University of Freiburg, Faculty of Medicine, Freiburg im Breisgau, Germany

**Aditya N. Sharma**
Institute of Neuroscience, Newcastle University, Newcastle upon Tyne, UK
Northumberland Tyne and Wear NHS Foundation Trust, Newcastle upon Tyne, UK
Academic Psychiatry, Wolfson Research Centre, Campus for Ageing and Vitality, Newcastle University, Newcastle upon Tyne NE4 5PL, UK

**Daniela Reich-Erkelenz, Sabrina K. Schaupp, Maria Hake, Monika Budde and Urs Heilbronner**
Institute of Psychiatric Phenomics and Genomics, University Hospital, LMU Munich, Nussbaumstrasse 7, 80336 Munich, Germany

**Ashley L. Comes**
Institute of Psychiatric Phenomics and Genomics, University Hospital, LMU Munich, Nussbaumstrasse 7, 80336 Munich, Germany
International Max Planck Research School for Translational Psychiatry (IMPRS-TP), 80804 Munich, Germany

**Darina Czamara**
Department of Translational Research in Psychiatry, Max Planck Institute of Psychiatry, 80804 Munich, Germany

**Kristina Adorjan, Sergi Papiol, Farah Klohn-Saghatolislam, Eva C. Schulte and Fanny Senner**
Institute of Psychiatric Phenomics and Genomics, University Hospital, LMU Munich, Nussbaumstrasse 7, 80336 Munich, Germany
Department of Psychiatry and Psychotherapy, University Hospital, LMU Munich, 80336 Munich, Germany

**Peter Falkai**
Department of Psychiatry and Psychotherapy, University Hospital, LMU Munich, 80336 Munich, Germany

**Heike Anderson-Schmidt**
Institute of Psychiatric Phenomics and Genomics, University Hospital, LMU Munich, Nussbaumstrasse 7, 80336 Munich, Germany
Department of Psychiatry and Psychotherapy, University Medical Center Göttingen, 37075 Göttingen, Germany

**Katrin Gade**
Department of Psychiatry and Psychotherapy, University Medical Center Göttingen, 37075 Göttingen, Germany

**Till F. M. Andlauer**
Department of Translational Research in Psychiatry, Max Planck Institute of Psychiatry, 80804 Munich, Germany
Department of Neurology, Klinikum rechts der Isar, School of Medicine, Technical University of Munich, 81675 Munich, Germany

**Janos L. Kalman**
Institute of Psychiatric Phenomics and Genomics, University Hospital, LMU Munich, Nussbaumstrasse 7, 80336 Munich, Germany
International Max Planck Research School for Translational Psychiatry (IMPRS-TP), 80804 Munich, Germany
Department of Psychiatry and Psychotherapy, University Hospital, LMU Munich, 80336 Munich, Germany

**Max Schmauß**
Department of Psychiatry and Psychotherapy, Bezirkskrankenhaus Augsburg, University of Augsburg, 86156 Augsburg, Germany

**Jörg Zimmermann**
Psychiatrieverbund Oldenburger Land gGmbH, Karl-Jaspers-Klinik, 26160 Bad Zwischenahn, Germany

**Jens Reimer**
Department of Psychiatry and Psychotherapy, University Medical Center Hamburg-Eppendorf, 20246 Hamburg, Germany

**Eva Reininghaus**
Department of Psychiatry and Psychotherapeutic Medicine, Research Unit for Bipolar Affective Disorder, Medical University of Graz, 8036 Graz, Austria

**Ion-George Anghelescu**
Department of Psychiatry, Dr. Frontheim-Mental Health, 38704 Liebenburg, Germany

**Carsten Konrad and Andreas Thiel**
Department of Psychiatry and Psychotherapy, Agaplesion Diakonieklinikum, 27356 Rotenburg, Germany

**Christian Figge**
Karl-Jaspers Clinic, European Medical School Oldenburg-Groningen, 26160 Oldenburg, Germany

**Martin von Hagen**
Clinic for Psychiatry and Psychotherapy, Clinical Center Werra-Meißner, 37269 Eschwege, Germany

**Manfred Koller**
Asklepios Specialized Hospital, 37081 Göttingen, Germany

**Detlef E. Dietrich**
AMEOS Clinical Center Hildesheim, 31135 Hildesheim, Germany
Center für Systems Neuroscience (ZSN) Hannover, 30559 Hannover, Germany
Department of Psychiatry, Medical School of Hannover, 30625 Hannover, Germany

**Sebastian Stierl**
Psychiatric Hospital Lüneburg, 21339 Lüneburg, Germany

**Harald Scherk**
AMEOS Clinical Center Osnabrück, 49088 Osnabrück, Germany

**Stephanie H. Witt and Marcella Rietschel**
Department of Genetic Epidemiology in Psychiatry, Central Institute of Mental Health, Medical Faculty Mannheim, University of Heidelberg, 68159 Mannheim, Germany

**Sugirthan Sivalingam, Franziska Degenhardt and Markus M. Nöthen**
Institute of Human Genetics, University of Bonn, School of Medicine & University Hospital Bonn, 53127 Bonn, Germany

**Andreas J. Forstner**
Institute of Human Genetics, University of Bonn, School of Medicine & University Hospital Bonn, 53127 Bonn, Germany
Center for Human Genetics, University of Marburg, 35033 Marburg, Germany
Department of Biomedicine, University of Basel, 4031 Basel, Switzerland
Department of Psychiatry (UPK), University of Basel, 4002 Basel, Switzerland

**Jens Wiltfang**
Department of Psychiatry and Psychotherapy, University Medical Center Göttingen, 37075 Göttingen, Germany
German Center for Neurodegenerative Diseases (DZNE), 37075 Göttingen, Germany
iBiMED, Medical Sciences Department, University of Aveiro, 3810-193 Aveiro, Portugal

**Niall M. McGowan and Amy C. Bilderbeck**
Department of Psychiatry, University of Oxford, Warneford Hospital, Oxford OX3 7JX, UK

**Molly Nichols**
Academic Centre, John Radcliffe Hospital, Oxford University Clinical School, Oxford OX3 9DU, UK

**Guy M. Goodwin**
Department of Psychiatry, University of Oxford, Warneford Hospital, Oxford OX3 7JX, UK
Oxford Health NHS Foundation Trust, Warneford Hospital, Oxford OX3 7JX, UK

**Kate E. A. Saunders**
Department of Psychiatry, University of Oxford, Warneford Hospital, Oxford OX3 7JX, UK1 Department of Psychiatry, University of Oxford, Warneford Hospital, Oxford OX3 7JX, UK
Oxford Health NHS Foundation Trust, Warneford Hospital, Oxford OX3 7JX, UK
NIHR Oxford Health Biomedical Research Centre, Oxford OX3 7JX, UK

**Rif S. El-Mallakh and Yonglin Gao**
Mood Disorders Research Program, Depression Center, Department of Psychiatry and Behavioral Sciences, University of Louisville School of Medicine, 401 East Chestnut Street, Suite 610, Louisville, KY 40202, USA

**Pan You**
Xiamen Xianyue Hospital, 399 Xianyue Road, Xiamen, China

**Marcel Kurtz, Pia Mohring and Katharina Förster**
Clinical Psychology and Behavioral Neuroscience, Faculty of Psychology, Technische Universität Dresden, Chemnitzer Str. 46, 01187 Dresden, Germany

**Philipp Kanske**
Max Planck Institute for Human Cognitive and Brain Sciences, Leipzig,Germany

**Abigail Ortiz and Benoit H. Mulsant**
Department of Psychiatry, University of Toronto, Toronto, ON, Canada
Centre for Addiction & Mental Health, CAMH 100 Stokes St, Rm 4229, Toronto, ON M6J 1H4, Canada

**Kamil Bradler**
ORCA Quantum Computing, Toronto, ON, Canada

**Maxine Mowete**
Department of Electrical Engineering, University of Ottawa, Ottawa, ON, Canada

**Stephane MacLean**
Institute for Mental Health Research, The Royal Ottawa Hospital, Ottawa, ON, Canada

**Julie Garnham and Claire Slaney**
Nova Scotia Health Authority, Halifax, NS, Canada

**Martin Alda**
Department of Psychiatry, Dalhousie University, Halifax, NS, Canada
National Institute of Mental Health, Klecany, Czech Republic

**Sheng-Yu Lee**
Department of Psychiatry, Kaohsiung Veterans General Hospital, Kaohsiung, Taiwan
Department of Psychiatry, School of Medicine, College of Medicine, Kaohsiung Medical University, Kaohsiung, Taiwan
Department of Psychiatry, College of Medicine, National Yang-Ming University, Taipei, Taiwan
Department of Psychiatry, National Cheng Kung University Hospital, College of Medicine, National Cheng Kung University, 138 Sheng-Li Road, Tainan 70428, Taiwan

**Tzu-Yun Wang, Po-See Chen, I-Hui Lee, Kao-Ching Chen, Yen-Kuang Yang and Ru-Band Lu**
Department of Psychiatry, National Cheng Kung University Hospital, College of Medicine, National Cheng Kung University, 138 Sheng-Li Road, Tainan 70428, Taiwan

**Shiou-Lan Chen**
Department of Neurology, School of Medicine, Kaohsiung Medical University, Kaohsiung, Taiwan

**Yun-Hsuan Chang**
Department of Psychology, College of Medical and Health Science, Asia University, Taichung, Taiwan

**San-Yuan Huang and Nian-Sheng Tzeng**
Department of Psychiatry, Tri-Service General Hospital, National Defense Medical Center, Taipei, Taiwan

**Liang-Jen Wang**
Department of Child and Adolescent Psychiatry, Kaohsiung Chang Gung Memorial Hospital and Chang Gung University College of Medicine, Kaohsiung, Taiwan

**Jau-Shyong Hong**
Laboratory of Toxicology and Pharmacology, NIH/NIEHS, Research Triangle Park, Durham, NC, USA
Yanjiao Furen Hospital, Hebei, China
Addiction Research Center, National Cheng Kung University, Tainan, Taiwan

**Diane Grillault Laroche**
INSERM U1144 - Optimisation Thérapeutique en Neuropsychopharmacologie, Université de Paris Descartes, Paris, France
AP-HP, DMU Neurosciences, GH Saint-Louis - Lariboisière - F. Widal, Hôpital Fernand Widal, Département de Psychiatrie et de Médecine Addictologique, Paris, France

**Frank Bellivier**
INSERM U1144 - Optimisation Thérapeutique en Neuropsychopharmacologie, Université de Paris Descartes, Paris, France
AP-HP, DMU Neurosciences, GH Saint-Louis - Lariboisière - F. Widal, Hôpital Fernand Widal, Département de Psychiatrie et de Médecine Addictologique, Paris, France
Faculté de Médecine, Université de Paris, Paris, France

**Bruno Etain**
INSERM U1144 - Optimisation Thérapeutique en Neuropsychopharmacologie, Université de Paris Descartes, Paris, France
AP-HP, DMU Neurosciences, GH Saint-Louis - Lariboisière - F. Widal, Hôpital Fernand Widal, Département de Psychiatrie et de Médecine Addictologique, Paris, France
Faculté de Médecine, Université de Paris, Paris, France
Centre for Affective Disorders, Institute of Psychiatry, Psychology and Neurosciences, London, UK

**Emanuel Severus**
Department of Psychiatry and Psychotherapy, University Hospital Carl Gustav Carus, TU Dresden, Dresden, Germany

**Jan Scott**
Faculté de Médecine, Université de Paris, Paris, France
Centre for Affective Disorders, Institute of Psychiatry, Psychology and Neurosciences, London, UK
Academic Psychiatry, Institute of Neuroscience, Newcastle University, Newcastle, UK

**Rosie H. Taylor, Andrea Ulrichsen and Rebecca Strawbridge**
Department of Psychological Medicine, Institute of Psychiatry, Psychology and Neuroscience, King's College London, London SE5 8AF, UK
South London & Maudsley NHS Foundation Trust, Maudsley Hospital, London, UK

**Michael Bauer**
Department of Psychiatry and Psychotherapy, Carl Gustav Carus University Hospital, Technische Universitat Dresden, Fetscherstrase 74, 01307 Dresden, Germany

**Karolina Leopold**
Department of Psychiatry and Psychotherapy, Carl Gustav Carus University Hospital, Technische Universitat Dresden, Fetscherstrase 74, 01307 Dresden, Germany
Department of Psychiatry, Psychotherapy and Psychosomatics, Vivantes Klinikum Am Urban, Berlin, Germany

**Veit Roessner**
Department of Childand Adolescent Psychiatry and Psychotherapy, Carl Gustav Carus University Hospital, Technische Universitat Dresden, Dresden, Germany

**Paolo Fusar-Poli**
Early Psychosis: Intervention and Clinical-Detection (EPIC) Lab, Institute of Psychiatry, Psychology and Neuroscience, King's College London, London, UK
Department of Brain and Behavioral Sciences, University of Pavia, Pavia, Italy

**Allan H. Young**
Department of Psychological Medicine, Institute of Psychiatry, Psychology and Neuroscience, King's College London & South London and Maudsley NHS Foundation Trust, Bethlem Royal Hospital, London, UK

**Christoph U. Correll**
Department of Child- and Adolescent Psychiatry and Psychotherapy, Charite Universitatsmedizin, Berlin, Germany
Department of Psychiatry, The Zucker Hillside Hospital, Northwell Health, Glen Oaks, NY, USA
Donald and Barbara Zucker School of Medicine At Hofstra/Northwell, Department of Psychiatry and Molecular Medicine, Hempstead, NY, USA

**Andrea Pfennig, Julia Martini, Anne Boehme, Steffi Pfeiffer, Christina Berndt, Maren Rottmann-Wolf, Cathrin Sauer and Philipp Ritter**
Department of Psychiatry and Psychotherapy, Carl Gustav Carus University Hospital, Technische Universität Dresden, Fetscherstraße 74, 01307 Dresden, Germany

**Andreas Bechdolf**
Department of Psychiatry, Psychotherapy and Psychosomatics, Vivantes Klinikum Am Urban, Berlin, Germany

**Martin Lambert**
Department of Psychiatry and Psychotherapy, University Medical Center Hamburg-Eppendorf, Hamburg, Germany

**Thomas Stamm**
Department of Psychiatry and Psychotherapy, Charité Universitätsmedizin Berlin, Berlin, Germany
Department of Psychiatry, Psychotherapy and Psychosomatic, Medical School Brandenburg, Neuruppin, Germany

**Sarah Kittel-Schneider**
Department of Psychiatry, Psychosomatics and Psychotherapy, University Hospital Frankfurt, Frankfurt, Germany

**Andreas J. Fallgatter**
Department of General Psychiatry and Psychotherapy, University Hospital Tübingen, Tübingen, Germany

**Parisa Vidafar**
Sleep and Circadian Research Laboratory, Department of Psychiatry, University of Michigan, Rachel Upjohn Building, 4250 Plymouth Rd, Ann Arbor, MI 48109, USA

**Helen J. Burgess**
Sleep and Circadian Research Laboratory, Department of Psychiatry, University of Michigan, Rachel Upjohn Building, 4250 Plymouth Rd, Ann Arbor, MI 48109, USA
Depression Center, Department of Psychiatry, University of Michigan, Ann Arbor, MI 48109, USA

**Anastasia K. Yocum and Melvin G. McInnis**
Depression Center, Department of Psychiatry, University of Michigan, Ann Arbor, MI 48109, USA

**Peisong Han**
Department of Biostatistics, School of Public Health, University of Michigan, Ann Arbor, MI 48109, USA

**Christie W. Musket**
Department of Psychology, University of Pittsburgh, Pittsburgh, USA

**Natasha S. Hansen and June Gruber**
Department of Psychology and Neuroscience, University of Colorado, Boulder, 345 UCB, Muenzinger D321C, Boulder, CO 80309-0345, USA

**Keith M. Welker**
Department of Psychology, University of Massachusetts, Boston, USA

**Kirsten E. Gilbert**
Department of Psychiatry, Washington University in St. Louis, St. Louis, USA

**Lisa Serravalle, Vanessa Iacono and Mark A. Ellenbogen**
Centre for Research in Human Development, Concordia University, Montréal, Canada

**Sheilagh Hodgins**
Département de Psychiatrie, Université de Montréal, Montréal, Canada
Department of Clinical Neuroscience, Karolinska Institute, Stockholm, Sweden

**Julia Drakopoulos, Timea Sparding and Erik Pålsson**
Department of Psychiatry and Neurochemistry, Institute of Neuroscience and Physiology, The Sahlgrenska Academy, University of Gothenburg, Sahlgrenska University Hospital, Blå Stråket 15, 413 45 Gothenburg, Sweden

**Mikael Landén**
Department of Psychiatry and Neurochemistry, Institute of Neuroscience and Physiology, The Sahlgrenska Academy, University of Gothenburg, Sahlgrenska University Hospital, Blå Stråket 15, 413 45 Gothenburg, Sweden
Department of Medical Epidemiology and Biostatistics, Karolinska Institutet, Stockholm, Sweden

**Caitlin Clements**
Department of Psychology, University of Pennsylvania, 3720 Walnut Street, Philadelphia, PA 19104, USA
Department of Medical Epidemiology and Biostatistics, Karolinska Institutet, Stockholm, Sweden
Center for Autism Research, The Children's Hospital of Philadelphia, 2716 South St, Philadelphia, PA 19104, USA

**Mette U. Fredskild, Sharleny Stanislaus, Klara Coello, Sigurd A. Melbye, Hanne Lie Kjærstad and Kimie Stefanie Ormstrup Sletved**
Copenhagen Affective Disorders Research Centre (CADIC), Psychiatric Centre Copenhagen, Department O, 6233, Rigshospitalet, Blegdamsvej 9, 2100 Copenhagen, Denmark

**Trisha Suppes**
Department of Psychiatry & Behavioral Sciences, Stanford University School of Medicine, Palo Alto, CA, USA

**Lars Vedel Kessing**
Copenhagen Affective Disorders Research Centre (CADIC), Psychiatric Centre Copenhagen, Department O, 6233, Rigshospitalet, Blegdamsvej 9, 2100 Copenhagen, Denmark
Department of Clinical Medicine, Faculty of Health and Medical Sciences, University of Copenhagen, Copenhagen, Denmark

**Maj Vinberg**
Copenhagen Affective Disorders Research Centre (CADIC), Psychiatric Centre Copenhagen, Department O, 6233, Rigshospitalet, Blegdamsvej 9, 2100 Copenhagen, Denmark
Department of Clinical Medicine, Faculty of Health and Medical Sciences, University of Copenhagen, Copenhagen, Denmark
Psychiatric Research Unit, Psychiatric Centre North Zealand, Hillerød, Denmark

**Arjan M. Van Alphen**
Department of Nephrology, Maasstad Hospital, Rotterdam, The Netherlands

**Tessa M. Bosch**
Department of Hospital Pharmacy, Maasstad Hospital, Rotterdam, The Netherlands

**Ralph W. Kupka**
Dept. of Psychiatry & Amsterdam Public Health Research Institute, Amsterdam UMC, Vrije Universiteit, Amsterdam, The Netherlands

**Rocco Hoekstra**
Outpatient Clinic for Bipolar Disorders, Antes Centre for Mental Health Care, Rotterdam, The Netherlands

**Norm O'Rourke and Yaacov G. Bachner**
Department of Public Health and Multidisciplinary Center for Research On Aging, Ben-Gurion University of the Negev, P.O. Box 653, 8410501 Béer Sheva, Israel

**Andrew Sixsmith**
STAR Institute, Simon Fraser University, Vancouver, BC, Canada

**Tal Michael**
School of Public Health, Faculty of Health Sciences, Ben-Gurion University of the Negev, Béer Sheva, Israel

# Index

www.ingramcontent.com/pod-product-compliance
Lightning Source LLC
LaVergne TN
LVHW060555210926
848485LV00005B/1319